C0-AOH-247

Advanced Digital Signal Processing

ELECTRICAL ENGINEERING AND ELECTRONICS

A Series of Reference Books and Textbooks

1. Rational Fault Analysis, *edited by Richard Saeks and S. R. Liberty*
2. Nonparametric Methods in Communications, *edited by P. Papantoni-Kazakos and Dimitri Kazakos*
3. Interactive Pattern Recognition, *Yi-tzuu Chien*
4. Solid-State Electronics, *Lawrence E. Murr*
5. Electronic, Magnetic, and Thermal Properties of Solid Materials, *Klaus Schröder*
6. Magnetic-Bubble Memory Technology, *Hsu Chang*
7. Transformer and Inductor Design Handbook, *Colonel Wm. T. McLyman*
8. Electromagnetics: Classical and Modern Theory and Applications, *Samuel Seely and Alexander D. Poularikas*
9. One-Dimensional Digital Signal Processing, *Chi-Tsong Chen*
10. Interconnected Dynamical Systems, *Raymond A. DeCarlo and Richard Saeks*
11. Modern Digital Control Systems, *Raymond G. Jacquot*
12. Hybrid Circuit Design and Manufacture, *Roydn D. Jones*
13. Magnetic Core Selection for Transformers and Inductors: A User's Guide to Practice and Specification, *Colonel Wm. T. McLyman*
14. Static and Rotating Electromagnetic Devices, *Richard H. Engelmann*
15. Energy-Efficient Electric Motors: Selection and Application, *John C. Andreas*
16. Electromagnetic Compossibility, *Heinz M. Schlicke*
17. Electronics: Models, Analysis, and Systems, *James G. Gottling*
18. Digital Filter Design Handbook, *Fred J. Taylor*
19. Multivariable Control: An Introduction, *P. K. Sinha*
20. Flexible Circuits: Design and Applications, *Steve Gurley, with contributions by Carl A. Edstrom, Jr., Ray D. Greenway, and William P. Kelly*
21. Circuit Interruption: Theory and Techniques, *Thomas E. Browne, Jr.*
22. Switch Mode Power Conversion: Basic Theory and Design, *K. Kit Sum*
23. Pattern Recognition: Applications to Large Data-Set Problems, *Sing-Tze Bow*
24. Custom-Specific Integrated Circuits: Design and Fabrication, *Stanley L. Hurst*
25. Digital Circuits: Logic and Design, *Ronald C. Emery*
26. Large-Scale Control Systems: Theories and Techniques, *Magdi S. Mahmoud, Mohamed F. Hassan, and Mohamed G. Darwish*
27. Microprocessor Software Project Management, *Eli T. Fathi and Cedric V. W. Armstrong (Sponsored by Ontario Centre for Microelectronics)*
28. Low Frequency Electromagnetic Design, *Michael P. Perry*
29. Multidimensional Systems: Techniques and Applications, *edited by Spyros G. Tzafestas*
30. AC Motors for High-Performance Applications: Analysis and Control, *Sakae Yamamura*
31. Ceramic Motors for Electronics: Processing, Properties, and Applications, *edited by Relva C. Buchanan*
32. Microcomputer Bus Structures and Bus Interface Design, *Arthur L. Dexter*
33. End User's Guide to Innovative Flexible Circuit Packaging, *Jay J. Miniet*
34. Reliability Engineering for Electronic Design, *Norman B. Fuqua*

35. Design Fundamentals for Low-Voltage Distribution and Control, *Frank W. Kussy and Jack L. Warren*
36. Encapsulation of Electronic Devices and Components, *Edward R. Salmon*
37. Protective Relaying: Principles and Applications, *J. Lewis Blackburn*
38. Testing Active and Passive Electronic Components, *Richard F. Powell*
39. Adaptive Control Systems: Techniques and Applications, *V. V. Chalam*
40. Computer-Aided Analysis of Power Electronic Systems, *Venkatachari Rajagopalan*
41. Integrated Circuit Quality and Reliability, *Eugene R. Hnatek*
42. Systolic Signal Processing Systems, *edited by Earl E. Swartzlander, Jr.*
43. Adaptive Digital Filters and Signal Analysis, *Maurice G. Bellanger*
44. Electronic Ceramics: Properties, Configuration, and Applications, *edited by Lionel M. Levinson*
45. Computer Systems Engineering Management, *Robert S. Alford*
46. Systems Modeling and Computer Simulation, *edited by Naim A. Kheir*
47. Rigid-Flex Printed Wiring Design for Production Readiness, *Walter S. Rigling*
48. Analog Methods for Computer-Aided Circuit Analysis and Diagnosis, *edited by Takao Ozawa*
49. Transformer and Inductor Design Handbook: Second Edition, Revised and Expanded, *Colonel Wm. T. McLyman*
50. Power System Grounding and Transients: An Introduction, *A. P. Sakis Meliopoulos*
51. Signal Processing Handbook, *edited by C. H. Chen*
52. Electronic Product Design for Automated Manufacturing, *H. Richard Stillwell*
53. Dynamic Models and Discrete Event Simulation, *William Delaney and Erminia Vaccari*
54. FET Technology and Application: An Introduction, *Edwin S. Oxner*
55. Digital Speech Processing, Synthesis, and Recognition, *Sadaoki Furui*
56. VLSI RISC Architecture and Organization, *Stephen B. Furber*
57. Surface Mount and Related Technologies, *Gerald Ginsberg*
58. Uninterruptible Power Supplies: Power Conditioners for Critical Equipment, *David C. Griffith*
59. Polyphase Induction Motors: Analysis, Design, and Application, *Paul L. Cochran*
60. Battery Technology Handbook, *edited by H. A. Kiehne*
61. Network Modeling, Simulation, and Analysis, *edited by Ricardo F. Garzia and Mario R. Garzia*
62. Linear Circuits, Systems, and Signal Processing: Advanced Theory and Applications, *edited by Nobuo Nagai*
63. High-Voltage Engineering: Theory and Practice, *edited by M. Khalifa*
64. Large-Scale Systems Control and Decision Making, *edited by Hiroyuki Tamura and Tsuneo Yoshikawa*
65. Industrial Power Distribution and Illuminating Systems, *Kao Chen*
66. Distributed Computer Control for Industrial Automation, *Dobrivoje Popovic and Vijay P. Bhatkar*

67. Computer-Aided Analysis of Active Circuits, *Adrian Ioinovici*
68. Designing with Analog Switches, *Steve Moore*
69. Contamination Effects on Electronic Products, *Carl J. Tautscher*
70. Computer-Operated Systems Control, *Magdi S. Mahmoud*
71. Integrated Microwave Circuits, *edited by Yoshihiro Konishi*
72. Ceramic Materials for Electronics: Processing, Properties, and Applications, Second Edition, Revised and Expanded, *edited by Relva C. Buchanan*
73. Electromagnetic Compatibility: Principles and Applications, *David A. Weston*
74. Intelligent Robotic Systems, *edited by Spyros G. Tzafestas*
75. Switching Phenomena in High-Voltage Circuit Breakers, *edited by Kunio Nakanishi*
76. Advances in Speech Signal Processing, *edited by Sadaoki Furui and M. Mohan Sondhi*
77. Pattern Recognition and Image Preprocessing, *Sing-Tze Bow*
78. Energy-Efficient Electric Motors: Selection and Application, Second Edition, *John C. Andreas*
79. Stochastic Large-Scale Engineering Systems, *edited by Spyros G. Tzafestas and Keigo Watanabe*
80. Two-Dimensional Digital Filters, *Wu-Sheng Lu and Andreas Antoniou*
81. Computer-Aided Analysis and Design of Switch-Mode Power Supplies, *Yim-Shu Lee*
82. Placement and Routing of Electronic Modules, *edited by Michael Pecht*
83. Applied Control: Current Trends and Modern Methodologies, *edited by Spyros G. Tzafestas*
84. Algorithms for Computer-Aided Design of Multivariable Control Systems, *Stanoje Bingulac and Hugh F. VanLandingham*
85. Symmetrical Components for Power Systems Engineering, *J. Lewis Blackburn*
86. Advanced Digital Signal Processing: Theory and Applications, *Glenn Zelniker and Fred J. Taylor*

Additional Volumes in Preparation

Neural Networks and Simulation Methods, *Jian-Kang Wu*

Advanced Digital Signal Processing

Theory and Applications

Glenn Zelniker
Z-Systems
Gainesville, Florida

Fred J. Taylor
University of Florida
Gainesville, Florida

Marcel Dekker, Inc. New York • Basel • Hong Kong

Library of Congress Cataloging-in-Publication Data

Zelniker, Glenn

Advanced digital signal processing: theory and applications / Glenn Zelniker, Fred J. Taylor.

p. cm. -- (Electrical engineering and electronics; 86)

Includes bibliographical references and index.

ISBN 0-8247-9145-2

1. Signal processing--Digital techniques. I. Taylor, Fred J. II. Title. III. Series.

TK5102.9.Z45 1994

621.382'2--dc20

93-20903

CIP

The publisher offers discounts on this book when ordered in bulk quantities. For more information, write to Special Sales/Professional Marketing at the address below.

This book is printed on acid-free paper.

MARCEL DEKKER, INC.
270 Madison Avenue, New York, New York 10016

Current printing (last digit):
10 9 8 7 6 5 4 3 2 1

PRINTED IN THE UNITED STATES OF AMERICA

PREFACE

The field of digital signal processing (DSP) has undergone tremendous changes, both theoretically and technologically, since its inception some twenty-odd years ago. In the early years, the primary focus of DSP researchers and engineers was on filter design and fast Fourier transform algorithms. Today, the cutting-edge DSP professional must be well-armed with background in such diverse areas as approximation theory, stochastic processes, matrix theory, and dynamical systems, to name but a few. These topics may seem to be the stuff of academic researchers, but the fact is they have found their way into the mainstream. Today, practicing engineers routinely have to design systems for optimal filtering, adaptive filtering, and spectral estimation.

Too often, acquiring background in some of the advanced techniques in DSP can be an intimidating exercise of sifting through unfamiliar mathematics in order to glean a recognizable morsel of information. This is by no means an indication on our part that mathematical sophistication is unwarranted. Rather, we are concerned about how the curious reader is supposed to *develop* this sophistication in the first place. Given the geometric increase in the number of publications in DSP every year, how is the reader to infer what constitutes essential background or important information? This is a question we are attempting to answer with this book. In it, the reader will find an in-depth introductory treatment of some current advanced topics in DSP, topics we find important as well as promising directions for future research. Our treatment of each topic is intended to convey to the reader the salient points, develop the mathematical machinery, provide an intuitive feel for what is happening, point out some of the pitfalls, and prepare the reader for further exploration, development, or implementation of the theory. Wherever possible, we also try to make a connection with applications. There is, of course, a certain amount of bias on the part of the authors. This is unavoidable; we can only indicate what *we* feel is important and worth pursuing.

We have tried to write the book so that it is accessible to readers with a wide range of backgrounds. As such, some of the first four chapters may be familiar to the reader who has had some exposure to the theory of discrete-time signals and systems. These chapters have been included for the sake of completeness and may certainly be omitted if the reader is already thoroughly conversant with the material. The first four chapters do contain some results with which the reader may not be familiar, even if he/she has had an introductory course in discrete-time signals and systems; in this case, we recommend a brief skimming of the material.

Chapters 1 through 4 cover topics such as convolution, impulse response, the $\mathcal{Z}$-transform, the discrete-time Fourier transform, frequency response, the sampling theorem, the discrete Fourier transform, fast Fourier transform algorithms, finite impulse response (FIR) digital filter design, and infinite impulse response (IIR) digital filter design. These topics often constitute an introductory course in digital signal processing, and for the most part are old and well-known. What is more, there exist numerous computer software packages which deal with this standard material. As such, we have chosen not to bog the reader down with endless computations and detailed numerical analyses. Rather, we try to place an emphasis on geometric intuition and an understanding of the fundamentals.

Chapter 5 provides an introductory treatment of stochastic processes, concentrating principally on wide-sense stationary (WSS) stochastic processes. We discuss several models for WSS stochastic processes, power spectral density, vector processes, and the important spectral factorization theorem. The material in this chapter is essential background for what follows in the remainder of the book.

Chapter 6 is about the state-variable representation of linear systems. This is an important topic because it allows the user to make the powerful connection between computational organization and system architecture. The state-variable representation is a mathematical description which has permeated control and system theory for years, yet it is often unfamiliar to the practicing DSP professional. We feel that it is extremely simple to learn, and a powerful and invaluable tool when making the choice between different filter architectures. Chapter 6 culminates with an examination of fixed-point digital filter design, which we feel is best discussed in the framework of state variables.

Chapter 7 covers the very large field of multi-rate signal processing. As the name implies, this field is concerned with systems in which there is more than one sampling rate. Multirate signal processing has found its way into nearly every applications area of DSP and is itself a topic worthy of deep study. Included in this chapter are introductions to the short-time Fourier transform and wavelet transform, and how they relate to multirate filter banks.

The primary topic of Chapter 8 is Wiener filtering. The Wiener filter is an important class of linear optimal filter and serves as a starting point for our later discussion of adaptive filtering. In this chapter, we will discuss the IIR Wiener filter, but will concentrate primarily on the FIR Wiener filter, including solution of the normal equations, lattice structures and the Levinson-Durbin algorithm, and applications such as channel equalization and linear prediction.

Chapter 9 gives an introduction to adaptive filtering. In this chapter, we will formulate a criterion for optimality for a class of adaptive algorithms known as *steepest descent* type algorithms. The most popular of these algorithms is known as the least-mean-squared (LMS) algorithm, and we will give a detailed analysis of the LMS algorithm in a wide variety of conditions. Chapter 10 is also about adaptive filtering, but examines a different class of algorithms which fall under the category of *least-squares* (LS) algorithms. While more computationally complex than the LMS algorithms, the LS algorithms will be seen to perform better than the LMS algorithms in many situations. We will study the recursive least-squares (RLS) algorithm as well as a number of fast least-squares (FLS) algorithms for efficient implementation of recursive least-squares adaptation.

The book concludes with Chapter 11, which discusses spectral estimation. Spectral estimation is concerned with estimating the spectral content of a stochastic process, and we will discuss techniques which are popular and have proved successful for practical spectral estimation. We will concentrate mainly on autoregressive (AR) spectral estimation techniques primarily because of their quality, simplicity, and relationship to the techniques we will cover earlier in the book. Additionally, we will study some high-resolution spectral estimation methods which are based on the singular value decomposition (SVD). SVD methods have found wide use in array signal processing and has been an area of great activity in the literature of late.

Finally, for completeness we have included an appendix which summarizes some of the mathematical material we have used throughout the book. The appendix covers matrix theory, including eigendecomposition, functions of a square matrix, quadratic forms, singular value decomposition, and pseudoinverse. Also included is an elementary introduction to stochastic processes.

Acknowledgments

G. Z. would like to thank: Ruth Dawe at Marcel Dekker for her patience during the preparation of this manuscript; Dr. Maurice Bellanger, Ahmad Ansari, Iztok Koren, Dr. Ross McElroy, Steve Varosi, Charles G. Crampton, Andrew Mitchell, George Larson, Ed Cometz, Dr. Pythagoras Mycat, Luke Smithwick, and Monica Murphy for their comments, suggestions, or help otherwise; Jon Mellott, John Ruckstuhl, and Erik Strom for technical assistance, especially with LaTeX and UNIX; Tim Tucker and Christine Tucker at Tucker-Davis Technologies for their generosity with toner and paper. Special thanks to all of my parents and grandparents. This book is dedicated to my wife, Patricia Ventura, with much appreciation for her comments, criticisms, patience, and companionship during the many long days spent writing this book.

Glenn Zelniker
Fred J. Taylor

Contents

Advanced Digital Signal Processing

Chapter 1

DISCRETE-TIME SIGNALS AND SYSTEMS

1.1 Discrete-Time Signals

Loosely speaking, a *discrete-time signal* is a sequence of numbers. In order to distinguish a complete signal from its individual elements, it will frequently be denoted by either a vector, $\boldsymbol{x}$ or by curly braces, as in $\{x(k)\}$. If the signal is obtained by sampling a continuous-time signal, $x(t)$, we sometimes make explicit reference to the sampling interval, T, and denote the signal by $\{x(kT)\}$. The k-th element of a signal $\boldsymbol{x}$ is denoted by $x(k)$.

One signal which we will use often is the *unit pulse*, $\{\delta(k)\}$ (also known as the *unit impulse*), which is described by

$$\delta(k) = \begin{cases} 1, & k = 0 \\ 0, & \text{otherwise.} \end{cases} \tag{1.1.1}$$

Another important signal is the *unit step*, $\{u(k)\}$, which is given by

$$u(k) = \begin{cases} 0, & k < 0 \\ 1, & k \geq 0. \end{cases} \tag{1.1.2}$$

In analogy with continuous-time Dirac impulses and step functions, it is readily verified that $u(k)$ is related to $\delta(k)$ by

$$u(k) = \sum_{n=-\infty}^{k} \delta(n).$$

Given a signal $\boldsymbol{x}$, we define the *delay* operator D^n as an operator which, when applied to $\boldsymbol{x}$, delays $\boldsymbol{x}$ by n samples. Formally,

$$(D^n \boldsymbol{x})(k) = x(k-n).$$

The delay operator allows us to represent arbitrary signals as sums of shifted and scaled unit pulses. We can write

$$x(k) = \sum_{n=-\infty}^{\infty} x(n)\delta(k-n), \tag{1.1.3}$$

which is easily shown by observing that $\delta(k-n)$ is nonzero only when $n = k$. We will find this representation very useful when examining the behavior of discrete-time systems.

1.2 Discrete-Time Systems

A useful interpretation of a discrete-time system, $\boldsymbol{S}$, is as a mapping which maps discrete-time signals to discrete-time signals. The domain of the map consists of input signals and the range of the map consists of output signals. Given an input signal $\boldsymbol{x}$, we will denote the output of the system $\boldsymbol{S}$ by $\boldsymbol{y} = \boldsymbol{S}(\boldsymbol{x})$.

To understand the concept of linearity, let $\boldsymbol{x}$ and $\boldsymbol{y}$ be two signals which are applied to the input of the system $\boldsymbol{S}$. Assume that the output in response to $\boldsymbol{x}$ is $\boldsymbol{S}(\boldsymbol{x})$ and that the output in response to $\boldsymbol{y}$ is $\boldsymbol{S}(\boldsymbol{y})$. If α and β are scalars, $\alpha\boldsymbol{x} + \beta\boldsymbol{y}$ is defined as the signal whose k-th element is given by

$$(\alpha\boldsymbol{x} + \beta\boldsymbol{y})(k) = \alpha x(k) + \beta y(k).$$

We then say that $\boldsymbol{S}$ is *linear* if for all $\boldsymbol{x}, \boldsymbol{y}, \alpha, \beta$ we have

$$\boldsymbol{S}(\alpha\boldsymbol{x} + \beta\boldsymbol{y}) = \alpha\boldsymbol{S}(\boldsymbol{x}) + \beta\boldsymbol{S}(\boldsymbol{y}).$$

If $\boldsymbol{S}$ is linear, it can be shown recursively that this superposition extends to arbitrary linear combinations of inputs. That is,

$$\boldsymbol{S}\left(\sum_i \alpha_i \boldsymbol{x}_i\right) = \sum_i \alpha_i \boldsymbol{S}(\boldsymbol{x}_i)$$

where the α_i are arbitrary scalars and the $\boldsymbol{x}_i$ are arbitrary signals.

Another important concept is *time-invariance*. Intuitively, a system is time-invariant if a time-shift applied to the input results in a corresponding time-shift of the output. Specifically, if the input $\{x(k)\}$ produces the output $\{y(k)\}$, delaying $\boldsymbol{x}$ by n samples and applying $\boldsymbol{S}$ should produce the output $\{y(k-n)\}$. More formally, a system $\boldsymbol{S}$ is time-invariant if the delay and system operators commute. In other words, for all inputs $\boldsymbol{x}$, we have

$$\boldsymbol{S}(\boldsymbol{D}^n(\boldsymbol{x})) = \boldsymbol{D}^m(\boldsymbol{S}(\boldsymbol{x})). \tag{1.2.1}$$

Causality will also play an important role in the development of the theory of discrete-time signals and systems. Causality essentially means an inability to anticipate the future. A causal system is defined in the following manner. Let $\boldsymbol{x}$ and $\boldsymbol{y}$ be inputs which are identical up until time $k = k_0$, *i.e.*,

$$x(k) = y(k), \quad k \leq k_0.$$

A system $\boldsymbol{S}$ is *causal* if

$$(\boldsymbol{S}(\boldsymbol{x}))(k) = (\boldsymbol{S}(\boldsymbol{y}))(k), \quad k \leq k_0.$$

For a system which is both linear and time invariant, the causality condition reduces to the requirement that for all inputs $\boldsymbol{x}$ for which $x(k) = 0$ whenever $k < 0$, the output of the system satisfies

$$(\boldsymbol{S}(\boldsymbol{x}))(k) = 0, \quad k < 0.$$

The most important class of systems to us are those which are both linear *and* time invariant, or *linear time-invariant* (LTI). We can examine how a LTI system responds to inputs. Let the system $\boldsymbol{S}$ be driven by the input $\boldsymbol{x}$. Recall that $\boldsymbol{x}$ can be written as

$$x(k) = \sum_{n=-\infty}^{\infty} x(n)\delta(k-n).$$

Because of linearity, the response $y(k)$ of $\boldsymbol{S}$ to $\boldsymbol{x}$ is given by

$$y(k) = (\boldsymbol{S}(\boldsymbol{x}))(k) = \boldsymbol{S}\left(\sum_{n=-\infty}^{\infty} x(n)\delta(k-n)\right) = \sum_{n=-\infty}^{\infty} x(n)\boldsymbol{S}(\delta(k-n)).$$

As a matter of convention, we will denote the output of a LTI system in response to a unit pulse by the sequence $\{h(k)\}$. Next, we use the property of time-invariance. If the response of $\boldsymbol{S}$ to the unit pulse is $\{h(k)\}$, by time-invariance the response of $\boldsymbol{S}$ to a delayed impulse, $\delta(k-n)$, is $\{h(k-n)\}$. Thus,

$$y(k) = \sum_{n=-\infty}^{\infty} x(n)h(k-n). \tag{1.2.2}$$

An equivalent expression for $y(k)$ is

$$y(k) = \sum_{n=-\infty}^{\infty} h(n)x(k-n). \tag{1.2.3}$$

Eqs. 1.2.2 and 1.2.3 are known as *linear convolution* (or *convolution*, for short), and express the response of a LTI system to an arbitrary input. Notice that the response is completely

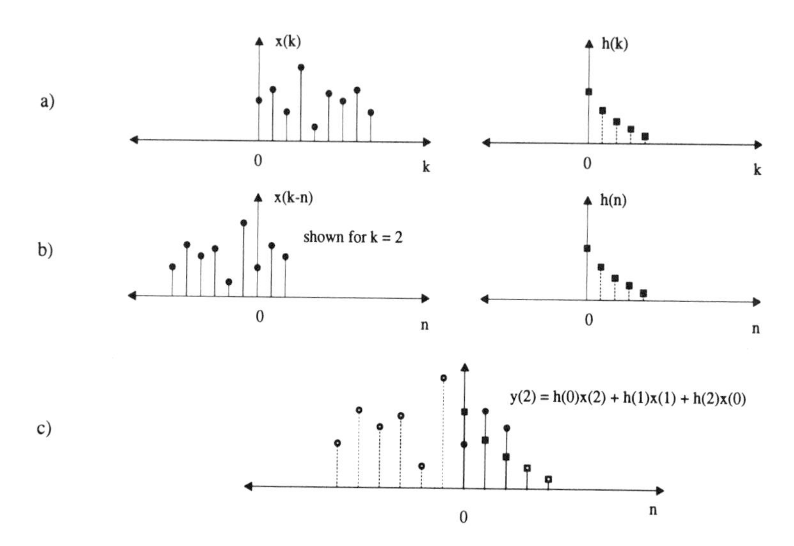

Figure 1.2.1: a) The sequences $h(k)$ and $x(k)$. b) The sequences $h(n)$ and $x(k-n)$ for $k=2$. c) Forming the product $h(n)x(k-n)$.

determined by the response of the system to a unit pulse input. The commonly used notation for convolution is "$*$" and we write

$$\boldsymbol{y} = \boldsymbol{h} * \boldsymbol{x}.$$

Let's take a closer look at Eq. 1.2.3. In order to calculate the output $\boldsymbol{y}$ at a given time k, we first form the sequence $\{h(n)\}$ by re-indexing with the dummy index n. Next, the time-reversed input sequence $\{x(-n)\}$ is formed by "flipping" the dummy-indexed sequence $\{x(n)\}$ about the point $n=0$. Next, $\{x(-n)\}$ is "dragged" k samples to the right, yielding the sequence $\{x(k-n)\}$. Finally, according to Eq. 1.2.3, the sequences $\{h(n)\}$ and $\{x(k-n)\}$ are multiplied pointwise and the product summed over the entire time axis. This process is illustrated in Figure 1.2.1.

Example 1.1

Suppose we are interested in evaluating the convolution, $\boldsymbol{y}$ of the sequences

$$\boldsymbol{h} = \{\ldots, 0, 0, h(0), h(1), h(2), 0, 0, \ldots\}$$

and

$$\boldsymbol{x} = \{\ldots, 0, 0, x(0), x(1), x(2), x(3), 0, 0, \ldots\}.$$

There is no output before $k = 0$. After $k = 0$, observe how the convolution works by following $x(i)$ along the diagonal of the following collection of equations.

$$\begin{array}{rcl} y(0) &=& h(0)x(0) \\ y(1) &=& h(0)x(1) + h(1)x(0) \\ y(2) &=& h(0)x(2) + h(1)x(1) + h(2)x(0) \\ y(3) &=& h(0)x(3) + h(1)x(2) + h(2)x(1) \\ y(4) &=& h(1)x(3) + h(2)x(2) \\ y(5) &=& h(2)x(3) \end{array}$$

After $k = 5$, we again have $y(k) = 0$.

Example 1.2

Suppose that the impulse response of a system is given by

$$h(k) = a^k u(k)$$

i.e.,

$$h(k) = \begin{cases} 0, & k < 0 \\ a^k, & k \geq 0 \end{cases}.$$

Assume that the input to the system is

$$x(k) = b^k u(k).$$

According to Eq. 1.2.3, the output is given by

$$y(k) = \sum_{n=-\infty}^{\infty} a^n u(n) b^{k-n} u(k-n).$$

But $u(n)$ is nonzero only for $n \geq 0$ and $u(k-n)$ is nonzero only for $k - n \geq 0$. In other words, the summand is nonzero only in the range $0 \leq n \leq k$ so that

$$y(k) = \sum_{n=0}^{k} a^n b^{k-n} = b^k \sum_{n=0}^{k} (a/b)^n.$$

We can use the formula for summation of a geometric series,

$$\sum_{n=0}^{N} x^n = \frac{1 - x^{N+1}}{1 - x}$$

to obtain

$$y(k) = b^k \frac{1 - (a/b)^{k+1}}{1 - (a/b)} u(k) = \frac{b^{k+1} - a^{k+1}}{b - a} u(k).$$

For the special case where $a = b$, we cannot use the geometric series formula, and instead must directly sum the series, which gives

$$y(k) = (k+1) b^k u(k).$$

We can see that the response to the impulse input plays a very important role in characterizing the behavior of LTI systems, but have yet to discuss how to actually evaluate the impulse response for an LTI system. This is because we have not yet given any notion of how to provide a description of the input/output relationship for LTI systems.

The most basic input/output description of a LTI system is the *standard difference equation* (SDE). The SDE gives a recursive description of the current output as a function of both current and past inputs and past outputs. The most general form of the SDE is

$$\sum_{n=0}^{N} a_n y(k-n) = \sum_{n=0}^{M} b_n x(k-n)$$

where we require $M \leq N$ for the system to be causal. This SDE can be iterate either forward or backward in time, depending on the nature of the input. To put the SDE into a form which is appropriate for iterating forward in time, we isolate the current output, $y(k)$, and force it to have a coefficient equal to one, which is accomplished by dividing the entire SDE by the leading coefficient a_0, giving

$$y(k) = -\sum_{n=1}^{N} \frac{a_n}{a_0} y(n-k) + \sum_{n=0}^{M} \frac{b_n}{a_0} x(k-n).$$

In order to solve the SDE for a known input $\boldsymbol{x}$, we must also have a collection of auxiliary initial conditions for the system from which the recursion is started. An example will best illustrate.

Example 1.3

Suppose a LTI system is described by the SDE

$$y(k) - ay(k-1) = x(k).$$

We are interested in evaluating the impulse response, which is the response to the input $\boldsymbol{x} = \{\delta(k)\}$. when the system is started from zero initial conditions, *i.e.*, $y(-1) = 0$. We first put the SDE in the form

$$y(k) = ay(k-1) + \delta(k)$$

and observe that the output is zero for all $k < 0$ because there is no input and zero initial conditions before that time. For $k = 0$, we have

$$y(0) = ay(-1) + \delta(0) = 1.$$

For $k = 1$, we have

$$y(1) = ay(0) + \delta(1) = ay(0) = a.$$

For $k = 2$,

$$y(2) = ay(1) + \delta(2) = a^2.$$

In general, we find

$$y(k) = a^k.$$

Thus, we have found that the impulse response is $h(k) = a^k u(k)$.

Similarly, a difference equation can be iterated backwards in time. In this case, we need to put the SDE in a form which is easily iterated backwards in time. This form is given by

$$y(k-N) = -\sum_{n=0}^{N-1} \frac{a_n}{a_N} y(n-k) + \sum_{n=0}^{M} \frac{b_n}{a_N} x(k-n).$$

Example 1.4

We return to the previous example, where the system is defined by the SDE

$$y(k) - ay(k-1) = x(k).$$

Suppose we are interested in iterating the SDE backwards from initial condition $y(0) = 1$ (which was obtained from the previous example) with unit pulse input. We first put the SDE in the form

$$y(k-1) = \frac{1}{a} y(k) - \frac{1}{a} \delta(k)$$

and begin the recursion backwards:

$$y(-1) = \frac{1}{a} y(0) - \frac{1}{a} \delta(0) = 0,$$

which is what we expected. Furthermore,

$$y(-2) = \frac{1}{a} y(-1) - \frac{1}{a} \delta(-1) = 0,$$

and we find in general that $y(k) = 0$ for all $k < 0$. A different choice of initial condition would have resulted in different behavior.

So far, we have only considered the response of LTI systems for the simple case of impulse inputs. For more complicated inputs, solving the SDE is more difficult. In general, the solution to the SDE consists of two parts: the homogeneous solution and the particular solution. The homogeneous solution, $y_h(k)$, corresponds to the solution to the homogeneous difference equation

$$\sum_{n=0}^{N} a_n y(k-n) = 0.$$

The particular solution, $y_p(k)$, depends on the particular input, $x(n)$.

It is possible to obtain the complete solution of the SDE for an arbitrary input by simple recursion of the SDE. Obtaining a closed-form solution, however, is more difficult. As a preface of what will follow later in the text, consider the homogeneous SDE

$$\sum_{n=0}^{N} a_n y(k-n) = 0.$$

Suppose the polynomial $a(z)$ is given by

$$a(z) = \sum_{n=0}^{N} a_n z^{-n}$$

and that $a(z)$ can be factored as

$$a(z) = (1 - z_1 z^{-1})(1 - z_2 z^{-1}) \cdots (1 - z_N z^{-1})$$

where the N roots $\boldsymbol{z}_i$ are distinct. It is readily shown that the solution to the homogeneous SDE is

$$y_h(k) = \sum_{n=1}^{N} \alpha_n z_n^k,$$

where the α_n are unknown coefficients which are determined by the initial conditions.

Interconnection of Systems

Simple systems can be interconnected to form more complicated systems. Figure 1.2.2 shows two basic types of interconnections: cascade and parallel. If the systems are LTI and described by impulse response sequences $\boldsymbol{h}_1$ and $\boldsymbol{h}_2$, respectively, the cascade combination is also LTI and is characterized by the impulse response sequence $\boldsymbol{h}_c$, where

$$\boldsymbol{h}_c = \boldsymbol{h}_1 * \boldsymbol{h}_2.$$

The parallel combination is also LTI, with impulse response

$$\boldsymbol{h}_p = \boldsymbol{h}_1 + \boldsymbol{h}_2.$$

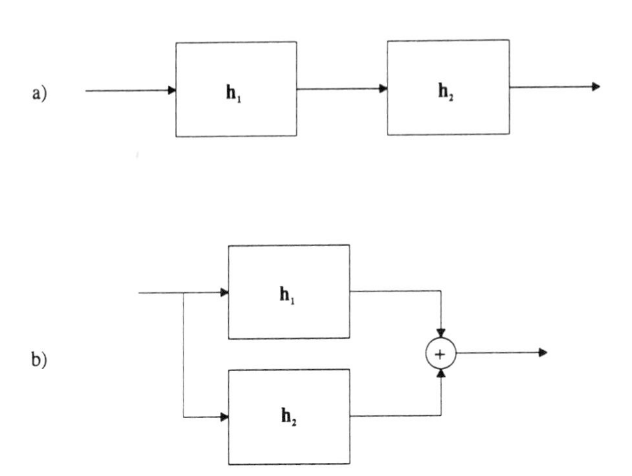

Figure 1.2.2: a) Cascade interconnection of LTI systems. b) Parallel interconnection of LTI systems.

1.3 Stability

A system is said to be bounded-input bounded-output (BIBO) stable if every bounded input sequence produces a bounded output sequence. An input sequence $\boldsymbol{x}$ is bounded if there exists a finite M such that

$$|x(k)| \leq M < \infty \qquad \text{for all } k.$$

The output sequence $\boldsymbol{y} = \boldsymbol{S}(\boldsymbol{x})$ is bounded if there exists a finite N such that

$$|y(k)| \leq N < \infty \qquad \text{for all } k.$$

Subsequent discussions of stability, fixed-point behavior, and statistical behavior will need the concept of a *norm*. The most important class of norms we will use are the so-called l^p norms. Given a sequence $\boldsymbol{x}$, the l^p norm of $\boldsymbol{x}$ is denoted by the symbol $||\cdot||_p$ and is defined by

$$||\boldsymbol{x}||_p = \left(\sum_{n=-\infty}^{\infty} |x(n)|^p \right)^{1/p}. \tag{1.3.1}$$

This definition can be shown to satisfy the properties required of a norm, namely that

1. $||\boldsymbol{x}||_p \geq 0$ with equality only for $\boldsymbol{x} = \boldsymbol{0}$

2. $||\boldsymbol{x}+\boldsymbol{y}||_p \leq ||\boldsymbol{x}||_p + ||\boldsymbol{y}||_p$ (triangle inequality)

3. $||\alpha\boldsymbol{x}||_p = |\alpha|||\boldsymbol{x}||_p$ for all scalars α.

The set of all sequences which have finite l^p norms can be given the structure of a vector space with the operations of pointwise addition and scalar multiplication. A sequence which has finite l^p norm is said to "be l^p" and we refer to the corresponding vector spaces as "l^p-spaces."

There are three such l^p-spaces which will be of interest to us: l^1, l^2, and l^∞. The vector space l^1 consists of all sequences $\boldsymbol{x}$ which satisfy

$$||\boldsymbol{x}||_1 = \sum_{n=-\infty}^{\infty} |x(n)| < \infty, \tag{1.3.2}$$

or sequences $\boldsymbol{x}$ which are *absolutely summable.* The vector space l^2 consists of all sequences $\boldsymbol{x}$ which satisfy

$$||\boldsymbol{x}||_2 = \left(\sum_{n=-\infty}^{\infty} |x(n)|^2\right)^{1/2} < \infty, \tag{1.3.3}$$

or sequences $\boldsymbol{x}$ which are *square summable.* It is common to refer to the squared l^2 norm of a signal $\boldsymbol{x}$ as its *energy*, denoted by E_x. That is,

$$E_x = \sum_{k=-\infty}^{\infty} |x(k)|^2. \tag{1.3.4}$$

If $E_x < \infty$, (*i.e.*, $\boldsymbol{x} \in l^2$), $\boldsymbol{x}$ is called a *finite energy signal.*

Suppose a sequence $\boldsymbol{x}$ is l^1. Then

$$||\boldsymbol{x}||_1^2 = \left(\sum_{k=-\infty}^{\infty} |x(k)|\right)^2 \geq \sum_{k=-\infty}^{\infty} |x(k)|^2 = ||\boldsymbol{x}||_2^2.$$

Thus

$$||\boldsymbol{x}||_2 \leq ||\boldsymbol{x}||_1.$$

Therefore, if $\boldsymbol{x} \in l^1$, then $\boldsymbol{x} \in l^2$. This means that

$$l^1 \subseteq l^2.$$

Actually, it is simple to come up with some simple sequences which are in l^2 but not l^1 (such as the sequence $\{1/k\}$), which means that

$$l^1 \subset l^2.$$

Finally, it can be shown that the l^∞ norm of a sequence $\boldsymbol{x}$ is given by

$$||\boldsymbol{x}||_\infty = \max_k |x(k)| \tag{1.3.5}$$

so that the vector space l^∞ consists of all sequences $\boldsymbol{x}$ which satisfy

$$||\boldsymbol{x}||_\infty = \max_k |x(k)| < \infty.$$

In the language of l^p spaces, we can rephrase the BIBO stability condition as follows. A system is BIBO stable if an l^∞ input produces an l^∞ output.

In the case of LTI systems, stability is easily characterized.

Theorem 1 *Assume that a LTI system is characterized by the impulse response sequence* $\boldsymbol{h}$. *Then the system is BIBO stable if and only if*

$$\sum_{n=-\infty}^{\infty} |h(n)| < \infty. \tag{1.3.6}$$

In other words, an LTI system is BIBO stable if and only if the impulse response $\boldsymbol{h} \in l^1$. To prove this, assume first that we are given an arbitrary bounded input, $\boldsymbol{x}$. Assume $\boldsymbol{x}$ is bounded by M, we have

$$|y(k)| = \left| \sum_{n=-\infty}^{\infty} h(n)x(k-n) \right|.$$

By the Cauchy-Schwartz inequality and the boundedness of $\boldsymbol{x}$, it follows that

$$|y(k)| < \sum_{n=-\infty}^{\infty} |h(n)||x(k-n)| \le M \sum_{n=-\infty}^{\infty} |h(n)|$$

so that if Eq. 1.3.6 holds, the output $\boldsymbol{y}$ will be bounded. To prove the "only if" part, assume by contradiction that Eq. 1.3.6 does not hold, *i.e.*, that

$$\sum_{n=-\infty}^{\infty} |h(n)| = \infty.$$

We will show that there exists a bounded input $\boldsymbol{x}$ that causes the output $\boldsymbol{y}$ to be unbounded. To this end, define the input sequence $\boldsymbol{x}$ by

$$x(k) = \frac{h(-k)}{|h(-k)|}$$

for nonzero $h(-k)$ and

$$x(k) = 0$$

when $h(-k) = 0$. Using the expression for convolution,

$$y(k) = \sum_{n=-\infty}^{\infty} h(n)x(k-n),$$

and we get

$$y(0) = \sum_{n=-\infty}^{\infty} h(n)x(-n) = \sum_{n=-\infty}^{\infty} h(n)\frac{h^*(n)}{|h(n)|},$$

which is seen to be equivalent to

$$y(0) = \sum_{n=-\infty}^{\infty} \frac{|h(n)|^2}{|h(n)|}$$

so that

$$y(0) = \sum_{n=-\infty}^{\infty} |h(n)| = \infty.$$

Thus, we have found a bounded input which produces an unbounded output. In other words, we have produced an l^∞ input which leads to an output which is not l^∞. This proves that if $\boldsymbol{h}$ is not l^1 (*i.e.*, absolutely summable), the system cannot be BIBO stable. Therefore, $\boldsymbol{h}$ is BIBO stable if and only if $\boldsymbol{h}$ is absolutely summable.

1.4 Correlation

Suppose we have two finite energy (l^2) signals $\boldsymbol{x}$ and $\boldsymbol{y}$. The *crosscorrelation* of $\boldsymbol{x}$ and $\boldsymbol{y}$ is the sequence $r_{xy}(k)$ defined by

$$r_{xy}(k) = \sum_{n=-\infty}^{\infty} x(n)y(n+k). \tag{1.4.1}$$

The value of k is known as the *lag* and $r_{xy}(k)$ is computed by shifting $\boldsymbol{y}$ k samples to the left, multiplying pointwise by $\boldsymbol{x}$, and summing over all indices. Similarly, the crosscorrelation of $\boldsymbol{y}$ and $\boldsymbol{x}$ is defined by

$$r_{yx} = \sum_{n=-\infty}^{\infty} y(n)x(n+k). \tag{1.4.2}$$

Comparing Eqs. 1.4.1 and 1.4.2, it can be seen that

$$r_{yx}(k) = r_{xy}(-k). \tag{1.4.3}$$

Notice that the structural form of crosscorrelation is similar to that of convolution, with the omission of the time-reversal step. It is easily shown, in fact, that

$$r_{xy}(k) = x(k) * y(-k).$$

Thus, a program which performs convolution can also be used to compute crosscorrelation.

In a manner similar to crosscorrelation, we define the *autocorrelation* of a signal $\boldsymbol{x}$ by the sequence $r_{xx}(k)$ where

$$r_{xx}(k) = \sum_{n=-\infty}^{\infty} x(n)x(n+k). \tag{1.4.4}$$

From the previous discussion, it immediately follows that

$$r_{xx}(k) = x(k) * x(-k).$$

As with the relationship in Eq. 1.4.3, the autocorrelation sequence is also even. That is,

$$r_{xx}(k) = r_{xx}(-k).$$

Notice from the definition that

$$r_{xx}(0) = \sum_{n=-\infty}^{\infty} |x(n)|^2 = E_x$$

so that the zeroth lag of the autocorrelation of the signal $\boldsymbol{x}$ (which exists since $\boldsymbol{x}$ is assumed to be l^2) is equal to its energy. Furthermore, it is easily shown that

$$|r_{xx}(k)| \leq r_{xx}(0)$$

so that the autocorrelation sequence is a maximum at the zeroth lag.

For the special case where $\boldsymbol{x}$ and $\boldsymbol{y}$ are causal and of finite duration, the crosscorrelation and autocorrelation will have finite limits on the summations. If $\boldsymbol{x}$ and $\boldsymbol{y}$ assume nonzero values only over the time range $0 \leq k \leq N$, we can write

$$r_{xy}(k) = \sum_{n=0}^{N-|k|} x(n)y(n+k) \tag{1.4.5}$$

and

$$r_{xx}(k) = \sum_{n=0}^{N-|k|} x(n)x(n+k). \tag{1.4.6}$$

If $\boldsymbol{x}$ and $\boldsymbol{y}$ are periodic, then they are not finite energy signals. In this case, we are concerned with *power* rather than energy. The power of a signal $\boldsymbol{x}$ is defined by

$$P_x = \lim_{M\to\infty} \frac{1}{2M+1} \sum_{n=-M}^{M} x^2(n).$$

If the limit is finite, the signal is said to be a finite power signal. Clearly, for a finite-energy signal, the power will be zero. With this in mind, the crosscorrelation of signals with finite power is given by

$$r_{xy}(k) = \lim_{M\to\infty} \frac{1}{2M+1} \sum_{n=-M}^{M} x(n)y(n+k)$$

and the autocorrelation by

$$r_{xx}(k) = \lim_{M\to\infty} \frac{1}{2M+1} \sum_{n=-M}^{M} x(n)x(n+k).$$

For periodic signals, the limit is equal to the average over one period. Thus, if the signals are periodic with period N, we have

$$r_{xy}(k) = \frac{1}{N} \sum_{n=0}^{N-1} x(n)y(n+k) \tag{1.4.7}$$

and the autocorrelation by

$$r_{xx}(k) = \frac{1}{N} \sum_{n=0}^{N-1} x(n)x(n+k). \tag{1.4.8}$$

Clearly, $r_{xy}(k)$ and $r_{xx}(k)$ are also periodic with period N.

Chapter 2

FREQUENCY-DOMAIN SIGNAL AND SYSTEM ANALYSIS

2.1 Introduction

The analysis of signals and systems in the frequency domain is a standard technique which has been used for many years in many branches of engineering. This is due largely to the mathematical simplicity it affords and the physical intuition it lends to the analysis. Many of the results we will use come from the theory of functions of a complex variable, which is a very old and elegant area of mathematics. For a solid introductory treatment, the reader is referred to [CB84].

In the previous chapter, it was shown that if $\{h(k)\}$ is the impulse response of a LTI system, the response to an input $\{x(k)\}$ is given by the convolution sum

$$y(k) = \sum_{n=-\infty}^{\infty} h(n)x(k-n). \tag{2.1.1}$$

Suppose that the input is of the form

$$x(k) = z^k,$$

where z is an arbitrary complex number. For example, if z is a real number a with $0 < a < 1$, $\boldsymbol{x}$ is a decaying exponential and if $z = e^{j\theta}$, $\boldsymbol{x}$ will be a complex exponential. From Eq. 2.1.1, the output, $y(k)$, is expressed by the convolution sum

$$y(k) = \sum_{n=-\infty}^{\infty} h(n)z^{k-n} = z^k \sum_{n=-\infty}^{\infty} h(n)z^{-n}.$$

Let us define $H(z)$ by

$$H(z) = \sum_{k=-\infty}^{\infty} h(k)z^{-k}.$$

Thus, for inputs of the form $x(k) = z^k$, the response of the system is

$$y(k) = H(z)z^k.$$

What this means is that for any input $x(k) = z_0^k$, the corresponding output is simply z_0^n scaled by the value of $H(z)$ evaluated at $z = z_0$. $H(z_0)$ is a complex number and hence has a magnitude and phase. Therefore, the output is the same exponential as the input, with scaled magnitude and some phase-shift determined by $H(z)$. Specifically, the magnitude is scaled by $|H(z)|$ and the phase is shifted by $\angle H(z)$. We say that z^n is an *eigenfunction* of the system defined by $h(k)$.

When z is constrained to lie on the unit circle, *i.e.*, $z = e^{j\theta}$, the $\mathcal{Z}$-transform reduces to the *discrete-time Fourier transform* (DTFT), which we will discuss in detail later in this chapter. We will develop the general theory of the $\mathcal{Z}$-transform, and all of the DTFT results will follow trivially. It is important, however, to bear in mind the connection between the $\mathcal{Z}$-transform and the DTFT. The $\mathcal{Z}$-transform corresponds to a more general class of inputs than the DTFT and will be used to analyze the transient and steady-state response of LTI systems to arbitrary inputs. The DTFT will be used specifically for sinusoidal input signals, and will be of particular importance to us when we discuss notions such as *frequency selectivity* and filtering.

2.2 $\mathcal{Z}$-Transform of Discrete-Time Signals

We will now examine the $\mathcal{Z}$-transform as an entity in its own right. Let $x(n)$ be a signal. The *bilateral* $\mathcal{Z}$-transform of $x(n)$ (henceforth referred to simply as the $\mathcal{Z}$-transform) is defined by

$$X(z) = \sum_{k=-\infty}^{\infty} x(k)z^{-k}. \tag{2.2.1}$$

We will frequently denote the $\mathcal{Z}$-transform of a signal $x(n)$ by

$$X(z) = \mathcal{Z}[x(n)].$$

The *unilateral* $\mathcal{Z}$-transform is defined by

$$X_u(z) = \sum_{k=0}^{\infty} x(k)z^{-k}$$

and is equivalent to the bilinear $\mathcal{Z}$-transform when $x(k) = 0$ for $n < 0$. We will almost always use the bilinear $\mathcal{Z}$-transform. However, the unilateral $\mathcal{Z}$-transform will be seen to be quite useful in solving difference equations with nonzero initial conditions.

The $\mathcal{Z}$-transform will not converge for all values of z. The values of z for which the sum converges is known as the *region of convergence* (ROC) of $X(z)$. Before a formal discussion of the ROC, we will illustrate with an example.

Example 2.1

Let

$$x(k) = a^k u(k).$$

From the definition of the $\mathcal{Z}$-transform , we have

$$X(z) = \sum_{k=-\infty}^{\infty} a^k u(k) z^{-k} = \sum_{k=0}^{\infty} a^k z^{-k}.$$

But

$$\sum_{k=0}^{\infty} a^k z^{-k} = \sum_{k=0}^{\infty} (a/z)^k$$

so that $X(z)$ converges if and only if $|a/z| < 1$, or

$$|z| > |a|.$$

Thus the region of convergence is the exterior of the circle in the complex plane defined by $|z| = |a|$ (see Figure 2.2.1). Notice that the unit circle is in the ROC only if $|a| < 1$. For any z in the ROC, $X(z)$ is given by

$$X(z) = \lim_{N\to\infty} \sum_{k=0}^{N} a^k z^{-k} = \lim_{N\to\infty} \frac{1-(a/z)^{N+1}}{1-a/z} = \frac{1}{1-az^{-1}}.$$

$X(z)$ can also be expressed as a ratio of polynomials in z rather than in z^{-1}, in which case

$$X(z) = \frac{1}{1-az^{-1}} = \frac{z}{z-a}.$$

The previous example suggests that the convergence of the $\mathcal{Z}$-transform only depends on the magnitude of z. Indeed, this is the case. Hence, the region of convergence will always have circular symmetry in the complex plane.

The absolute summability of a sequence can also be determined from the region of convergence. If the sequence of interest is the impulse response of a system, we showed that absolute summability corresponds to system stability. Absolute summability of a sequence $\{x(k)\}$ means that

$$\sum_{k=-\infty}^{\infty} |x(k)| < \infty.$$

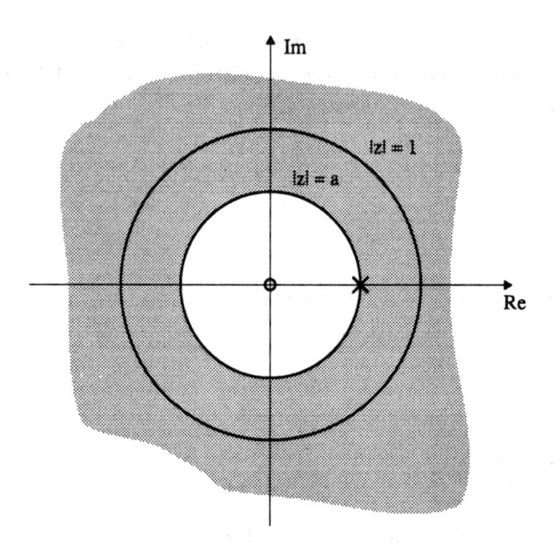

Figure 2.2.1: Region of convergence for Example 2.1.

How can this condition be described in terms of $X(z)$? Suppose first that the $\{x(k)\}$ is absolutely summable. Let z be a point on the unit circle, *i.e.*, $|z| = 1$. We wish to show that z is in the region of convergence. This means that we would like to show that

$$\left| \sum_{k=-\infty}^{\infty} x(k) z^{-k} \right| < \infty.$$

But

$$\left| \sum_{k=-\infty}^{\infty} x(k) z^{-k} \right| \leq \sum_{k=-\infty}^{\infty} |x(k)||z|^{-k}$$

and we have assumed that $|z| = 1$, so that

$$\left| \sum_{k=-\infty}^{\infty} x(k) z^{-k} \right| < \sum_{k=-\infty}^{\infty} |x(k)| < \infty.$$

This means that if $x(k)$ is absolutely summable, the unit circle belongs to the ROC of $X(z)$. Conversely, assume that the unit circle $|z| = 1$ is in the region of convergence of $X(z)$. The $\mathcal{Z}$-transform $X(z)$ satisfies

$$|X(z)| < \infty$$

only if

$$\sum_{k=-\infty}^{\infty} |x(k)||z|^{-k} < \infty.$$

In other words, the $\mathcal{Z}$-transform converges only if the sequence $\{x(k)|z|^{-k}\}$ is absolutely summable. Since $|z| = 1$ by assumption, this is equivalent to the absolute summability of $\{x(k)\}$. Therefore, absolute summability of a sequence $\{x(k)\}$ is equivalent to the requirement that the ROC of $X(z)$ include the unit circle.

For the special case where $X(z)$ is a rational function (as will almost always be the case in this text), the values of z for which the numerator vanishes are known as the *zeros* of $X(z)$, and the values of z for which the denominator of $X(z)$ vanishes are known as the *poles* of $X(z)$. We will frequently compute $\mathcal{Z}$-transforms which are rational functions expressed in z^{-1}. To examine the pole-zero distribution, we must be able to obtain an equivalent expression in z. If $X(z)$ is rational and expressed in terms of z^{-1}, it will be the ratio of two polynomials in z^{-1}:

$$X(z) = \frac{b_0 + b_1 z^{-1} + \cdots + b_M z^{-M}}{a_0 + a_1 z^{-1} + \cdots + a_N z^{-N}}.$$

If we multiply both the numerator and denominator by $z^N z^M$, we obtain

$$X(z) = \frac{z^N(b_0 z^M + b_1 z^{M-1} + \cdots + b_M)}{z^M(a_0 z^N + a_1 z^{N-1} + \cdots + a_N)}.$$

This shows that $X(z)$ will have M zeros and N poles in the complex plane plus an additional $|N - M|$ poles or zeros at the origin, depending on whether M or N is greater. In other words, there are the same number of poles and zeros in the finite z-plane.

Returning to our above example, we see that $X(z)$ has one zero at $z = 0$ and a pole at $z = a$. The ROC for $X(z)$ was determined by the value of the pole. We will see that the locations of the poles play an important role in determining the ROC, in general. Let us now consider another example.

Example 2.2

Suppose $x(k)$ is given by

$$x(k) = \left(\frac{1}{3}\right)^k u(k) + \left(\frac{1}{2}\right)^k u(k).$$

Then the $\mathcal{Z}$-transform is computed as

$$X(z) = \sum_{k=-\infty}^{\infty} \left[\left(\frac{1}{3}\right)^k u(k) + \left(\frac{1}{2}\right)^k u(k)\right] z^{-k}$$

or,

$$X(z) = \sum_{k=0}^{\infty} \left(\frac{1}{3}\right)^k z^{-k} + \sum_{k=0}^{\infty} \left(\frac{1}{2}\right)^k z^{-k}.$$

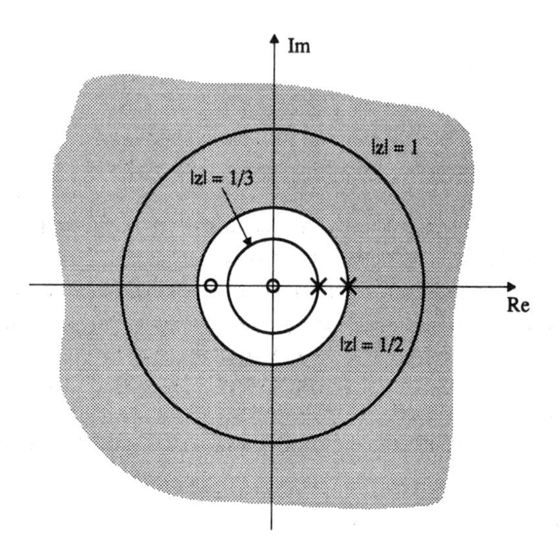

Figure 2.2.2: Pole-zero plot and region of convergence for Example 2.2.

We already know that the summation on the left converges only for values of z in the region $|z| > \frac{1}{3}$ and that the summation on the right converges only for values of z in the region $|z| > \frac{1}{2}$. For the entire expression to converge, then, z must be in the intersection of the two regions, which is given by $|z| > \frac{1}{2}$. In this case, we have

$$X(z) = \frac{1}{1 - \frac{1}{3}z^{-1}} + \frac{1}{1 - \frac{1}{2}z^{-1}} = \frac{2 + \frac{5}{6}z^{-1}}{(1 + \frac{1}{3}z^{-1})(1 + \frac{1}{2}z^{-1})}$$

or,

$$X(z) = \frac{z(2z + \frac{5}{6})}{(z + \frac{1}{3})(z + \frac{1}{2})}.$$

Notice that $X(z)$ has zeros at $z = 0, z = -\frac{5}{12}$ and poles at $z = -\frac{1}{3}, z = -\frac{1}{2}$. The region of convergence is the exterior of the circle with radius determined by the pole of largest magnitude (see Figure 2.2.2).

The previous example suggests the following important property.

Property 1 *If $x(n)$ is a right-sided signal, R_x, the region of convergence of the $\mathcal{Z}$-transform $X(z)$ is the exterior of the circle in the complex plane, centered at the origin, with radius given by the pole of largest magnitude. The point $z = \infty$ belongs to R_x only if $x(k) = 0$ for all $k < 0$ (i.e., $x(k)$ causal).*

It is easy to see why we must require a right-sided $x(k)$ to be causal if $\infty \in R_x$. Suppose $x(k_0) \neq 0$ for some $k_0 < 0$. Then $X(z)$ will include some term $z^{-k_0} = z^{|k_0|}$, which diverges as z approaches infinity. An example will clarify.

Example 2.3

Let

$$x(k) = a^k u(k) + \delta(k+1),$$

which is right-sided but non-causal. Then

$$X(z) = \sum_{k=-\infty}^{\infty} (a^k u(k) + \delta(k+1))z^{-k} = \sum_{k=-\infty}^{\infty} a^k u(k) + \sum_{k=-\infty}^{\infty} \delta(k+1)z^{-k}.$$

But we already know that

$$\sum_{k=-\infty}^{\infty} a^k u(k) = \frac{1}{1-az^{-1}}$$

with region of convergence $|z| > |a|$. Also,

$$\sum_{k=-\infty}^{\infty} \delta(k+1)z^{-k} = z$$

with region of convergence $|z| < \infty$ so that

$$X(z) = \frac{1}{1-az^{-1}} + z$$

with region of convergence

$$R_x = |a| < |z| < \infty.$$

We will now consider the $\mathcal{Z}$-transform of a left-sided signal. This example will point out the significance of the region of convergence in $\mathcal{Z}$-transform analysis.

Example 2.4

Let

$$x(k) = -a^k u(-k-1).$$

Then

$$X(z) = \sum_{k=-\infty}^{\infty} -a^k u(-k-1)z^{-k} = \sum_{k=-\infty}^{-1} -a^k z^{-k}.$$

But

$$-\sum_{k=-\infty}^{-1} a^k z^{-k} = 1 - \sum_{k=0}^{\infty} a^{-k} z^k = 1 - \sum_{k=0}^{\infty} (z/a)^k$$

so that $X(z)$ converges if and only if $|z/a| < 1$, or

$$|z| < |a|.$$

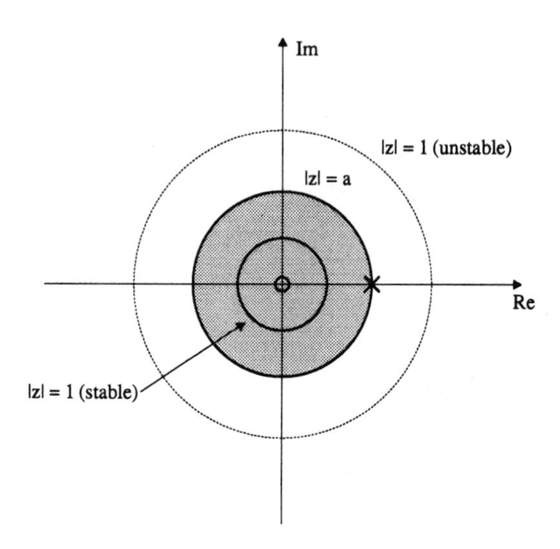

Figure 2.2.3: Pole-zero plot and region of convergence for Example 2.4.

Thus the region of convergence is the interior of the circle in the complex plane defined by $|z| = |a|$ (see Figure 2.2.3). Notice that $x(k)$ is stable only if $|a| > 1$. For any z in the ROC, $X(z)$ is given by

$$X(z) = 1 - \lim_{N\to\infty} \sum_{k=0}^{N} a^{-k} z^{k} = \lim_{N\to\infty} \frac{1 - (z/a)^{N+1}}{1 - z/a} = \frac{1}{1 - az^{-1}}$$

or

$$X(z) = \frac{1}{1 - az^{-1}} = \frac{z}{z - a}.$$

Notice that this expression is identical to the $\mathcal{Z}$-transform in Example 2.1. This indicates the importance of specifying the region of convergence along with the $\mathcal{Z}$-transform. In other words, it is impossible to determine the signal corresponding to a particular $\mathcal{Z}$-transform if the region of convergence is not specified; several different signals can give rise to the same $\mathcal{Z}$-transform.

In direct analogy with the right-sided case, we can establish a relationship between the pole locations and the ROC for left-sided signals as follows.

Property 2 *If $x(k)$ is a left-sided signal, R_x, the region of convergence of the $\mathcal{Z}$-transform $X(z)$ is the interior of the circle in the complex plane, centered at the origin, with radius given by the pole of smallest magnitude. The point $z = 0$ belongs to R_x only $x(k) = 0$ for all $k > 0$ (i.e., $x(k)$ anti-causal).*

This time, it is easy to see why we must require a left-sided $x(k)$ to be anti-causal if $0 \in R_x$. Suppose $x(k_0) \neq 0$ for some $k_0 > 0$. Then $X(z)$ will include some term z^{-k_0}, which diverges as z approaches zero.

We have already seen that the ROC of a left-sided or right-sided signal is either the interior or exterior of a circle in the complex plane. There is one more important case to consider: two-sided signals. Recall that a two-sided signal is a signal which is neither left-sided nor right-sided.

Example 2.5

Let

$$x(k) = \left(\frac{1}{2}\right)^k u(k) - \left(\frac{3}{2}\right)^k u(-k-1).$$

This signal consists of a purely causal part and a purely anti-causal part. Then

$$X(z) = \sum_{k=0}^{\infty} \left(\frac{1}{2}\right)^k z^{-k} - \sum_{k=-\infty}^{-1} \left(\frac{3}{2}\right)^k z^{-k}.$$

We have already seen that the sum on the left converges to

$$\frac{1}{(1-\frac{1}{2}z^{-1})}$$

provided that $|z| > \frac{1}{2}$. The sum on the right converges to

$$\frac{1}{(1-\frac{3}{2}z^{-1})}$$

provided that $|z| < \frac{3}{2}$. Thus,

$$X(z) = \frac{(2-\frac{5}{6}z^{-1})}{(1-\frac{1}{2}z^{-1})(1-\frac{1}{3}z^{-1})},$$

or

$$X(z) = \frac{z(2z-\frac{5}{6})}{(z-\frac{1}{2})(z-\frac{1}{3})}$$

with region of convergence

$$\frac{1}{2} < |z| < \frac{3}{2}.$$

Notice that the ROC is ring-shaped, bounded on the interior and exterior by poles (see Figure 2.2.4).

The situation in general is as follows.

Property 3 *If $x(k)$ is a two-sided signal, R_x, the region of convergence of the $\mathcal{Z}$-transform $X(z)$ is a ring in the complex plane, centered at the origin. The ring is bounded on the interior by a pole and on the exterior by a pole. No pole may belong to the region of convergence.*

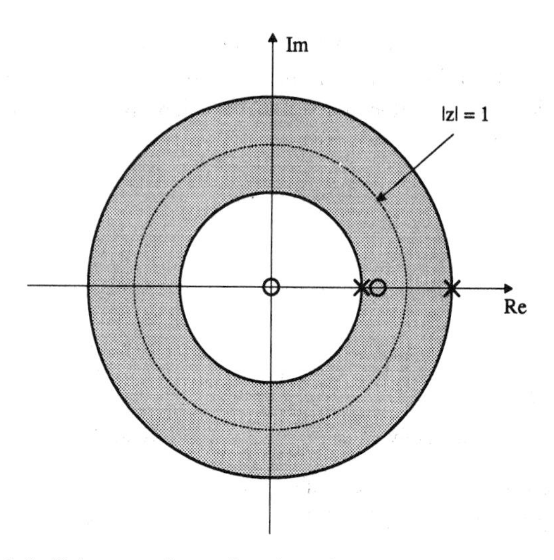

Figure 2.2.4: Pole-zero plot and region of convergence for Example 2.5.

Finally, we need to consider the case where $x(k)$ is nonzero for only a finite number of samples.

Property 4 *Let $x(k)$ be nonzero for only a finite number of samples, i.e., there exist finite M, N such that $x(k) = 0$ for all $k < M$ and $x(k) = 0$ for all $k > N$. Then the region of convergence of $X(z)$ is the entire complex plane with the possible deletion of zero or infinity as follows: If $M < 0$ then $0 \notin ROC$. If $N > 0$ then $\infty \notin ROC$.*

Example 2.6

Let $x(k)$ be the signal consisting of three samples, given by

$$x(k) = 2\delta(k+1) + \delta(k) + 3\delta(k-1).$$

Then

$$X(z) = 2z + 1 + 2z^{-1},$$

which clearly converges for all values of z except zero and infinity.

2.3 $\mathcal{Z}$-Transform Properties

The $\mathcal{Z}$-transform has a number of important properties which make it very useful for the analysis of linear discrete-time systems.

• **Linearity**

It follows from the defining equation that if $x_1(k)$ and $x_2(k)$ have $\mathcal{Z}$-transforms $X_1(z)$ and $X_2(z)$, respectively, that for any constants a and b,

$$\mathcal{Z}[ax_1(k) + bx_2(k)] = aX_1(z) + bX_2(z). \quad (2.3.1)$$

Example 2.7

Let $x(k) = (\cos(\theta_0 k))u(k)$. We can use Euler's identity and the linearity property to obtain the $\mathcal{Z}$-transform as follows.

$$\cos(\theta_0 k) = \frac{1}{2}(e^{j\theta_0 k} + e^{-j\theta_0 k})$$

so that

$$X(z) = \frac{1}{2}\sum_{k=0}^{\infty} e^{j\theta_0 k} z^{-k} + \frac{1}{2}\sum_{k=0}^{\infty} e^{-j\theta_0 k} z^{-k}$$

which gives

$$X(z) = \frac{1/2}{1 - e^{j\theta_0 k} z^{-1}} + \frac{1/2}{1 - e^{-j\theta_0 k} z^{-1}}.$$

with region of convergence $|z| > 1$. Simplifying, we have

$$X(z) = \frac{1 - \frac{1}{2}z^{-1}(e^{-j\theta_0} + e^{j\theta_0})}{1 - (e^{j\theta_0} + e^{-j\theta_0})z^{-1} + z^{-2}},$$

or

$$X(z) = \frac{1 - (\cos(\theta_0))z^{-1}}{1 - (2\cos(\theta_0))z^{-1} + z^{-2}}.$$

- **Time Shifting**

Suppose we time-shift a signal $x(k)$ by k_0 samples. It is simple to show (this is left to the reader) that

$$\mathcal{Z}[x(k - k_0)] = z^{-k_0} X(z). \quad (2.3.2)$$

Example 2.8

Let $x(k) = \delta(k - 5)$. The $\mathcal{Z}$-transform of $\delta(k)$ is given by

$$X(z) = \sum_{k=-\infty}^{\infty} \delta(k) z^{-k} = 1$$

so that

$$\mathcal{Z}[\delta(k - 5)] = z^{-5} X(z) = z^{-5}.$$

- **Modulation**

Consider modulating $x(k)$ by the sequence z_0^k. Then

$$\mathcal{Z}[z_0^k x(k)] = \sum_{k=-\infty}^{\infty} x(k) z_0^k z^{-k}.$$

But

$$\sum_{k=-\infty}^{\infty} x(k) z_0^k z^{-k} = \sum_{k=-\infty}^{\infty} x(k) \left(\frac{z}{z_0}\right)^k.$$

This is simply the $\mathcal{Z}$-transform of $x(k)$ evaluated at z/z_0 so that

$$\mathcal{Z}[z_0^k x(k)] = X(z/z_0). \tag{2.3.3}$$

- **Complex Conjugation**

If $x(k)$ is a signal, consider the $\mathcal{Z}$-transform of $x^*(k)$, the complex conjugate of $x(k)$. We have

$$\mathcal{Z}[x^*(k)] = \sum_{k=-\infty}^{\infty} x^*(k) z^{-k}.$$

But

$$\sum_{k=-\infty}^{\infty} x^*(k) z^{-k} = \left(\sum_{k=-\infty}^{\infty} x(k)(z^*)^{-k}\right)^* = X^*(z^*). \tag{2.3.4}$$

- **Multiplication by n**

To derive the next property, suppose $x(k)$ has $\mathcal{Z}$-transform $X(z)$. If we differentiate the expression for $X(z)$, we get

$$\frac{dX(z)}{dz} = \sum_{k=-\infty}^{\infty} (-kx(k)) z^{k-1},$$

so that

$$-z\frac{dX(z)}{dz} = \sum_{k=-\infty}^{\infty} kx(k) z^{-k},$$

which is clearly the $\mathcal{Z}$-transform of $kx(k)$. We thus have

$$\mathcal{Z}[kx(k)] = -z\frac{dX(z)}{dz}. \tag{2.3.5}$$

Example 2.9

Suppose $x(k) = a^k u(k)$, which has $\mathcal{Z}$-transform

$$X(z) = \frac{1}{1 - az^{-1}} = \frac{z}{z-a}.$$

Then $ka^k u(k)$ has $\mathcal{Z}$-transform given by

$$\mathcal{Z}[ka^k u(k)] = -z\frac{d}{dz}\left(\frac{z}{z-a}\right) = \frac{az}{(z-a)^2}.$$

• **Convolution**

The following property is perhaps the most important property of the $\mathcal{Z}$-transform. Suppose $x_1(k)$ and $x_2(k)$ have $\mathcal{Z}$-transforms $X_1(z)$ and $X_2(z)$, respectively. Define $w(k)$ as the convolution of $x_1(k)$ and $x_2(k)$. That is,

$$w(k) = \sum_{n=-\infty}^{\infty} x_1(n)x_2(k-n).$$

Then

$$W(z) = \sum_{k=-\infty}^{\infty} w(k)z^{-k} = \sum_{k=-\infty}^{\infty} z^{-k}\left[\sum_{n=-\infty}^{\infty} x_1(n)x_2(k-n)\right]. \tag{2.3.6}$$

Reversing the order of summation of Eq. 2.3.6,

$$W(z) = \sum_{n=-\infty}^{\infty} x_1(n)\left[\sum_{k=-\infty}^{\infty} z^{-k}x_2(k-n)\right]. \tag{2.3.7}$$

We recognize the inner summation of Eq. 2.3.7 as the $\mathcal{Z}$-transform of $x_2(k-n)$, which is just $z^{-n}X_2(z)$, so that

$$W(z) = X_2(z)\sum_{k=-\infty}^{\infty} z^{-k}x_1(k). \tag{2.3.8}$$

Thus, for z in the ROCs of both $X_1(z)$ and $X_2(z)$, Eq. 2.3.8 becomes

$$W(z) = \mathcal{Z}[x_1(k) * x_2(k)] = X_1(z)X_2(z). \tag{2.3.9}$$

What this says is that convolution in the time-domain corresponds to simple multiplication of $\mathcal{Z}$-transforms where the ROC contains the intersection of the ROCs of $X_1(z)$ and $X_2(z)$. If a pole at the edge of the ROC of either $X_1(z)$ or $X_2(z)$ is canceled by a zero, the ROC can possibly be larger.

Example 2.10

Suppose we wish to find an expression for the convolution of the two exponential sequences $x_1(k) = \left(\frac{1}{2}\right)^k u(k)$ and $x_2(k) = \left(\frac{1}{3}\right)^k u(k)$. $x_1(k)$ has $\mathcal{Z}$-transform

$$X_1(z) = \frac{z}{z-\frac{1}{2}}$$

and $x_2(k)$ has $\mathcal{Z}$-transform

$$X_2(z) = \frac{z}{z-\frac{1}{3}}.$$

It follows from the convolution property of the $\mathcal{Z}$-transform that

$$\mathcal{Z}[x_1(k) * x_2(k)] = \frac{z^2}{(z-\frac{1}{2})(z-\frac{1}{3})}.$$

In order to recover a time-domain expression for the result, we must first learn how to invert the $\mathcal{Z}$-transform, which is the subject of the next section.

• Correlation

Recall that for a sequence $x(k)$, the autocorrelation sequence, $r_{xx}(k)$ is defined by

$$r_{xx}(k) = \sum_{n=-\infty}^{\infty} x^*(n)x(k+n).$$

The $\mathcal{Z}$-transform, $R_{xx}(z)$, of $r_{xx}(k)$ is computed according to

$$R_{xx}(z) = \sum_{k=-\infty}^{\infty} r_{xx}(k)z^{-k} = \sum_{k=-\infty}^{\infty} z^{-k} \sum_{n=-\infty}^{\infty} x^*(n)x(k+n). \tag{2.3.10}$$

Reversing the order of summation of Eq. 2.3.10,

$$R_{xx}(z) = \sum_{n=-\infty}^{\infty} x^*(n) \sum_{k=-\infty}^{\infty} z^{-k}x(k+n). \tag{2.3.11}$$

The inner summation of Eq. 2.3.11 is recognized as the $\mathcal{Z}$-transform of $x(k+n)$, which is just $z^n X(z)$, so that

$$R_{xx}(z) = X(z) \sum_{n=-\infty}^{\infty} x^*(n)z^n. \tag{2.3.12}$$

But

$$\sum_{n=-\infty}^{\infty} x^*(n)z^n = \sum_{n=-\infty}^{\infty} x^*(n)(1/z)^{-n}, \tag{2.3.13}$$

which is just the $\mathcal{Z}$-transform of $x^*(k)$ evaluated at $1/z$. We already know that

$$\mathcal{Z}[x^*(k)] = X^*(z^*)$$

so that

$$\sum_{n=-\infty}^{\infty} x^*(n)(1/z)^{-n} = X^*(1/z^*).$$

Thus,

$$R_{xx}(z) = X(z)X^*(1/z^*). \tag{2.3.14}$$

• **Initial value theorem**
Suppose $x(k)$ is a causal signal. Then $|z| = \infty$ is in the ROC of $X(z)$. Thus,

$$\lim_{z\to\infty} \sum_{k=0}^{\infty} x(k)z^{-k} = x(0). \tag{2.3.15}$$

Therefore, for causal signals, the initial value of $x(k)$ can be computed from the $\mathcal{Z}$-transform according to

$$x(0) = \lim_{z\to\infty} X(z).$$

Example 2.11

Let $X(z)$ be given by

$$X(z) = \frac{1}{1 - az^{-1}}, \quad |z| > |a|.$$

Then $x(k)$ is causal and

$$x(0) = \lim_{z\to\infty} \frac{1}{1 - az^{-1}} = 1,$$

which is easily verified since $x(k)$ is easily seen to be given by $a^k u(k)$.

We have provided a listing of important $\mathcal{Z}$-transform pairs in Table 2.1 and a collection of important properties in Table 2.2.

2.4 Inverting the $\mathcal{Z}$-Transform

Inversion of the $\mathcal{Z}$-transform is formally defined in terms of a complex contour integral. We will not discuss the general theory of contour integration, but instead will concentrate on contour integration of rational functions. For the general case, the reader is again referred to [CB84].

A major result from the theory of complex variables is Cauchy's integral theorem, which is as follows.

Theorem 2 (Cauchy's Integral Theorem) *The contour integral*

$$\frac{1}{2\pi j} \oint_\Gamma z^{k-1} dz,$$

where Γ is a counter-clockwise contour in the complex plane which encircles the origin, takes on the value zero for all $k \neq 0$. When $k = 0$, the value of the integral is one.

We are not yet concerned with how to evaluate a complex contour integral. This will be discussed soon. Cauchy's integral theorem can be used to derive the inverse $\mathcal{Z}$-transform. Consider the expression

$$\hat{x}(k) = \frac{1}{2\pi j} \oint_C X(z) z^{k-1}\, dz \tag{2.4.1}$$

where C is in the region of convergence of the $\mathcal{Z}$-transform $X(z)$. We have used the symbol $\hat{x}(k)$ to indicate that we are not certain if $\hat{x}(k)$ is the true inverse $\mathcal{Z}$-transform.

Let us substitute the expression for $X(z)$ (Eq. 2.4.1) into Eq. 2.4.1:

$$\hat{x}(k) = \frac{1}{2\pi j} \oint \left[\sum_{n=-\infty}^{\infty} x(n) z^{-n} \right] z^{k-1}\, dz. \tag{2.4.2}$$

Interchanging the order of summation and integration in Eq. 2.4.2 (which is permissible because of the uniform convergence of the $\mathcal{Z}$-transform), we have

$$\hat{x}(k) = \sum_{n=-\infty}^{\infty} \left[\frac{1}{2\pi j} \oint_C x(n) z^{k-n-1}\, dz \right]. \tag{2.4.3}$$

Because of Cauchy's integral theorem, the value of the integral in Eq. 2.4.3 is zero for all n except $n = k$ so that

$$\hat{x}(k) = \sum_{n=-\infty}^{\infty} x(n) \delta(k-n) = x(k). \tag{2.4.4}$$

Therefore, $\hat{x}(k) = x(k)$, and the inverse $\mathcal{Z}$-transform is given by

$$x(k) = \frac{1}{2\pi j} \oint_C X(z) z^{k-1}\, dz \tag{2.4.5}$$

where C is a counter-clockwise contour in the region of convergence of $X(z)$.

We must now discuss how to actually evaluate the contour integral defining the inverse $\mathcal{Z}$-transform. Fortunately, there is another important result from the theory of complex variables which makes the evaluation of contour integrals very simple.

Assume that $F(z)$ is a rational function of z. This means that we can write $F(z)$ as the ratio of two polynomials, $n(z)$ and $d(z)$, *i.e.*,

$$F(z) = \frac{n(z)}{d(z)}.$$

The denominator, $d(z)$ can be factored according to

$$d(z) = \prod_{i=1}^{L} (z - r_i)^{m_i}$$

where the r_i are the L *distinct* roots of $a(z)$ and the m_i are the multiplicities of the roots. The *method of residues* then states that

$$\frac{1}{2\pi j}\oint_C F(z)\,dz = \sum_i \rho_{r_i} \tag{2.4.6}$$

where the ρ_{r_i} are the *residues of* $F(z)$ *at the poles* r_i *which are interior to* C. The residue ρ_i is computed according to

$$\rho_i = \frac{1}{(m_i-1)!}\left(\frac{d^{m_i-1}}{dz^{m_i-1}}\left[(z-r_i)^{m_i}F(z)\right]\right)\Bigg|_{z=r_i}. \tag{2.4.7}$$

An example will best illustrate.

Example 2.12

This example illustrates contour integration by the method of residues but does not yet correspond to $\mathcal{Z}$-transform inversion. Suppose

$$F(z) = \frac{1}{(z+1)(z+2)^2}$$

and we wish to evaluate

$$\frac{1}{2\pi j}\oint_{|z|=3} F(z)\,dz.$$

According to Eq. 2.4.6, since both poles are interior to the contour of integration, we have

$$\frac{1}{2\pi j}\oint_C F(z)\,dz = \rho_{-1} + \rho_{-2}$$

where, by Eq. 2.4.7

$$\rho_{-1} = \frac{1}{0!}\left(\frac{d^0}{dz^0}[(z+1)F(z)]\right)\Bigg|_{z=-1} = 1$$

and

$$\rho_{-2} = \frac{1}{1!}\left(\frac{d}{dz}[(z+2)^2F(z)]\right)\Big|_{z=-2} = \frac{-1}{(z+1)^2}\Bigg|_{z=-2} = -1.$$

We then have

$$\frac{1}{2\pi j}\oint_{|z|=3} F(z)\,dz = \rho_{-1} + \rho_{-2} = 1 - 1 = 0.$$

To relate the residue method of contour integration to $\mathcal{Z}$-transform inversion, simply let $F(z)$ be the rational function $z^{k-1}X(z)$. It is particularly important that the region of convergence be specified so that an appropriate contour may be chosen.

Example 2.13

Let

$$X(z) = \frac{z}{z-a}$$

with region of convergence

$$|z| > a.$$

The inverse $\mathcal{Z}$-transform is then given by

$$x(n) = \frac{1}{2\pi j}\oint_C X(z)z^{k-1}\,dz = \frac{1}{2\pi j}\oint_C \frac{z^k}{z-a}\,dz.$$

For $k < 0$, $z^{k-1}X(z)$ has a pole at $z = a$ and n poles at $z = 0$. Choose a contour of integration, C, with radius greater than a so that all of the poles lie inside this contour. Let's consider the case $k = -2$ first. Then

$$z^{k-1}X(z) = \frac{1}{z^2(z-a)}.$$

There will be two residues: one at $z = a$ and one at $z = 0$. According to Eq. 2.4.7,

$$\rho_a = \left.\frac{1}{z^2}\right|_{z=a} = \frac{1}{a^2}$$

and

$$\rho_0 = \left.\frac{d}{dz}\left(\frac{1}{z-a}\right)\right|_{z=0} = -\frac{1}{a^2}$$

so that

$$x(-2) = \rho_a + \rho_0 = 0.$$

Similarly, we can easily show for any $k < 0$ that $x(k) = 0$, as expected.

For any $k \geq 0$, there is one pole at $z = a$ and k zeros at the origin. In this case,

$$x(k) = \frac{1}{2\pi j}\oint_C \frac{x^k}{z-a}\,dz = \rho_a.$$

But by Eq. 2.4.7,

$$\rho_a = z^k|_{z=a} = a^k$$

so that

$$x(k) = a^k, \quad k \geq 0.$$

2.5 Partial Fraction Expansion

The method of partial fractions is often used to invert the $\mathcal{Z}$-transform. This method is popular because it reduces the inversion of the $\mathcal{Z}$-transform to a kind of "template matching." That is, $X(z)$ is reduced to a sum of terms of the form

$$\frac{Az}{z-r}$$

which are easily inverted using a table of transforms. Assume $F(z)$ is expressed as a ratio of polynomials in z, *i.e.*,

$$F(z) = \frac{n(z)}{d(z)}$$

If $n(z)$ is of higher degree than $d(z)$, reduce $F(z)$ to a *proper* fraction plus a polynomial part, *i.e.*,

$$F(z) = p(z) + \frac{q(z)}{d(z)}.$$

Now, we need to examine the factorization of $d(z)$. The multiplicities of the roots are important in the partial fraction expansion. Thus, assume that there are L *distinct* roots,

$$r_1, r_2, \ldots, r_L,$$

with multiplicities

$$m_1, m_2, \ldots, m_L,$$

respectively. Obviously,

$$m_1 + m_2 + \cdots + m_L = N$$

where N is the degree of $d(z)$. Then

$$d(z) = \prod_{i=1}^{L}(z-r_i)^{m_i} = (z-r_1)^{m_1}(z-r_2)^{m_2}\cdots(z-r_L)^{m_L}.$$

Each term $(z-r_i)^{m_i}$ has associated with it m_i partial fraction coefficients, $A_1^{(i)}, A_2^{(i)}, \ldots, A_{m_i}^{(i)}$, and the partial fraction expansion of $q(z)/d(z)$ is of the form

$$\sum_{i=1}^{L}\left[\sum_{j=1}^{m_i}\frac{A_j^{(i)}}{(z-r_i)^j}\right]. \tag{2.5.1}$$

The problem now is to find all of the $A_j^{(i)}$. The formula is quite simple. For $i = 1, 2, \ldots, L$, define the function $\Phi_i(z)$ by

$$\Phi_i(z) = \frac{(z - r_i)^{m_i} q(z)}{d(z)}, \tag{2.5.2}$$

which is just $q(z)/d(z)$ with the term $(z - r_i)^{m_i}$ removed from the denominator. Now, for each root r_i, start with the partial fraction coefficient corresponding to $(z - r_i)^{m_i}$ and compute $A_{m_i}^{(i)}$ according to

$$A_{m_i}^{(i)} = \Phi_i(z)|_{z=r_i}. \tag{2.5.3}$$

Now, work backwards. $A_{m_i-1}^{(i)}$ is given by

$$A_{m_i-1}^{(i)} = \left.\frac{d\Phi_i(z)}{dz}\right|_{z=r_i}. \tag{2.5.4}$$

In general, $A_j^{(i)}$ is computed according to

$$A_j^{(i)} = \frac{1}{(m_i - j)!} \left.\frac{d^j \Phi_i(z)}{dz^j}\right|_{z=r_i}, \quad i = 1, 2, \ldots, L, \quad j = 1, 2, \ldots, m_i. \tag{2.5.5}$$

Now, let's see how to relate this to the inversion of $\mathcal{Z}$-transforms. We choose to work with polynomials in z rather than in z^{-1}. For reasons which will become obvious later, we will frequently choose to work with $X(z)/z$ rather than with $X(z)$ directly.

Example 2.14

Let

$$X(z) = \frac{z^6 + 4z^5 + z^3 + 2z^2 + 6z + 1}{(z + 1)(z - 1)^2}.$$

Then

$$F(z) = \frac{X(z)}{z} = \frac{z^6 + 4z^5 + z^3 + 2z^2 + 6z + 1}{z(z + 1)(z - 1)^2}.$$

The numerator is of higher degree than the denominator, so we perform long division to obtain

$$F(z) = z^2 + 5z + 6 + \frac{11z^3 + 3z^2 + 1}{z(z + 1)(z - 1)^2}.$$

We must now perform partial fraction expansion on the fractional part above. Let's identify the parameters with the previous discussion. The degree of the denominator is four. If we let

$$r_1 = 0, \quad r_2 = -1, \quad r_3 = 1,$$

we have

$$m_1 = 1, \quad m_2 = 1, \quad m_3 = 2,$$

and $m_1 + m_2 + m_3 = 4$.

The expansion will be of the form

$$\frac{11z^3 + 3z^2 + 1}{z(z+1)(z-1)^2} = \frac{A_1^{(1)}}{z} + \frac{A_1^{(2)}}{(z+1)} + \frac{A_1^{(3)}}{(z-1)} + \frac{A_2^{(3)}}{(z-1)^2}.$$

$A_1^{(1)}$ is found according to

$$A_1^{(1)} = \Phi_1(z)|_{z=0} = \left.\frac{11z^3 + 3z^2 + 1}{(z+1)(z-1)^2}\right|_{z=0} = 1.$$

We find $A_1^{(2)}$ by

$$A_1^{(2)} = \Phi_2(z)|_{z=-1} = \left.\frac{11z^3 + 3z^2 + 1}{z(z-1)^2}\right|_{z=-1} = 1.75$$

Now we must deal with the multiple pole at $z = 1$. We start from the highest power and work backwards. $A_2^{(3)}$ is found according to

$$A_2^{(3)} = \Phi_3(z)|_{z=1} = \left.\frac{11z^3 + 3z^2 + 1}{z(z+1)}\right|_{z=1} = 7.5$$

Finally, we find $A_1^{(3)}$ by

$$A_1^{(3)} = \left.\frac{d\Phi_3(z)}{dz}\right|_{z=1} = \frac{1}{1!}\frac{d}{dz}\left.\left(\frac{11z^3 + 3z^2 + 1}{z(z+1)}\right)\right|_{z=1}.$$

But

$$\frac{d\Phi_3(z)}{dz} = \frac{11z^4 + 22z^3 + 3z^2 - 2z - 1}{z^2(z+1)^2}$$

so that

$$A_1^{(3)} = 8.25$$

We thus have

$$\frac{X(z)}{z} = z^2 + 5z + 6 + \frac{1}{z} + \frac{1.75}{(z+1)} + \frac{8.25}{(z-1)} + \frac{7.5}{(z-1)^2}.$$

Now we will see why we divided by z. Since $X(z)/z$ is as shown above, it follows that

$$X(z) = z^3 + 5z^2 + 6z + 1 + \frac{1.75z}{(z+1)} + \frac{8.25z}{(z-1)} + \frac{7.5z}{(z-1)^2}.$$

If the region of convergence is specified as

$$|z| > 1,$$

then the signal is right-sided, and is given by

$$\begin{aligned} x(n) &= \delta(n+3) + 5\delta(n+2) + 6\delta(n+1) + \delta(n) + 1.75(-1)^n u(n) \\ &\quad + 8.25u(n) + 7.5nu(n). \end{aligned}$$

If, instead, the region of convergence had been given as $|z| < 1$, then the signal is left-sided and is expressed by

$$\begin{aligned} x(n) &= \delta(n+3) + 5\delta(n+2) + 6\delta(n+1) + \delta(n) - 1.75(-1)^n u(-n-1) \\ &\quad - 8.25u(-n-1) - 7.5nu(-n-1). \end{aligned}$$

2.6 Transfer Function and System Response

In the previous chapter, we introduced the standard difference equation representation of a linear time-invariant system. We can apply our $\mathcal{Z}$-transform results to the solution of these difference equations.

Recall that the standard difference equation is given by

$$\sum_{n=0}^{N} a_n y(k-n) = \sum_{n=0}^{M} b_n x(k-n)$$

where $x(k)$ is the input and $y(k)$ is the output. Assume that all initial conditions are zero; the system is started from rest. Applying both the the linearity and time-shifting properties of the $\mathcal{Z}$-transform to the standard difference equation,

$$\sum_{n=0}^{N} a_n z^{-n} X(z) = \sum_{n=0}^{N} b_n z^{-n} Y(z),$$

or,

$$Y(z) = \frac{\sum_{n=0}^{M} b_n z^{-n}}{\sum_{n=0}^{N} a_n z^{-n}} X(z). \tag{2.6.1}$$

If we define the *transfer function*, $H(z)$ by

$$H(z) = \frac{Y(z)}{X(z)} = \frac{\sum_{n=0}^{M} b_n z^{-n}}{\sum_{n=0}^{N} a_n z^{-n}}, \tag{2.6.2}$$

then

$$Y(z) = H(z)X(z). \tag{2.6.3}$$

Equation 2.6.3 relates the $\mathcal{Z}$-transform of the output to the $\mathcal{Z}$-transform of the input. Now, let $x(k) = \delta(k)$ so that $X(z) = 1$. Then

$$Y(z) = H(z)$$

and $H(z)$ is clearly the $\mathcal{Z}$-transform of the impulse response, $h(k)$. Thus, to find the impulse response of a system from the standard difference equation, we can find $H(z)$ and invert the $\mathcal{Z}$-transform to obtain $h(k)$.

In deriving this result, we made no assumptions about stability or causality; all that was assumed was linearity and time-invariance. What this means is that from the difference equation we can obtain an expression for the transfer function of the system but not the ROC. All that is required for Eq. 2.6.3 to be true is that the ROCs of $X(z)$ and $Y(z)$ overlap. We do know that the ROC of $H(z)$ must be ring-shaped and bounded by poles. A number of possible choices for the ROC will satisfy this constraint. If we assume that the system is causal, then $h(k)$ will be right-sided and hence the ROC of $H(z)$ must be outside the pole of largest magnitude. If we assume that the system is stable, the ROC must include the unit circle.

Example 2.15

Consider the system described by the difference equation

$$y(k) = x(k) + ay(k-1).$$

This is a recursive system whose present output depends on the past output and the present input. Taking the $\mathcal{Z}$-transform we have

$$Y(z) = X(z) + az^{-1}Y(z)$$

so that

$$H(z) = \frac{1}{1 - az^{-1}}.$$

There are two possible choices for the ROC:

$$|z| > a$$

and

$$|z| < a.$$

Let's choose the first ROC, $|z| > a$. Then the inverse $\mathcal{Z}$-transform gives

$$h(k) = a^k u(k),$$

and if $|a| < 1$, the system is stable and causal. If $|a| > 1$, the system is unstable and causal. For the second ROC, we have

$$h(k) = -a^{k-1} u(k-1),$$

and if $|a| > 1$, the system is stable and noncausal. If $|a| < 1$, the system is unstable and noncausal. Notice that for all of these cases, the ROCs of $X(z)$ and $Y(z)$ overlap.

For most of our applications, we will be interested in systems which are stable and causal. The previous example showed that stability and causality are not always compatible requirements. We need a condition which characterizes *both* stability and causality. This is simple to describe: in order for an LTI system to be both causal and stable, all of the poles of $H(z)$ must lie inside the unit circle.

2.7 The Unilateral $\mathcal{Z}$-Transform

When analyzing systems with nonzero initial conditions which are driven by causal inputs, we need to modify the previous procedure by using the *unilateral* $\mathcal{Z}$-transform. The unilateral $\mathcal{Z}$-transform of a signal $x(k)$ is defined by

$$X_u(z) = \sum_{k=0}^{\infty} x(k) z^{-k}. \tag{2.7.1}$$

For causal signals, the bilateral and unilateral $\mathcal{Z}$-transforms are identical. All of the properties of the bilinear $\mathcal{Z}$-transform hold for the unilateral $\mathcal{Z}$-transform, but the time-shifting property must be modified somewhat. To this end, consider a sequence $x(k)$ with unilateral $\mathcal{Z}$-transform $X_u(z)$. Let

$$y(k) = x(k-1).$$

Then

$$Y_u(z) = \sum_{k=0}^{\infty} x(k-1) z^{-k} = x(-1) + \sum_{k=1}^{\infty} x(k-1) z^{-k}.$$

If we let $m = k - 1$, then

$$Y_u(z) = x(-1) + z^{-1} \sum_{m=0}^{\infty} x(m) z^{-m}$$

so that

$$Y_u(z) = x(-1) + z^{-1} X_u(z).$$

In general, we find that if $y(k) = x(k - m)$, then

$$Y_u(z) = x(-m) + z^{-1} x(-m+1) + \cdots + z^{-m+1} x(-1) + z^{-m} X_u(z). \tag{2.7.2}$$

Example 2.16

Consider the system described by the standard difference equation

$$y(k) - 2y(k-1) = x(k)$$

with input

$$x(k) = u(k)$$

and initial condition

$$y(-1) = 1.$$

Applying Eq. 2.7.2, we have

$$Y_u(z) - 2(y(-1) + z^{-1} Y_u(z)) = X_u(z)$$

which yields

$$Y_u(z) = \frac{2}{1 - 2z^{-1}} + \frac{1}{(1 - z^{-1})(1 - 2z^{-1})}.$$

After some manipulation, we obtain

$$Y_u(z) = \frac{4}{1 - 2z^{-1}} + \frac{1}{1 - z^{-1}}.$$

Because all of the signals involved were right-sided, the inverse unilateral $\mathcal{Z}$-transform is the same as the inverse bilateral $\mathcal{Z}$-transform , so that

$$y(k) = 4(2)^k u(k) + u(k).$$

Inverse systems

Given an impulse response $\boldsymbol{h}$, we wish to find the sequence $\boldsymbol{h}_i$ such that

$$\boldsymbol{h} * \boldsymbol{h}_i = \delta,$$

the unit pulse. This problem is equivalent to finding the system $H_i(z)$, which when cascaded with $H(z)$ gives

$$H(z)H_i(z) = 1,$$

which implies that

$$H_i(z) = \frac{1}{H(z)}. \tag{2.7.3}$$

One problem remains, however. We do not know when $H_i(z)$ actually exists. Fortunately, for LTI systems, $H(z)$ is a rational function so that $H_i(z)$ will always exist. It is immediately obvious that if $H(z)$ is a rational function of z, the poles of $H(z)$ become the zeros of $H_i(z)$ and the zeros of $H(z)$ become the poles of $H_i(z)$. What remains to be seen is whether this inverse system is stable or causal.

For the relation $H_i(z)H(z) = 1$ to hold, all that is required is that the ROCs of $H(z)$ and $H_i(z)$ overlap. Some examples will best illustrate.

Example 2.17

Suppose $H(z)$ is given by

$$H(z) = \frac{1 - 0.5z^{-1}}{1 - 0.75z^{-1}}$$

with ROC $|z| > 0.75$ (*i.e.*, $H(z)$ is stable and causal). $H_i(z)$ is given by

$$H_i(z) = \frac{1 - 0.75z^{-1}}{1 - 0.5z^{-1}}$$

and there are two possibilities for the ROC of $H_i(z)$. The first choice, $|z| < 0.5$, does not overlap the ROC of $H(z)$ and is discarded. The second choice, $|z| > 0.5$, does overlap the ROC of $H(z)$ and leads to a causal, stable inverse system.

Suppose, instead, that

$$H(z) = \frac{1 - 4z^{-1}}{1 - 0.5z^{-1}}$$

with ROC $|z| > 0.5$. The inverse system is given by

$$H_i(z) = \frac{1 - 0.5z^{-1}}{1 - 4z^{-1}}$$

and there are two possible ROCs: $|z| < 4$ and $|z| > 4$. The case $|z| < 4$ overlaps the ROC of $H(z)$ and corresponds to a stable, noncausal system. The case $|z| > 4$ *also* overlaps the ROC of $H(z)$ and corresponds to an unstable causal system. Thus, we have two valid inverse systems.

This example should give a clue as to the requirement a system must satisfy to guarantee the existence of a stable and causal inverse. The requirement is simple: *a linear system $H(z)$ is stable and causal and has a stable and causal inverse if and only if all of its poles and zeros are inside the unit circle.* For reasons which will become clear later, such systems are referred to as *minimum phase systems.*

2.8 Complex Convolution and Parseval's Theorem

Now that we understand contour integration, we can present some more very important results which pertain to the $\mathcal{Z}$-transform . We already know that convolution in the time domain corresponds to multiplication of $\mathcal{Z}$-transforms. This time, let $x_1(k)$ and $x_2(k)$ be signals and define $w(k)$ by

$$w(k) = x_1(k)x_2(k).$$

Then

$$W(z) = \sum_{k=-\infty}^{\infty} x_1(k)x_2(k)z^{-k}. \tag{2.8.1}$$

Using Eq. 2.4.5 to express $x_1(k)$,

$$x_1(k) = \frac{1}{2\pi j}\oint_C X_1(v)v^{k-1}\,dv \tag{2.8.2}$$

where C lies in the region of convergence of $X_1(z)$. Substitution of Eq. 2.8.2 into Eq. 2.8.1 yields

$$W(z) = \frac{1}{2\pi j}\sum_{k=-\infty}^{\infty}\left[\oint_C X_1(v)v^{k-1}\,dv\right]. \tag{2.8.3}$$

Now, reverse the order of summation and integration in Eq. 2.8.3 to obtain

$$W(z) = \frac{1}{2\pi j}\oint_C X_1(v)\left[\sum_{k=-\infty}^{\infty} x_2(n)(z/v)^{-k}\right]v^{-1}\,dv. \tag{2.8.4}$$

The term in brackets is recognized as the $\mathcal{Z}$-transform of $x_2(k)$ evaluated at (z/v) so that

$$W(z) = \frac{1}{2\pi j}\oint_C X_1(v)X_2(z/v)v^{-1}\,dv. \tag{2.8.5}$$

where C is a contour in the overlap of the ROCs of $X_1(v)$ and $X_2(z/v)$. Equation 2.8.5 is known as the *complex convolution theorem.* Complex convolution has a relatively simple interpretation in the context of discrete time Fourier transforms, which will be presented later in this chapter.

Example 2.18

Let $x_1(k) = u(k)$ and $x_2(k) = 2^k u(k)$. Then the $\mathcal{Z}$-transforms of $x_1(k)$ and $x_2(k)$ are

$$X_1(z) = \frac{z}{z-1}, \quad |z| > 1$$

and

$$X_2(z) = \frac{z}{z-2}, \quad |z| > 2.$$

Substituting the above into Eq. 2.8.5, we obtain

$$W(z) = \frac{1}{2\pi j}\oint_C \frac{z}{(v-1)(z-2v)}\,dv.$$

The problem is in determining the contour C, which must lie in the overlap of the ROCs of $X_1(v)$ and $X_2(z/v)$. The ROC of $X_1(v)$ is $|v| > 1$ and the ROC of $X_2(z/v)$ is $|z/v| > 2$, or $|v| < |z|/2$. The integrand has poles at $v = 1$ and $v = z/2$, so the contour C only encloses the pole at $v = 1$ (see Figure 2.8.1). Thus, by the method of residues, we need only consider the residue at $v = 1$, and

$$W(z) = \left.\frac{z}{z-2v}\right|_{v=1} = \frac{z}{z-2}$$

which is what was expected.

Another important quantity is the summation

$$\sum_{k=-\infty}^{\infty} x_1(k)x_2^*(k)$$

of signals $x_1(k)$ and $x_2(k)$. Recall from Eq. 2.8.5 that

$$\sum_{k=-\infty}^{\infty} x_1(k)x_2(k)z^{-k} = \frac{1}{2\pi j}\oint_C X_1(v)X_2(z/v)v^{-1}\,dv. \tag{2.8.6}$$

From the complex conjugation property of the $\mathcal{Z}$-transform (Eq. 2.3.4),

$$\mathcal{Z}[x_2^*(k)] = X_2^*(z^*)$$

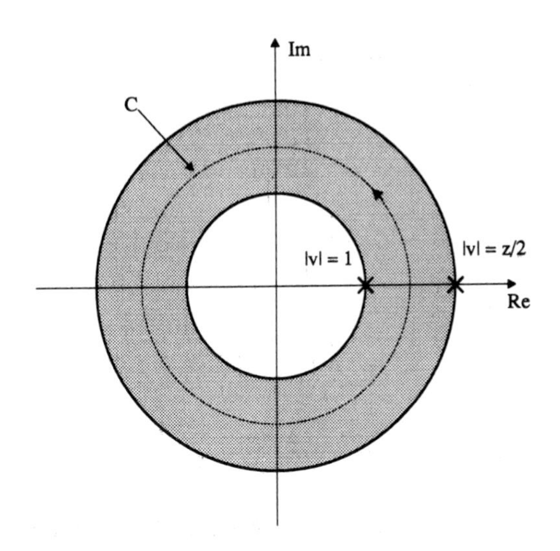

Figure 2.8.1: Contour of integration for Example 2.18.

so that Eq. 2.8.6 becomes

$$\sum_{k=-\infty}^{\infty} x_1(k)x_2^*(k)z^{-k} = \frac{1}{2\pi j} X_1(v)X_2^*(z^*/v^*)v^{-1}\, dv. \tag{2.8.7}$$

If Eq. 2.8.7 is evaluated at $z = 1$,

$$\sum_{k=-\infty}^{\infty} x_1(k)x_2^*(k) = \frac{1}{2\pi j} \oint_C X_1(v)X_2^*(1/v^*)v^{-1}\, dv. \tag{2.8.8}$$

where C is a contour in the overlap of the ROCs of $X_1(v)$ and $X_2^*(1/v^*)$. Equation 2.8.8 is known as *Parseval's Theorem* and has a simple interpretation on the unit circle which will be discussed later in this chapter.

Example 2.19

Suppose we wish to use Parseval's theorem to compute for real a the value of

$$\sum_{k=0}^{\infty}(a^2)^k, \quad |a| < 1.$$

Let $x_1(k) = x_2(k) = a^k u(k)$. Then Eq. 2.8.8 states that

$$\sum_{k=0}^{\infty}(a^2)^k = \frac{1}{2\pi j}\oint_C X_1(v)X_1^*(1/v^*)v^{-1}\,dv.$$

We have

$$X_1(v) = \frac{v}{v-a}$$

and

$$X_2^*(1/v^*) = \frac{1}{1-av}$$

so that

$$\sum_{k=0}^{\infty}(a^2)^k = \frac{1}{2\pi j}\oint_C \frac{1}{(v-a)(1-av)}\,dv.$$

The contour C must lie in the overlap of the ROCs of $X_1(v)$ and $X_1^*(1/v^*)$. Since the ROC of $X_1(z)$ is $|z|>|a|$, we find that C must lie in the region

$$|a| < |v| < \frac{1}{|a|}.$$

The integrand has poles at $v=a$ and $v=1/a$, and only the pole at $v=a$ is enclosed by the contour C. Thus, by the method of residues, the integral is equal to the residue at $v=a$, *i.e.*,

$$\frac{1}{2\pi j}\oint_C \frac{1}{(v-a)(1-av)}\,dv = \left.\frac{1}{1-av}\right|_{v=a} = \frac{1}{1-a^2}.$$

Thus,

$$\sum_{k=0}^{\infty}(a^2)^k = \frac{1}{1-a^2}.$$

In this case, it would have been easier to sum the series directly.

Analytic continuation

An important concept in the study of linear systems is *analytic continuation.* Briefly explained, if $A(z)$ and $B(z)$ are rational functions of z for which $A(e^{j\theta}) = B(e^{j\theta})$ then $A(z)=B(z)$. In other words, the rational functions are identical (in actuality, this property holds for more general analytic functions). This powerful property allows us to extend results which hold on the unit circle to the entire complex plane.

Time Function	$\mathcal{Z}$-Transform	ROC
$\delta(k)$	1	All z
$u(k)$	$\dfrac{1}{1-z^{-1}}$	$\|z\| > 1$
$-u(-k-1)$	$\dfrac{1}{1-z^{-1}}$	$\|z\| < 1$
$a^k u(k)$	$\dfrac{1}{1-az^{-1}}$	$\|z\| > \|a\|$
$-a^k u(-k-1)$	$\dfrac{1}{1-az^{-1}}$	$\|z\| < \|a\|$
$ka^k u(k)$	$\dfrac{az^{-1}}{(1-az^{-1})^2}$	$\|z\| > \|a\|$
$-ka^k u(-k-1)$	$\dfrac{az^{-1}}{(1-az^{-1})^2}$	$\|z\| < \|a\|$
$(\cos(\theta_0 k))u(k)$	$\dfrac{1-(\cos(\theta_0))z^{-1}}{1-(2\cos(\theta_0))z^{-1}+z^{-2}}$	$\|z\| > 1$
$(\sin(\theta_0 k))u(k)$	$\dfrac{(\sin(\theta_0))z^{-1}}{1-(2\cos(\theta_0))z^{-1}+z^{-2}}$	$\|z\| > 1$
$(r^k \cos(\theta_0 k))u(k)$	$\dfrac{1-(r\cos(\theta_0))z^{-1}}{1-(2r\cos(\theta_0))z^{-1}+r^2z^{-2}}$	$\|z\| > r$
$(r^k \sin(\theta_0 k))u(k)$	$\dfrac{(r\sin(\theta_0))z^{-1}}{1-(2r\cos(\theta_0))z^{-1}+r^2z^{-2}}$	$\|z\| > r$

Table 2.1: Important $\mathcal{Z}$-transform pairs

Operation	Time Function	$\mathcal{Z}$-Transform
Definition	$x(k)$	$X(z) = \sum_{k=-\infty}^{\infty} x(k)z^{-k}$
Inversion	$\frac{1}{2\pi j}\oint_C X(z)z^{k-1}\,dz$	$X(z)$
Linearity	$ax_1(k) + bx_2(k)$	$aX_1(z) + bX_2(z)$
Convolution	$x_1(k) * x_2(k)$	$X_1(z)X_2(z)$
Multiplication of sequences	$x_1(k)x_2(k)$	$\frac{1}{2\pi j}\oint_C X_1(v)X_2\left(\frac{z}{v}\right)v^{-1}\,dv$
Time delay	$x(k-k_0)$	$z^{-k_0}X(z)$
Modulation	$z_0^k x(k)$	$X\left(\frac{z}{z_0}\right)$
Multiplication by k	$kx(k)$	$-z\frac{dX(z)}{dz}$
Time reversal	$x(-k)$	$X\left(\frac{1}{z}\right)$
Conjugation	$x^*(k)$	$X^*(z^*)$
Correlation	$\sum_{n=-\infty}^{\infty} x^*(n)x(k+n)$	$X(z)X^*\left(\frac{1}{z^*}\right)$
Initial value	$x(0)$	$\lim_{z\to\infty} X(z)$

Table 2.2: Important $\mathcal{Z}$-transform properties

2.9 Frequency Response of LTI Systems

We have previously shown for linear time-invariant (LTI) systems that the representation of an input signal as a weighted sum of shifted impulses leads naturally to the convolution representation. There are other valuable representations for discrete-time signals, as well. As with continuous-time signals, sinusoidal sequences are extremely valuable for representation and analysis of discrete-time signals and systems. The reason for this is because sinusoids are eigenfunctions of LTI systems. To demonstrate this fact, assume we have a LTI system with impulse response $\{h(k)\}$. The response to an input $x(k) = e^{j\theta k}$ is given by the convolution sum

$$y(k) = \sum_{n=-\infty}^{\infty} h(n)e^{j\theta(k-n)} = e^{j\theta k}\left(\sum_{n=-\infty}^{\infty} h(n)e^{-j\theta n}\right).$$

We define the *frequency response* $H(e^{j\theta})$ by

$$H(e^{j\theta}) = \sum_{n=-\infty}^{\infty} h(n)e^{-j\theta n}. \tag{2.9.1}$$

Notice that Eq. 2.9.1 is simply the $\mathcal{Z}$-transform of $h(k)$ evaluated at $z = e^{j\theta}$. If the sum in Eq. 2.9.1 converges, it follows that

$$y(k) = H(e^{j\theta})e^{j\theta k}.$$

As we will see, Eq. 2.9.1 will converge if the sequence $\boldsymbol{h}$ is l^1 (*i.e.*, $\boldsymbol{h}$ is the impulse response of a BIBO stable system. When this is true, $e^{j\theta k}$ is an eigenfunction of the system with eigenvalue $H(e^{j\theta})$. The output is also a complex exponential of the same frequency, but has amplitude equal to $|H(e^{j\theta})|$ and a phase which is shifted by $\arg(H(e^{j\theta}))$. We refer to $H(e^{j\theta})$ as the *frequency response* of the system. Likewise, $|H(e^{j\theta})|$ is known as the *magnitude frequency response* and $\angle H(e^{j\theta})$ as the *phase response.* Frequently, we will denote the phase response by the function φ where

$$\varphi(H(e^{j\theta})) = \arg H(e^{j\theta}). \tag{2.9.2}$$

Another quantity of interest is the *group delay.* The group delay provides a measure of the linearity (or nonlinearity) of the phase. The group delay is defined by

$$\operatorname{grd}(H(e^{j\theta})) = -\frac{d\varphi(H(e^{j\theta}))}{d\theta}. \tag{2.9.3}$$

It can be seen that when the phase response of a system is a linear function of θ, the group delay is constant. The group delay will be examined in detail later.

Because of linearity, if we know how to decompose a signal $x(k)$ as a weighted sum of complex exponentials,

$$x(k) = \sum_n x_n e^{j\theta_n k},$$

the output is given by

$$y(k) = \sum_n x_n H(e^{j\theta_n}) e^{j\theta_n k}.$$

Example 2.20

Suppose the impulse response of a LTI system is $\{h(k)\}$. Let $x(k) = \cos(\theta_0 k)$. Then $x(k)$ can be decomposed as the sum of two complex exponentials,

$$x(k) = \frac{1}{2}e^{j\theta_0 k} + \frac{1}{2}e^{-j\theta_0 k}.$$

It follows that the response of the system to $x(k)$ is given by

$$y(k) = \frac{1}{2}(H(e^{j\theta_0})e^{j\theta_0 k} + H(e^{-j\theta_0})e^{-j\theta_0 k}).$$

We will see that if $h(k)$ is real, $H(e^{-j\theta_0}) = H^*(e^{j\theta_0})$ so that

$$y(k) = |H(e^{j\theta_0})| \cos(\theta_0 k + \varphi(H(e^{j\theta_0}))).$$

Thus, the output of the system is also a cosine, but with magnitude $H(e^{j\theta_0})$ and phase $\varphi(H(e^{j\theta_0}))$.

It immediately follows from the definition that $H(e^{j\theta})$ is periodic in θ with period 2π. In other words,

$$H(e^{j(\theta+2\pi l)}) = H(e^{j\theta})$$

for all integers l. This is due to the periodicity of the sequence $e^{j\theta k}$. Because of this periodicity, we need only specify the frequency response of the system over a single period. We will usually choose the region

$$-\pi \leq \theta \leq \pi.$$

If we further assume that the impulse response is real, it follows that

$$H^*(e^{j\theta}) = \left(\sum_{k=-\infty}^{\infty} h(k)e^{-j\theta k}\right)^* = \sum_{k=-\infty}^{\infty} h(k)e^{jk\theta}. \tag{2.9.4}$$

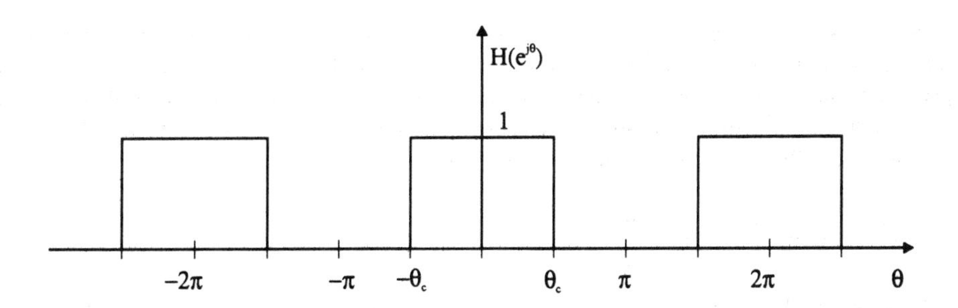

Figure 2.9.1: Frequency response of an ideal lowpass filter.

Thus,

$$H^*(e^{j\theta}) = H(e^{-j\theta}),$$

which implies that

$$|H(e^{j\theta})| = |H(e^{-j\theta})| \tag{2.9.5}$$

and

$$\varphi(H(e^{j\theta})) = -\varphi(H(e^{-j\theta})). \tag{2.9.6}$$

Therefore, the magnitude response is an even function of θ and the phase response is an odd function of θ. Consequently, for real $\boldsymbol{h}$, the magnitude and phase need only be plotted over the range $0 \leq \theta \leq \pi$.

Example 2.21

Consider the *ideal lowpass filter* with cutoff frequency θ_c, which has frequency response given by

$$H(e^{j\theta}) = \begin{cases} 1, & |\theta| \leq \theta_c \\ 0, & \theta_c < |\theta| < \pi \end{cases}$$

Figure 2.9.1 shows the frequency response, including the periodic images centered at -2π and 2π. This filter passes all frequencies in the range $|\theta| < \theta_c$ and completely attenuates all frequencies outside this range.

One of the most important concepts in digital filtering is *frequency selectivity.* It should be familiar to anyone who has experience working with analog filters that the main purpose of filtering is to alter the frequency content of a signal by either attenuation or gain. That is, we are interested in either emphasizing or de-emphasizing certain bands of frequency content of an input signal. The basis for this interpretation is the Fourier transform, which lets us represent a signal as a superposition of weighted sinusoids. A fundamental skill in digital filter design, then, is an understanding of how filters modify sinusoidal input signals.

Suppose a LTI system is described by the SDE

$$y(k) + \sum_{n=1}^{N} a_n y(k-n) = \sum_{n=0}^{M} b_n x(k-n)$$

(we have assumed that $a_0 = 1$, a condition which can always be forced by dividing the entire SDE by a_0 if it is not equal to one). Recall from the definition of frequency response that the when the input is the complex exponential $x(k) = e^{j\theta k}$, the output is

$$y(k) = H(e^{j\theta})e^{j\theta k}.$$

Also, by time-invariance, the response to the time-shifted input $e^{j(k-n)\theta}$ will be $H(e^{j\theta})e^{j(k-n)\theta}$. Finally, because of linearity, when $x(k) = e^{j\theta k}$, the SDE can be written as

$$H(e^{j\theta})e^{j\theta k} + \sum_{n=1}^{N} a_n H(e^{j\theta})e^{j(k-n)\theta} = \sum_{n=0}^{M} b_n e^{j(k-n)\theta}.$$

Notice that we can factor $H(e^{j\theta})$ and $e^{j\theta k}$ from the entire SDE and obtain a closed-form expression for $H(e^{j\theta})$ as

$$H(e^{j\theta}) = \frac{b_0 + b_1 e^{-j\theta} + \cdots + b_M e^{-jM\theta}}{1 + a_1 e^{-j\theta} + \cdots + a_N e^{-jM\theta}}. \tag{2.9.7}$$

Thus, we have shown that the frequency response of a LTI system is expressible as a ratio of polynomials in $e^{j\theta}$.

Geometric evaluation of $H(e^{j\theta})$

Recall that the $\mathcal{Z}$-transform description of a LTI system is obtained as the $\mathcal{Z}$-transform of the SDE and we obtained

$$H(z) = \frac{b_0 + b_1 z^{-1} + \cdots + b_M z^{-M}}{1 + a_1 z^{-1} + \cdots + a_N z^{-N}} = \frac{b(z)}{a(z)}. \tag{2.9.8}$$

Comparing Eqs. 2.9.7 and 2.9.8, it is seen that the frequency response of a BIBO-stable LTI system is obtainable by evaluating $H(z)$ on the unit circle:

$$H(e^{j\theta}) = H(z)\big|_{z=e^{j\theta}}.$$

For the $\mathcal{Z}$-transform, we have the relation

$$Y(z) = H(z)X(z).$$

We should expect that there is a similar relation

$$Y(e^{j\theta}) = H(e^{j\theta})X(e^{j\theta}) \tag{2.9.9}$$

where the meaning of $X(e^{j\theta})$ will be made more precise soon. Intuitively, $X(e^{j\theta})$ is a function which gives a measure of the frequency content of $x(k)$ at each frequency θ (this should be familiar to anyone who has studied Fourier analysis). According to Eq. 2.9.9, the frequency content of the output, $Y(e^{j\theta})$, is obtained by multiplying $H(e^{j\theta})$ and $X(e^{j\theta})$. To eliminate frequency components at $\theta = \theta_0$, we would like $H(e^{j\theta_0})$ to be small. The opposite is true for frequencies we would like to boost. Hence, the behavior of $H(z)$ on the unit circle is of central importance to our study of digital filtering.

To this end, we can rewrite $H(z)$ as the ratio of polynomials in z rather than in z^{-1}. We have

$$H(z) = \frac{z^{N-M}(b_0 z^M + b_1 z^{M-1} + \cdots + b_M)}{a_0 z^N + a_1 z^{N-1} + \cdots + a_N}.$$

Now, rewrite the numerator and denominator in factored form as

$$H(z) = \frac{z^{N-M}\prod_{k=1}^{M}(z - z_k)}{\prod_{k=1}^{N}(z - p_k)}$$

where the z_k are the M roots of $b(z)$ and the p_k are the N roots of $a(z)$. Let $z = e^{j\theta}$ be some point on the unit circle. It then follows that

$$H(e^{j\theta}) = \frac{e^{j(N-M)\theta}\prod_{k=1}^{M}(e^{j\theta} - z_k)}{\prod_{k=1}^{N}(e^{j\theta} - p_k)}.$$

The term $(e^{j\theta} - z_k)$ is simply a vector directed from the point z_k to the point $e^{j\theta}$. This vector has an associated magnitude B_k and phase θ_k. Similarly for $(e^{j\theta} - p_k)$. Let us write

$$e^{j\theta} - z_k = B_k e^{j\theta_k}$$

and

$$e^{j\theta} - p_k = A_k e^{j\phi_k}.$$

The magnitude of $e^{j(N-M)\theta}$ is clearly unity, so the magnitude of $H(e^{j\theta})$ is given by

$$|H(e^{j\theta})| = \frac{\prod_{k=1}^{M} B_k}{\prod_{k=1}^{N} A_k}.$$

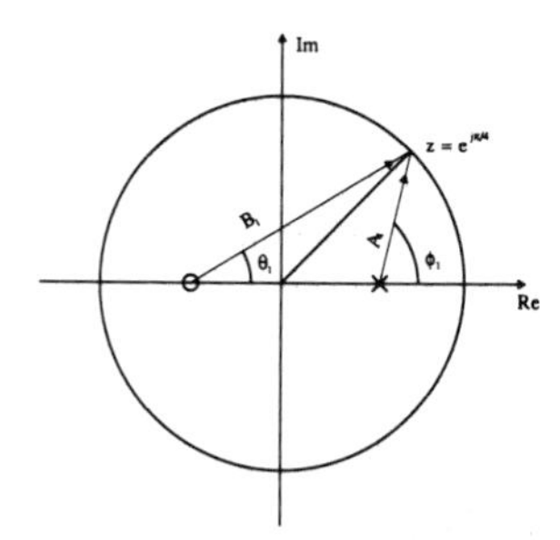

Figure 2.9.2: Pole-zero plot and associated vectors for $H(z) = (z+0.5)/(z-0.5)$.

The phase contribution from the term $e^{j(N-M)\theta}$ is just $(N-M)\theta$ so that the phase of $H(e^{j\theta})$ is given by

$$\varphi(H(e^{j\theta})) = (N-M)\theta + \sum_{k=1}^{M} \theta_k - \sum_{k=1}^{N} \phi_k.$$

Example 2.22

Let

$$H(z) = \frac{z+0.5}{z-0.5}.$$

Then

$$H(e^{j\theta}) = \frac{(e^{j\theta}+0.5)}{(e^{j\theta}-0.5)}.$$

Let

$$e^{j\theta} + 0.5 = B_1 e^{j\theta_1}$$

be the vector from $z_1 = -0.5$ to the point $e^{j\theta}$ and let

$$e^{j\theta} - 0.5 = A_1 e^{j\phi_1}$$

be the vector from the point $p_1 = 0.5$ to the point $e^{j\theta}$. The situation where $\theta = \pi/4$ is shown in Figure 2.9.2. Notice that over the range $0 \leq \theta \leq \pi$, angle θ_1 is always less than angle ϕ_1. Since the overall phase is given by $\theta_1 - \phi_1$, the phase over the range $0 \leq \theta \leq \pi$ is negative.

An important skill is qualitative evaluation of frequency response from a pole-zero diagram. Because of the availability of computer software for rigorous analysis, minute detail is not as significant as it once was. However, it is still important to be able to give rough estimates of magnitude and phase without having to perform a detailed analysis.

There are some heuristics which can be provided. Intuitively, to yield a locally maximal magnitude at $e^{j\theta_0}$, one should place a pole close to this point. The reasoning behind this is that as θ approaches θ_0, the distance A_k to this pole is becoming small so that division by A_k will yield a large magnitude. An example will clarify.

Example 2.23

Suppose

$$H(z) = \frac{1}{(1 - re^{j\alpha}z^{-1})(1 - re^{-j\alpha}z^{-1})} = \frac{z^2}{z^2 - 2rz\cos\alpha + r^2}.$$

There are two zeros at the origin an poles at $re^{\pm j\alpha}$. Intuitively, we expect the maximal gain of the filter to occur at $\theta = \pm\alpha$, which are the points on the unit circle closest to the poles. Also, as r approaches 1, the distance between the pole and the unit circle is smaller so that the gain at $\theta = \alpha$ grows larger.

2.10 Allpass Systems

Consider the stable first-order system with transfer function

$$H_{ap}(z) = \frac{1 - a^* z}{z - a}.$$

$H_{ap}(z)$ has a zero at $z = 1/a^*$ and a pole at $z = a$. The pole and zero are at *conjugate reciprocal* locations. Let's look at the frequency response of $H_{ap}(z)$. We have

$$H_{ap}(e^{j\theta}) = \frac{1 - a^* e^{j\theta}}{e^{j\theta} - a}. \tag{2.10.1}$$

If $e^{j\theta}$ is factored out of the numerator of Eq. 2.10.1, then

$$H_{ap}(e^{j\theta}) = e^{j\theta}\frac{e^{-j\theta} - a^*}{e^{j\theta} - a}. \tag{2.10.2}$$

The magnitude frequency response is then given by

$$|H_{ap}(e^{j\theta})| = |e^{j\theta}|\frac{|e^{-j\theta} - a^*|}{|e^{j\theta} - a|}.$$

But $|e^{j\theta}| = 1$ so that

$$|H_{ap}(e^{j\theta})| = \left| \frac{e^{-j\theta} - a^*}{e^{j\theta} - a} \right|,$$

and the numerator and denominator are conjugates of one another, which means that

$$|H_{ap}(e^{j\theta})| = 1.$$

In other words, the magnitude frequency response of $|H_{ap}(z)|$ is constant and independent of θ. For this reason, $H_{ap}(z)$ is called an *allpass* filter. If a system $H(z)$ is cascaded with an allpass system, the magnitude response will not be altered. This makes allpass filters useful for phase and group delay compensation. In other words, if the phase or group delay response of a system $H(z)$ are undesirable, the system can be cascaded with an allpass system which has additive phase or group delay and brings the phase or group delay closer to some desired response.

It is clear that a cascade of allpass systems is still allpass. What will always be true for an allpass system of arbitrary order is that its poles and zeros are located at conjugate reciprocal locations. The most general form for an allpass system is

$$H_{ap}(z) = \prod_{i=1}^{N_r} \left(\frac{1 - a_i z}{z - a_i} \right) \left(\prod_{i=1}^{N_c} \frac{(1 - b_i^* z)(1 - b_i z)}{(z - b_i)(z - b_i^*)} \right) \tag{2.10.3}$$

where N_r is the number of real poles and N_c is the number of complex pole pairs. In order to ensure stability of a causal allpass system, it is required that all of the poles be inside the unit circle. Because the zeros are at conjugate reciprocal locations, all of the zeros of a causal stable allpass system will be *outside* the unit circle.

To examine the frequency response of a general allpass system, it suffices to examine the frequency response of first order allpass system, since any allpass system can be generated as a cascade of first order allpass systems. We have already shown that the magnitude response is always equal to one. For a first order allpass system with a pole at $a = re^{j\theta_0}$, it can be shown that

$$\varphi(H_{ap}(e^{j\theta})) = -\theta - 2\tan^{-1}\left(\frac{r\sin(\theta - \theta_0)}{1 - r\cos(\theta - \theta_0)} \right).$$

Recall that the group delay of a system $H(z)$ was defined as

$$\text{grd}(H(e^{j\theta})) = -\frac{d}{d\theta}\left(\varphi(H(e^{j\theta}))\right). \tag{2.10.4}$$

It can be shown with some simple manipulation that

$$\text{grd}(H_{ap}(e^{j\theta})) = \frac{1 - r^2}{|1 - re^{j\theta_0}e^{-j\theta}|^2}.$$

For a stable allpass system, we will always have $|r| < 1$, from which it follows that the group delay of a stable allpass system *is always nonnegative.* Next, we consider the phase of the allpass system. Because of Eq. 2.10.4, it follows that

$$\varphi(H_{ap}(e^{j\theta})) = -\int_0^\theta \operatorname{grd}(H_{ap}(e^{j\phi})\, d\phi + \varphi(H_{ap}(e^{j0})). \tag{2.10.5}$$

From the expression for $H_{ap}(z)$ in Eq. 2.10.3, it is clear that

$$H_{ap}(e^{j0}) = 1$$

so that $\varphi(H_{ap}(e^{j0})) = 0$ and Eq. 2.10.5 becomes

$$\varphi(H_{ap}(e^{j\theta})) = -\int_0^\theta \operatorname{grd}(H_{ap}(e^{j\phi})\, d\phi. \tag{2.10.6}$$

Because of the nonnegativity of the integrand, it follows that the phase of an allpass system *is always nonpositive.* It is fairly simple to show that the phase of the stable first-order allpass system sweeps through a range of 2π as θ goes from $-\pi$ to π.

Thusfar, we have seen that the magnitude response of an allpass system is unity everywhere, the group delay is nonnegative, and the phase is nonpositive. Although we derived these facts for first order allpass systems, they hold for allpass systems of any order. This is because magnitude response is multiplicative and phase and group delay are additive.

2.11 Minimum-Phase Systems

Recall that we defined a causal minimum-phase system as a causal system with all of its poles and zeros inside the unit circle. This ensured that the inverse system would also be stable and causal. The reason we called such systems *minimum-phase* is not clear from the definition, but will become clear soon.

We begin with an important assertion: Any rational transfer function, $H(z)$ can be factored as

$$H(z) = H_{min}(z)H_{ap}(z) \tag{2.11.1}$$

where $H_{min}(z)$ is minimum-phase and $H_{ap}(z)$ is allpass. To show that this is true, assume that $H(z)$ is nonminimum-phase and has a single zero outside the unit circle at $z = 1/a^*$, where $|a| < 1$. Then we can write

$$H(z) = H_1(z)(1 - a^* z), \tag{2.11.2}$$

where, $H_1(z)$ is minimum phase (because we have removed the offending zero from $H(z)$). Equivalently, $H(z)$ can be expressed as

$$H(z) = H_1(z)(1 - a^* z)\frac{(z-a)}{(z-a)},$$

or

$$H(z) = H_1(z)(z-a)\frac{(1 - a^* z)}{(z-a)}. \tag{2.11.3}$$

Now, because $H_1(z)$ is minimum phase and $(z-a)$ contributes a zero inside the unit circle, their product is minimum phase. Thus, define $H_{min}(z)$ by

$$H_{min}(z) = H_1(z)(z-a). \tag{2.11.4}$$

The rest of Eq. 2.11.3 is recognized as an allpass system. That is,

$$H_{ap}(z) = \frac{1 - a^* z}{z - a}. \tag{2.11.5}$$

Therefore,

$$H(z) = H_{min}(z)H_{ap}(z), \tag{2.11.6}$$

as was asserted.

Let's re-iterate how the factorization was performed for the simple case of a single zero outside the unit circle. First, the zero was reflected to a conjugate reciprocal location inside the unit circle. Next, a pole was placed at the same location inside the unit circle to cancel the new zero. The new pole and the zero outside the unit circle were attributed to the allpass system and the original transfer function (without the zero outside the unit circle) and the new reflected zero inside the unit circle were attributed to the minimum-phase system. This is illustrated in Fig. 2.11.1.

Because of the factorization in Eq. 2.11.6,

$$H(z) = H_{min}(z)H_{ap}(z),$$

it follows that

$$|H(e^{j\theta})| = |H_{min}(e^{j\theta})||H_{ap}(e^{j\theta})| = |H_{min}(e^{j\theta})|. \tag{2.11.7}$$

Thus, the minimum-phase system has the same magnitude response as the original system $H(z)$.

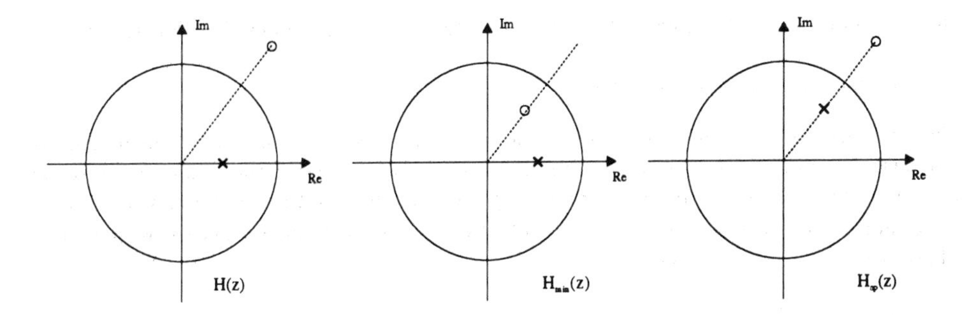

Figure 2.11.1: Factorizing a nonminimum-phase transfer function into the product of minimum-phase and allpass transfer functions.

For a nonminimum-phase system with multiple zeros outside the unit circle, the above procedure is repeated one zero at a time to yield the same type of factorization. Again, we will have

$$H(z) = H_{min}(z)H_{ap}(z)$$

and

$$|H(e^{j\theta})| = |H_{min}(e^{j\theta})|.$$

Furthermore, if $H_1(z)$ and $H_2(z)$ are systems with the same magnitude response, the ratio $H_1(z)/H_2(z)$ is allpass. Thus, if $H_1(z)$ is minimum phase, we can write

$$H_2(z) = H_1(z)H_{ap}(z)$$

where $H_1(z)$ is minimum phase. This relationship has some important implications on the phase response and the group delay of nonminimum-phase systems. For example, suppose $H_1(z)$ and $H_2(z)$ have the same magnitude response, where $H_1(z)$ is minimum phase and $H_2(z)$ is nonminimum-phase. If the frequency response is written as

$$H_2(e^{j\theta}) = H_1(e^{j\theta})H_{ap}(e^{j\theta}),$$

it follows that

$$\varphi(H_2(e^{j\theta})) = \varphi(H_1(e^{j\theta})) + \varphi(H_{ap}(e^{j\theta})).$$

Recall, however, that the phase of an allpass system is always nonpositive. For this reason,

$$\varphi(H_2(e^{j\theta})) \leq \varphi(H_1(e^{j\theta})) \quad \text{for all } \theta.$$

This is where the term *minimum phase* comes from: if two systems have the same magnitude response and one of the systems is minimum phase, the phase of the nonminimum-phase system is always more negative (has *more lag*) than the phase of the minimum phase system.

Geometrically, it is simple to understand why a zero outside the unit circle leads to more phase lag. Consider the systems

$$H_1(z) = \frac{z+a}{z}$$

and

$$H_2(z) = \frac{1+az}{z}$$

where $|a| < 1$. These two systems have the same magnitude response (because $H_2(z)/H_1(z)$ is allpass) and $H_2(z)$ is nonminimum-phase. The pole-zero plots for $H_1(z)$ and $H_2(z)$ are shown in Fig. 2.11.2. For any point $e^{j\theta}$ on the unit circle, it can be seen that the phase contribution from the zero outside the unit circle is less than the phase contribution from the zero inside the unit circle. Therefore, the phase *lag* of system $H_2(z)$ will be greater than that of $H_1(z)$.

A similar relationship can be derived for the group delay. Again, suppose $H_1(z)$ and $H_2(z)$ have the same magnitude response, where $H_1(z)$ is minimum phase and $H_2(z)$ is nonminimum-phase. The group delay is given by

$$\text{grd}(H_2(e^{j\theta})) = \text{grd}(H_1(e^{j\theta})) + \text{grd}(H_{ap}(e^{j\theta})).$$

Recall that the group delay of an allpass system was shown to be nonnegative. Therefore,

$$\text{grd}(H_2(e^{j\theta})) \geq \text{grd}(H_1(e^{j\theta}))$$

and the group delay of the nonminimum phase system is greater than the group delay of the minimum phase system.

Example 2.24

Suppose $H(z)$ is given by

$$H(z) = \frac{(z-\frac{1}{8})(z-2)}{(z-\frac{1}{4})(z-\frac{1}{3})}.$$

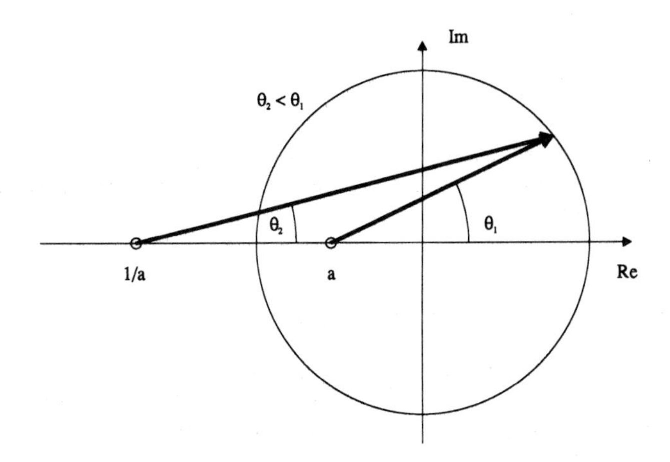

Figure 2.11.2: Zero outside unit circle contributes less phase than zero inside unit circle, resulting in greater phase lag.

Clearly, $H(z)$ is nonminimum-phase because there is a zero at $1/a = 2$, or $a = 1/2$. To perform the factorization into the product of a minimum phase system and an allpass system, we wish to extract a term $(1 - \frac{1}{2}z)$ from the numerator, which gives

$$H(z) = \frac{(-2)(z - \frac{1}{8})}{(z - \frac{1}{4})(z - \frac{1}{3})} \cdot (1 - \frac{1}{2}z).$$

Next, we write

$$H(z) = \frac{(-2)(z - \frac{1}{8})}{(z - \frac{1}{4})(z - \frac{1}{3})} \cdot (1 - \frac{1}{2}z) \cdot \frac{(z - \frac{1}{2})}{(z - \frac{1}{2})}$$

which can also be written as

$$H(z) = \frac{(-2)(z - \frac{1}{2})(z - \frac{1}{8})}{(z - \frac{1}{4})(z - \frac{1}{3})} \cdot \frac{(1 - \frac{1}{2}z)}{(z - \frac{1}{2})}.$$

Clearly, then

$$H(z) = H_{min}(z)H_{ap}(z)$$

where

$$H_{min}(z) = \frac{(-2)(z - \frac{1}{2})(z - \frac{1}{8})}{(z - \frac{1}{4})(z - \frac{1}{3})}$$

and

$$H_{ap}(z) = \frac{(1 - \frac{1}{2}z)}{(z - \frac{1}{2})}.$$

Figure 2.11.3 shows the magnitude, phase, and group delays of $H(z)$ and $H_{min}(z)$. As we expect, the magnitude responses are identical, and the phase and group delay of $H_{min}(z)$ are smaller than those of $H(z)$.

Time-domain characterization of minimum phase

So far, we have only given frequency-domain interpretations of what minimum phase means. There are also some useful time-domain characterizations of minimum phase. Suppose $H_1(z)$ and $H_2(z)$ are two systems with the same magnitude response, and one is known to be minimum phase, whereas the other is nonminimum-phase. In the time domain, how can we determine which is which? To wit, assume $H_1(z)$ is the minimum phase system. We can then write

$$H_2(z) = H_1(z)H_{ap}(z). \tag{2.11.8}$$

Assume for now that the allpass system is first-order, given by

$$H_{ap}(z) = \frac{1 - a^*z}{z - a}$$

where

$$|a| < 1.$$

Let's look at the impulse response of each system. From Eq. 2.11.8 and the initial value theorem, it follows that

$$h_2(0) = \lim_{z \to \infty} H_1(z)H_{ap}(z) \tag{2.11.9}$$

so that

$$|h_2(0)| = |\lim_{z \to \infty} H_1(z)||\lim_{z \to \infty} H_{ap}(z)|.$$

Therefore,

$$|h_2(0)| = |h_1(0)||\lim_{z \to \infty} H_{ap}(z)|. \tag{2.11.10}$$

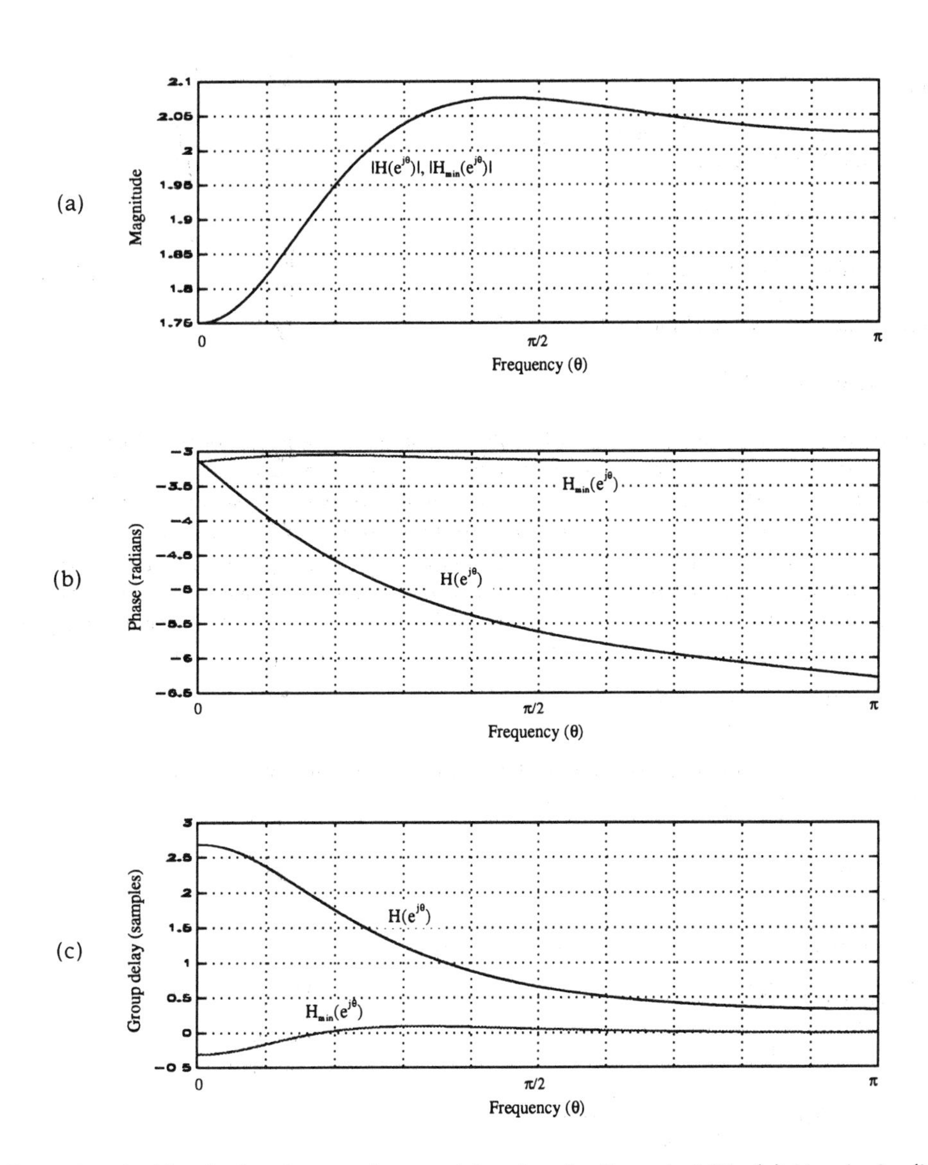

Figure 2.11.3: Magnitude, phase, and group delay plots for Example 2.24: (a) Magnitude; (b) phase; (c) group delay.

But

$$\lim_{z\to\infty} H_{ap}(z) = \lim_{z\to\infty} \frac{1 - a^* z}{z - a} = -a^*$$

and Eq. 2.11.10 becomes

$$|h_2(0)| = |h_1(0)||-a^*| = |a||h_1(0)|. \tag{2.11.11}$$

Because $|a| < 1$, we conclude that

$$|h_1(0)| > |h_2(0)|.$$

This argument was based on a first-order allpass system. Since higher-order allpass systems can be realized as a cascade of first order allpass systems, we have the following result: *if two systems have the same magnitude response and one is known to be minimum phase, the system with the larger magnitude zeroth impulse response is minimum phase.*

Actually, there is a generalization to the above. Minimum phase systems are said to possess the attribute of *minimum energy delay.* If $H_1(z)$ and $H_2(z)$ have the same magnitude response, where $H_1(z)$ is minimum phase and $H_2(z)$ is not, it can be shown that for any N,

$$\sum_{k=0}^{N} |h_1(k)|^2 > \sum_{k=0}^{N} |h_2(k)|^2.$$

In other words, minimum phase systems tend to have their energy concentrated toward the beginning of their impulse responses. The quantity

$$\sum_{k=0}^{N} |h(k)|^2$$

is known as the *partial energy*, denoted by $E_N(h(k))$

Example 2.25

Suppose $H_1(z)$ and $H_2(z)$ are given by

$$H_1(z) = \frac{(-2)(z - \frac{1}{2})(z - \frac{1}{8})}{(z - \frac{1}{4})(z - \frac{1}{3})}$$

and

$$H_2(z) = \frac{(z - \frac{1}{8})(z - 2)}{(z - \frac{1}{4})(z - \frac{1}{3})}.$$

We saw in the previous example that $H_2(z) = H_1(z)H_{ap}(z)$ where $H_1(z)$ is minimum-phase. Thus, $H_1(z)$ and $H_2(z)$ have the same magnitude response and $H_2(z)$ is nonminimum-phase.

Computing the initial values, we have

$$h_1(0) = \lim_{z\to\infty} H_1(z) = -2$$

and

$$h_2(0) = \lim_{z\to\infty} H_2(z) = 1.$$

Thus,

$$|h_1(0)| > |h_2(0)|,$$

as expected. The partial energies, $E_N(h_1(k))$ and $E_N(h_2(k))$ are as follows:

$$E_N(h_1(k)) = 1.0000, 3.3767, 3.9134, 4.0028, 4.0156, 4.0173, 4.0175, 4.0176, \ldots$$

and

$$E_N(h_2(k)) = 4.0000, 4.0069, 4.0150, 4.0171, 4.0175, 4.0176, 4.0176, 4.0176, \ldots.$$

Notice that the partial energy is always greater for $h_2(k)$, as expected.

A curious property of stable nonminimum-phase systems is that they are capable of "blocking" certain unstable inputs. That is, there are unbounded inputs which produce bounded outputs. To see this, assume $H(z)$ is stable but has a single zero outside the unit circle at $z = a$, where $|a| > 1$. Then $H(z)$ can be factored as

$$H(z) = H_1(z)(1 - az^{-1})$$

where $H_1(z)$ is minimum-phase. Suppose we apply the unbounded input

$$x(k) = a^k u(k)$$

to the system. The output has a $\mathcal{Z}$-transform given by

$$Y(z) = H(z)X(z) = H_1(z)\frac{1 - az^{-1}}{1 - az^{-1}} = H_1(z).$$

Therefore,

$$y(k) = h_1(k)$$

and since $h_1(k)$ is the impulse response of a stable system, it is bounded.

Another curious property of allpass filters is *losslessness*. Let $H(z)$ be a stable allpass filter and let $x(k)$ be and arbitrary input. It then follows that the output of the system satisfies

$$|Y(e^{j\theta})| = |X(e^{j\theta})|.$$

Therefore,

$$\frac{1}{2\pi}\int_{-\pi}^{\pi}|Y(e^{j\theta})|^2\,d\theta = \frac{1}{2\pi}\int_{-\pi}^{\pi}|X(e^{j\theta})|^2\,d\theta$$

and using Parseval's theorem, we can write

$$\sum_{k=-\infty}^{\infty} y^2(k) = \sum_{k=-\infty}^{\infty} x^2(k)$$

for *any* input $x(k)$. This means that the energy appearing at the output of the allpass system is the same as that appearing at the input; hence the term *lossless*.

2.12 The Discrete-Time Fourier Transform

The discrete-time Fourier transform (DTFT) of a sequence $x(k)$ is defined by

$$X(e^{j\theta}) = \sum_{k=-\infty}^{\infty} x(k)e^{-jk\theta}. \tag{2.12.1}$$

It can be seen that the DTFT is a special case of the $\mathcal{Z}$-transform when z is on the unit circle, *i.e.*,

$$z = e^{j\theta}.$$

A sufficient condition for the existence of the DTFT of $x(k)$ is that the unit circle is in the region of convergence of $X(z)$. This corresponds to absolute summability of $x(k)$, *i.e.*,

$$\sum_{k=-\infty}^{\infty} |x(k)| < \infty,$$

(or, $\boldsymbol{x} \in l^1$). Because all stable sequences are absolutely summable (by definition), all stable sequences have a DTFT.

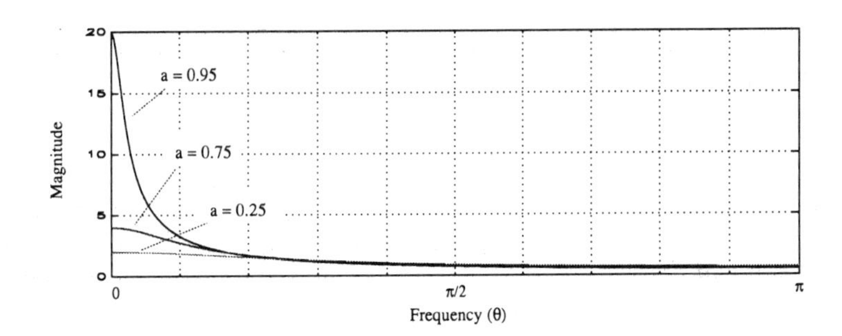

Figure 2.12.1: Magnitude of DTFT for $x(k) = a^k u(k)$.

We will see that even if absolute summability is not satisfied, we can still provide a meaningful interpretation of the DTFT (more on this later). When $x(k)$ is absolutely summable, however, it follows that

$$X(e^{j\theta}) = X(z)|_{z=e^{j\theta}} = \sum_{k=-\infty}^{\infty} x(k)e^{-j\theta k}. \tag{2.12.2}$$

At this point, we can make the connection between frequency response and the DTFT. We know that a system $H(z)$ is stable if and only if its impulse response $h(k)$ is absolutely summable. Thus, the DTFT of the impulse response $h(k)$ will exist. Referring to Eqs. 2.9.1 and 2.12.1, it is clear that the frequency response of a system is simply the DTFT of its impulse response.

Example 2.26

Suppose $x(k)$ is a right-sided exponential sequence

$$x(k) = a^k u(k), \quad |a| < 1.$$

We know that the region of convergence of the $\mathcal{Z}$-transform $X(z)$ is the region in the complex plane described by $|z| > |a|$. Because $|a| < 1$, the unit circle is included in the region of convergence so that the sequence is absolutely summable. Thus, the DTFT exists and is given by

$$X(e^{j\theta}) = X(z)|_{z=e^{j\theta}} = \frac{1}{1 - ae^{j\theta}}.$$

The magnitude of $X(e^{j\theta})$ for several values of α is shown in Figure 2.12.1.

Because we will be using the DTFT as a transform representation of discrete-time sequences, we need to establish an inversion formula which allows a sequence to be recovered from its DTFT. Inversion of the DTFT is a special case of $\mathcal{Z}$-transform inversion. Recall from Eq. 2.4.5 that

$$x(k) = \frac{1}{2\pi j} \oint_C X(z) z^{k-1}\, dz.$$

To eliminate the need for contour integration, we can parameterize the unit circle as follows. Start with the point $z = -1$, which corresponds to $\theta = -\pi$, and traverse the unit circle counter-clockwise until the point $z = -1$ is again reached. This corresponds to $\theta = \pi$. We can then parameterize the counter-clockwise unit circle as

$$z = e^{j\theta}, \quad -\pi \leq \theta \leq \pi.$$

It also follows that

$$dz = j e^{j\theta}\, d\theta$$

so that

$$x(k) = \frac{1}{2\pi} \int_{-\pi}^{\pi} X(e^{j\theta}) e^{jk\theta}\, d\theta. \tag{2.12.3}$$

This is the inversion formula for the DTFT.

As we have already mentioned, absolute summability is only a *sufficiency* requirement for the existence of the DTFT. If we are willing to relax the requirement of uniform convergence of the defining sum, a broader class of admissible signals arises. One such class are the *finite energy signals*, which are signals that satisfy

$$\sum_{k=-\infty}^{\infty} |x(k)|^2 < \infty$$

which we denote by $\boldsymbol{x} \in l^2$. Assume that $\boldsymbol{x}$ is finite energy and consider the approximation

$$X_M(e^{j\theta}) = \sum_{k=-M}^{M} x(k) e^{-j\theta k}.$$

It can be shown that there exists some function $X(e^{j\theta})$ such that

$$\lim_{M\to\infty} \int_{-\pi}^{\pi} |X(e^{j\theta}) - X_M(e^{j\theta})|^2\, d\theta = 0.$$

This is known as *mean-square convergence*, and in this case, we will accept $X(e^{j\theta})$ as the DTFT of $x(k)$. For signals which are not absolutely summable, it is usually difficult to determine the DTFT by direct evaluation. Fortunately, we can usually verify whether $X(e^{j\theta})$ is a valid DTFT for $\{x(k)\}$ by inverting the DTFT.

Example 2.27

Let $H(e^{j\theta})$ be an ideal lowpass filter with cutoff frequency θ_c, *i.e.*,

$$H(e^{j\theta}) = \begin{cases} 1, & |\theta| \leq \theta_c \\ 0 & \theta_c < |\theta| < \pi \end{cases}$$

The impulse response is found by inverting the DTFT as per Eq. 2.12.3:

$$h(k) = \frac{1}{2\pi} \int_{-\pi}^{\pi} e^{j\theta k}\, d\theta = \frac{1}{2\pi} \int_{-\theta_c}^{\theta_c} e^{j\theta k}\, d\theta$$

which yields

$$h(k) = \frac{\sin \theta_c n}{\pi k}.$$

This is a non-causal impulse response which is not absolutely summable, and the DTFT defined by

$$\sum_{k=-\infty}^{\infty} \frac{\sin \theta_c k}{\pi k} e^{j\theta k}$$

does not converge uniformly for all θ. If $H_M(e^{j\theta})$ is given by

$$\sum_{k=-M}^{M} \frac{\sin \theta_c k}{\pi k} e^{j\theta k},$$

we do have mean-square convergence. This mean-square convergence is shown in Fig. 2.12.2. Notice the oscillatory behavior of the approximations at the points of discontinuity. This is known as *Gibbs' phenomenon.*

We will also encounter sequences which are not finite energy sequences. We can still define a useful DTFT by appealing to the theory of distributions. These DTFTs will involve impulses at certain frequencies and can still be manipulated as ordinary DTFTs.

Example 2.28

Let $x(k) = 1$ for all k. Clearly, $x(k)$ is neither absolutely summable nor finite-energy. Suppose we define the DTFT of $x(k)$ as

$$X(e^{j\theta}) = \sum_{r=-\infty}^{\infty} 2\pi\delta(\theta + 2\pi r).$$

Applying the inverse DTFT, Eq. 2.12.3, we have

$$x(k) = \frac{1}{2\pi} \int_{-\pi}^{\pi} 2\pi \left(\sum_{r=-\infty}^{\infty} \delta(\theta + 2\pi r) \right) e^{j\theta k}\, d\theta.$$

Because the shifted impulses are outside the frequency range $|\theta| < \pi$, it follows that

$$x(k) = \int_{-\pi}^{\pi} \delta(\theta) e^{j\theta k}\, d\theta = \int_{-\pi}^{\pi} \delta(\theta) e^{j\theta 0}\, d\theta = \int_{-\pi}^{\pi} \delta(\theta)\, d\theta = 1,$$

which is what we expected.

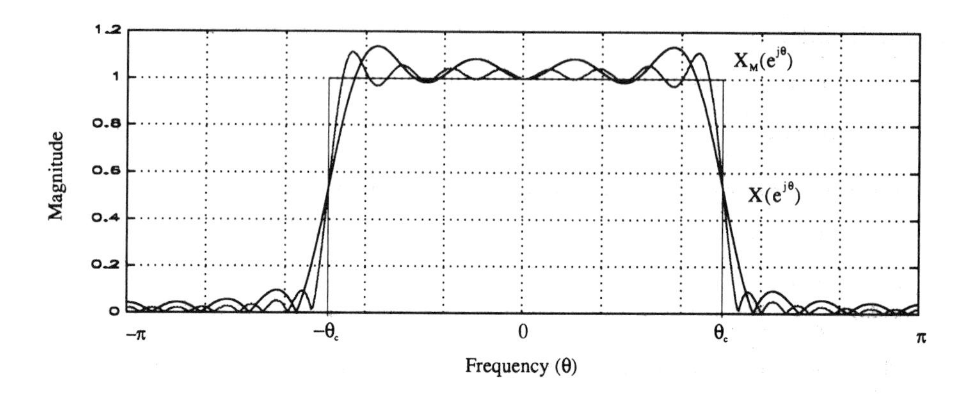

Figure 2.12.2: Mean-square convergence of the DTFT.

We have provided a list of important DTFT pairs in 2.14. Many of these pairs can be obtained by applying the properties of the DTFT which we will soon discuss to the basic DTFT pairs. Complicated DTFTs can often be inverted by using partial fractions as with the $\mathcal{Z}$-transform.

Because of its relationship to the $\mathcal{Z}$-transform, the DTFT shares many of the properties we have discussed for the $\mathcal{Z}$-transform. What follows is an explanation of the most important properties. In what follows, we will be using the notation $\mathcal{F}[\cdot]$ to indicate the DTFT.

- **Linearity**

It follows from the defining equation that if $x_1(k)$ and $x_2(k)$ have DTFTs $X_1(e^{j\theta})$ and $X_2(e^{j\theta})$, respectively, that for any constants a and b, we have

$$\mathcal{F}[ax_1(k) + bx_2(k)] = aX_1(e^{j\theta}) + bX_2(e^{j\theta}). \tag{2.12.4}$$

- **Time Shifting**

Suppose we time-shift a signal $x(k)$ by k_0 samples. Then

$$\mathcal{F}[x(k - k_0)] = e^{-j\theta k_0} X(e^{j\theta}). \tag{2.12.5}$$

- **Complex Conjugation**

If $\{x(k)\}$ has DTFT $X(e^{j\theta})$, then

$$\mathcal{F}[x^*(k)] = X^*(e^{-j\theta}). \tag{2.12.6}$$

- **Modulation**

Consider modulating $x(k)$ by the sequence $e^{j\theta k_0}$. Then

$$\mathcal{F}[e^{j\theta_0 k} x(k)] = X(e^{j(\theta - \theta_0)}). \tag{2.12.7}$$

Example 2.29

Suppose $x(k) = e^{j\theta_0 k}$. We know that the DTFT of the sequence $x_1(k) = 1$ is

$$X_1(e^{j\theta}) = \sum_{r=-\infty}^{\infty} 2\pi\delta(\theta + 2\pi r).$$

But

$$x(k) = e^{j\theta_0 k} x_1(k)$$

so that by the modulation property,

$$X(e^{j\theta}) = \sum_{r=-\infty}^{\infty} 2\pi\delta(\theta - \theta_0 + 2\pi r).$$

Example 2.30

If $x(k) = \cos(\theta_0 k)$, we can use the linearity property and the modulation property to find $X(e^{j\theta})$. Because

$$\cos(\theta_0 k) = \frac{e^{j\theta_0 k} + e^{-j\theta_0 k}}{2},$$

we have

$$X(e^{j\theta}) = \sum_{r=-\infty}^{\infty} \pi(\delta(\theta - \theta_0 + 2\pi r) + \delta(\theta + \theta_0 + 2\pi r)).$$

In digital communication systems, a discrete-time signal can be transmitted by amplitude modulating it with a local oscillator, converting to an analog signal by D/A conversion, transmitting over an analog communication channel, and then digitizing again at the receiver end. The received discrete-time signal can then be demodulated digitally to recover the original signal. Formally, if $x(k)$ is the original signal, the amplitude-modulated signal is given by

$$x_m(k) = x(k) cos(\theta_c k)$$

where θ_c is called the *carrier frequency.* Using Euler's identity, we have

$$x_m(k) = \frac{1}{2}x(k)e^{j\theta_c k} + \frac{1}{2}x(k)e^{-j\theta_c k}$$

so that

$$X_m(e^{j\theta}) = \frac{1}{2}X(e^{j(\theta-\theta_c)}) + \frac{1}{2}X(e^{j(\theta+\theta_c)}). \tag{2.12.8}$$

The spectrum of the modulated signal is shown in Fig. 2.12.3b. Notice that it consists of two frequency-shifted copies of $X(e^{j\theta})$, one by θ_c and one by $-\theta_c$, each of whose magnitude is half that of $X(e^{j\theta})$. The amplitude-modulated signal is then converted to analog an transmitted over the analog channel.

At the receiver end, after the signal has been converted back to digital, the spectrum is again equal to $X_m(e^{j\theta})$. In order to recover the original signal, we again multiply by a local oscillator with frequency θ_c, giving the demodulated signal

$$x_d(k) = x_m(k)\cos(k\theta_c).$$

In order to recover the original signal $x(k)$, consider the spectrum of the demodulated signal, $X_d(e^{j\theta})$. Using the modulation theorem, we have

$$X_d(e^{j\theta}) = \frac{1}{2}X_m(e^{j(\theta-\theta_c)}) + \frac{1}{2}X_m(e^{j(\theta+\theta_c)}).$$

Referring to Fig. 2.12.3c, it is seen that this sum of frequency-shifted copies of $X_m(e^{j\theta})$ results in a baseband image and two bandpass images, located at $\pm 2\theta_c$. Therefore, if $x_d(k)$ is filtered by a lowpass filter which removes these bandpass images and scales by two, the original signal $x(k)$ results. This is shown in Fig. 2.12.3d. Analytically, we could have determined this by using

$$x_d(k) = x_m(k)\cos(\theta_c k) = x(k)\cos^2(\theta_c k).$$

Using the identity

$$\cos^2(\theta_c k) = \frac{1+\cos(2\theta_c k)}{2},$$

we get

$$x_d(k) = \frac{1}{2}x(k) + \frac{1}{2}x(k)\cos(2\theta_c k).$$

Hence,

$$X_d(e^{j\theta}) = \frac{1}{2}X(e^{j\theta}) + \frac{1}{4}X(e^{j(\theta-2\theta_c)}) + \frac{1}{4}X(e^{j(\theta+2\theta_c)}).$$

If the images of $X(e^{j\theta})$ centered at $\pm 2\theta_c$ are removed with a lowpass filter with gain 2, $x(k)$ is recovered.

• **Multiplication by k**
If $x(k)$ has DTFT $X(e^{j\theta})$ then

$$\mathcal{F}[kx(k)] = -j\frac{dX(e^{j\theta})}{d\theta}. \tag{2.12.9}$$

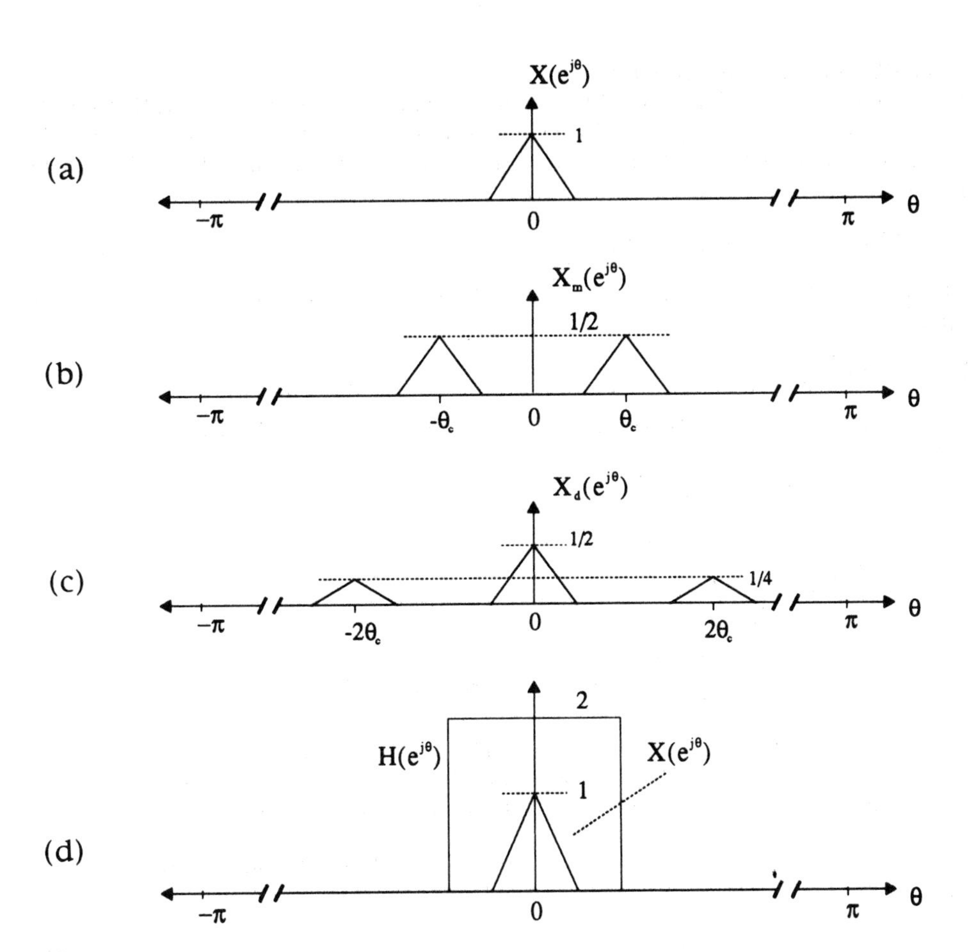

Figure 2.12.3: Amplitude modulation/demodulation: (a) Original signal, $X(e^{j\theta})$; (b) amplitude modulated signal $X_m(e^{j\theta})$; (c) demodulated signal $X_d(e^{j\theta})$; (d) lowpass filter and recovered signal, $X(e^{j\theta})$.

• DTFT Convolution Property

We know that if $\boldsymbol{x}_1$ and $\boldsymbol{x}_2$ have $\mathcal{Z}$-transforms $X_1(z)$ and $X_2(z)$, respectively, that the $\mathcal{Z}$-transform of $\boldsymbol{x}_1 * \boldsymbol{x}_2$ is $X_1(z)X_2(z)$. There is an analogous property for the DTFT. Let $x_1(k)$ and $x_2(k)$ have DTFTs $X_1(e^{j\theta})$ and $X_2(e^{j\theta})$, respectively. Then the DTFT of $x_1(k) * x_2(k)$ is given by

$$\mathcal{F}[x_1(k) * x_2(k)] = X_1(e^{j\theta})X_2(e^{j\theta}). \tag{2.12.10}$$

This property is *extremely* important because it gives us the basis for frequency selective filtering.

Example 2.31

Let $H(e^{j\theta})$ be an *ideal lowpass filter* with cut-off frequency $\theta_c = \pi/2$. That is,

$$H(e^{j\theta}) = \begin{cases} 1, & |\theta| \leq \theta_c \\ 0 & \theta_c < |\theta| < \pi \end{cases}$$

Suppose we apply the input

$$x(k) = \cos(3\pi k/4)$$

which has DTFT

$$X(e^{j\theta}) = \frac{1}{2} \sum_{n=-\infty}^{\infty} \delta(\theta - 3\pi/4 + 2\pi n) + \delta(\theta + 3\pi/4 + 2\pi n).$$

Notice that $X(e^{j\theta})$ is non-zero only in the stopband of the low-pass filter. Thus, because the output of the lowpass filter is given by $Y(e^{j\theta}) = H(e^{j\theta})X(e^{j\theta})$, the sinusoid is completely annihilated and the output of the filter is zero. This is shown in Figure 5.

Recall from Eq. 2.8.5 that the $\mathcal{Z}$-transform of the product of two sequences is expressed by

$$W(z) = \frac{1}{2\pi j} \oint_C X_1(v)X_2(z/v)v^{-1}\, dv, \tag{2.12.11}$$

which is rather cryptic in appearance. Its interpretation is simplified when one allows z and v to lie on the unit circle. This corresponds to the DTFT and is permissible when the unit circle is in the region of convergence. In this case, let

$$z = e^{j\theta}$$

and

$$v = e^{j\varphi}.$$

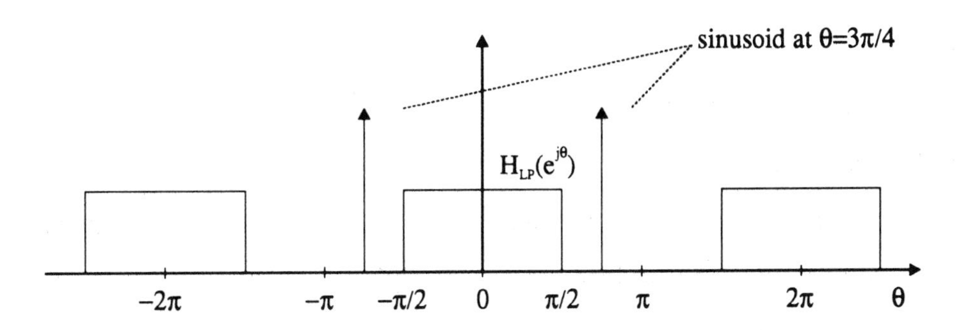

Figure 2.12.4: Ideal low-pass filtering from Example 2.31.

Making the substitutions for z and v in Eq. 2.12.11,

$$W(e^{j\theta}) = \frac{1}{2\pi}\int_{-\pi}^{\pi} X_1(e^{j\phi})X_2(e^{j(\theta-\varphi)})\,d\varphi. \tag{2.12.12}$$

Equation 2.12.12 is known as *periodic convolution.*

If the unit circle is in the region of convergence, let $v = e^{j\theta}$. Then

$$\sum_{k=-\infty}^{\infty} x_1(k)x_2^*(k) = \frac{1}{2\pi}\int_{-\pi}^{\pi} X_1(e^{j\theta})X_2^*(e^{j\theta})\,d\theta. \tag{2.12.13}$$

For the special case $x_2(k) = x_1(k)$, we have the following elegant result:

$$\sum_{k=-\infty}^{\infty} x(k)x^*(k) = \sum_{k=-\infty}^{\infty} |x(k)|^2 = \frac{1}{2\pi}\int_{-\pi}^{\pi} |X(e^{j\theta})|^2\,d\theta.$$

This is a special form of Parseval's Theorem which shows that energy can be computed in either the time or the frequency domain.

• **Correlation**

According to Eq. 2.3.14, if

$$r_{xx}(k) = \sum_{n=-\infty}^{\infty} x(n+k)x(k)$$

then

$$R_{xx}(z) = X(z)X^*(1/z^*).$$

It then follows that

$$R_{xx}(e^{j\theta}) = X(e^{j\theta})X^*(e^{j\theta}) = |X(e^{j\theta})|^2. \tag{2.12.14}$$

Applying the inverse DTFT, we have

$$r_{xx}(k) = \frac{1}{2\pi}\int_{-\pi}^{\pi} |X(e^{j\theta})|^2 e^{j\theta k}\, d\theta. \tag{2.12.15}$$

It was previously shown that $r_{xx}(0) = E_x$. Thus, Parseval's theorem can also be derived from the Eq. 2.12.15, giving

$$E_x = r_{xx}(0) = \frac{1}{2\pi}\int_{-\pi}^{\pi} |X(e^{j\theta})|^2\, d\theta.$$

The function $R_{xx}(e^{j\theta}) = |X(e^{j\theta})|^2$ is known as the *energy spectral density* and indicates the energy distribution of the signal in the frequency domain.

2.13 The Hilbert Transform

We have seen that amplitude modulating a baseband signal with a sinusoid of frequency θ_c results in a bandpass signal which has images of the baseband signal at both $\pm\theta_c$. If the original signal has a baseband bandwidth of B, the bandpass signal has a bandwidth of $2B$. Transmitting this signal requires twice the bandwidth of the original signal. We can achieve a substantial reduction in the necessary bandwidth if we exploit the symmetry of the baseband spectrum. This is the idea behind the Hilbert transform.

The transfer function of the *ideal Hilbert transformer* (see Fig. 2.13.1a) is given by

$$H(e^{j\theta}) = \begin{cases} j, & -\pi \le \theta < 0 \\ -j, & 0 \le \theta \le \pi \end{cases} \tag{2.13.1}$$

The ideal Hilbert transformer is physically unrealizable, but good approximations can be achieved in practice. Let $m(k)$ be a real baseband signal with DTFT $M(e^{j\theta})$ as shown in Fig. 2.13.1b. The frequency θ_B is defined as the baseband bandwidth of $m(k)$. Define $\hat{m}(k)$ as the Hilbert-transformed signal

$$\hat{m}(k) = m(k) * h(k). \tag{2.13.2}$$

The Hilbert-transformed signal $\hat{m}(k)$ has a DTFT $\hat{M}(e^{j\theta})$ which has the same magnitude as $M(e^{j\theta})$ but has a phase which is shifted by 90 degrees for negative frequencies and by -90 degrees for positive frequencies. Suppose the signal $x_u(k)$ is formed by

$$x_u(k) = m(k)\cos(\theta_c k) - \hat{m}(k)\sin(\theta_c k) \tag{2.13.3}$$

by using the arrangement shown in Fig. 2.13.2. We claim that $x_u(k)$ occupies half as much bandwidth as an amplitude modulated version of $m(k)$. To see this, define the complex signal $u(k)$ by

$$u(k) = m(k) + j\hat{m}(k). \tag{2.13.4}$$

Then $x_u(k)$ can be represented by

$$x_u(k) = \text{Re}[u(k)e^{j\theta_c k}]. \tag{2.13.5}$$

The signal $u(k)$ has a DTFT $U(e^{j\theta})$ which is given by

$$U(e^{j\theta}) = M(e^{j\theta}) + j\hat{M}(e^{j\theta}) = M(e^{j\theta})[1 + jH(e^{j\theta})], \tag{2.13.6}$$

which, by Eq. 2.13.1, becomes

$$U(e^{j\theta}) = \begin{cases} 0, & -\pi \le \theta < 0 \\ 2M(e^{j\theta}), & 0 \le \theta \le \pi \end{cases} \tag{2.13.7}$$

The spectrum $U(e^{j\theta})$ is shown in Fig. 2.13.1c. Notice that it consists of only the upper half of $M(e^{j\theta})$. Now, to determine $X_u(e^{j\theta})$, recall that

$$\text{Re}[z] = \frac{1}{2}(z + z^*)$$

so that

$$x_u(k) = \text{Re}[u(k)e^{j\theta_c k}] = \frac{1}{2}u(k)e^{j\theta_c k} + \frac{1}{2}u^*(k)e^{-j\theta_c k}.$$

Using Eq. 2.12.6,

$$u^*(k) \overset{DTFT}{\longleftrightarrow} U^*(e^{-j\theta}),$$

and the DTFT is easily evaluated as

$$X_u(e^{j\theta}) = \frac{1}{2}[U(e^{j(\theta-\theta_c)}) + U^*(e^{j(-\theta-\theta_c)})].$$

The spectrum $U(e^{j(\theta-\theta_c)})$ is simply $U(e^{j\theta})$ shifted to the right by θ_c. The spectrum $U(e^{j(-\theta-\theta_c)})$ is formed by first "flipping" $U(e^{j\theta})$ about $\theta = 0$ and shifting to the left by θ_c. Because of Eq. 2.13.7, we now have

$$X_u(e^{j\theta}) = \begin{cases} M(e^{j(\theta-\theta_c)}), & \omega_c \leq |\theta| \leq \theta_c + \theta_B \\ 0, & \text{otherwise} \end{cases} \tag{2.13.8}$$

The spectrum $X_u(e^{j\theta})$, shown in Fig. 2.13.1d, is referred to as an *upper sideband* spectrum. Notice that the bandwidth of this signal is half of what would be obtained had $m(k)$ been amplitude modulated directly. A *lower sideband* spectrum would have been obtained if we had used $u^*(k)$ rather than $u(k)$. Collectively, these are known as *single sideband spectra.*

To recover the signal $m(k)$ from the upper sideband signal $x_u(k)$, we can modulate by $\cos(\theta_c k)$. We get

$$x_u(k)\cos(\theta_c k) = m(k)\cos^2(\theta_c k) - \hat{m}(k)\sin(\theta_c k)\cos(\theta_c k)$$

which, after some simplification, becomes

$$x_u(k)\cos(\theta_c k) = \frac{1}{2}m(k) + \frac{1}{2}m(k)\cos(2\theta_c k) - \frac{1}{2}\hat{m}(k)\sin(2\theta_c k).$$

Therefore, if we filter the output of the demodulator by a lowpass filter with gain two which rejects the bandpass components at $\pm 2\theta_c$, we can recover $m(k)$. If needed, $\hat{m}(k)$ can be recovered in a similar manner by instead modulating $x_u(k)$ by $\sin(\theta_c k)$. This is shown in Fig. 2.13.2.

The procedure for generating single sideband signals and recovering information from them suggests another scheme for bandwidth compression known as *quadrature amplitude modulation* (QAM). Suppose $m_1(k)$ and $m_2(k)$ are two signals and we form the QAM signal $x(k)$ by

$$x(k) = m_1(k)\cos(\theta_c k) + m_2(k)\sin(\theta_c k)$$

as shown in Fig. 2.13.3a. The carrier $\cos(\theta_c k)$ is known as the *in-phase* carrier and the phase-shifted carrier $\sin(\theta_c k)$ is known as the *quadrature* carrier. We can expand the expression for $x(k)$ as

$$x(k) = \frac{1}{2}m_1(k)[e^{j\theta_c k} + e^{-j\theta_c k}] - j\frac{1}{2}m_2(k)[e^{j\theta_c k} - e^{-j\theta_c k}].$$

Using the modulation theorem, the QAM signal $x(k)$ has a DTFT given by

$$X(e^{j\theta}) = \frac{1}{2}[M_1(e^{j(\theta+\theta_c)}) + M_1(e^{j(\theta-\theta_c)}) + jM_2(e^{j(\theta+\theta_c)}) - jM_2(e^{j(\theta-\theta_c)})].$$

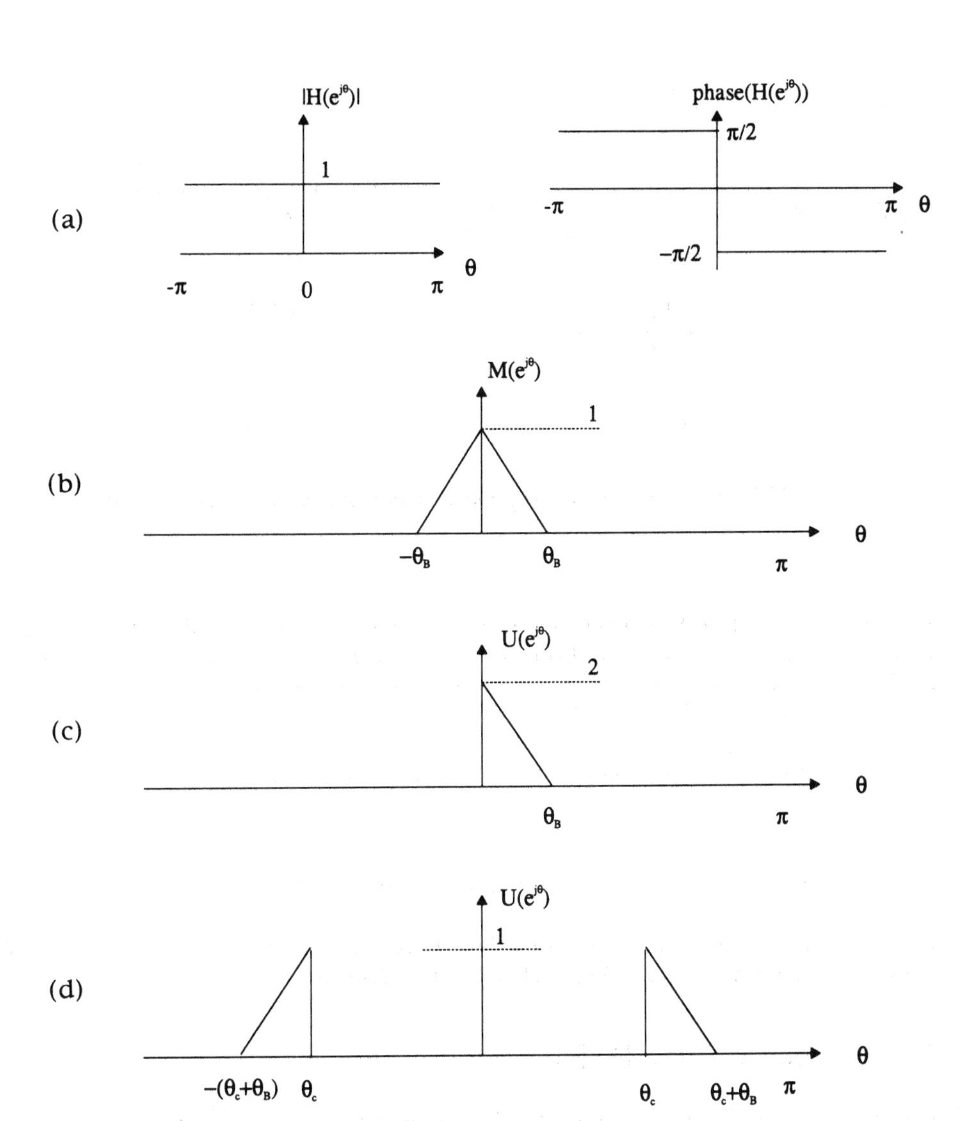

Figure 2.13.1: (a) Magnitude and phase response of ideal Hilbert transformer; (b) baseband spectrum $M(e^{j\theta})$; (c) spectrum of complex signal, $u(k)$; (d) upper-sideband spectrum $X_u(e^{j\theta})$.

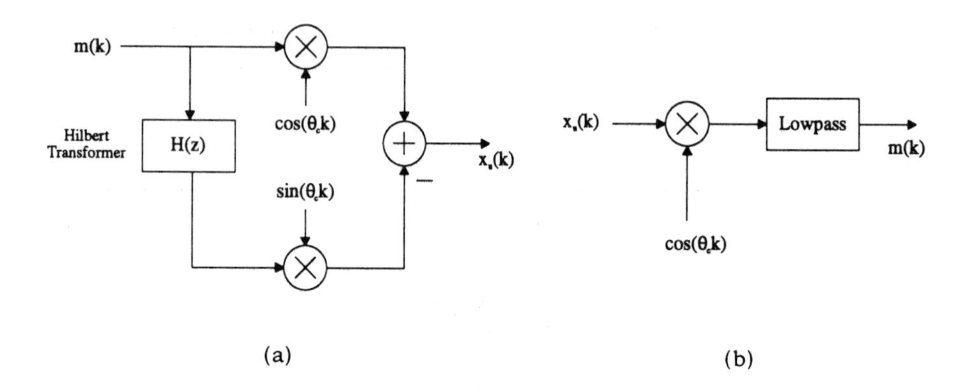

Figure 2.13.2: (a) Generation and (b) demodulation of a single sideband signal.

Observe that the bandwidth of $x(k)$ is not greater than the larger of the bandwidths of $m_1(k)$ and $m_2(k)$. Even though the spectral components of $m_1(k)$ and $m_2(k)$ overlap in $x(k)$, we can still reconstruct $m_1(k)$ and $m_2(k)$. To recover the signals $m_1(k)$ and $m_2(k)$ from the QAM signal $x(k)$, notice that

$$x(k)\cos(\theta_c k) = \frac{1}{2}\left[m_1(k) + m_1(k)\cos(2\theta_c k) + m_2(k)\sin(2\theta_c k)\right]$$

and

$$x(k)\sin(\theta_c k) = \frac{1}{2}\left[m_2(k) + m_1(k)\sin(2\theta_c k) - m_2(k)\cos(2\theta_c k)\right].$$

The signals $m_1(k)$ and $m_2(k)$ can be recovered by lowpass filtering $x(k)\cos(\theta_c k)$ and $x(k)\sin(\theta_c k$ to reject the bandpass terms at $\pm 2\theta_c$, as shown in Fig. 2.13.3b.

2.14 Symmetry of the DTFT

There are a number of symmetry properties for the discrete-time Fourier transform. These properties are often very useful in gaining insight into a system's behavior. We briefly summarize some of the more important properties in this section.

An *even* sequence is defined as a sequence $x(k)$ which satisfies

$$x_e(k) = x_e^*(-k).$$

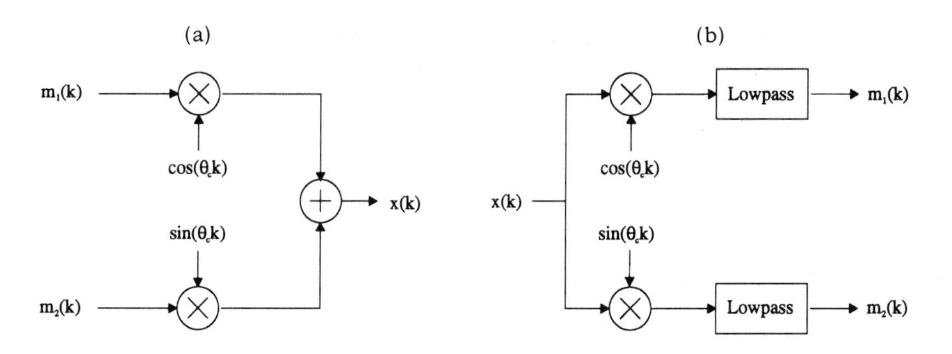

Figure 2.13.3: (a) Generation and (b) demodulation of a quadrature amplitude modulated (QAM) signal.

When $x(k)$ is real, this condition reduces to

$$x_e(k) = x_e(-k).$$

Similarly, an *odd sequence* is a sequence $x_o(k)$ for which

$$x_o(k) = -x_o^*(-k)$$

and a real odd sequence satisfies

$$x_o(k) = -x_o(-k).$$

It is simple to show that any sequence $x(k)$ can be decomposed as the sum of even and odd sequences. If $x_e(k)$ and $x_o(k)$ are given by

$$x_e(k) = \frac{1}{2}(x(k) + x^*(-k))$$

and

$$x_o(k) = \frac{1}{2}(x(k) - x^*(-k)),$$

respectively, it follows that

$$x(k) = x_e(k) + x_o(k).$$

It is readily verified that $x_e(k)$ and $x_o(k)$ as given above are indeed even and odd, respectively.

The function $X_e(e^{j\theta})$ is called *conjugate-symmetric* if

$$X_e(e^{j\theta}) = X_e^*(e^{-j\theta}).$$

$X_o(e^{j\theta})$ is called *conjugate-antisymmetric* if

$$X_o(e^{j\theta}) = -X_o^*(e^{-j\theta}).$$

A DTFT $X(e^{j\theta})$ can be decomposed into the sum of conjugate-symmetric and conjugate-antisymmetric functions. This decomposition is given by

$$X(e^{j\theta}) = X_e(e^{j\theta}) + X_o(e^{j\theta})$$

where

$$X_e(e^{j\theta}) = \frac{1}{2}(X(e^{j\theta}) + X^*(e^{-j\theta}))$$

and

$$X_o(e^{j\theta}) = \frac{1}{2}(X(e^{j\theta}) - X^*(e^{-j\theta})).$$

Again, it is readily verified that $X_e(e^{j\theta})$ and $X_o(e^{j\theta})$ are conjugate-symmetric and conjugate-antisymmetric, respectively.

Many useful symmetry properties of the DTFT can be obtained from even-odd decompositions of the time series and the DTFT. Some of these properties are given in Table 2.4. From these properties, we can make the following observations:

1. If $x(k)$ is real and even, then $X(e^{j\theta})$ will be purely real.
2. If $x(k)$ is real and odd, then $X(e^{j\theta})$ will be purely imaginary.

We can illustrate some of these properties by example.

Example 2.32

Consider the *ideal Hilbert transformer*, whose transfer function is given by

$$H(e^{j\theta}) = \begin{cases} -j, & -\pi < \theta < 0 \\ j, & 0 \le \theta < \pi \end{cases}$$

The inverse DTFT is given by

$$h(k) = -\frac{1}{2\pi}\int_{-\pi}^{0} je^{j\theta k}\,d\theta + \frac{1}{2\pi}\int_{0}^{\pi} je^{j\theta k}\,d\theta,$$

which gives

$$h(k) = \frac{1}{\pi k}(\cos(\pi k) - 1).$$

Therefore,

$$h(k) = \begin{cases} -2/(\pi k), & k \text{ odd} \\ 0, & k \text{ even} \end{cases}$$

This is an example of a sequence which is real and odd and has a DTFT which is purely imaginary.

Example 2.33

We have already showed that

$$x(k) = \frac{\sin(\theta_c k)}{\pi k}$$

has the DTFT

$$X(e^{j\theta}) = \begin{cases} 1, & |\theta| < \theta_c \\ 0, & \theta_c < |\theta| < \pi. \end{cases}$$

The sequence $x(k)$ is clearly real and even, and we can see that the DTFT is purely real.

Until now, we have discussed several methods for obtaining the frequency response of a LTI system. These have included using the $\mathcal{Z}$-transform, direct evaluation of the DTFT from the system's impulse response, and using the eigenfunction property of linear systems. Consider now the following method. Suppose the system's SDE representation is

$$y(k) + \sum_{n=1}^{N} a_n y(k-n) = \sum_{n=0}^{M} b_n x(k-n).$$

If the input is $x(k) = \delta(k)$, the output $y(k)$ will be the impulse response sequence, $h(k)$ so that

$$h(k) + \sum_{n=1}^{N} a_n h(k-n) = \sum_{n=0}^{M} b_n \delta(k-n). \tag{2.14.1}$$

Recall that

$$\delta(k) \stackrel{DTFT}{\longleftrightarrow} 1$$

Time Function	DTFT
$\delta(k)$	1
$u(k)$	$\dfrac{1}{1-e^{-j\theta}} + \sum_{r=-\infty}^{\infty} \pi\delta(\theta + 2\pi r)$
1	$\sum_{r=-\infty}^{\infty} 2\pi\delta(\theta + 2\pi r)$
$a^k u(k)$	$\dfrac{1}{1-ae^{-j\theta}}$
$e^{j\theta_0 k}$	$\sum_{r=-\infty}^{\infty} 2\pi\delta(\theta - \theta_0 + 2\pi r)$
$\cos(\theta_0 k)$	$\pi \sum_{r=-\infty}^{\infty} [\delta(\theta - \theta_0 + 2\pi r) + \delta(\theta + \theta_0 + 2\pi r)]$
$\dfrac{\sin(\theta_c k)}{\pi k}$	$X(e^{j\theta}) = \begin{cases} 1, & \|\theta\| < \theta_c \\ 0, & \theta_c < \|\theta\| \leq \pi \end{cases}$
$w_N(k)$	$e^{-j(N+1)\theta/2}\dfrac{\sin(N\theta/2)}{\sin(\theta/2)}$
$x^*(k)$	$X^*(e^{-j\theta})$
$x^*(-k)$	$X^*(e^{j\theta})$
$\mathrm{Re}(x(k))$	$X_e(e^{j\theta})$
$j\mathrm{Im}(x(k))$	$X_o(e^{j\theta})$
$x_e(k)$	$\mathrm{Re}(X(e^{j\theta}))$
$x_o(k)$	$j\mathrm{Im}(X(e^{j\theta}))$

Table 2.3: Important DTFT pairs

Operation	Time Function	DTFT
Linearity	$ax_1(k) + bx_2(k)$	$aX_1(e^{j\theta}) + bX_2(e^{j\theta})$
Convolution	$x_1(k) * x_2(k)$	$X_1(e^{j\theta})X_2(e^{j\theta})$
Multiplication of sequences	$x_1(k)x_2(k)$	$\frac{1}{2\pi}\int_{-\pi}^{\pi} X_1(e^{j\phi})X_2(e^{j(\theta-\phi)})\,d\phi$
Time delay	$x(k-k_0)$	$e^{-j\theta k_0}X(e^{j\theta})$
Modulation	$e^{j\theta_0 k}x(k)$	$X(e^{j(\theta-\theta_0)})$
Multiplication by k	$kx(k)$	$-j\frac{dX(e^{j\theta})}{d\theta}$
Time reversal	$x(-k)$	$X(e^{-j\theta})$

Table 2.4: Important DTFT properties

and

$$h(k) \overset{DTFT}{\longleftrightarrow} H(e^{j\theta}).$$

Because of the time-shifting property of the DTFT, we also have

$$\delta(k-n) \longleftrightarrow e^{jn\theta}$$

and

$$h(k-n) \overset{DTFT}{\longleftrightarrow} e^{jn\theta}H(e^{j\theta}).$$

Applying the linearity and time-shifting properties together, the DTFT of Eq. 2.14.1 is

$$H(e^{j\theta}) + \sum_{n=1}^{N} a_n e^{jn\theta}H(e^{j\theta}) = \sum_{n=0}^{M} b_n e^{jn\theta}. \tag{2.14.2}$$

We then solve Eq. 2.14.2 for $H(e^{j\theta})$, which gives

$$H(e^{j\theta}) = \frac{\sum_{n=0}^{M} b_n e^{jn\theta}}{1 + \sum_{n=1}^{N} a_n e^{jn\theta}}. \tag{2.14.3}$$

2.15 Windowing

We have seen how to compute the DTFT of several infinite-time signals, such as $a^n u(n)$ or $\cos(\theta_0 n)$. What we now must do is study the effect of time-limiting these infinite-duration signals. Rather than study this effect in the time domain (which is rather trivial), we are interested in the manner in which truncating the signal will affect the signal's DTFT. This is accomplished by using the multiplication-in-time/convolution-in-frequency property of the DTFT.

Define the N-point *rectangular window*, $w_N(k)$ by

$$w_N(k) = \begin{cases} 1, & n \leq N-1 \\ 0, & \text{otherwise} \end{cases}$$

The DTFT of $w_N(k)$ is given by

$$W_N(e^{j\theta}) = \sum_{k=0}^{N-1} 1 \cdot e^{j\theta k} = \frac{1 - e^{jN\theta}}{1 - e^{j\theta}}. \tag{2.15.1}$$

Equation 2.15.1 can be rewritten as

$$W_N(e^{j\theta}) = \frac{e^{-jN\theta/2}(e^{jN\theta/2} - e^{-jN\theta/2})}{e^{-j\theta/2}(e^{j\theta/2} - e^{-j\theta/2})}$$

which is the same as

$$W_N(e^{j\theta}) = e^{-j(N-1)\theta/2} \frac{\sin(N\theta/2)}{\sin(\theta/2)}. \tag{2.15.2}$$

If N is odd, the *symmetric* (about $k = 0$) rectangular window of length N by

$$v_N(k) = \begin{cases} 1, & |k| \leq (N-1)/2 \\ 0, & \text{otherwise} \end{cases}$$

The symmetric window $v_N(k)$ is obtained by advancing $w_N(k)$ in time by $(N-1)/2$ samples. Thus,

$$v_N(k) = w_N(k + \frac{(N-1)}{2}).$$

Because of the time-shift property of the DTFT, it follows that

$$V_N(e^{j\theta}) = e^{j(N-1)\theta/2} W_N(e^{j\theta})$$

so that

$$V_N(e^{j\theta}) = \frac{\sin(N\theta/2)}{\sin(\theta/2)}. \tag{2.15.3}$$

Thus, the magnitude of $v_N(k)$ and $w_N(k)$ are identical. Only the phase has been shifted.

A plot of the symmetric window spectrum is shown in Fig. 2.15.1. The magnitude at $\theta = 0$ is obtained using L'Hospital's rule and is easily shown to be equal to N. This quantity is known as the *mainlobe amplitude*. Furthermore, there are zero-crossings whenever $\sin(N\theta/2)$ is equal to zero. This occurs when

$$\theta = \frac{2k\pi}{N}, \quad k = \pm 1, \pm 2, \ldots.$$

The width of the main lobe between zero crossings on the left and right is known as the *mainlobe width*. Thus, the rectangular window has a mainlobe width of $4\pi/N$. If N is large, the next maximum of the DTFT occurs when

$$\frac{N\theta}{2} = \frac{3\pi}{2},$$

which gives $\theta = 3\pi/N$. The magnitude at $\theta = 3\pi/N$ is given by

$$|V_N(e^{j3\pi/N})| = \frac{|\sin(3\pi/2)|}{|\sin(3\pi/2N)|}.$$

For large N, $\sin(\pi/2N) \approx 3\pi/2N$ so that

$$|V_N(e^{j\pi/N})| \approx \frac{2N}{3\pi}.$$

This quantity is known as the *sidelobe amplitude*. The ratio of the sidelobe amplitude to the mainlobe amplitude is an important figure of merit for windows. For the rectangular window, this ratio is seen to equal

$$R \approx \frac{2N/3\pi}{N} = \frac{3\pi}{2}.$$

This ratio is essentially independent of N and indicates that the sidelobe/mainlobe amplitude ratio never decreases below -13.6 dB.

Let's study the effect of applying a symmetric rectangular window to an infinite-duration signal. Suppose $x(k)$ is given by

$$x(k) = \cos(\theta_0 k).$$

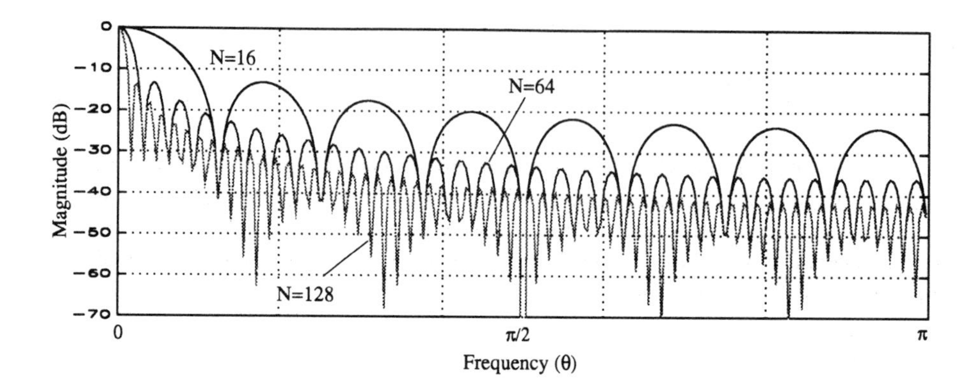

Figure 2.15.1: Magnitude spectrum of the symmetric rectangular window $v_N(k)$.

Define the windowed cosine sequence $x_v(k)$ by

$$x_v(k) = v_N(k)\cos(\theta_0 k) = \begin{cases} \cos(\theta_0 k), & |k| \le (N+1)/2 \\ 0, & |k| > (N+1)/2. \end{cases}$$

How can we determine $X_v(e^{j\theta})$? Recall that the DTFT of the product of two signals is given by the periodic convolution of their DTFTs. Thus,

$$X_v(e^{j\theta}) = \frac{1}{2\pi}\int_{-\pi}^{\pi} X(e^{j\phi})V_N(e^{j(\theta-\phi)})\,d\phi.$$

More easily, this can also be interpreted in the context of modulation. Because $x(k)$ is a cosine sequence, $x_v(k)$ corresponds to the sequence $v_N(k)$ modulated by $x(k)$. Hence, by the modulation theorem,

$$X_v(e^{j\theta}) = \frac{1}{2}\left(V_N(e^{j(\theta-\theta_0)}) + V_N(e^{j(\theta+\theta_0)})\right).$$

Notice that $X_v(e^{j\theta})$ is simply a frequency-shifted version of $V_N(e^{j\theta})$.

Example 2.34

Let $h(k)$ be the impulse response of the ideal lowpass filter with cutoff frequency θ_c. Then

$$h(k) = \frac{\sin(\theta_c k)}{\pi k}.$$

Suppose we symmetrically truncate the sequence to length N by applying the rectangular window $v_N(k)$. Then

$$h_N(k) = h(k)v_N(k).$$

What has happened to the magnitude response? We have the relationship

$$H_N(e^{j\theta}) = \frac{1}{2\pi}\int_{-\pi}^{\pi} H(e^{j\phi})V_N(e^{j(\theta-\phi)})\,d\phi.$$

Because of the rectangular nature of $H(e^{j\theta})$, it follows that

$$H_N(e^{j\theta}) = \frac{1}{2\pi}\int_{-\theta_c}^{\theta_c} V_N(e^{j(\theta-\phi)})\,d\phi.$$

Therefore, the value of $H_N(e^{j\theta})$ at a given value of θ is given by the integral of the shifted window spectrum between $-\theta_c$ and θ_c. For the ideal case where the window has an impulsive spectrum, this will produce the proper result. However, the window spectrum has a sinc profile and hence "blurs" the ideal spectrum. Intuitively, if the mainlobe width of the window is extremely narrow relative to θ_c, this blurring will be minimized. Recall, however, that the sidelobe amplitude is only roughly 14 dB below the mainlobe amplitude for all N. Therefore, the crisp transition of the ideal lowpass will be "smeared" by the sidelobes. This is sometimes referred to as *window leakage.* Figure 2.15.2 shows the effect of windowing an ideal lowpass filter with $\theta_c = \pi/2$ for window lengths $N = 16, 64, 128$. Notice that even for large N there will still be ringing near the transition band. This is a manifestation of Gibbs phenomenon.

2.16 Sampling Continuous-Time Signals

We have not yet discussed how to process continuous-time signals with digital signal processing techniques. All of our results so far have been based on discrete-time signals and systems. What must be developed now is the mathematical machinery for dealing with the process of *sampling,* whereby a continuous-time signal is converted to a discrete-time signal. One of the fundamental results which (arguably) makes digital signal processing possible is *Shannon's sampling theorem.*

Theorem 3 (Shannon Sampling Theorem) *Let $x_c(t)$ be a continuous-time signal whose Fourier transform is bandlimited to ω_N, i.e.,*

$$X_c(j\omega) = 0, \quad |\omega| > \omega_N.$$

Then $x_c(t)$ is completely determined by its samples,

$$\ldots, x_c(-2T), x_c(-T), x_c(0), x_c(T), x_c(2T), \ldots$$

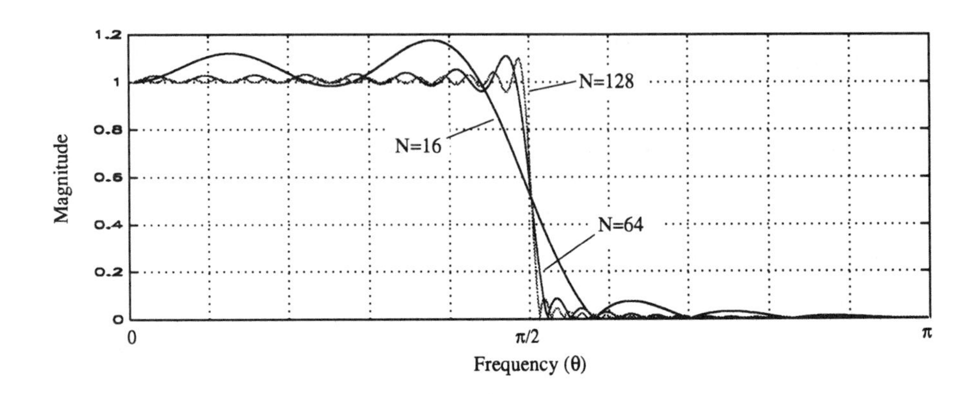

Figure 2.15.2: The effect of applying symmetric rectangular windows of length 16,64,and 128 to an ideal lowpass filter.

if

$$\omega_s = \frac{2\pi}{T} > 2\omega_N.$$

The proof of this fundamental result is constructive. Assume $x_c(t)$ is bandlimited to ω_N. The first step is to modulate $x_c(t)$ by a periodic impulse train of period T. The impulse train is given by

$$s(t) = \sum_{k=-\infty}^{\infty} \delta(t - kT)$$

and the modulated signal is given by $x_s(t)$ where

$$x_s(t) = x_c(t) \sum_{k=-\infty}^{\infty} \delta(t - kT). \tag{2.16.1}$$

Using the sifting property for Dirac functions, an alternate expression for $x_s(t)$ is

$$x_s(t) = \sum_{k=-\infty}^{\infty} x_c(kT)\delta(t - kT). \tag{2.16.2}$$

The Fourier transform of $x_s(t)$ is given by the convolution theorem for Fourier transforms:

$$X_s(j\omega) = \frac{1}{2\pi} X_c(j\omega) * S(j\omega).$$

It can be shown that

$$S(j\omega) = \frac{2\pi}{T} \sum_{k=-\infty}^{\infty} \delta(\omega - \omega_s)$$

so that

$$X_s(j\omega) = \frac{1}{2\pi} X_c(j\omega) * \left(\frac{2\pi}{T} \sum_{k=-\infty}^{\infty} \delta(\omega - \omega_s) \right).$$

Thus,

$$X_s(j\omega) = \frac{1}{T} \sum_{k=-\infty}^{\infty} X_c(j(\omega - k\omega_s)). \tag{2.16.3}$$

Let's take a closer look at Eq. 2.16.3. This equation states that the spectrum $X_s(j\omega)$ is given by summing shifted copies of $X_c(j\omega)$. This is illustrated in Fig. 2.16.1. It can be seen that there is no overlap in the shifted replicas of $X_c(j\omega)$ if

$$\omega_s - \omega_N > \omega_N,$$

or

$$\omega_s > 2\omega_N.$$

It is clear that if this condition is met, $x_c(t)$ can be recovered by an ideal lowpass filter. This lowpass filter should have a cutoff frequency ω_c such that

$$\omega_N < \omega_c < \omega_s - \omega_N.$$

One particular choice of ω_c which satisfies these requirements is

$$\omega_c = \frac{\omega_s}{2}.$$

Also, in order to compensate for the $1/T$ in Eq. 2.16.3, the lowpass filter should have a gain of T. Call this ideal lowpass filter $h_r(t)$ (the subscript r indicates "reconstruction"). It then follows that the output of the reconstruction filter will be

$$X_r(j\omega) = H_r(j\omega) X_s(j\omega)$$

and

$$x_r(t) = x_s(t) * h_r(t). \tag{2.16.4}$$

It then follows that

$$x_r(t) = x_c(t).$$

The reconstruction process is also illustrated in Fig. 2.16.1.

If the condition $\omega_s > 2\omega_N$ is not met, the shifted copies of $X_c(j\omega)$ will overlap and the spectrum $X_s(j\omega)$ will be distorted. In this case, it will not be possible to recover the original signal by lowpass filtering. This phenomenon is known as *aliasing*. The origin of the term aliasing can be understood in terms of sampling and reconstruction of a sinusoidal signal. Let $x_c(t)$ be given by

$$x_c(t) = \cos(\omega_N t).$$

Assume that the sampling frequency is such that

$$\omega_s < 2\omega_N.$$

It can be seen in Fig. 2.16.2 that the sampled signal $x_s(t)$ will have spectral components at $\omega_s - \omega_N$ and $\omega_s + \omega_N$. If the reconstruction filter has cutoff frequency $\omega_c = \omega_N$, the reconstructed signal will be given by

$$x_r(t) = \cos((\omega_s - \omega_N)t).$$

Thus, the original signal has assumed the "alias" of a sinusoid with a different frequency. This is illustrated in Fig. 2.16.2.

If a continuous-time signal $x_c(t)$ has frequency content above the frequency $\omega_s/2$, it must first be lowpass-filtered in the analog domain to attenuate all frequency content above $\omega_s/2$ and *then* sampled. While this will destroy all frequency information beyond $\omega_s/2$, the low-frequency information will be preserved. Such a procedure is warranted when certain high-frequency information is not of interested. For example, in digital processing of telephone signals, only the frequency range between 0 and approximately 4 KHz is needed for intelligibility. There *is* frequency content beyond 4 KHz, but it can be removed by analog lowpass filtering and the signal then sampled at 8 KHz or higher. Figure 2.16.3 illustrates the effect of aliasing when a signal is not bandlimited to $\omega_s/2$ before sampling. Notice that the frequency-shifted copies of $X_c(j\omega)$ overlap since the condition $\omega_s - \omega_N > \omega_N$ is not met. Consequently, when the frequency-shifted copies of $X_c(j\omega)$ are summed to form $X_s(j\omega)$, severe distortion can result. In general, this distortion can not be eliminated. If, instead, the

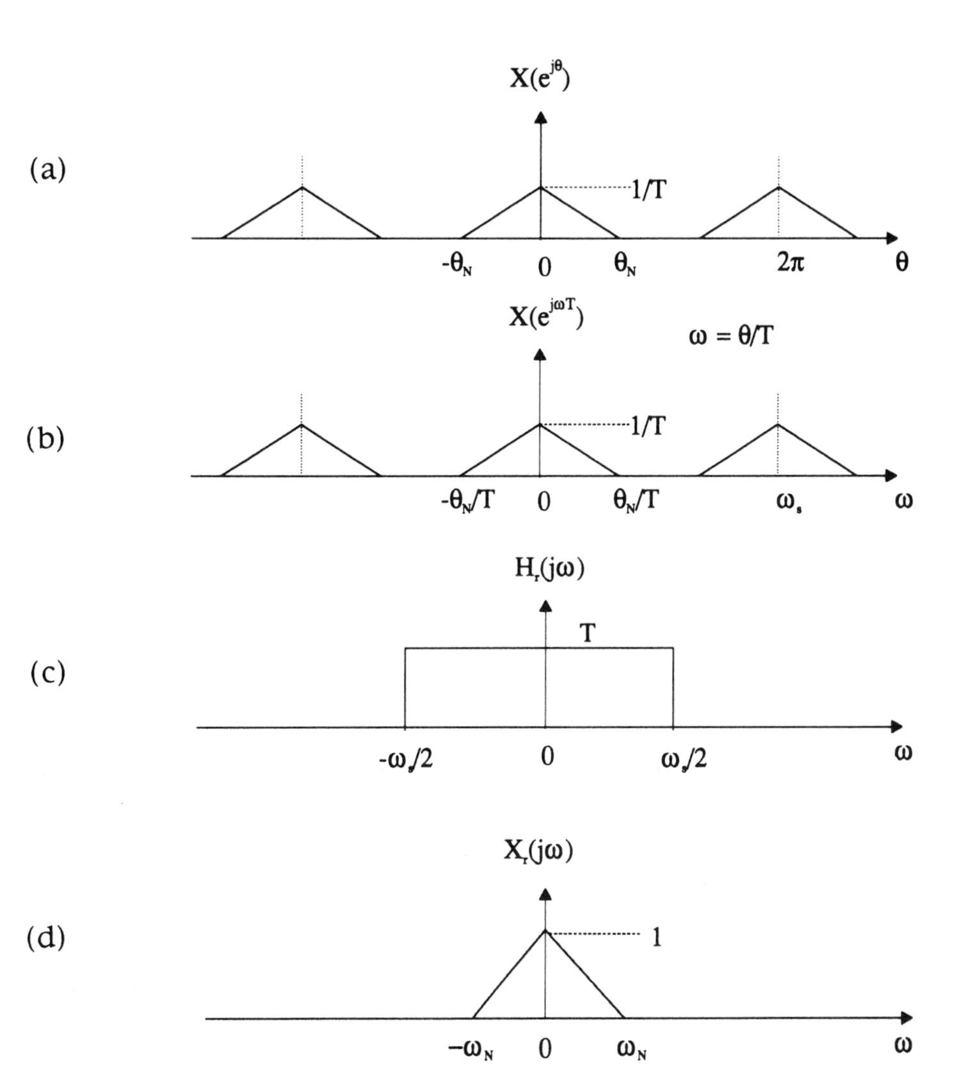

Figure 2.16.1: (a) Spectrum of bandlimited signal; (b) $X_s(j\omega)$. (c) reconstruction filter $H_r(j\omega)$; (d) output of reconstruction filter.

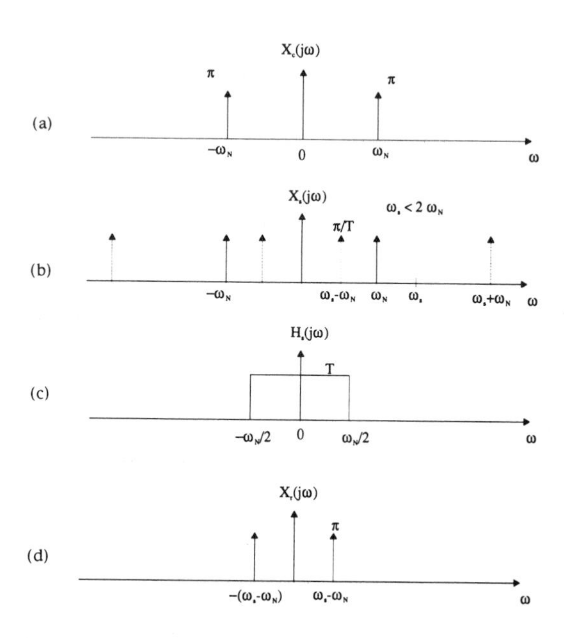

Figure 2.16.2: (a) Spectrum of sinusoid with frequency ω_N; (b) $X_s(j\omega)$; (c) reconstruction filter $H_r(j\omega)$; (d) output of reconstruction filter.

signal $x_c(t)$ had been bandlimited to $\omega_s/2$ before sampling, the low-frequency information in the signal $x_c(t)$ is preserved in $x_s(t)$ and can be recovered.

Now that we have obtained an expression for the Fourier transform of the *continuous-time* modulated impulse train, we can derive the DTFT of the sequence whose samples correspond to $x_c(kT)$. The discrete-time signal $x(k)$ is defined by

$$x(k) = x_c(kT),$$

we seek an expression for the spectrum $X(e^{j\theta})$. Taking the Fourier transform of Eq. 2.16.2, we have

$$X_s(j\omega) = \sum_{k=-\infty}^{\infty} x_c(kT)e^{-jk\omega T}. \tag{2.16.5}$$

By definition,

$$X(e^{j\theta}) = \sum_{k=-\infty}^{\infty} x(k)e^{-jk\theta}. \tag{2.16.6}$$

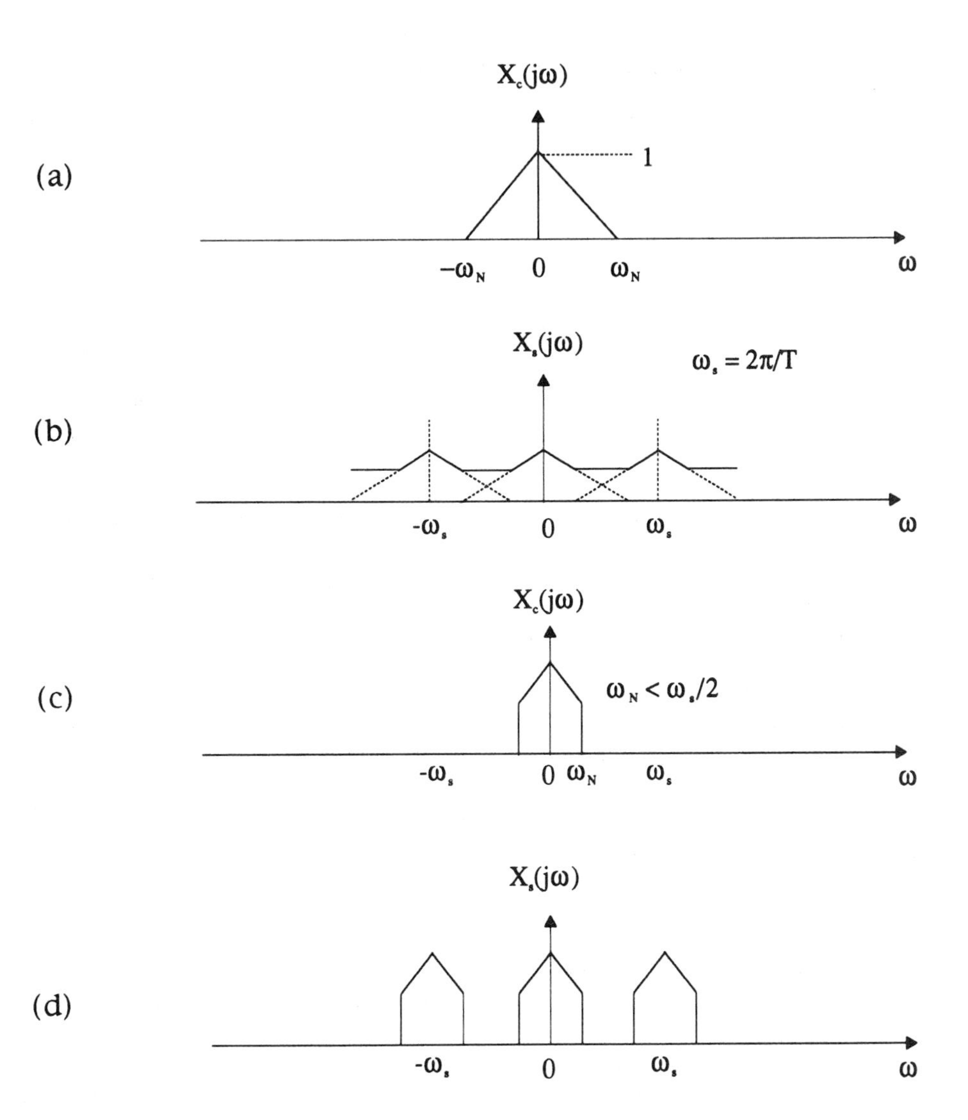

Figure 2.16.3: (a) $X_c(j\omega)$; (b) $X_s(j\omega)$ for $\omega_s < 2\omega_N$; (c) $X_c(j\omega)$ after band-limiting to $\omega_s/2$; (d) $X_s(j\omega)$ corresponding to band-limited $X_c(j\omega)$.

Comparing Eqs. 2.16.6 and 2.16.5, it can be seen that

$$X_s(j\omega) = X(e^{j\theta})\Big|_{\theta=\omega T} = X(e^{j\omega T}). \tag{2.16.7}$$

Therefore, we have the pair of relations

$$X(e^{j\omega T}) = \frac{1}{T}\sum_{k=-\infty}^{\infty} X_c(j(\omega - k\omega_s))$$

and

$$X(e^{j\theta}) = \frac{1}{T}\sum_{k=-\infty}^{\infty} X_c\left(j(\frac{\theta}{T} - \frac{2\pi k}{T})\right).$$

Equation 2.16.7 states that $X(e^{j\theta})$ is obtained from $X_S(j\omega)$ simply by scaling the frequency axis according to the rule

$$\theta = \omega T.$$

This normalization results in the analog frequency $\omega = \omega_s$ being mapped to the digital frequency $\theta = 2\pi$. The purpose of scaling the frequency axis is to implicitly account for the spacing between time samples. Figure 2.16.5 depicts the sampling and frequency normalization process in the frequency domain.

It should be kept in mind that the process of modulating $x_c(t)$ by the impulse train $s(t)$ is purely for mathematical convenience; it allows us to obtain the expression for $X(e^{j\theta})$ simply. In practice, the instantaneous samples $x_c(kT)$ are obtained directly from $x_c(t)$ using sample-and-hold devices followed by an analog-to-digital converter. The conversion of a continuous-time signal $x_c(t)$ to a discrete-time signal $x(k)$ is known as *continuous-to-discrete* (C/D) conversion. Ideal C/D conversion is depicted in Fig. 2.16.4.

In practice, the signal $x_c(t)$ can assume a continuum of amplitudes whereas the samples $x(k)$ are limited to a finite precision due to the digital devices used to sample and process signals. A discrete-time signal which assumes a discrete number of amplitudes is known as a *digital* signal, and the process of converting $x_c(t)$ to a digital signal $x(k)$ is known as *analog-to-digital* (A/D) conversion.

The process of converting a discrete-time signal $x(k)$ to the reconstructed continuous-time signal $x_r(t)$ is known as *discrete-to-continuous conversion* (D/C) and is depicted in Fig. 2.16.6. We have seen that the original continuous-time signal $x_c(t)$ could be recovered from the impulsive signal $x_s(t)$ by filtering with an ideal reconstruction filter. This can be used as an intermediate step in reconstructing $x_c(t)$ from $x(k)$. The sequence $x(k)$ is input to a system which converts samples to impulses. This system converts the sequence $x(k)$ to the modulated impulse train $x_s(t)$,

$$x_s(t) = \sum_{k=-\infty}^{\infty} x(k)\delta(t - kT).$$

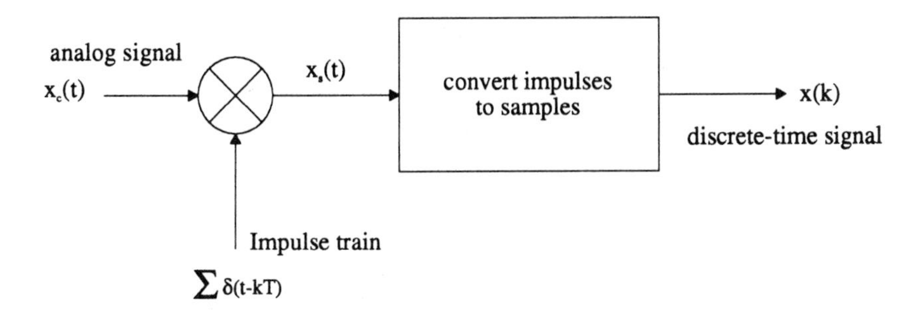

Figure 2.16.4: Ideal C/D conversion.

Next, the signal $x_s(t)$ is passed through the ideal reconstruction filter $h_r(t)$, which produces the output $x_r(t)$ according to

$$x_r(t) = h_r(t) * x_s(t).$$

In other words,

$$x_r(t) = h_r(t) * \left(\sum_{k=-\infty}^{\infty} x(k)\delta(t - kT) \right). \tag{2.16.8}$$

Therefore,

$$x_r(t) = \sum_{k=-\infty}^{\infty} x(k)h_r(t - kT). \tag{2.16.9}$$

Again, when digital signals are involved, the reconstruction process is known as *digital-to-analog* (D/A) conversion.

In order to examine the reconstruction process in the frequency domain, we need to take the Fourier transform of Eq. 2.16.8. Using the Fourier transform pair

$$h_r(t - kT) \longleftrightarrow e^{-j\omega kT} H_r(j\omega),$$

we have

$$X_r(j\omega) = H_r(j\omega) \sum_{k=-\infty}^{\infty} x(k)e^{-jk\omega T}.$$

We immediately recognize the summation as $X(e^{j\omega T})$, hence

$$X_r(j\omega) = H_r(j\omega)X(e^{j\omega T}). \tag{2.16.10}$$

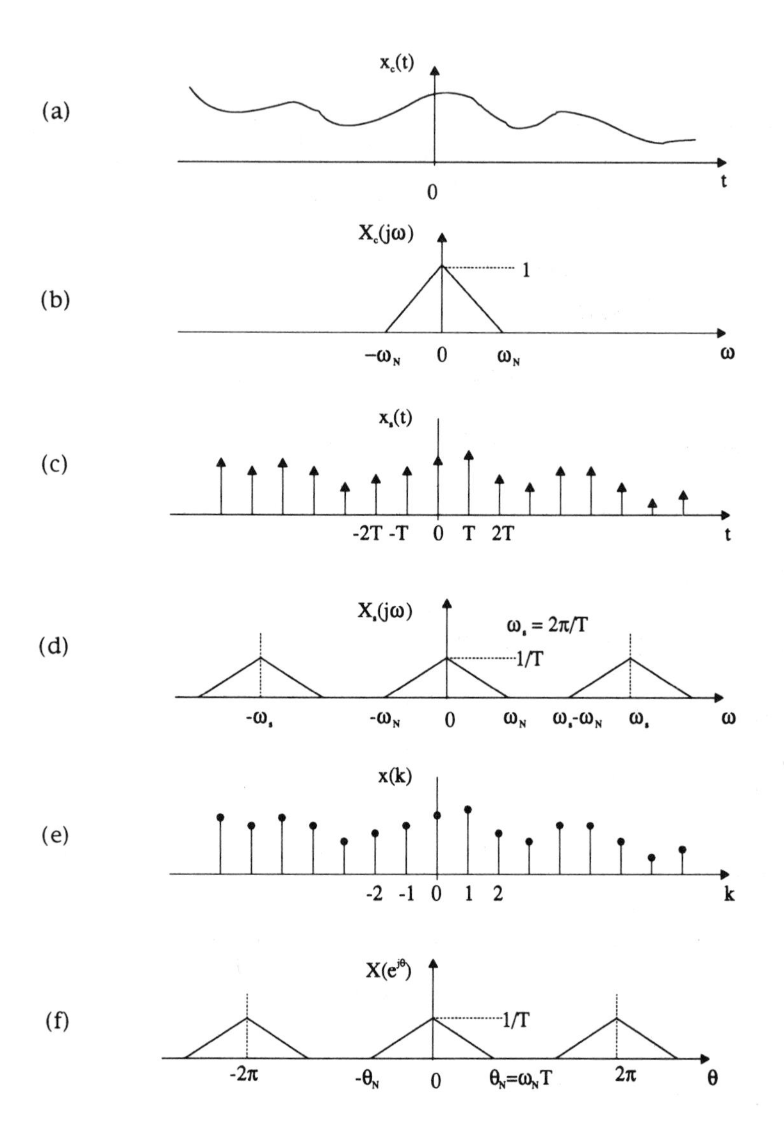

Figure 2.16.5: (a) Continuous-time signal $x_c(t)$; (b) spectrum of continuous signal, $X_c(j\omega)$; (c) $x_s(t)$; (d) $X_s(j\omega)$; (e) $x(k) = x_c(kT)$; (f) $X(e^{j\theta})$.

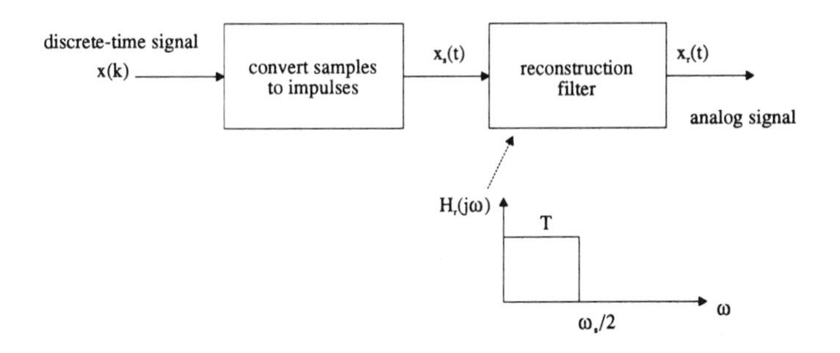

Figure 2.16.6: Ideal D/C conversion.

The spectrum $X(e^{j\omega T})$ is simply $X(e^{j\theta})$ "renormalized" with $\theta = \omega T$. Therefore, the lowpass filter $H_r(j\omega)$ simply removes the images of $X(e^{j\omega T})$ beyond the baseband, as shown in Fig. 2.16.7.

The sampling and reconstruction procedure has thusfar been examined only in the frequency domain. It may seem odd at first that a continuous-time signal can be specified from a collection of points which is "thin" compared to the continuum of time points over which the signal is defined. How, then, is the signal actually reconstructed? In other words, how can we obtain the value of $x_c(t)$ at a time instant not captured by the sampling process? The answer lies in the reconstruction function $h_r(t)$. The reconstruction filter acts as an "interpolator" which provides the continuum of signal values between samples. Recall that $h_r(t)$ is an ideal lowpass filter with gain T and cutoff frequency

$$\omega_c = \frac{\omega_s}{2} = \frac{\pi}{T}.$$

The function $h_r(t)$ is given by the inverse Fourier transform

$$h_r(t) = \frac{1}{2\pi}\int_{-\infty}^{\infty} H_r(j\omega)e^{j\omega t}\,d\omega = \frac{T}{2\pi}\int_{-\pi/T}^{\pi/T} e^{j\omega t}\,d\omega$$

which gives

$$h_r(t) = \frac{\sin(\pi t/T)}{\pi t/T}.$$

Substituting the above into Eq. 2.16.9,

$$x_r(t) = \sum_{k=-\infty}^{\infty} x(k)\frac{\sin(\pi(t-kT)/T)}{\pi(t-kT)/T}.$$

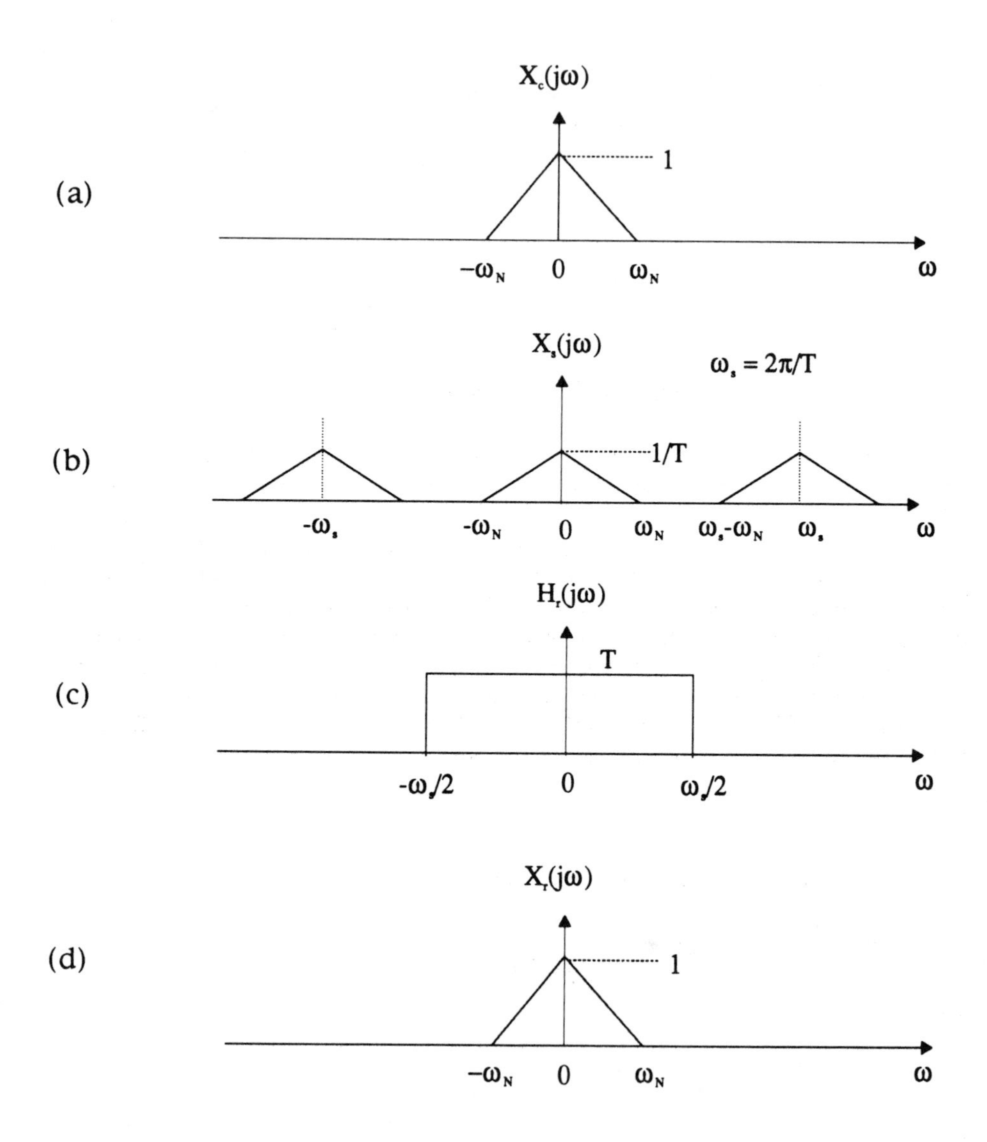

Figure 2.16.7: Ideal D/C conversion: (a) $X(e^{j\theta})$; (b) $X(e^{j\omega T})$; (c) $H_r(j\omega)$; (d) $X_r(j\omega)$.

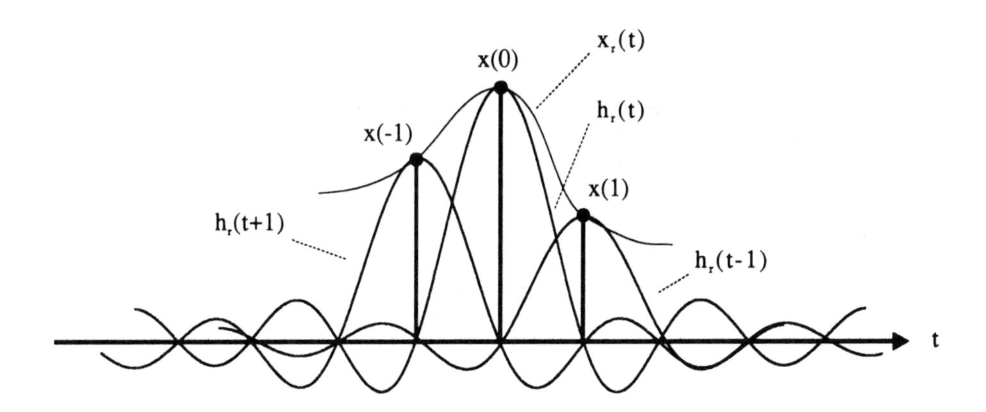

Figure 2.16.8: Interpolation of a band-limited signal $x_c(t)$ using samples $x(k)$ and ideal reconstruction filter $h_r(t)$.

Let's take a closer look at the function $h_r(t)$. This is a sinc function with unity magnitude at $t = 0$ and zero magnitude at $t = nT$, $n \neq 0$. Therefore, the time-shifted function, $h_r(t-kT)$, has unity magnitude at $t = kT$ and passes through zero at all other multiples of T. It thus follows that $x_r(t)$ and $x_c(t)$ agree at the sample instants kT. At values of t between samples, the scaled, time shifted versions of $h_r(t)$ add up to the proper value, $x_c(t)$. This is depicted in Fig. 2.16.8.

We can see that ideal D/C conversion consists of a step which first converts discrete samples to a modulated impulse train. In practice, this is physically impossible. One practical technique uses the samples as the input to a zero-order hold (ZOH) device which converts the samples to a "staircase" approximation of a continuous signal, as shown in Fig. 2.16.9a, followed by a lowpass filter. Let's analyze the effect this has on the reconstruction process. The ZOH converts a discrete-time impulse $\delta(k)$ to a rectangular pulse $h_{zoh}(t)$ as shown in Fig. 2.16.9b. Therefore, the staircase response of the ZOH to the signal $x(k)$ is given by

$$y(t) = \sum_{k=-\infty}^{\infty} x(k) h_{zoh}(t - kT). \tag{2.16.11}$$

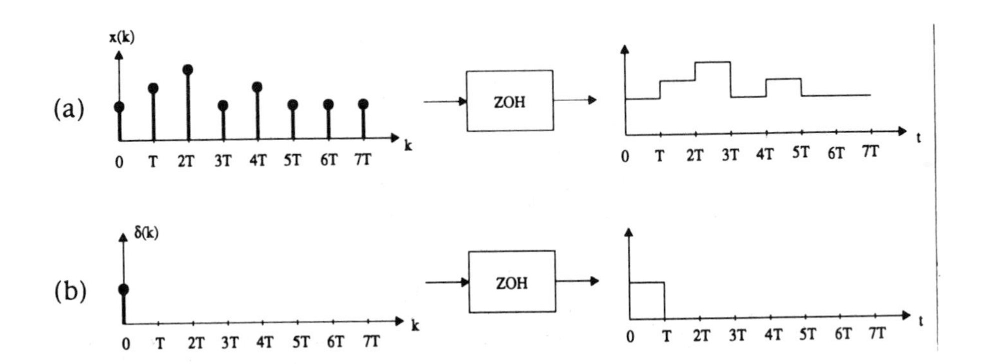

Figure 2.16.9: (a) Staircase approximation produced using ZOH; (b) ZOH response.

The magnitude of $H_{zoh}(j\omega)$ is simple to evaluate. Since $h_{zoh}(t)$ is a rectangular pulse of width T, the magnitude of its Fourier transform is given by

$$|H_{zoh}(j\omega)| = \left|\frac{2\sin(\omega T/2)}{\omega}\right|.$$

This is a sinc function with unity magnitude at $\omega = 0$ and nulls at $\omega = 2\pi k/T = k\omega_s$, $k = 1, 2, \ldots$. As can be seen in Fig. 2.16.10b. The Fourier transform of the time-shifted ZOH response $h_{zoh}(t - kT)$ is given by $e^{-j\omega kT}H_{zoh}(j\omega)$ so that the staircase waveform $y(t)$ as given by Eq. 2.16.11 has a Fourier transform given by

$$Y(j\omega) = \sum_{k=-\infty}^{\infty} x(k)e^{-j\omega kT}H_{zoh}(j\omega) = H_{zoh}(j\omega)\sum_{k=-\infty}^{\infty} x(k)e^{-j\omega kT}. \tag{2.16.12}$$

The summation on the right is recognized as $X(e^{j\omega T})$ so that

$$Y(j\omega) = H_{zoh}(j\omega)X(e^{j\omega T}). \tag{2.16.13}$$

Therefore, the ZOH acts as a lowpass filter which attenuates the images of $X(e^{j\omega T})$ outside the baseband, as shown in Fig. 2.16.10c. Finally, the remaining high frequency components are removed by lowpass filtering, giving $x_r(t)$ as shown in Fig. 2.16.10d. Notice that the ZOH induces a sinc-type rolloff in the reconstructed signal. A refinement to the ZOH reconstruction scheme compensates for this rolloff, which is fairly simple to perform in the discrete-time domain.

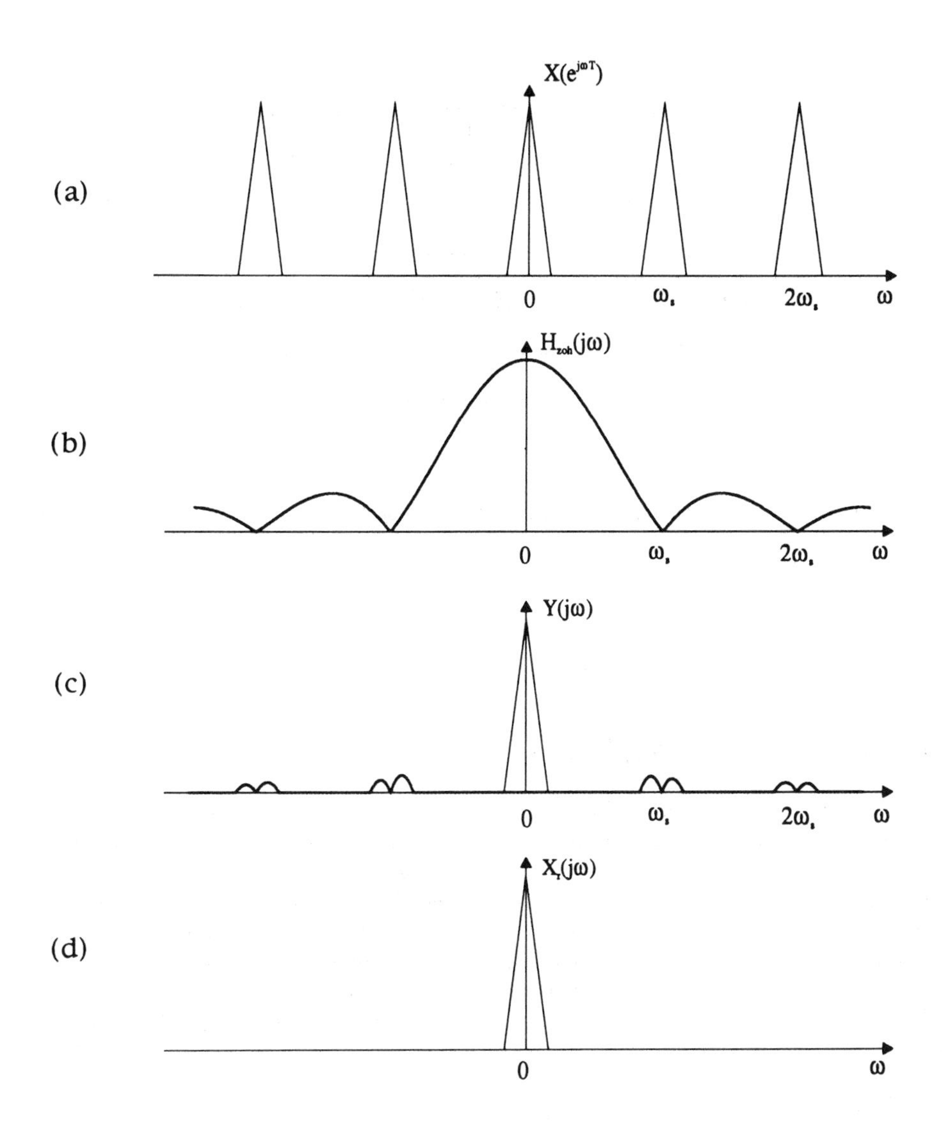

Figure 2.16.10: ZOH reconstruction: (a) $X(e^{j\omega T})$; (b) ZOH magnitude response $|H_{zoh}(j\omega)|$; (c) spectrum $Y(j\omega)$ of staircase approximation $y(t)$; (d) smoothed output, $X_r(j\omega)$.

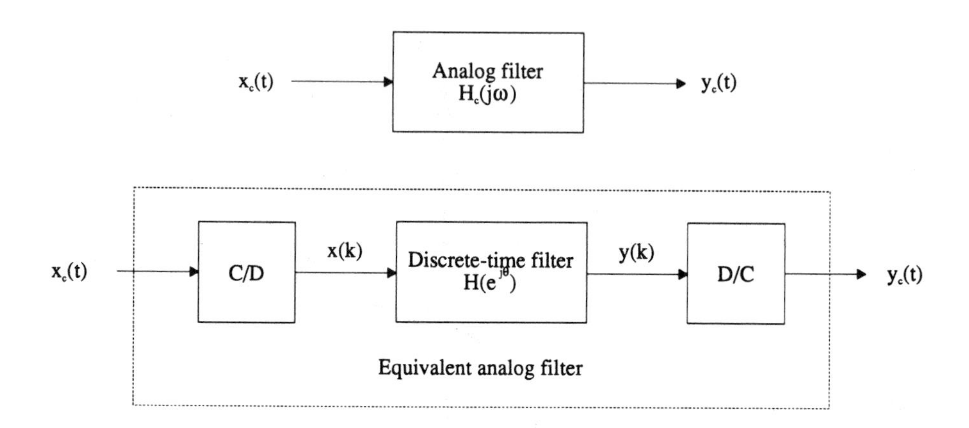

Figure 2.17.1: Equivalent analog filtering.

2.17 Equivalent Analog Filters

In the previous section, we derived a frequency-domain expression for a discrete-time signal which is a sampled version of a continuous-time signal. The problem we now wish to consider is that of deriving an *equivalent analog filter*. Specifically, consider the configuration shown in Fig. 2.17.1. The bandlimited continuous-time signal $x_c(t)$ is to be filtered by the analog filter, $h_c(t)$, resulting in the analog output $y_c(t)$. What we wish to do is replace the analog filter $h_c(t)$ with a C/D converter, a digital filter $H(e^{j\theta})$ and a D/C converter. The problem which must be solved is how to choose the digital filter $H(e^{j\theta})$ such that the output of the D/C converter is the same as would be obtained using the analog filter. In other words, we desire

$$y_r(t) = y_c(t).$$

The key to solving this problem is representing the various signals in the frequency domain. Assume that $x_c(t)$ is bandlimited to ω_N. The sampled input signal $x(k)$ is given by

$$x(k) = x_c(kT)$$

and we have shown that the DTFT of $x(k)$ is related to the spectrum $X_c(j\omega)$ by

$$X(e^{j\theta}) = \frac{1}{T}\sum_{k=-\infty}^{\infty} X_c\left(j(\frac{\theta}{T} - \frac{2\pi k}{T})\right).$$

If the digital filter has frequency response $H(e^{j\theta})$, the output, $y(k)$ of the digital filter has DTFT

$$Y(e^{j\theta}) = H(e^{j\theta})X(e^{j\theta}). \tag{2.17.1}$$

Next, we convert the signal $y(k)$ to the analog output $y_r(t)$ using the D/C converter. As usual, let the reconstruction filter be an ideal lowpass filter with cutoff frequency $\omega_c = \omega_s/2 = \pi/T$ and gain T. Recall from Eq. 2.16.10 that the Fourier transform of the reconstructed output is given by

$$Y_r(j\omega) = H_r(j\omega)Y(e^{j\omega T}).$$

Substituting Eq. 2.17.1 into the above produces

$$Y_r(j\omega) = H_r(j\omega)H(e^{j\omega T})X(e^{j\omega T}).$$

Remember that the effect of the reconstruction filter is to extract the base period of $X(e^{j\theta})$ and scale by T. Thus, because $x_c(t)$ was bandlimited to $\omega_s/2$, we have

$$H_r(j\omega)X(e^{j\omega T}) = X_r(j\omega)$$

and thus

$$Y_r(j\omega) = \begin{cases} H(e^{j\omega T})X_c(j\omega), & |\omega| < \omega_s/2 \\ 0, & |\omega| \geq \omega_s/2. \end{cases}$$

Therefore, if $x_c(t)$ is bandlimited to $\omega_s/2$, the effect of the digital filter combined with the C/D and D/C systems is to provide filtering over the range of frequencies from 0 to $\omega_s/2$. If we define the *equivalent analog filter*, $H_{eq}(j\omega)$ by

$$H_{eq}(j\omega) = \begin{cases} H(e^{j\omega T}), & |\omega| < \omega_s/2 \\ 0, & |\omega| \geq \omega_s/2 \end{cases},$$

we can then write

$$Y_r(j\omega) = H_{eq}(j\omega)X_c(j\omega).$$

The solution to our equivalent analog filtering problem is now trivial. The digital filter is chosen such that

$$H(e^{j\theta}) = H_c(j\theta/T). \tag{2.17.2}$$

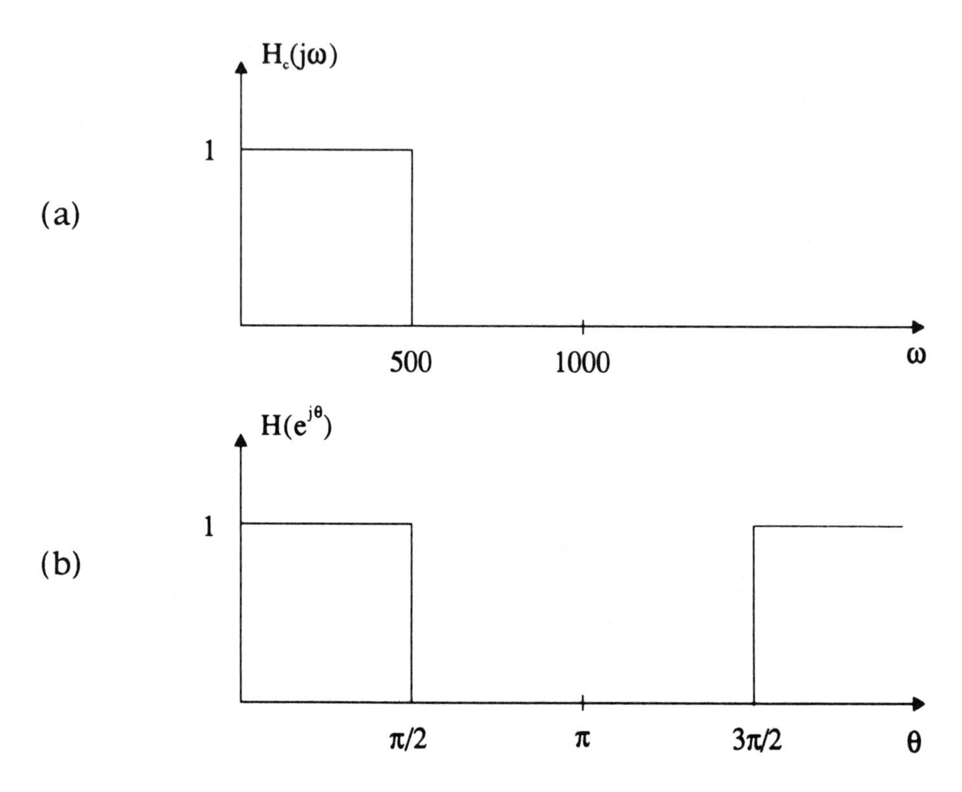

Figure 2.17.2: (a) Ideal analog lowpass filter; (b) digital filter frequency response.

Example 2.35

Let's use the equivalent analog filter method to design an ideal discrete-time lowpass filter. Assume we wish to bandlimit an analog signal with bandwidth $\omega_N = 1000$ to a bandwidth of $\omega_p = 500$. Let's take $\omega_s = 2\omega_N = 2000$ rad/s. All that remains to be specified is the digital filter $H(e^{j\theta})$. Equation 2.17.2 states that we must choose $H(e^{j\theta})$ according to

$$H(e^{j\theta}) = H_c(j\theta/T).$$

where $H_c(j\omega)$ is an ideal lowpass filter with a cutoff frequency of 500 rad/s. Thus, the digital filter $H(e^{j\theta})$ is simply a frequency-scaled version of the analog filter $H_c(j\omega)$. The cutoff frequency for the digital filter is thus given by the relation

$$\omega_1 = \frac{\theta_1}{T},$$

which gives

$$\theta_1 = \omega_1 T = \frac{2\pi\omega_1}{\omega_s}.$$

Therefore,

$$\theta_c = \frac{2\pi 500}{2000} = \frac{\pi}{2}.$$

With the digital filter thus specified, the combination of C/D, digital filter, and D/C will implement the ideal analog lowpass filter. The various spectra are shown in Fig. 2.17.2.

Chapter 3

THE DISCRETE FOURIER TRANSFORM

3.1 Introduction

So far, we have represented discrete-time signals and systems in terms of Fourier and $\mathcal{Z}$-transforms. These frameworks are quite suitable when the signals to be analyzed are finite-duration, and often lead to simple closed-form solutions. In practice, all signals will be finite-duration for one reason or another. In this case, there is a representation known as the *discrete Fourier transform* (DFT). Whereas the DTFT is a continuous function of frequency, the DFT is itself a sequence whose samples correspond to the DTFT of the finite-duration signal. Because there are highly efficient algorithms for computation of the DFT (the so-called *fast Fourier transform algorithms*), the DFT has become a critical tool for digital signal processing.

There is a very important connection between the DFT analysis of finite-duration signals and Fourier series representation of periodic discrete-time signals. For this reason, we will first discuss the discrete Fourier series.

3.2 Discrete Fourier Series

Periodic continuous-time signals are known to have a representation as an infinite sum of harmonically related sinusoids. Specifically, if $x(t)$ is periodic with period ω_0, we can write

$$x(t) = \sum_{k=-\infty}^{\infty} c_k e^{-jk\omega_0 t}. \tag{3.2.1}$$

This is known as a Fourier series representation, and the c_k are called the Fourier coefficients of $x(t)$. Because the functions $\{e^{-jk\omega_0 t}\}$ are complete and orthonormal over the range $[0, T_0]$, the c_k are computed by projection onto the basis functions $\{e^{-jk\omega_0 t}\}$ according to

$$c_k = \int_0^{T_0} x(t)e^{jk\omega_0 t}\,dt. \tag{3.2.2}$$

Equations 3.2.1 and 3.2.2 constitute synthesis and analysis equations, respectively, for periodic continuous-time signals.

If the continuous-time signal is not periodic, the appropriate Fourier representation is the Fourier transform, which represents the continuous-time signal as an integral over a continuum of frequencies from $-\infty$ to ∞. Similarly, the appropriate Fourier representation for aperiodic discrete-time signals is the DTFT, which represents the sequence as an integral over a continuum of frequencies, this time from $-\pi$ to π. In analogy, we should expect that periodic *discrete-time* signals should have a Fourier representation which consists of a linear combination of complex exponentials. Indeed, this is the case.

Assume that $x_p(k)$ is periodic with period N, which means that $x_p(k) = x_p(k+lN)$ for all integers l. We will show that $x_p(k)$ has a representation of the form

$$x_p(k) = \frac{1}{N}\sum_n X_p(n)e^{j2\pi kn/N}. \tag{3.2.3}$$

This is a decomposition into a linear combination of complex exponentials, where the $X_p(n)$, are known as the *discrete Fourier series* (DFS) coefficients for $x_p(k)$. With regard to the range of summation in Eq. 3.2.3, notice that

$$e^{j2\pi(n+lN)k/N} = e^{j2\pi n/N}$$

so that complex exponentials with frequencies differing by a multiple of 2π are indistinguishable. For this reason, we can rewrite Eq. 3.2.3 as

$$x_p(k) = \frac{1}{N}\sum_{n=0}^{N-1} X_p(n)e^{j2\pi kn/N}. \tag{3.2.4}$$

Equation 3.2.4 is the DFS synthesis equation for $x_p(k)$. we now need is a formula for computing the DFS coefficients, $X_p(n)$.

The first step in deriving the formula for the DFS coefficients is showing that the functions $\{e^{j2\pi kn/N}\}$ are orthogonal over a period. Consider first the summation

$$\sum_{n=0}^{N-1} z_1^n z_2^{-n} = \frac{1-z_1^N z_2^{-N}}{1-z_1 z_2^{-1}}. \tag{3.2.5}$$

Let $z_1 = e^{j2\pi p/N}$ and $z_2 = e^{j2\pi q/N}$. Then

$$z_1^N = z_2^N = 1$$

and the summation can be rewritten as

$$\sum_{n=0}^{N-1} e^{j2\pi(p-q)n/N} = 0$$

unless the denominator vanishes as well. The denominator vanishes when

$$e^{j2\pi(p-q)/N} = 1,$$

which means that $p - q = mN$. In this case, Eq. 3.2.5 sums to N. Therefore,

$$\sum_{n=0}^{N-1} e^{j2\pi(p-q)n/N} = \begin{cases} 1, & p-q = mN \\ 0, & \text{otherwise} \end{cases} \tag{3.2.6}$$

and we have shown that the complex exponentials are orthogonal over a period. Now, multiply both sides of Eq. 3.2.3 by $e^{-j2\pi kr/N}$ and sum over k for one period, giving

$$\sum_{k=0}^{N-1} x_p(k)e^{-j2\pi kr/N} = \sum_{k=0}^{N-1} \frac{1}{N} X_p(n) \sum_{n=0}^{N-1} e^{j2\pi(n-r)k/N}.$$

Reversing the order of summation, we have

$$\sum_{k=0}^{N-1} x_p(k)e^{-j2\pi kr/N} = \sum_{n=0}^{N-1} X_p(n) \left(\frac{1}{N} \sum_{k=0}^{N-1} e^{j2\pi(n-r)k/N} \right).$$

According to Eq. 3.2.6, the term inside the parentheses is equal to $\delta(n-r)$ over the range of summation so that

$$\sum_{k=0}^{N-1} x_p(k)e^{-j2\pi kr/N} = \sum_{n=0}^{N-1} X_p(n)\delta(n-r) = X_p(r).$$

This is the formula we were looking for. It is common practice to denote the quantity $e^{-j2\pi/N}$ by the symbol W_N. The DFS is thus defined by the *analysis* equation:

$$X_p(n) = \sum_{k=0}^{N-1} x_p(k) W_N^{-nk} \tag{3.2.7}$$

and the *synthesis* equation:

$$x_p(k) = \frac{1}{N} \sum_{n=0}^{N-1} X_p(n) W_N^{kn}. \tag{3.2.8}$$

Let's stop and assess what we have developed thusfar. Equation 3.2.8 indicates that a periodic discrete-time signal $x_p(k)$ with period N can be represented as a weighted sum of N complex exponentials where the weights of the exponential modes are given by the DFS coefficients. That is,

$$x_p(k) = \frac{1}{N}\left(X_p(0)(W_N^0)^k + X_p(1)(W_N^1)^k + X_p(2)(W_N^2)^k + \cdots + X_p(N-1)(W_N^{N-1})^k\right)$$

where each term $(W_N^n)^k$ is a complex exponential of the form

$$(W_N^n)^k = (e^{j2\pi n/N})^k.$$

The DFS coefficients are determined by a simple inner product, given by Eq. 3.2.7. Because of the periodicity of the sequences $(W_N^{-n})^k$ in Eq. 3.2.7, the DFS coefficients $X_p(n)$ are also periodic with period N. Only one period of the DFS coefficients is needed for the synthesis of $x_p(k)$, however.

We can now make an important connection between the DFS of a periodic sequence and the DTFT of a finite duration sequence. Let $x_p(k)$ be periodic with period N and define the sequence $x(k)$ by

$$x(k) = \begin{cases} x_p(k), & k = 0, 1, \ldots N-1 \\ 0, & \text{otherwise.} \end{cases} \tag{3.2.9}$$

That is, $x(k)$ is a finite-duration sequence which is formed by extracting a single period of $x_p(k)$. The DTFT of $x(k)$ is given by

$$X(e^{j\theta}) = \sum_{k=0}^{N-1} x(k)e^{-jk\theta},$$

which, because of Eq. 3.2.9, can also be written as

$$X(e^{j\theta}) = \sum_{k=0}^{N-1} x_p(k)e^{-jk\theta}.$$

Comparing the above with Eq. 3.2.7, it can be seen that

$$X_p(n) = X(e^{j\theta})\Big|_{\theta=2\pi n/N} = X(W_N^n).$$

In other words, the N DFS coefficients of the periodic sequence $x_p(k)$ match the DTFT of the finite-duration sequence $x(k)$ at the N discrete frequencies

$$\theta_n = \frac{2\pi n}{N}, \quad n = 0, 1, \ldots, N-1.$$

The angular spacing between the discrete frequencies θ_n is known as the *frequency resolution* and is equal to $2\pi/N$.

Conversely, this important connection can be used to obtain the "outline" or "envelope" of the spectrum of a finite-duration sequence, $x(k)$. Given a finite-duration sequence $x(k)$ of length N, we can form the periodic sequence $x_p(k)$ by

$$x_p(k) = \sum_{r=-\infty}^{\infty} x(k - rN). \tag{3.2.10}$$

This is known as *periodic extension* and simply consists of adding time-shifted non-overlapping replicas of $x(k)$. The sequences $x_p(k)$ and $x(k)$ now satisfy Eq. 3.2.9 so that the N DFS coefficients $X_p(n)$ match the DTFT of $x(k)$ at the N frequencies $2\pi n/N$, $n = 0, 1, \ldots, N-1$.

Example 3.1

Let $x(k)$ be the seven-point finite-duration sequence

$$x(k) = \begin{cases} 1, & 0 \leq k \leq 6 \\ 0, & \text{otherwise.} \end{cases}$$

The magnitude spectrum $|X(e^{j\theta})|$ is shown in Fig. 3.2.1. The periodic extension $x_p(k)$ with period $N = 7$ is simply equal to one everywhere. The DFS coefficients are computed according to

$$X_p(n) = \sum_{k=0}^{6} x(k) W_7^{nk} = \sum_{k=0}^{6} W_7^{nk}.$$

For $n = 0$, we have

$$X_p(0) = \sum_{k=0}^{6} W_7^{0k} = 7.$$

For $n \neq 0$, we use the formula for summation of a geometric series, giving

$$X_p(n) = \frac{1 - W_7^{7n}}{1 - W_7^n}.$$

Because $(W_7^7)^n = 1$ for all $n \neq 0$, we have

$$X_p(n) = 0.$$

Thus,

$$X_p(n) = \begin{cases} 1, & n = 0 \\ 0, & n = 1, 2, \ldots, 6 \end{cases}$$

Notice that the DFS coefficients agree with $X(e^{j\theta})$ at the N frequencies $2\pi n/7$. This is shown in Fig. 3.2.1.

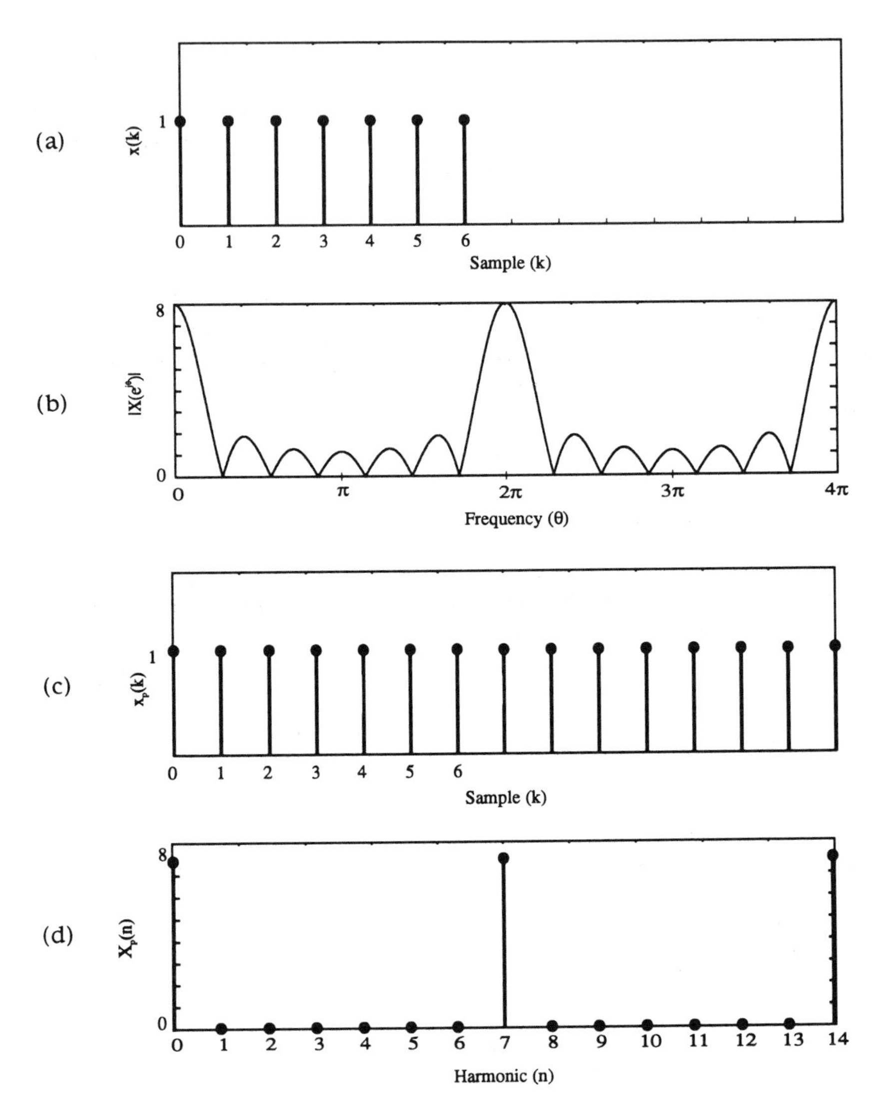

Figure 3.2.1: (a) Finite-duration sequence $x(k)$; (b) magnitude of $X(e^{j\theta})$; (c) periodically extended sequence $x_p(k)$; (d) magnitudes of DFS coefficients $X_p(n)$.

The problem with the above example is that the "snapshots" of the DTFT given by the N DFS coefficients do not give a very useful picture of the true spectrum. Namely, all but the zeroth DFS coefficient correspond to frequencies where the spectrum has nulls. There is a solution to this problem, however. Given a finite-duration sequence $x(k)$ of length N, we can "zero-pad" $x(k)$ to create a new sequence $\hat{x}(k)$ where

$$\hat{x}(k) = \begin{cases} x(k), & k = 0, 1, \ldots, N-1 \\ 0, & k = N, N+1, \ldots, M-1 \end{cases}$$

The new sequence $\hat{x}(k)$ is finite-duration of length M where M can be chosen arbitrarily. It is important to recognize that

$$\hat{X}(e^{j\theta}) = X(e^{j\theta}).$$

Now, we form the periodic sequence $\hat{x}_p(k)$ by periodically extending $\hat{x}(k)$ which gives a sequence with period M, where $M > N$. The DFS coefficients of $\hat{x}_p(k)$ are given by

$$\hat{X}_p(n) = \sum_{k=0}^{M-1} \hat{x}_p(k) W_M^{nk} = \sum_{k=0}^{M-1} \hat{x}(k) W_M^{nk}.$$

As before, the M DFS coefficients $\hat{X}_p(n)$ agree with the spectrum $\hat{X}(e^{j\theta})$ at the M frequencies $2\pi n/M$ which have angular spacing $2\pi/M$. But $\hat{X}(e^{j\theta}) = X(e^{j\theta})$ so that we now have M samples of the spectrum $X(e^{j\theta})$. The only additional expense is in computing the additional $M - N$ DFS coefficients.

Example 3.2

Again, let $x(k)$ be given by

$$x(k) = \begin{cases} 1, & 0 \le k \le 6 \\ 0, & \text{otherwise.} \end{cases}$$

This time, we will zero-pad the sequence to length 28, giving $\hat{x}(k)$, shown in Fig. 3.2.2. The periodic extension $\hat{x}_p$ is also shown in Fig. 3.2.2. The 28 DFS coefficients $\hat{X}_p(n)$ corresponding to the 28 discrete frequencies $2\pi n/28$, $n = 0, 1, \ldots, 27$ are computed according to

$$\hat{X}_p(n) = \sum_{k=0}^{27} \hat{x}_p(k) W_{28}^{nk} = \sum_{k=0}^{6} W_{28}^{nk}.$$

The magnitudes of the DFS coefficients are shown in Fig. 3.2.2. Notice that the frequency resolution has been enhanced over the previous example from $2\pi/7$ to $2\pi/28$. What results is a better picture of the true spectrum $X(e^{j\theta})$.

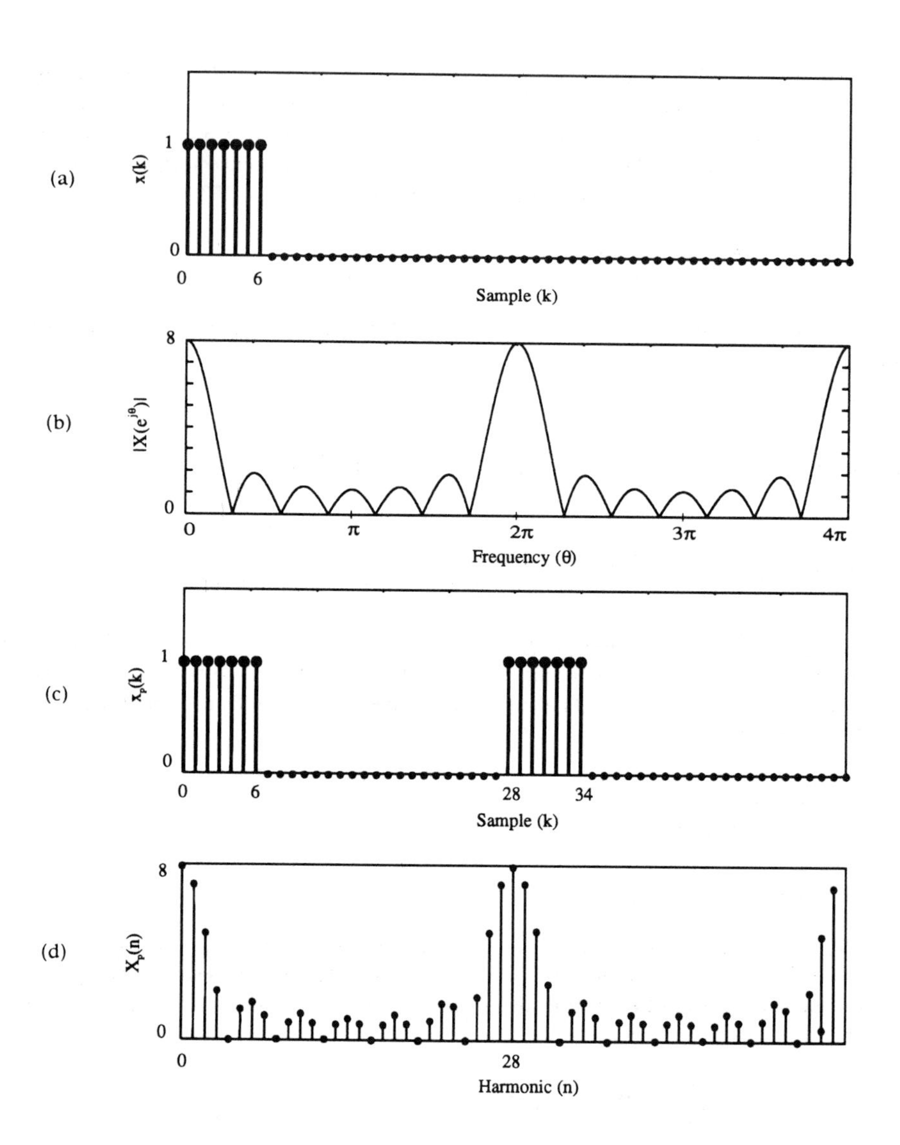

Figure 3.2.2: (a) Finite-duration sequence $x(k)$; (b) magnitude of $X(e^{j\theta})$; (c) periodically extended zero-padded sequence; (d) magnitude of DFS coefficients.

Properties of the DFS

Just as with the DTFT and the $\mathcal{Z}$-transform, there are a number of useful properties of the DFS. Unless otherwise noted, it will be assumed that all sequences are periodic with period N.

- **Linearity**

If $x_p(k)$ and $y_p(k)$ are both periodic with period N and have DFS coefficients $X_p(n)$ and $Y_p(n)$, respectively, then

$$ax_p(k) + by_p(k) \stackrel{DFS}{\longleftrightarrow} aX_p(n) + bY_p(n).$$

This is easily shown from the definition.

- **Time-Shift**

Suppose $x_p(k)$ has DFS coefficients $X_p(n)$ and we wish to find the DFS coefficients of the time-shifted sequence $x_p(k-m)$. From the definition,

$$x_p(k-m) \stackrel{DFS}{\longleftrightarrow} \sum_{k=0}^{N-1} x_p(k-m)W_N^{nk}.$$

If we make the substitution $r = k - m$, we have

$$\sum_{k=0}^{N-1} x_p(k-m)W_N^{nk} = W_N^{nm} \sum_{r=-m}^{N-m-1} x_p(r)W_N^{nr}. \tag{3.2.11}$$

The summation on the right can be broken into two parts, giving

$$\sum_{r=-m}^{N-m-1} x_p(r)W_N^{nr} = \sum_{r=-m}^{-1} x_p(r)W_N^{nr} + \sum_{r=0}^{N-m-1} x_p(r)W_N^{nr}.$$

Because of the periodicity of $x_p(r)$ and W_N^{nr}, we can add N to r above, which gives

$$\sum_{r=-m}^{N-m-1} x_p(r)W_N^{nr} = \sum_{r=N-m}^{N-1} x_p(r)W_N^{nr} + \sum_{r=0}^{N-m-1} x_p(r)W_N^{nr},$$

so that

$$\sum_{r=-m}^{N-m-1} x_p(r)W_N^{nr} = \sum_{r=0}^{N-1} x_p(r)W_N^{nr} = X_p(n).$$

Substituting the above into Eq. 3.2.11, we have the DFS pair

$$x_p(k-m) \stackrel{DFS}{\longleftrightarrow} W_N^{nm} X_p(n). \tag{3.2.12}$$

Equation 3.2.12 expresses the DFS time-shift property and indicates that the DFS coefficients of the time-shifted sequence are given by modulating the DFS coefficients of the unshifted sequence by the complex exponential W_N^{nm}.

• Modulation

Let $x_p(k)$ have DFS coefficients $X_p(n)$. Then

$$W_N^{-nm} x_p(k) \stackrel{DFS}{\longleftrightarrow} X_p(n-m).$$

Notice the duality between this property and the time-shift property in Eq. 3.2.12. Because $X_p(n)$ is periodic with period N, the value of $X_p(n)$ for an index outside the range $0 \le n \le N-1$ corresponds to the value of $X_p(n)$ for an index *in* the range $0 \le n \le N-1$ which is given by the least positive remainder when divided by N. In other words, if $N = 7$, the $X_p(8) = X_p(1)$. Similarly, $X_p(15) = X_p(1)$. The situation for negative indices is similar. For example, $X_p(-3) = X_p(4)$ because

$$-3 = 7 \cdot (-1) + 4.$$

Formally, we say that these indices are *congruent modulo N*.

•Periodic Convolution

We have already seen how to perform the convolution of two aperiodic sequences. This will henceforth be referred to as *linear convolution.* For periodic sequences $x_p(k), y_p(k)$, we define the *periodic convolution* $z_p(k)$ of $x_p(k)$ and $y_p(k)$ by

$$z_p(k) = \sum_{m=0}^{N-1} x_p(m) y_p(k-m). \tag{3.2.13}$$

which is also equivalent to

$$z_p(k) = \sum_{m=0}^{N-1} x_p(k-m) y_p(m).$$

Notice that this is nearly identical to linear convolution except that the sum runs over only one period. To obtain the DFS coefficients of $z_p(k)$, we apply the definition of DFS to Eq. 3.3.6 which gives

$$Z_p(n) = \sum_{k=0}^{N-1} W_N^{nk} \left(\sum_{m=0}^{N-1} x_p(m) y_p(k-m) \right)$$

Interchanging the order of summation,

$$Z_p(n) = \sum_{m=0}^{N-1} x_p(m) \left(\sum_{k=0}^{N-1} y_p(k-m) W_N^{nk} \right).$$

The inner summation is simply the DFS of $y_p(k-m)$, which we know has DFS coefficients $W_N^{nm} Y_p(n)$. Thus,

$$Z_p(n) = Y_p(n) \sum_{m=0}^{N-1} x_p(m) W_N^{mn} = X_p(n) Y_p(n).$$

Thus,

$$\sum_{m=0}^{N-1} x_p(m) y_p(k-m) \overset{DFS}{\longleftrightarrow} X_p(n) Y_p(n). \tag{3.2.14}$$

Equation 3.2.14 states that the DFS coefficients of the periodic convolution of two sequences are given by the products of the DFS coefficients of the two sequences.

Let's look at how periodic convolution is performed. We start with two periodic sequences $x_p(k)$ and $y_p(k)$ and then re-index with the new index m to form $x_p(m)$ and $y_p(m)$. Next, the sequence $y_p(m)$ is flipped about the point $m = 0$ to give $y_p(-m)$. Then $y_p(-m)$ is dragged to the right by k, giving $y_p(k-m)$. Finally, the sequences $x_p(m)$ and $y_p(k-m)$ are multiplied "pointwise" over the range $0 \leq m \leq N-1$ and summed to give $z_p(k)$. This is illustrated in Fig. 3.2.3. Notice that as $y_p(-m)$ is slid to the right, the values of $y_p(k-m)$ which move to the right past the point $m = N-1$ come in from the left of the point $m = 0$. This is because of the periodicity of the sequences $x_p(k)$ and $y_p(k)$. This property makes $z_p(k)$ periodic with period N, as well.

•Multiplication of Sequences

From the DTFT, the DTFT of the product of two sequences was given by the periodic frequency-domain convolution of the DTFTs of the two sequences. We should anticipate a similar relationship for the DFS. Indeed, there is such a property for the DFS, and it is extremely similar in form to the DFS convolution property expressed in Eq. 3.2.14. If $x_p(k)$ and $y_p(k)$ have DFS coefficients $X_p(n)$ and $Y_p(n)$, respectively, then

$$x_p(k) y_p(k) \overset{DFS}{\longleftrightarrow} \frac{1}{N} \sum_{m=0}^{N-1} X_p(m) Y_p(n-m). \tag{3.2.15}$$

In other words, the DFS coefficients of the product sequence are given by the periodic convolution of the DFS coefficients of the individual sequences (with the additional $1/N$ factor). Again, note the structural similarity to the DFS convolution property.

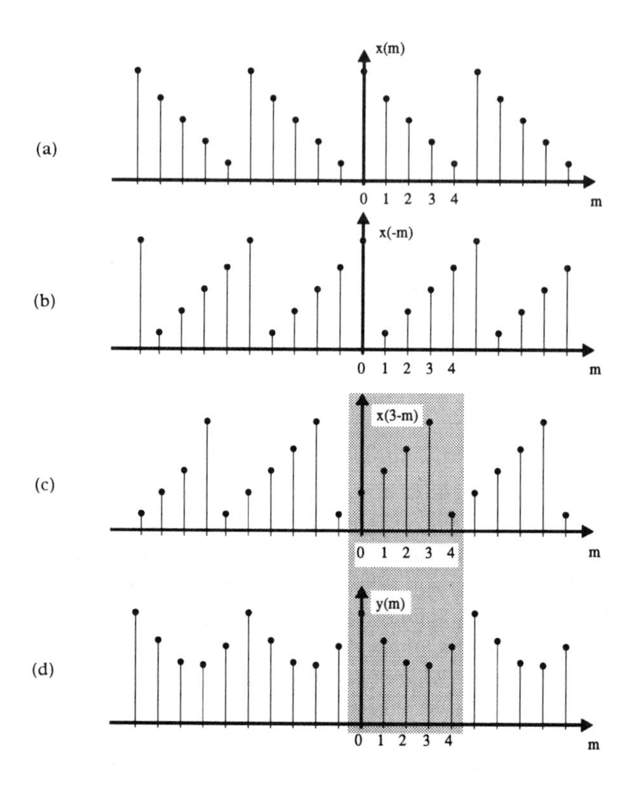

Figure 3.2.3: Illustration of periodic convolution: (a) $x(m)$; (b) $x(-m)$; (c) $x(k-m)$ for $k=3$; (d) $y(m)$ (region of overlap with $x(k-m)$ is shown in shaded area).

• Miscellaneous Symmetry Properties

Suppose $x_p(k)$ has DFS coefficients $X_p(n)$. The DFS coefficients of the conjugate sequence, $x_p^*(k)$, are found by

$$x_p^*(k) \stackrel{DFS}{\longleftrightarrow} \sum_{k=0}^{N-1} x_p^*(k) W_N^{nk}.$$

Next, by definition,

$$(W_N^{nk})^* = W_N^{-nk}$$

so that

$$\sum_{k=0}^{N-1} x_p^*(k) W_N^{nk} = \left(\sum_{k=0}^{N-1} x_p(k) W_N^{-nk} \right)^*.$$

The summation on the right is simply $X_p(-n)$ which means that

$$x_p^*(k) \stackrel{DFS}{\longleftrightarrow} X_p^*(-n). \tag{3.2.16}$$

This time, consider the time-reversed, conjugated sequence $x_p^*(-k)$. In a manner similar to the above, we can show that

$$x_p^*(-k) \stackrel{DFS}{\longleftrightarrow} X_p^*(n). \tag{3.2.17}$$

Equations 3.2.16 and 3.2.17 can be used to derive a number of other useful properties of the DFS. For instance, consider the *even* part of a sequence $x_p(k)$, given by

$$x_p^{(e)}(k) = \frac{1}{2}(x_p(k) + x_p^*(-k)).$$

Using Eq. 3.2.17, we have

$$x_p^{(e)}(k) \stackrel{DFS}{\longleftrightarrow} \frac{1}{2}(X_p(n) + X_p^*(n))$$

so that

$$x_p^{(e)}(k) \stackrel{DFS}{\longleftrightarrow} \mathrm{Re}(X_p(n)). \tag{3.2.18}$$

Similarly, the *odd* part of $x_p(k)$ is defined by

$$x_p^{(o)}(k) = \frac{1}{2}(x_p(k) - x_p(-k)),$$

and again using Eq. 3.2.17, we have

$$x_p^{(e)}(k) \stackrel{DFS}{\longleftrightarrow} \frac{1}{2}(X_p(n) - X_p^*(n))$$

so that

$$x_p^{(o)}(k) \stackrel{DFS}{\longleftrightarrow} j\mathrm{Im}(X_p(n)). \tag{3.2.19}$$

Next, we consider the real and imaginary parts of a sequence $x_p(k)$. Because

$$\mathrm{Re}(x_p(k)) = \frac{1}{2}(x_p(k) + x_p^*(k)),$$

we use Eq. 3.2.16 to give

$$\mathrm{Re}(x_p(k)) \stackrel{DFS}{\longleftrightarrow} \frac{1}{2}(X_p(n) + X_p^*(-n)),$$

which, by definition, is the even part of $X_p(n)$. Thus,

$$\mathrm{Re}(x_p(k)) \stackrel{DFS}{\longleftrightarrow} X_p^{(e)}(n) \tag{3.2.20}$$

Finally, the imaginary part of $x_p(k)$ has DFS coefficients given by

$$\mathrm{Im}(x_p(k)) \stackrel{DFS}{\longleftrightarrow} X_p^{(o)}(n). \tag{3.2.21}$$

We have summarized some of the important DFS properties in Table 3.1.

Sequence	*DFS Coefficients*
$x_p(k)$	$X_p(n)$
$ax_p(k) + by_p(k)$	$aX_p(n) + bY_p(n)$
$x_p(k-m)$	$W_N^{nm} X_p(n)$
$W_N^{-mk} x_p(k)$	$X_p(n-m)$
$\sum_{m=0}^{N-1} x_p(m) y_p(k-m)$	$X_p(n) Y_p(n)$
$x_p(k) y_p(k)$	$\frac{1}{N} \sum_{m=0}^{N-1} X_p(m) Y_p(n-m)$
$x_p^*(k)$	$X_p^*(-n)$
$x_p^*(-k)$	$X_p^*(n)$
$x_p^{(e)}(k)$	$\mathrm{Re}(X_p(n))$
$x_p^{(o)}(k)$	$\mathrm{Im}(X_p(n))$
$\mathrm{Re}(x_p(k))$	$X_p^{(e)}(n)$
$\mathrm{Im}(x_p(k))$	$X_p^{(o)}(n)$

Table 3.1: Important DFS properties

3.3 The Discrete Fourier Transform

In the previous section we showed how to compute the discrete Fourier series (DFS) coefficients for a periodic sequence $x_p(k)$ as well as some important properties of the DFS. More importantly, we saw that the DFS could be used to obtain samples of the DTFT of a finite-duration sequence. This was done by first periodically extending the finite duration sequence and then computing the DFS. The DFS coefficients of the periodically extended sequence then correspond to samples of the finite duration sequence.

The discrete Fourier transform (DFT) is easily understood using the ideas we developed when discussing the DFS. Whereas the DFS takes an infinite-duration periodic sequence and produces a set of DFS coefficients, the DFT is applied directly to finite-duration sequences. To be precise, let $x(k)$ be a finite duration sequence which is nonzero only over the range $0 \leq k \leq N-1$. The DFT of $x(k)$ is also a sequence of length N which is given by the *DFT analysis equation*

$$X(n) = \sum_{k=0}^{N-1} x(k) W_N^{nk}, \quad n = 0, 1, \ldots, N-1. \tag{3.3.1}$$

The DTFT of $x(k)$ is given by

$$X(e^{j\theta}) = \sum_{k=0}^{N-1} x(k) e^{-jk\theta},$$

and comparing the above with Eq. 3.3.1, it immediately follows that

$$X(n) = X(e^{j\theta})\Big|_{\theta=2\pi n/N} = X(W_N^n).$$

Thus, the DFT produces N samples of the DTFT of $x(k)$ spaced equally around the unit circle with angular separation $2\pi/N$. Notice the similarity with the DFS. The difference is that the sequence $x(k)$ is finite-duration as is the DFT $X(n)$.

Because the DFT values $X(n)$ are samples of the DTFT $X(e^{j\theta})$, the magnitude and phase of $X(n)$ will certainly agree with the magnitude and phase of $X(e^{j\theta})$ at the N frequencies $2\pi n/N$. To be precise, $X(n)$ will in general be complex and can be written as

$$X(n) = X_R(n) + jX_I(n)$$

and

$$|X(e^{j2\pi n/N})| = |X(n)| = \sqrt{X_R^2(n) + X_I^2(n)}$$

and

$$\angle X(e^{j2\pi n/N}) = \angle X(n) = tan^{-1}\left(\frac{X_I(n)}{X_R(n)}\right).$$

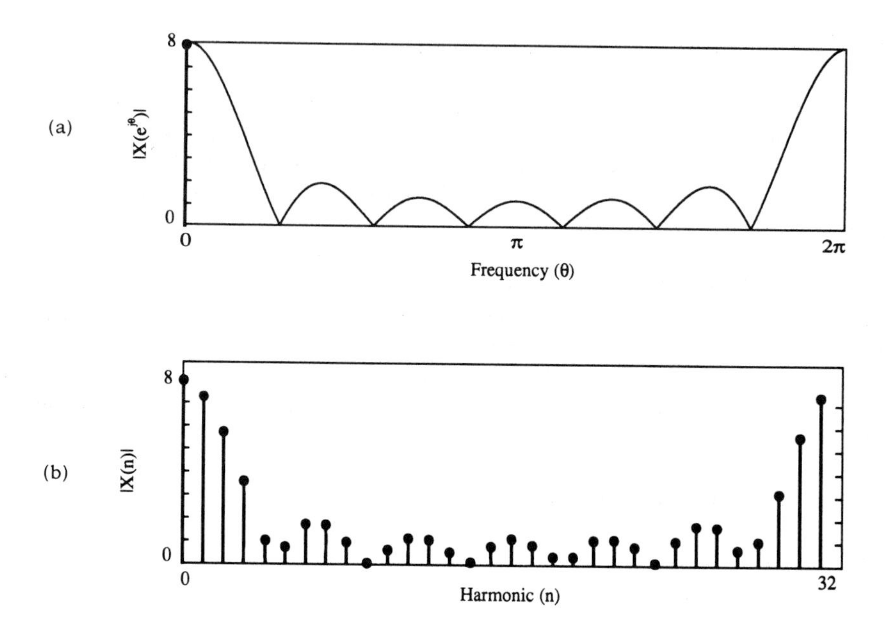

Figure 3.3.1: (a) Magnitude of $X(e^{j\theta})$; (b) magnitude of DFT.

As with the DFS, we can obtain enhanced frequency resolution by zero-padding the length N sequence $x(k)$ to length M where $M > N$. This will give M samples of $X(e^{j\theta})$ which are spaced in frequency by $2\pi/M$, which is smaller than $2\pi/N$.

Example 3.3

Let $x(k)$ be given by

$$\{x(k)\} = \{1, 1, 1, 1, 1, 1, 1, 1\}.$$

The magnitude of the DTFT $X(e^{j\theta})$ is shown in Fig. 3.3.1. The sequence $x(k)$ is zero-padded to length 32 and the DFT computed. The resulting magnitude of the 32 DFT points are also shown in Fig. 3.3.1. Notice that the DFT points match exactly the DTFT at the frequencies $2\pi n/32$, $n = 0, 1, \ldots, 31$.

The DFT will provide a collection of *exact* samples of the DTFT of a finite-duration signal. What can we do to analyze the DTFT of an infinite-duration signal using the DFT? The only solution is to truncate the signal to a finite length using a window in the time domain. In the frequency domain, we have seen that this has the effect of blurring the true spectrum by convolving the true DTFT with the DTFT of the window. Thus, the DFT of the truncated signal corresponds to samples of the blurred spectrum. The effects of this blurring can, of course, be controlled by the choice of window, which will be discussed in a later chapter. What we can do, however, is increase the window length. For now, we assume a rectangular which corresponds to simple truncation in the time domain.

Example 3.4

Let $x(k)$ be given by

$$x(k) = (0.95)^k u(k),$$

which has DTFT given by

$$X(e^{j\theta}) = \frac{1}{1 - 0.95e^{-j\theta}},$$

shown in Fig. 3.3.2a. Suppose we truncate $x(k)$ to length 32 and compute the DFT. The magnitude of the DFT is shown in Fig. 3.3.2b. Notice that the DFT does not have precisely the envelope of the DTFT because of the effect of truncation. Instead, the DFT has the envelope of the rectangular-windowed spectrum. If the window length is increased to 128, the DFT in Fig. 3.3.2c results. Notice that this gives a more accurate picture of the unwindowed spectrum.

A logical question is how original sequence $x(k)$ can be recovered from the DFT $X(n)$. A little thought will produce the answer. If the sequence $x(k)$ is periodically extended to the sequence $x_p(k)$ as in Eq. 3.2.10, the DFS coefficients $X_p(n)$ over a single period are precisely the DFT values $X(n)$, namely

$$X(n) = X_p(n), \quad 0 \leq n \leq N-1. \tag{3.3.2}$$

Furthermore, $x_p(k)$ can be recovered from $X_p(n)$ by

$$x_p(k) = \frac{1}{N} \sum_{n=0}^{N-1} X_p(n) W_N^{-nk}.$$

This relationship is valid for all k. Because of Eq. 3.3.2, we have

$$x_p(k) = \frac{1}{N} \sum_{n=0}^{N-1} X(n) W_N^{-nk}.$$

Finally, *by construction* $x_p(k)$ and $x(k)$ satisfy

$$x(k) = x_p(k), \quad 0 \leq k \leq N-1$$

so that

$$x(k) = \frac{1}{N} \sum_{n=0}^{N-1} X(n) W_N^{-nk}, \quad k = 0, 1, \ldots, N-1. \tag{3.3.3}$$

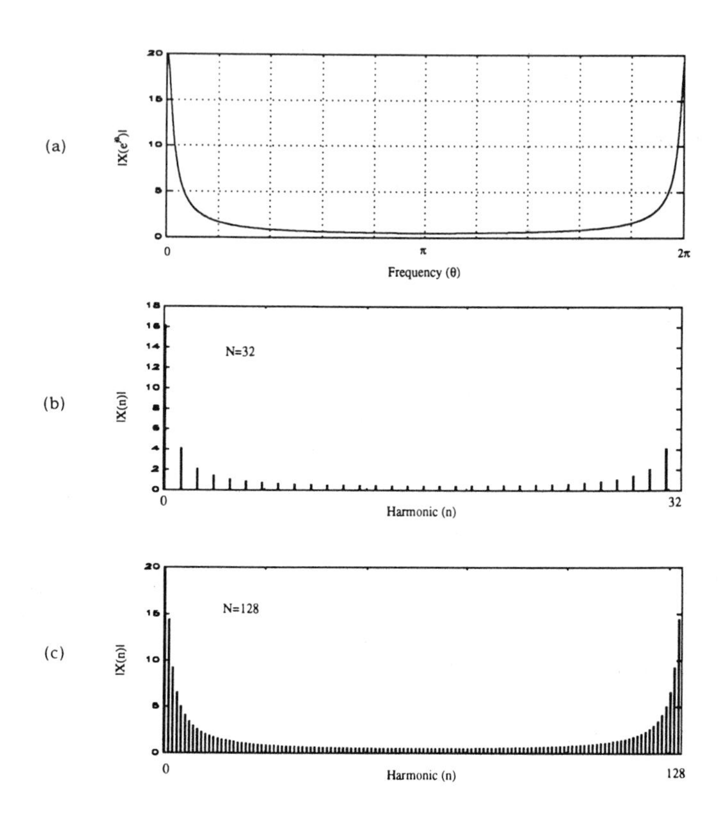

Figure 3.3.2: (a) DTFT of unwindowed infinite-duration signal; (b) DFT of 32-point rectangularly windowed signal; (c) DFT of 128-point rectangularly windowed signal.

Equation 3.3.3 is the inversion formula for the DFT, also referred to as the *DFT synthesis equation.*

In summary, given the finite-duration sequence $x(k)$ of length N, we have

$$X(n) = \sum_{k=0}^{N-1} x(k) W_N^{nk}, n = 0, 1, \ldots, N-1 \tag{3.3.4}$$

which is the equation for the DFT, and

$$x(k) = \frac{1}{N} \sum_{n=0}^{N-1} X(n) W_N^{-nk}, \quad k = 0, 1, \ldots, N-1, \tag{3.3.5}$$

which is the equation for the *inverse* discrete Fourier transform (IDFT).

3.3.1 DFT Properties

The DFT has a collection of properties which are nearly identical to those of the DFS with the understanding that we are now working with finite-duration sequences. In our discussion of the DFS, we alluded to the notion of indices being equivalent relative to the integer N. This was because of the N-periodicity of the sequences $x_p(k)$ and $X_p(n)$. The DFS properties are easily extended to the DFT if we realize that $x(k)$ and $X(n)$ are now ***finite-duration*** of length N. Thus, any reference to k or n outside the range $0 \le k, n \le N-1$ must be interpreted appropriately. The appropriate interpretation is to regard the indices ***modulo N***. This means that an index is to be interpreted as the *least positive remainder when divided by N*.

For example, consider the sequence $x(k)$ when $N = 5$ given by

$$\{x(0), x(1), x(2), x(3), x(4)\}.$$

Suppose we are interested in the sequence $x(k-1)$. For $k = 0$, we run into trouble since there is no $x(-1)$. Rather, we are interested in $x(k - 1 \bmod 5)$. Because

$$-1 \bmod 5 = 4,$$

the sequence $x(k-1)$ is given by

$$\{x(4), x(0), x(1), x(2), x(3)\}$$

which is seen to be a right-circular shift of $x(k)$ with the rightmost value, $x(4)$, shifted out from the right and in from the left. Similarly, $x(k + 1 \bmod 5)$ is the sequence

$$\{x(1), x(2), x(3), x(4), x(0)\}$$

which is a left-circular shift with the leftmost value, $x(0)$, shifted out from the left and in from the right.

This circular shifting is easily understood in the context of periodic signals. If $x(m)$ is finite-duration of length N, we can form the periodic extension, $x_p(m)$ according to Eq. 3.2.10. Then $x(k - m \bmod N)$ is given by first forming the *linear shift* $x_p(k-m)$ and then retaining only those values of $x_p(k-m)$ which lie in the range $0 \le k \le N$. This is illustrated in Fig. 3.3.3.

With the above caveat in mind, here is a listing of DFT properties, the proofs of which are easily obtainable from the corresponding DFS proofs. It will be assumed that unless otherwise noted, all sequences are finite-duration of length N.

- **Linearity**

If $x(k)$ and $y(k)$ are both finite duration with DFTs $X(n)$ and $Y(n)$, respectively, then

$$ax(k) + by(k) \overset{DFT}{\longleftrightarrow} aX(n) + bY(n).$$

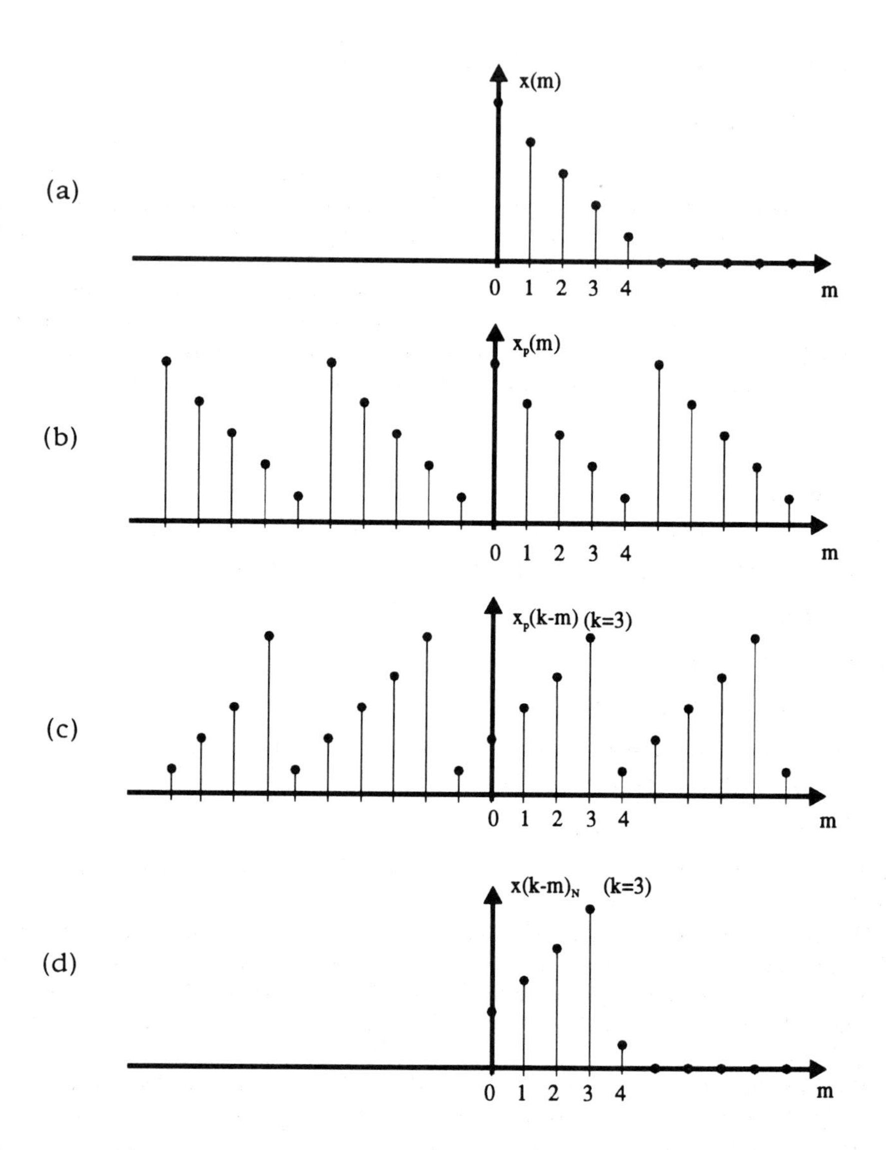

Figure 3.3.3: Visualizing cyclic shifts: (a) Finite-duration $x(m)$; (b) periodic extension, $x_p(m)$; (c) linear shift $x_p(k-m)$; (d) cyclically shifted finite-duration signal, $x(k-m \text{ mod } N)$.

This assumes that the sequences are of the same length. If not, the sequence of shorter duration must be zero-padded to the length of the longer sequence.

• Time-Shift

Suppose $x(k)$ has DFT $X(n)$ and we wish to find the DFT of the cyclically-shifted sequence $x(k-m \bmod N)$. Then

$$x(k-m \bmod N) \stackrel{DFT}{\longleftrightarrow} W_N^{nm} X(n).$$

There is no need to account for the modulo N correction in the sequence W_N^{nm} because it is periodic with period N.

• Modulation

Let $x(k)$ have DFT $X(n)$. Then

$$W_N^{-nm} x(k) \stackrel{DFT}{\longleftrightarrow} X(n-m \bmod N).$$

Again, there is no need to correct the indices of the complex exponential W_N^{-nk}.

• Cyclic Convolution

For periodic sequences $x_p(k), y_p(k)$, we saw how to perform *periodic convolution.* For *finite duration* sequences, we have an operation which is nearly identical and is known as *cyclic convolution.* We define the cyclic convolution $z(k)$ of $x(k)$ and $y(k)$ by

$$z(k) = \sum_{m=0}^{N-1} x(m) y(k-m \bmod N). \tag{3.3.6}$$

Cyclic convolution will be denoted by the symbol "$\otimes$", as in

$$z(k) = x(k) \otimes y(k).$$

Notice that cyclic convolution is nearly identical to periodic convolution except for the mod-N operation. The DFT of the cyclic convolution of two sequences is given by

$$\sum_{m=0}^{N-1} x(m) y(k-m \bmod N) \stackrel{DFT}{\longleftrightarrow} X(n)Y(n). \tag{3.3.7}$$

or by

$$\sum_{m=0}^{N-1} x(k-m \bmod N) y(m) \stackrel{DFT}{\longleftrightarrow} X(n)Y(n).$$

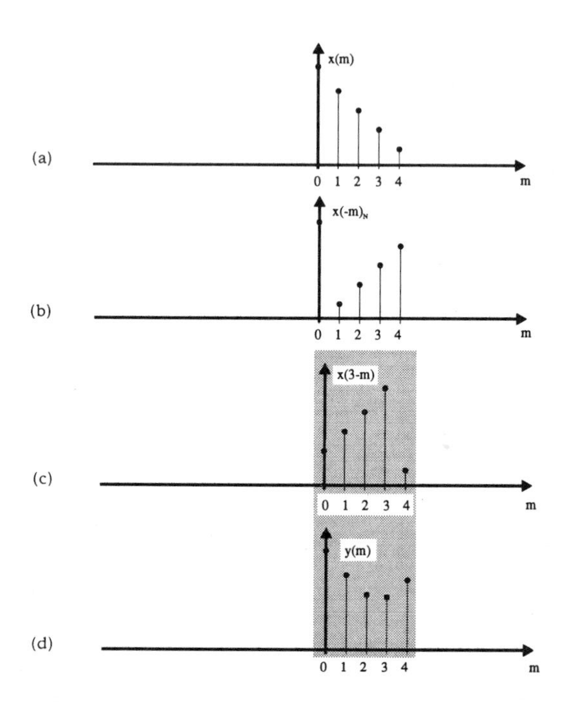

Figure 3.3.4: Illustration of cyclic convolution: (a) $x(m)$; (b) $x(-m \bmod N)$; (c) $x(k-m \bmod N)$ for $k=3$; (d) $y(m)$ (overlap with $x(k-m \bmod N)$ shown in shaded region).

Equation 3.3.7 states that the DFT of the cyclic convolution of two sequences is given by the product of the DFTS of the two sequences.

Let's look at how cyclic convolution is performed. We start with $x(k)$ and $y(k)$ and then re-index with the new index m giving $x(m)$ and $y(m)$. Next, $x(-m \bmod N)$ is formed. This is done according to

$$x(-0 \bmod N) = x(0)$$

and

$$x(-m \bmod N) = x(N-m), \quad n = 1, 2, \ldots, N-1.$$

Finally, $x(-m \bmod N)$ is cyclically shifted to the right by k, multiplied pointwise by $y(m)$ and summed. This is depicted in Fig. 3.3.4.

Cyclic convolution is easily visualized if it is represented in matrix form. Suppose $f(k)$ and $g(k)$ are both of length three, where

$$\{f(k)\} = \{f(0), f(1), f(2)\}$$

and

$$\{g(k)\} = \{g(0), g(1), g(2)\}.$$

Let $y(k) = f(k) \otimes g(k)$. Then

$$y(k) = \sum_{m=0}^{2} f(m)g(k - m \bmod 3).$$

Let's compute each term of $y(k)$. We have

$$y(0) = \sum_{m=0}^{2} f(k)g(-k \bmod 3) = f(0)g(0) + f(1)g(2) + f(2)g(1).$$

Similarly,

$$y(1) = f(0)g(1) + f(1)g(0) + f(2)g(2)$$

and

$$y(2) = f(0)g(2) + f(1)g(1) + f(2)g(0).$$

These three expressions can be combined into the matrix equation

$$\begin{pmatrix} y(0) \\ y(1) \\ y(2) \end{pmatrix} = \begin{pmatrix} g(0) & g(2) & g(1) \\ g(1) & g(0) & g(2) \\ g(2) & g(1) & g(0) \end{pmatrix} \begin{pmatrix} f(0) \\ f(1) \\ f(2) \end{pmatrix}. \tag{3.3.8}$$

More compactly, we may write

$$\boldsymbol{y} = \boldsymbol{G}\boldsymbol{f}.$$

Examining the matrix $\boldsymbol{G}$ in Eq. 3.3.8, we see that it has a highly regular structure. Specifically, the first column of $\boldsymbol{G}$ is given by the sequence $\{g(k)\}$. Subsequent columns are obtained by a cyclic shift of the previous column. This will be the case in general.

Example 3.5

Suppose we wish to perform the cyclic convolution $\boldsymbol{y}$ of the sequences

$$\boldsymbol{f} = \{1, 2, 3\}$$

and

$$\boldsymbol{g} = \{1, 2, 1\}.$$

We use the matrix representation

$$\begin{pmatrix} y(0) \\ y(1) \\ y(2) \end{pmatrix} = \begin{pmatrix} 1 & 1 & 2 \\ 2 & 1 & 1 \\ 1 & 2 & 1 \end{pmatrix} \begin{pmatrix} 1 \\ 2 \\ 3 \end{pmatrix}$$

which gives

$$\boldsymbol{y} = \{9, 7, 8\}.$$

We have seen that for signals $f(k)$ and $g(k)$, the linear convolution $y(k)$ can be computed using $\mathcal{Z}$-transforms by computing the product of the $\mathcal{Z}$-transforms, $Y(z) = F(z)G(z)$. It turns out that the cyclic convolution can be computed according to

$$f(k) \otimes g(k) \longleftrightarrow F(z)G(z) \bmod (z^{-N} - 1)$$

where the "mod$(z^{-N} - 1)$" corresponds to polynomial reduction modulo $(z^{-N} - 1)$. For example, suppose

$$\boldsymbol{f} = \{1, 2, 3\} \quad \text{and} \quad \boldsymbol{g} = \{1, 2, 1\}.$$

Then

$$Y(z) = F(z)G(z) =$$
$$(1 + 2z^{-1} + 3z^{-2})(1 + 2z^{-1} + z^{-2}) = 1 + 4z^{-1} + 8z^{-2} + 8z^{-3} + 3z^{-4}.$$

Now, to reduce the polynomial $F(z)G(z)$ modulo $(z^{-3} - 1)$, we make the identification $z^{-3} = 1$, which when multiplied on both sides by z^{-1} further implies that $z^{-4} = z^{-1}z^{-3} = z^{-1}$. Therefore,

$$F(z)G(z) \bmod (z^{-3} - 1) = 1 + 4z^{-1} + 8z^{-2} + 8z^{-1} + 3z^{-2}$$

which gives

$$Y(z) = 9 + 7z^{-1} + 8z^{-2},$$

giving $\boldsymbol{y} = \{9, 7, 8\}$, which is what we expected.

Now that we know how to perform cyclic convolution, it is reasonable to wonder why it is used. It turns out that cyclic convolution can be used to perform linear convolution, which in turn can be computed by using the DFT. Although this may seem like a roundabout way to perform linear convolution, there exist many efficient algorithms for computing the DFT so that for long signals, this is often the preferred method to compute linear convolution.

Assume that $f(k)$ and $g(k)$ are finite-duration signals of length M and N, respectively. The linear convolution, $y(k)$, can be computed by $\mathcal{Z}$-transforms according to

$$Y(z) = F(z)G(z).$$

Because $F(z)$ is a polynomial of degree $M-1$ and $G(z)$ is a polynomial of degree $N-1$, their product $Y(z)$ will be of degree at most $M+N-2$. Thus, $y(k)$ has length at most $M+N-1$. Therefore, suppose both sequences are zero-padded to length $M+N-1$ and consider computing the cyclic convolution using the product of the $\mathcal{Z}$-transforms followed by polynomial reduction modulo the polynomial $(z^{-(N+M-1)}-1)$. Zero-padding the sequences does not change the fact that the product of the $\mathcal{Z}$-transforms is of degree no higher than $M+N-2$ and reduction modulo $(z^{-(N+M-1)}-1)$ will have no effect on the product. Therefore, the cyclic and linear convolutions will yield the same results.

We can gain some useful insight into the structure of convolution by putting the convolution in matrix form. An example will best illustrate. Suppose $f(k)$ and $g(k)$ are both of length three. By definition,

$$y(k)=\sum_{m=-\infty}^{\infty} f(m)g(k-m).$$

The sequence $y(k)$ will be of length at most $3+3-1=5$, and we have

$$\begin{aligned}
y(0) &= f(0)g(0) + \\
y(1) &= f(0)g(1) + f(1)g(0) \\
y(2) &= f(0)g(2) + f(1)g(1) + f(2)g(1) \\
y(3) &= f(1)g(2) + f(2)g(1) \\
y(4) &= f(2)g(2)
\end{aligned}$$

This can be put in matrix form as

$$\begin{pmatrix} y(0) \\ y(1) \\ y(2) \end{pmatrix} = \begin{pmatrix} g(0) & 0 & 0 \\ g(1) & g(0) & 0 \\ g(2) & g(1) & g(0) \\ 0 & g(2) & g(1) \\ 0 & 0 & g(2) \end{pmatrix} \begin{pmatrix} f(0) \\ f(1) \\ f(2) \end{pmatrix}, \tag{3.3.9}$$

which we denote by

$$\boldsymbol{y}=\boldsymbol{G}\boldsymbol{f}.$$

Here is how to perform the same convolution using cyclic convolution. Zero-pad both $f(k)$ and $g(k)$ to length $3+3-1=5$ to form the new sequences $\hat{f}(k)$ and $\hat{g}(k)$. We already saw how to put a cyclic convolution into matrix form: the matrix has as its n-th column the sequence $\hat{g}(k)$ cyclically shifted by n. The cyclic convolution $\hat{y}(k)$ of $\hat{f}(k)$ and $\hat{g}(k)$ will also be of length 5. We have

$$\begin{pmatrix} \hat{y}(0) \\ \hat{y}(1) \\ \hat{y}(2) \\ \hat{y}(3) \\ \hat{y}(5) \end{pmatrix} = \left(\begin{array}{ccc|cc} g(0) & 0 & 0 & g(2) & g(1) \\ g(1) & g(0) & 0 & 0 & g(2) \\ g(2) & g(1) & g(0) & 0 & 0 \\ 0 & g(2) & g(1) & g(0) & 0 \\ 0 & 0 & g(2) & g(1) & g(0) \end{array}\right) \begin{pmatrix} f(0) \\ f(1) \\ f(2) \\ 0 \\ 0 \end{pmatrix}. \tag{3.3.10}$$

We can write this compactly as

$$\hat{\boldsymbol{y}} = \hat{\boldsymbol{G}}\hat{\boldsymbol{f}}. \tag{3.3.11}$$

The matrix $\hat{\boldsymbol{G}}$ is a partitioned matrix which contains as a submatrix $\boldsymbol{G}$ from Eq. 3.3.9. We can thus write

$$\hat{\boldsymbol{G}} = [\boldsymbol{G} \;\; \boldsymbol{X}]$$

where $\boldsymbol{X}$ is the right half of the partitioned matrix $\hat{\boldsymbol{G}}$. The vector $\boldsymbol{f}$ can be partitioned as

$$\hat{\boldsymbol{f}} = \begin{pmatrix} \boldsymbol{f} \\ \boldsymbol{0} \end{pmatrix}.$$

Thus, Eq. 3.3.11 can be expressed by

$$\hat{\boldsymbol{y}} = [\boldsymbol{G} \;\; \boldsymbol{X}] \begin{pmatrix} \boldsymbol{f} \\ \boldsymbol{0} \end{pmatrix}$$

which means that

$$\hat{\boldsymbol{y}} = \boldsymbol{G}\boldsymbol{f} + \boldsymbol{X}\boldsymbol{0} = \boldsymbol{G}\boldsymbol{f} = \boldsymbol{y}.$$

Therefore, the cyclic convolution produces the same result as linear convolution when the sequences are both zero-padded to their maximal length.

Example 3.6

Let's use cyclic convolution to compute the linear convolution, $\boldsymbol{y}$ of

$$\boldsymbol{f} = \{1, 2, 3\}$$

and

$$\boldsymbol{g} = \{1, 2, 1\}.$$

We first zero-pad both sequences to length $3 + 3 - 1 = 5$, giving

$$\hat{\boldsymbol{f}} = \{1, 2, 3, 0, 0\}$$

and

$$\hat{g} = \{1, 2, 1, 0, 0\}.$$

The cyclic convolution $\hat{f}(k) \otimes \hat{g}(k)$ is then put in the matrix form

$$\hat{y} = \begin{pmatrix} 1 & 0 & 0 & 1 & 2 \\ 2 & 1 & 0 & 0 & 1 \\ 1 & 2 & 1 & 0 & 0 \\ 0 & 1 & 2 & 1 & 0 \\ 0 & 0 & 1 & 2 & 1 \end{pmatrix} \begin{pmatrix} 1 \\ 2 \\ 3 \\ 0 \\ 0 \end{pmatrix}$$

which gives

$$\hat{y} = \{1, 4, 8, 8, 3\}.$$

It is easily verified that this produces the proper result for the linear convolution.

In summary, to perform the linear convolution of sequences $f(k)$ and $g(k)$ of length M and N, respectively, we zero-pad both $f(k)$ and $g(k)$ to length $M + N - 1$ and perform the cyclic convolution of the zero-padded sequences. The cyclic convolution will then agree with the linear convolution. If $f(k)$ and $g(k)$ are zero-padded to a length greater than $M + N - 1$ and cyclically convolved, the first $M + N - 1$ values of the cyclic convolution will *still* agree with the linear convolution and the remaining values will all be equal to zero. This is important because some of the fast algorithms we will use for computing the DFT require that the sequences to be of a particular length (a power of two, for example).

To perform linear convolution of $f(k)$ and $g(k)$ by DFTs, we first zero-pad the two sequences to length $M+N-1$ and take the DFT of each zero-padded sequence. The DFTs are then multiplied together pointwise (because of Eq. 3.3.7). We then apply the IDFT equation which gives the proper time series. This is illustrated in Fig. 3.3.5. Notice that this scheme requires a total of two DFTs, $M + N - 1$ pointwise multiplications, and one IDFT. We will soon see that this can be made to require much less multiplication than direct evaluation of the convolution sum.

• Multiplication of Sequences

If $x(k)$ and $y(k)$ have DFTs $X(n)$ and $Y(n)$, respectively, then

$$x(k)y(k) \overset{DFT}{\longleftrightarrow} \frac{1}{N} \sum_{m=0}^{N-1} X(m)Y(n - m \bmod N). \tag{3.3.12}$$

Note the structural similarity to the DFT convolution property.

• Miscellaneous Symmetry Properties

Suppose $x(k)$ has DFT $X(n)$. The DFT of the conjugate sequence $x^*(k)$ is given by

$$x^*(k) \overset{DFS}{\longleftrightarrow} X^*(-n \bmod N). \tag{3.3.13}$$

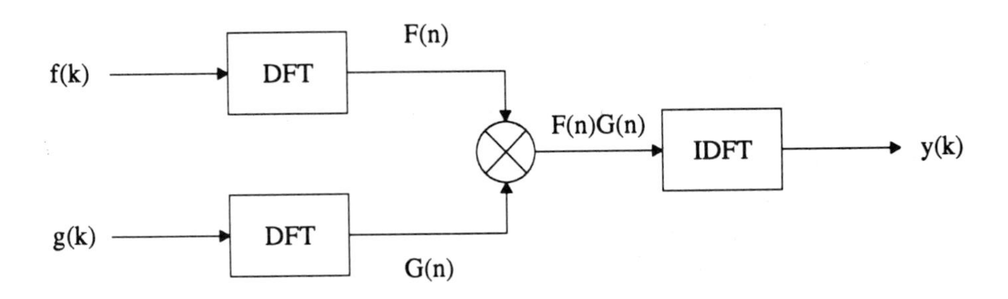

Figure 3.3.5: Using the DFT to compute linear convolution.

Similarly,

$$x^*(-k \bmod N) \overset{DFS}{\longleftrightarrow} X^*(n). \tag{3.3.14}$$

Just as with the DFS, Equations 3.3.13 and 3.3.14 can be used to derive a number of other useful DFT properties. If $x^{(e)}(k)$ is given by

$$x^{(e)}(k) = \frac{1}{2}(x(k) + x^*(-k \bmod N))$$

then

$$x^{(e)}(k) \overset{DFT}{\longleftrightarrow} \frac{1}{2}(X(n) + X^*(n))$$

so that

$$x^{(e)}(k) \overset{DFT}{\longleftrightarrow} \mathrm{Re}(X(n)). \tag{3.3.15}$$

With $x^{(o)}(k)$ given by

$$x^{(o)}(k) = \frac{1}{2}(x(k) - x(-k \bmod N)),$$

we get

$$x^{(o)}(k) \overset{DFT}{\longleftrightarrow} j\mathrm{Im}(X(n)). \tag{3.3.16}$$

Finally,

$$\mathrm{Re}(x(k)) \stackrel{DFT}{\longleftrightarrow} \frac{1}{2}(X(n) + X^*(-n \bmod N)) = X^{(e)}(n) \tag{3.3.17}$$

and

$$\mathrm{Im}(x(k)) \stackrel{DFT}{\longleftrightarrow} \frac{1}{2}(X(n) - X^*(-n \bmod N) = X^{(o)}(n). \tag{3.3.18}$$

If $x(k)$ is real, then

$$X^*(n) = \sum_{k=0}^{N-1} x(k)(W_N^{nk})^*.$$

But

$$(W_N^{nk})^* = W_N^{(N-n)k} = W_N^{(-n \mathrm{mod} N)k}$$

which means that

$$X^*(n) = X(-n \bmod N).$$

In a similar fashion, we can show that if $x(k)$ is imaginary, then

$$X^*(n) = -X(-n \bmod N).$$

There is one more property we need to explore: the DFT version of Parseval's theorem. In so doing, we will introduce a matrix notation for the DFT. In addition to making the derivation of Parseval's theorem quite simple, the matrix notation provides a clear and concise framework which will prove valuable in later chapters.

To begin, Define the vector $\boldsymbol{x}$ and $\boldsymbol{X}$ by

$$\boldsymbol{x} = \begin{pmatrix} x(0) \\ x(1) \\ \vdots \\ x(N-1) \end{pmatrix}, \quad \boldsymbol{X} = \begin{pmatrix} X(0) \\ X(1) \\ \vdots \\ X(N-1) \end{pmatrix}.$$

According to Eq. 3.3.4, we can write

$$\boldsymbol{X} = \boldsymbol{V}\boldsymbol{x} \tag{3.3.19}$$

where $\boldsymbol{V}$ is an $N \times N$ matrix whose n, k element is given by

$$[\boldsymbol{V}]_{n,k} = W_N^{nk}.$$

If $\boldsymbol{V}$ is invertible, we can recover $\boldsymbol{x}$ from $\boldsymbol{X}$ by

$$\boldsymbol{x} = \boldsymbol{V}^{-1}\boldsymbol{X}.$$

We should expect that $\boldsymbol{V}$ is invertible since there is an equation for the IDFT. In fact, according to Eq. 3.3.5, we can write

$$\boldsymbol{x} = \frac{1}{N}\boldsymbol{U}\boldsymbol{X} \tag{3.3.20}$$

where $\boldsymbol{U}$ is an $N \times N$ matrix whose n,k element is given by

$$[\boldsymbol{U}]_{n,k} = W_N^{-nk}.$$

Thus,

$$[\boldsymbol{U}]_{n,k} = ([\boldsymbol{V}]_{n,k})^*.$$

Combining Eqs. 3.3.19 and 3.3.20, we have

$$\boldsymbol{X} = \frac{1}{N}\boldsymbol{V}\boldsymbol{U}\boldsymbol{X}$$

and

$$\boldsymbol{x} = \frac{1}{N}\boldsymbol{U}\boldsymbol{V}\boldsymbol{x}.$$

Thus,

$$\boldsymbol{U}\boldsymbol{V} = \boldsymbol{V}\boldsymbol{U} = N\boldsymbol{I}.$$

This is simply a restatement of the orthogonality property of the sequences W_N^{nk} and W_N^{mk}. We therefore have

$$\boldsymbol{V}^{-1} = \frac{1}{N}\boldsymbol{U} = \frac{1}{N}\boldsymbol{V}^H \tag{3.3.21}$$

which implies that

$$\boldsymbol{V}^H\boldsymbol{V} = N\boldsymbol{I}$$

where $\boldsymbol{V}^H$ is the conjugate-transpose of $\boldsymbol{V}$.

We can use Eq. 3.3.21 to derive some useful properties of the DFT. For example, suppose we have sequences $x(k)$ and $y(k)$ of length N with

$$\boldsymbol{x} \overset{DFT}{\longleftrightarrow} \boldsymbol{X} = \boldsymbol{V}\boldsymbol{x}$$

and

$$\boldsymbol{y} \stackrel{DFT}{\longleftrightarrow} \boldsymbol{Y} = \boldsymbol{V}\boldsymbol{y}.$$

Suppose we form the sum

$$\frac{1}{N}\sum_{n=0}^{N-1} X(n)Y^*(n) = \frac{1}{N}\boldsymbol{Y}^H\boldsymbol{X}.$$

But

$$\boldsymbol{Y}^H\boldsymbol{X} = \boldsymbol{y}^H\boldsymbol{V}^H\boldsymbol{V}\boldsymbol{x}$$

and according to Eq. 3.3.21, $\boldsymbol{V}^H\boldsymbol{V} = N\boldsymbol{I}$. Thus,

$$\boldsymbol{Y}^H\boldsymbol{X} = N\boldsymbol{y}^H\boldsymbol{x} = N\sum_{k=0}^{N-1} x(k)y^*(k)$$

so that

$$\frac{1}{N}\sum_{n=0}^{N-1} X(n)Y^*(n) = \sum_{k=0}^{N-1} x(k)y^*(k). \tag{3.3.22}$$

Equation 3.3.22 is a DFT expression of Parseval's theorem. For the special case where $x(k) = y(k)$, we have

$$\frac{1}{N}\sum_{n=0}^{N-1} |X(n)|^2 = \sum_{k=0}^{N-1} |x(k)|^2. \tag{3.3.23}$$

Thus, the energy in a finite duration signal can be computed in either directly in the time domain or indirectly in the frequency domain using the DFT values.

For a more sophisticated view of the Parseval theorem for the DFT, we can appeal to the theory of vector spaces. The DFT matrix $\boldsymbol{V}$ has orthogonal columns and the DFT mapping $\boldsymbol{X} = \boldsymbol{V}\boldsymbol{x}$ can be interpreted as linear transformation from C^N to C^N. In the time domain, the energy is computed as the inner product $\boldsymbol{x}^H\boldsymbol{x}$ and in the frequency domain the energy is computed as the inner product $\boldsymbol{X}^H\boldsymbol{X}$ (up to the scale factor $1/N$ which could have been absorbed into the matrix $\boldsymbol{V}$). Because $\boldsymbol{V}$ has orthogonal columns, the linear transformation $\boldsymbol{V}$ preserves inner products (a property of so-called *unitary* matrices).

Table 3.1 gives a brief summary of some important DFT properties.

Sequence	*DFT*
$x(k)$	$X(n)$
$ax(k) + by(k)$	$aX(n) + bY(n)$
$x(k - m \bmod N)$	$W_N^{nm} X(n)$
$W_N^{-mk} x(k)$	$X(n - m \bmod N)$
$\sum_{m=0}^{N-1} x(m)y(k - m \bmod N)$	$X(n)Y(n)$
$x(k)y(k)$	$\frac{1}{N} \sum_{m=0}^{N-1} X(m)Y(n - m \bmod N)$
$x^*(k)$	$X^*(-n \bmod N)$
$x^*(-k \bmod N)$	$X^*(n)$
$x^{(e)}(k)$	$\mathrm{Re}(X(n))$
$x^{(o)}(k)$	$\mathrm{Im}(X(n))$
$\mathrm{Re}(x(k))$	$X^{(e)}(n)$
$\mathrm{Im}(x(k))$	$X^{(o)}(n)$
Symmetry Properties	
$x(k)$ real	$X^*(n) = X(-n \bmod N)$
$x(k)$ imaginary	$X^*(n) = -X(-n \bmod N)$
$x(k) = x^*(-k \bmod N)$	$X(n)$ real
$x(k) = -x^*(-k \bmod N)$	$X(n)$ imaginary

Table 3.2: Important DFT properties

3.4 Block Processing of FIR Filters

We have already seen how cyclic convolution can be used to perform the linear convolution of two finite-duration sequences. We can also use cyclic convolution to perform the linear convolution of a finite-duration sequence and an infinite-duration sequence by ***block processing.*** This is the kind of situation which arises when an input signal is arriving in real-time and must be filtered by an FIR of length N. Because the FIR is described by the input/output equation

$$y(k) = \sum_{m=0}^{N-1} h(m)x(k-m)$$

we can see that the computation of each output point requires a total of L multiplications and additions. Thus, to process a block of N output samples, we must perform NL multiplications and additions. For large L and N, this can be very burdensome. We have already alluded to the fact that there are fast algorithms for computing the DFT, which can in turn compute cyclic convolution. In fact, for large L and N, this is the preferred way to work.

Let $h(k)$ be the coefficients of an FIR of length L and let $u(k)$ be an infinite-duration input signal. Let $v(k)$ be a finite-duration segment of $u(k)$ of length N. Without loss of generality, we let

$$v(k) = u(k), \quad k = 0, 1, \ldots, N-1$$

where N is chosen to be greater than L. Now, let's compare the linear convolution of $h(k) * v(k)$ with the cyclic convolution $h(k) \otimes v(k)$, where $h(k)$ has been zero-padded to length N. The linear convolution will be a sequence of length $L + N - 2$ which can be visualized by the usual "flip and drag" computation method. To visualize the cyclic convolution, we can periodically extend both $h(k)$ and $v(k)$ and regard the cyclic convolution as a single period of a periodic convolution. When $h_p(m)$ is flipped and dragged, there is no overlap with the periodic images of $v_p(m)$ outside the range $0 \leq m \leq N-1$ only when the value of k satisfies

$$L - 1 \leq k \leq N - 1$$

Therefore, the linear and cyclic convolutions will be the same for k in this range. Hence, we can perform the cyclic convolution and keep only the $N - L - 1$ last values. These output values are placed in an output buffer and we move on to a new block of input data. This is known as the *overlap-save* method of block convolution processing. When the DFT is used to compute the cyclic convolution, substantial savings can result.

3.5 Fast Fourier Transform Algorithms

Direct evaluation of the discrete Fourier transform is a computationally intensive task. For each harmonic index n, the sum-of-products

$$X(n) = \sum_{k=0}^{N-1} x(k)W_N^{nk}$$

must be computed. Each harmonic $X(n)$ requires N multiplications and $N-1$ additions. If the time series $\{x(k)\}$ is complex, each complex multiply consists of four real multiplies and two real adds. For the complete N-point DFT, N^2 complex multiplications must be performed (this total includes trivial multiplications by $\pm 1, \pm j$ which for large N constitute a small percentage of the multiplications). Historically, multiplication has been a difficult task for general-purpose digital computers because they usually lack dedicated hardware multipliers. Modern DSP microprocessors, however, have multiplier/accumulators which are capable of single-cycle multiplication/accumulation. Nonetheless, the usual metric of computational complexity for Fourier transform is the number of multiplications.

There are many algorithms for the fast computation of the DFT. Collectively, these are known as fast Fourier transform (FFT) algorithms. Most FFT algorithms exploit the symmetry inherent in the expression for the DFT to allow the DFT to be computed with *significantly* fewer multiplications than direct evaluation of the DFT. These algorithms have made real-time spectral analysis a practical reality and have had much to do with the popularity of DSP today. Much of the pioneering work in the field of fast Fourier transforms can be credited to Cooley and Tukey [CT65], who popularized the ubiquitous radix-2 FFT, and to I. J. Good [Goo71], who developed one of the first number-theoretic approaches to DFT computation (Good's work actually predated that of Cooley and Tukey).

3.5.1 The Radix-2 FFT

Recall that

$$X(n) = \sum_{k=0}^{N-1} x(k)W_N^{-nk}.$$

The computation of each harmonic requires N complex multiplications. Therefore, the entire DFT requires N^2 complex multiplications. Let's see how this can be reduced. Suppose the blocklength N is a power of two, *i.e.*,

$$N = 2^K$$

for some integer K. Divide the sequence $x(k)$ into two subsequences, one consisting of the even indices and one consisting of the odd indices:

$$a(k) = x(2k), \quad k = 0, 1, \ldots, N/2 - 1,$$

and

$$b(k) = x(2k+1), \quad k = 0, 1, \ldots, N/2 - 1.$$

We can then write

$$X(n) = \sum_{k=0}^{N/2-1} x(2k) W_N^{-(2n)k} + \sum_{k=0}^{N/2-1} x(2k+1) W_N^{-(2n+1)k},$$

which can be rewritten using the sequences $a(k)$ and $b(k)$ as

$$X(n) = \sum_{k=0}^{N/2-1} a(k) W_N^{-2nk} + W_N^{-n} \sum_{k=0}^{N/2-1} b(k) W_N^{-2nk}.$$

Now, recall that

$$W_N = e^{j2\pi/N}.$$

Therefore,

$$W_N^2 = e^{j2\pi/(N/2)} = W_{N/2}$$

and we can express $X(n)$ as

$$X(n) = \sum_{k=0}^{N/2-1} a(k) W_{N/2}^{-nk} + W_N^{-n} \sum_{k=0}^{N/2-1} b(k) W_{N/2}^{-nk}.$$

The summations above are recognized as the $N/2$-point DFTs of the sequences $a(k)$ and $b(k)$, respectively, which we denote by

$$A(n) = \sum_{k=0}^{N/2-1} a(k) W_{N/2}^{-nk}, \quad n = 0, 1, \ldots, N/2 - 1$$

and

$$B(n) = \sum_{k=0}^{N/2-1} b(k) W_{N/2}^{-nk}, \quad n = 0, 1, \ldots, N/2 - 1.$$

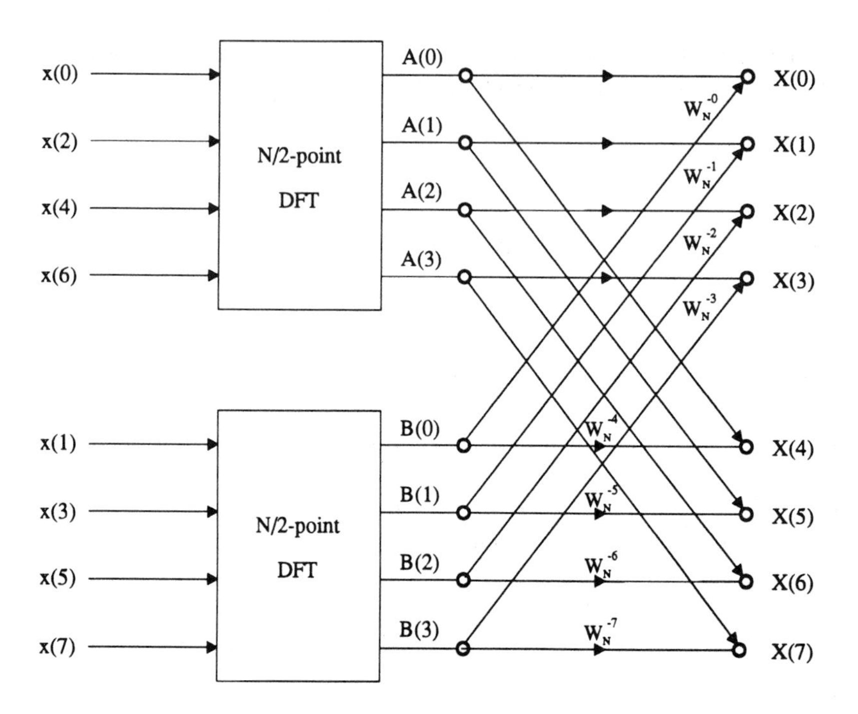

Figure 3.5.1: Decomposing an eight-point DFT into two four-point DFTs.

Hence,

$$X(n) = A(n) + W_N^{-n} B(n), \quad n = 0, 1, \ldots, N/2 - 1.$$

How about the harmonics between $N/2$ and $N - 1$? Because $A(n)$ and $B(n)$ are $N/2$-point DFTs, they are periodic with period $N/2$. Therefore,

$$X(n) = A(n - N/2) + W_N^{-n} B(n - N/2), \quad n = N/2, N/2 + 1, \ldots, N - 1.$$

The decomposition of an eight-point DFT into two four-point DFTs is shown in Fig. 3.5.1. Notice the symmetry of the computations. The powers of W_N which multiply the $B(n)$ are known as *twiddle factors.*

Let's analyze the reduction in multiplicative complexity thusfar. The $N/2$-point DFTs each require $(N/2)^2$ complex multiplications and there are an additional N twiddle factor multiplications. Therefore, the new complexity is

$$2(N/2)^2 + N = N^2/2 + N$$

complex multiplications. While this may not seem like a drastic reduction in complexity, we can continue the decomposition at a second level of depth. Because N is a power of two, we can decompose each $N/2$-point DFT into two $N/4$-point DFTs. We will only give the details for the DFT $A(n)$.

The sequence $a(k)$ can be decomposed into even and odd parts as

$$r(k) = a(2k), \quad k = 0, 1, \ldots, N/4 - 1$$

and

$$s(k) = a(2k+1), \quad k = 0, 1, \ldots, N/4 - 1.$$

We can then express $A(n)$ as

$$A(n) = \sum_{k=0}^{N/4-1} a(2k) W_{N/2}^{-n(2k)} + \sum_{k=0}^{N/4-1} a(2k+1) W_{N/2}^{-n(2k+1)}.$$

This time, we use the fact that

$$W_{N/2}^2 = W_{N/4}$$

to determine that

$$A(n) = \sum_{k=0}^{N/4-1} r(k) W_{N/4}^{-nk} + W_{N/2}^{-n} \sum_{k=0}^{N/4-1} s(k) W_{N/4}^{-nk}.$$

This time, the summations are recognized as $N/4$-point DFTs $R(n)$ and $S(n)$,

$$R(n) = \sum_{k=0}^{N/4-1} r(k) W_{N/4}^{-nk}, \quad n = 0, 1, \ldots N/4 - 1$$

and

$$S(n) = \sum_{k=0}^{N/4-1} s(k) W_{N/4}^{-nk}, \quad n = 0, 1, \ldots, N/4 - 1.$$

Thus,

$$A(n) = R(n) + W_{N/2}^{-n} S(n), \quad n = 0, 1, \ldots, N/4 - 1.$$

We still need the values of $A(n)$ for indices between $N/4$ and $N/2 - 1$. Because $R(n)$ and $S(n)$ are $N/4$-periodic, we have

$$A(n) = R(n - N/4) + W_{N/2}^{-n} S(n - N/4), \quad n = N/4, N/4 + 1, \ldots, N/2 - 1.$$

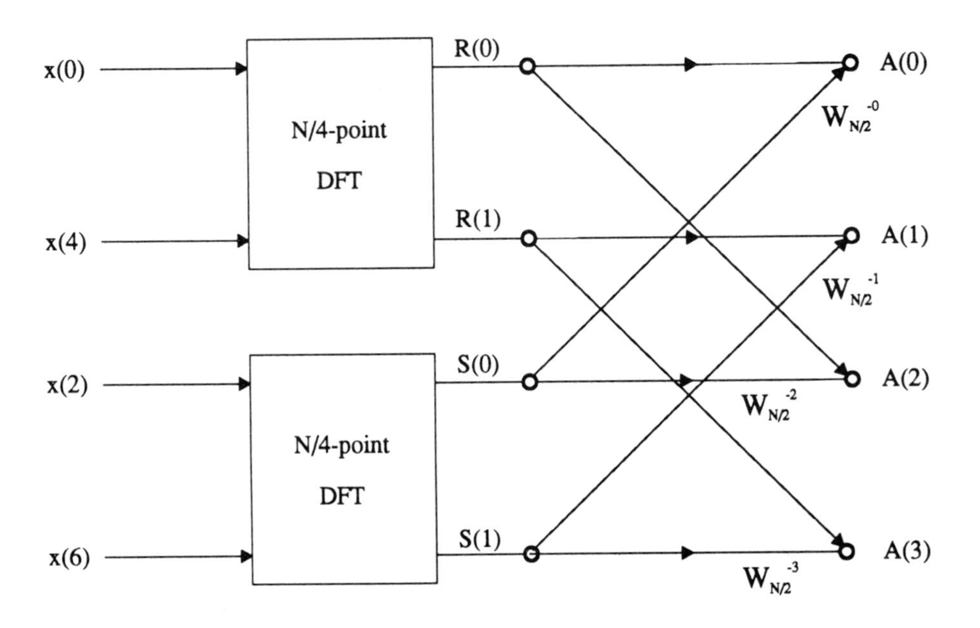

Figure 3.5.2: Decomposing a four-point DFT into two 2-point DFTs.

These expressions give the decomposition of the $N/2$-point DFT $A(n)$ as two $N/4$-point DFTs which are pieced together with a set of twiddle factors. The decomposition of the four-point DFT $A(n)$ is shown in Fig. 3.5.2. For the eight-point DFT we are considering, an identical decomposition is performed for the four-point DFT $B(n)$.

The process of "decimating" the sequence continues until we are left with nothing but two-point DFTs. The expression for a two-point DFT is quite simple. We have

$$Q(n) = q(0) + q(1)W_2^{-n}.$$

Because $W_2 = -1$, it follows that

$$\begin{aligned} Q(0) &= q(0) + q(1) \\ Q(1) &= q(0) - q(1). \end{aligned}$$

The structure for computing a two-point DFT is known as an "FFT butterfly" and is shown in Fig. 3.5.3.

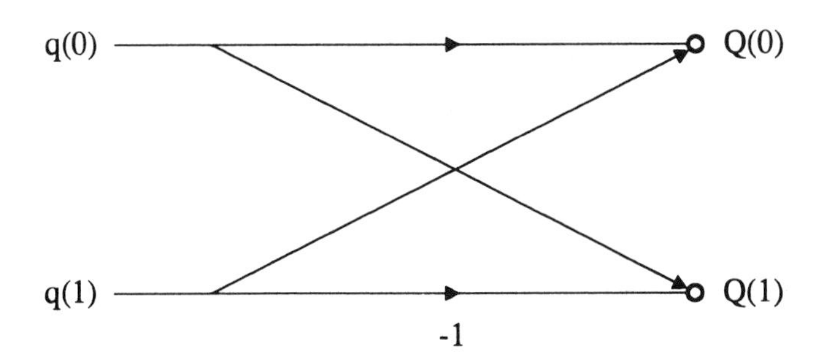

Figure 3.5.3: An FFT butterfly.

For the two-point DFTs, we partition the four-point DFTs into odd and even parts. The four-point sequences for the four-point DFTs were obtained by partitioning the eight-point DFTs into odd and even parts. In general, we find that the inputs to the two-point DFTs are given by $x(m)$ and $x(m+N/2)$. This partitioning is shown in Fig. 3.5.4.

The entire decomposition of an eight-point DFT is shown in Fig. 3.5.5. Referring to the order of the sequence $x(k)$ at the left side of the figure, it can be seen that the indices are scrambled. Although the new ordering may seem somewhat confusing, there is actually a well-defined structure to the ordering. Let's trace the path of $x(0)$ from the beginning of the algorithm to the end. We began by separating the sequence into even and odd indices. The data point $x(0)$ became the zeroth point of the sequence $a(k)$. Then the sequence $a(k)$ was separated into even and odd parts, and $a(0)$ became the zeroth point of the sequence $r(k)$ and thus appears at the top left. In general, we successively sort the sequences by an "even-odd-even-etc." type of ordering. The data point $x(k)$ is determined to have odd or even index according to the least significant bit of the index. The next level of even/odd is determined by the next bit of significance, and so on. To find the location of a data point $x(k)$ at the left-hand side of the FFT, we begin by writing the index k in binary and reversing the order of the bits. The "bit-reversed" index indicates the position of $x(k)$. For example, let's locate $x(3)$. We have

$$3 \sim 011.$$

The bit reversal of 011 is 110, which corresponds to the decimal 6. Therefore, $x(3)$ appears as the seventh element of the bit-reversed input to the FFT.

Referring to Fig. 3.5.5, we see that the FFT is naturally partitioned into stages. Assume that the sequence $x(k)$ is stored in bit-reversed order in memory. At the first stage, there are are $N/2$ butterfly operations. Two data points are removed from memory, a butterfly operation is performed, and the transformed data points are then returned to *the same* memory locations. This is known as *in-place* computation. This process is repeated until an

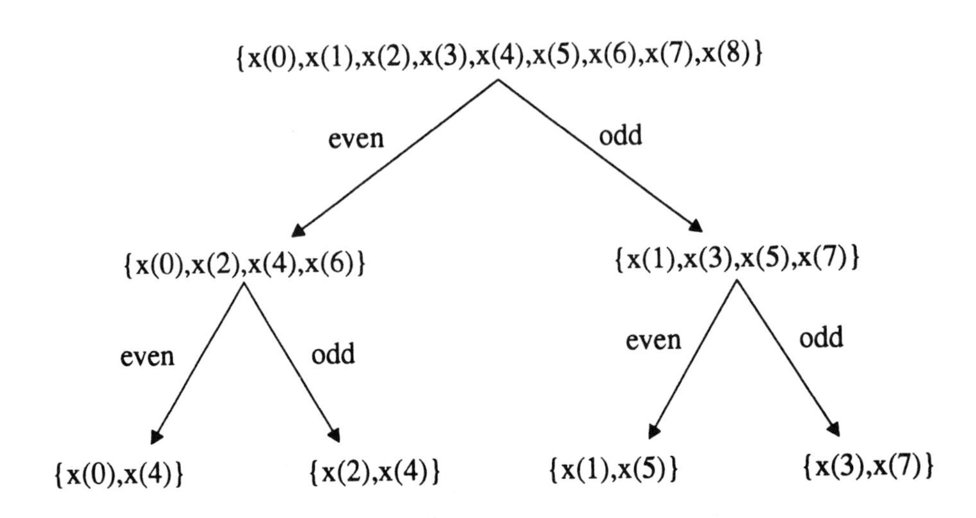

Figure 3.5.4: Partitioning of sequences for an eight-point FFT.

entire first stage is completed. At the second stage, we similarly perform two-point in-place butterfly operations (where the butterfly operations are now performed on different data pairs than before, but still in-place). We continue processing stages until the transform is finished. In Fig. 3.5.5, the twiddle factors are all expressed in terms of W_N rather than in terms of $W_{N/2}$ and $W_{N/4}$ so that the twiddle factor pattern can be seen easily.

The multiplicative complexity of the radix-2 FFT algorithm is simple to compute. There are $\log_2 N$ stages, each of which requires N complex multiplications. Therefore, there are a total of

$$N \log_2 N$$

complex multiplications for the entire FFT. This can represent a *substantial* reduction in complexity. Consider, for example, the case $N = 1024$. Direct evaluation of the DFT requires $N^2 = 2^{20}$ complex multiplications. Using the radix-2 FFT, the complexity is reduced to $N \log_2 N = 10240$ multiplications. This is a reduction by more than a factor of 100. The acceleration in computation time is even more pronounced for larger N.

In actuality, we can do even better. In general, each butterfly operation is of the form shown in Fig. 3.5.6a. The powers of W_N in each butterfly are separated by $N/2$. That is, each butterfly requires two multiplications: one by W_N^r and one by $W_N^{r+N/2}$. Because

$$W_N^{r+N/2} = W_N^{N/2} W_N^r = -W_N^r,$$

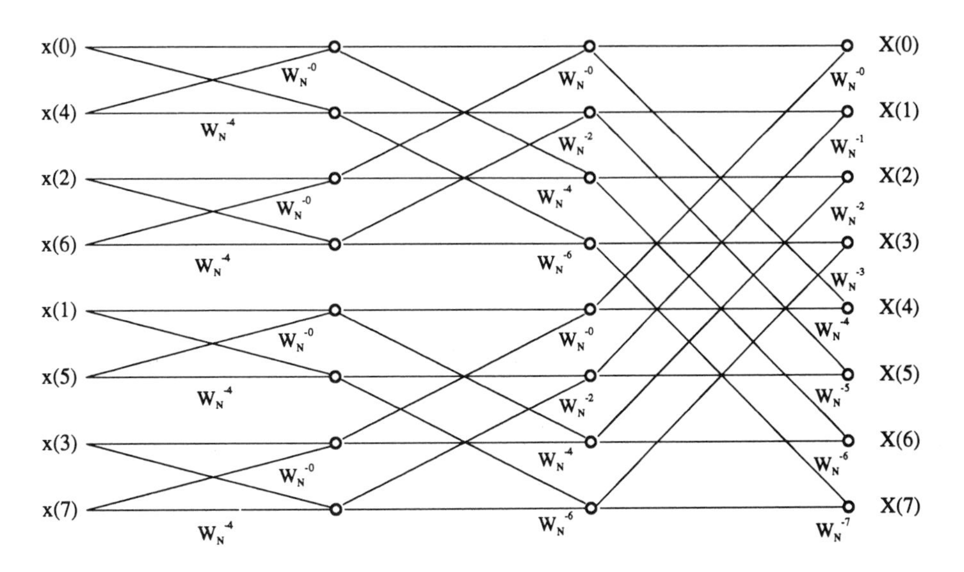

Figure 3.5.5: Eight-point radix-2 decimation-in-time FFT.

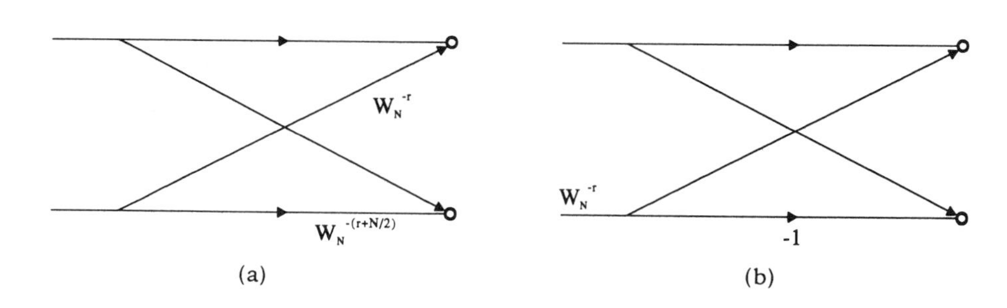

Figure 3.5.6: Simplifying the two-point FFT butterfly operation: (a) Original two-point butterfly; (b) simplified butterfly.

the butterfly in Fig. 3.5.6a can be replaced by the butterfly in Fig. 3.5.6b. The new butterfly requires only one multiplication. The eight-point FFT with the new butterfly structure is shown in Fig. 3.5.7. Notice that it consists of four 2-point DFTs at each stage, followed by four twiddle-factor multiplications. In general, we find that the overall multiplicative complexity has been reduced to

$$\frac{N}{2}\log_2 N$$

complex multiplications for the entire FFT.

Another radix-2 FFT algorithm is obtained if we perform the above derivation, but perform the sorting based on the harmonic index n rather than on the time index k. This algorithm is known as the radix-2 *decimation-in-frequency* algorithm. The decimation-in-frequency has the same computational complexity as the decimation-in-time algorithm and offers no particular advantages over the decimation-in-time algorithm. An eight-point radix-2 decimation-in-frequency FFT is shown in Fig. 3.5.8. Notice that the time series $x(k)$ appears at the left in normal and that the harmonics $X(n)$ now appear in bit-reversed order. As before, the computations can occur in-place.

There are transpositions of both the decimation-in-time and decimation-in-frequency algorithms which are capable of accepting the time series in unpermuted order and delivering the harmonics in unpermuted order. In-place computation is not possible with these rearrangements, so they are not as popular as their bit-reversed counterparts.

3.5.2 The Cooley-Tukey FFT

The Cooley-Tukey FFT is a generalization of the radix-2 and radix-4 FFTs. The Cooley-Tukey FFT allows us to decompose a DFT with composite blocklength into a collection

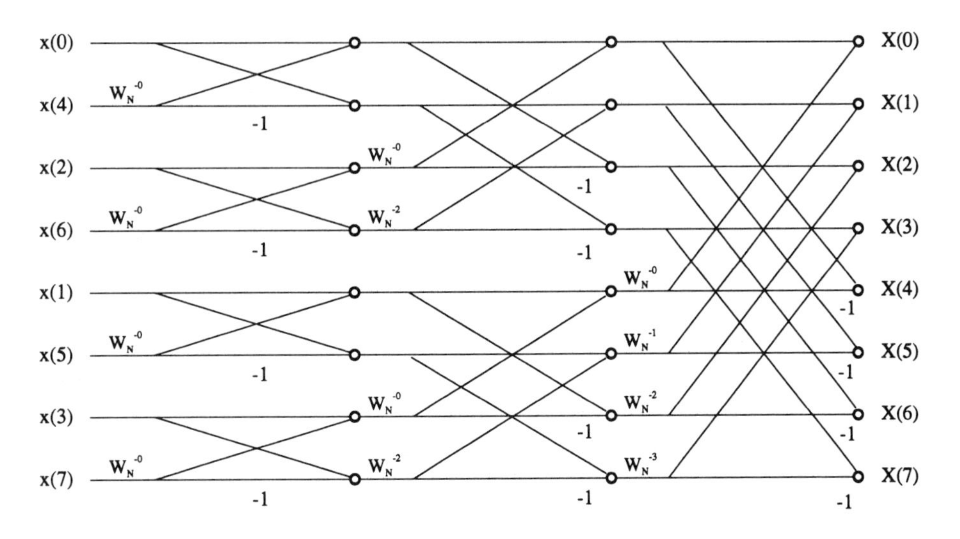

Figure 3.5.7: Simplified eight-point FFT.

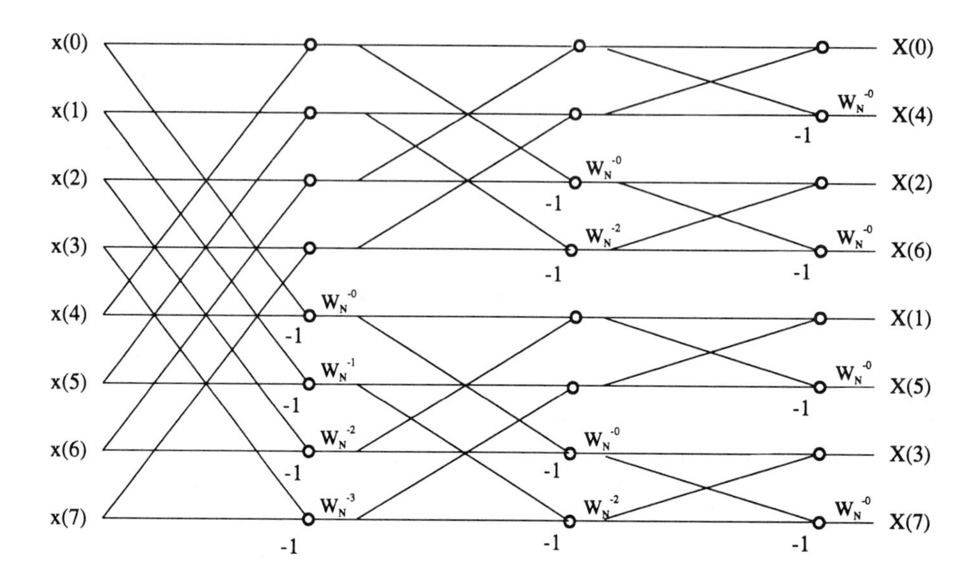

Figure 3.5.8: Eight-point radix-2 decimation-in-frequency FFT.

of smaller DFTs which are then pieced together with twiddle factors, much in the same manner we have seen already. Whereas the FFTs we have studied thusfar can be applied to blocklengths which are a power of two or four, the Cooley-Tukey FFT can be applied to any blocklength which is a composite number. Any of the FFTs which we have discussed can be obtained by repeated application of the Cooley-Tukey FFT.

Assume that $x(k)$ is a sequence of length N and N can be factored as

$$N = N_1 N_2.$$

Recall that the DFT of $x(k)$ is expressed as

$$X(n) = \sum_{k=0}^{N-1} x(k) W_N^{nk}.$$

The index k can be expressed by its remainder and quotient when divided by N_1 as

$$k = k_1 + N_1 k_2, \quad k_1 = 0, 1, \ldots, N_1 - 1 \quad \text{and} \quad k_2 = 0, 1, \ldots, N_2 - 1. \tag{3.5.1}$$

Similarly, we can express n by its remainder and quotient when divided by N_2 as

$$n = N_2 n_1 + n_2, \quad n_1 = 0, 1, \ldots, N_1 - 1 \quad \text{and} \quad n_2 = 0, 1, \ldots, N_2 - 1. \tag{3.5.2}$$

The sequence $x(k)$ can be regarded as a two-dimensional sequence $x(k_1, k_2)$ where

$$x(k_1, k_2) = x(k_1 + N_1 k_2)$$

and we can do the same for $X(n)$, where

$$X(n_1, n_2) = X(N_2 n_1 + n_2).$$

The sequences $x(k_1, k_2)$ and $X(n_1, n_2)$ are shown in Fig. 3.5.9 for the case $N = 15$ where $N_1 = 3, N_2 = 5$. This procedure is known as *index shuffling*.

The DFT can be written as

$$X(n_1, n_2) = \sum_{k_1=0}^{N_1-1} \sum_{k_2=0}^{N_2-1} x(k_1, k_2) W_N^{nk}.$$

According to Eqs. 3.5.1 and 3.5.2,

$$nk = N_2 n_1 k_1 + N_1 k_2 n_2 + N_1 N_2 n_1 k_1 + n_2 k_1.$$

Using the fact that $N = N_1 N_2$, we have

$$W_N^{nk} = W_N^{N_2 n_1 k_1} W_N^{N_1 k_2 n_2} W_N^{N n_1 k_1} W_N^{n_2 k_1}.$$

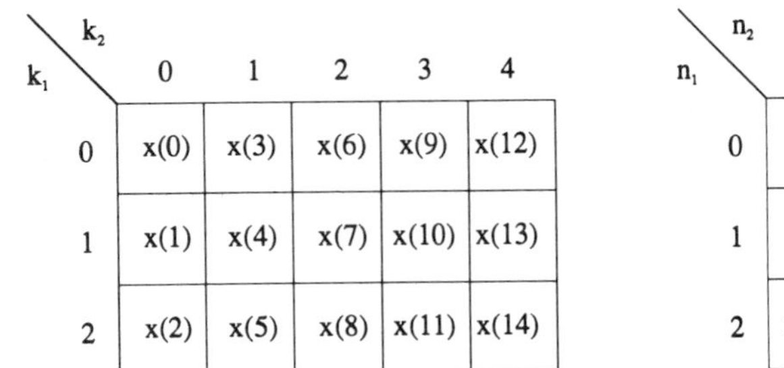

Figure 3.5.9: Index shuffling for Cooley-Tukey FFT when $N = 15$, $N_1 = 3$, $N_2 = 5$.

Also, $W_N^N = 1$, and we have the pair of relationships

$$W_N^{N_1} = W_{N_2} \quad \text{and} \quad W_N^{N_2} = W_{N_1}.$$

Therefore,

$$W_N^{nk} = W_{N_1}^{n_1 k_1} W_{N_2}^{k_2 n_2} W_N^{n_2 k_1}$$

and we can write the DFT as

$$X(n_1, n_2) = \sum_{k_1=0}^{N_1-1} W_{N_1}^{n_1 k_1} \left[W_N^{n_2 k_1} \sum_{k_2=0}^{N_2-1} x(k_1, k_2) W_{N_2}^{k_2 n_2}. \right].$$

Let's examine this equation in detail. The inner summation is an N_2-point DFT which is performed on the k_1-th row of the two-dimensional sequence $x(k_1, k_2)$. There are N_1 such DFTs, one for each n_1. Thus, a DFT is performed on each row of $x(k_1, k_2)$. This generates an intermediate array, $G(k_1, n_2)$. Next, the entire array is multiplied element-by-element by the twiddle factors $W_N^{k_1 n_2}$, giving the intermediate array $H(k_1, n_2)$. Finally, the outer summation is an N_1-point DFT on the n_1-th column of $H(k_1, n_2)$. There are N_2 such DFTs, one for each n_1. We are then left with the two-dimensional array $X(n_1, n_2)$, and the output DFT harmonics are extracted from the two-dimensional array $X(n_1, n_2)$ according to Eq. 3.5.2.

To analyze the computational complexity of the Cooley-Tukey FFT, each inner DFT requires $(N_2)^2$ multiplications for a total of $N_1(N_2)^2$ multiplications. Each outer DFT requires

$(N_1)^2$ multiplications for a total of $N_2(N_1)^2$ multiplications. Finally, there are $N_1N_2 = N$ twiddle factor multiplications so that the overall computational complexity of the Cooley-Tukey FFT is

$$N_1(N_2)^2 + N_2(N_1)^2 + N = N(N_1 + N_2 + 1)$$

complex multiplications. Even for moderate N, this can represent a substantial reduction in total multiplications.

Where the Cooley-Tukey FFT becomes truly powerful is when it is applied repeatedly to successively smaller blocklengths. For instance, when N is a power of two, we can decompose N as

$$N = 2 \cdot \frac{N}{2}$$

and apply the Cooley-Tukey FFT with $N_1 = 2$ and $N_2 = N/2$. The Cooley-Tukey FFT can be used to further decompose the $N/2$-point DFT into $N/4$-point and two-point DFTs, and so on until only two-point DFTs remain. This is how the radix-2 FFT can be obtained from the Cooley-Tukey FFT. It is interesting to note that the decimation-in-time algorithm results from the choice $N_1 = 2$ and the decimation-in-frequency algorithm is obtained if we take $N_1 = N/2$.

As another example of repeated application of the Cooley-Tukey FFT, suppose $N = 100$. The 100-point DFT can be decomposed into 25-point and 4-point DFTs. Each 25-point DFT can further be decomposed as a collection of 5-point DFTs. The four- and five-point DFTs can be implemented directly. This is shown schematically in Fig. 3.5.10.

A substantial reduction in multiplicative complexity results if the blocklength N is a power of four (or has a power of four as one of its divisors). In this case, the N-point DFT can be decomposed into many four-point DFTs. To see why this is advantageous, let's examine the expression for a four-point DFT. We have

$$X(n) = \sum_{k=0}^{3} x(k)W_4^{nk}.$$

Since

$$W_4 = j,$$

the four point DFT is given by

$$\begin{aligned} X(0) &= x(0) + x(1) + x(2) + x(3) \\ X(1) &= x(0) + jx(1) - x(2) - jx(3) \\ X(2) &= x(0) - x(1) + x(2) - x(3) \\ X(3) &= x(0) - jx(1) - x(2) + jx(3). \end{aligned}$$

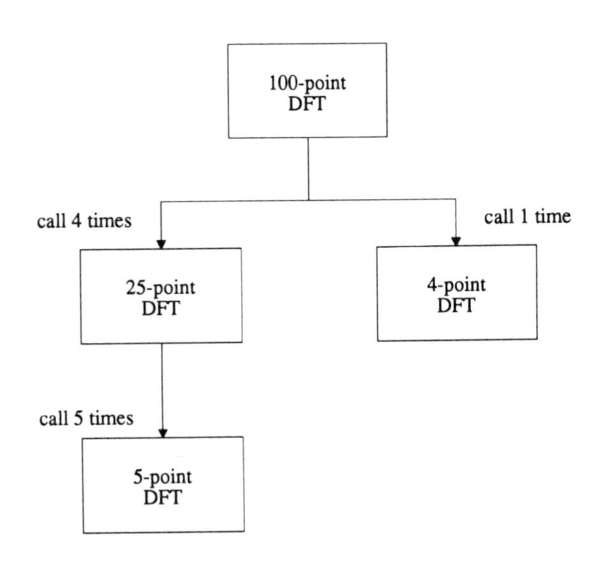

Figure 3.5.10: Using the Cooley-Tukey FFT to perform a 100-point DFT.

Notice that the only multiplications involved in the computation of the four-point DFT are by ± 1 and $\pm j$. These multiplications can be implemented purely by negation and by swapping real and imaginary parts. Therefore, the four-point DFTs which constitute the overall N-point DFT require *no multiplications* and the only multiplications required are by the twiddle factors. For the case where N is a power of four, this decomposition results in the *radix-4 FFT*.

3.5.3 The Chinese Remainder Theorem

The Chinese remainder theorem (CRT) [Bla85] is an ancient result from the theory of numbers which will is used as the basis of many fast algorithms for convolution and computing DFTs.

Recall that two integers m and n are called *congruent modulo* N if they have the same remainder when divided by N. This is denoted by

$$m \equiv n \bmod N \tag{3.5.3}$$

and is sometimes abbreviated by $m \equiv n$ when the reference to N is clear. If $m \equiv n$, it follows that

$$m - n = kN$$

for some integer k.

Given integers n and N, the division algorithm states that we can write

$$n = qN + r \tag{3.5.4}$$

where $0 \leq r \leq r - 1$. The integer q is called the quotient and the integer r is called the remainder. The remainder will always be taken as the least positive integer satisfying Eq. 3.5.4. According to Eq. 3.5.3, it follows that

$$n \equiv r \bmod N.$$

We will refer to the operation of extracting the remainder simply by "mod." Namely, by $n \bmod N$, we mean the least positive remainder, r, when n is divided by N.

The *multiplicative inverse* of m modulo N is defined as the integer n which satisfies

$$mn \equiv 1 \bmod N. \tag{3.5.5}$$

This means that

$$mn - 1 = kN \tag{3.5.6}$$

for some integer k. The multiplicative inverse of m modulo N will exist whenever m and N are *relatively prime*, meaning the greatest common divisor of m and N is 1. For example, the multiplicative inverse of 3 modulo 5 is 2 since

$$3 \cdot 2 \equiv 1 \bmod 5.$$

Consider the following problem. We have integers N_1 and N_2 and remainders r_1 and r_2. How can we determine the integer x such that r_1 and r_2 are the remainders when x is divided by N_1 and N_2, respectively? The solution is simple. Define the integers M_1 and M_2 by

$$M_1 N_2 \equiv 1 \bmod N_1 \tag{3.5.7}$$

and

$$M_2 N_1 \equiv 1 \bmod N_2. \tag{3.5.8}$$

The solution x is then computed by

$$x = (M_1 N_2 r_1 + M_2 N_1 r_2) \bmod N_1 N_2. \tag{3.5.9}$$

This method of reconstructing x from its remainders is known as the Chinese remainder theorem.

For example, consider the case $N_1 = 5$ and $N_2 = 7$. Suppose we have the remainders $r_1 = 2, r_2 = 3$. In this case, the solution x could probably be computed by brute force or by an educated guess, but the solution is more difficult for larger numbers. First, we need to solve Eq. 3.5.7 for M_1,

$$M_1 \cdot 7 \equiv 1 \bmod 5,$$

which gives

$$M_1 = 3.$$

Next, Eq. 3.5.8 is solved for M_2 as

$$M_2 \cdot 5 \equiv 1 \bmod 7,$$

which gives

$$M_2 = 3.$$

The solution x is then found using Eq. 3.5.9, giving

$$x = (3 \cdot 7 \cdot 2 + 3 \cdot 5 \cdot 3) \bmod 5 \cdot 7,$$

or

$$x = 87 \bmod 35 = 17,$$

which can be verified rather easily. It should be mentioned here that the Chinese remainder theorem can be used to find an integer from its remainders modulo *any number* of pairwise relatively prime integers, not just two as we have shown here.

3.5.4 The Good-Thomas FFT

The Good-Thomas FFT algorithm is a variation of the Cooley-Tukey FFT algorithm. This time, assume that the blocklength N can be factored as the product of two relatively prime integers N_1 and N_2. That is,

$$N = N_1 N_2, \quad gcd(N_1, N_2) = 1.$$

The key to the Good-Thomas algorithm is determining a pair of index mappings for k and n such that the twiddle factors vanish. Suppose the indices k_1 and k_2 are defined as the integers which satisfy

$$(N_2 k_1 + N_1 k_2) \bmod N = k. \tag{3.5.10}$$

Let's determine how to choose k_1 and k_2. According to the Chinese remainder theorem, k can be recovered from its residues modulo N_1 and N_2 according to

$$k = [M_1 N_2 (k \bmod N_1) + M_2 N_1 (k \bmod N_2)] \bmod N \tag{3.5.11}$$

where M_1 is the multiplicative inverse of N_2 modulo N_1 and M_2 is the multiplicative inverse of N_1 modulo N_2. Comparing Eqs. 3.5.10 and 3.5.11, we see that

$$k_1 = (M_1 k) \bmod N_1 \quad \text{and} \quad k_2 = (M_2 k) \bmod N_2. \tag{3.5.12}$$

Equation 3.5.12 explicitly indicates how to derive the two-dimensional indices k_1 and k_2 from the one-dimensional index k.

Next, consider the harmonic index n. Assume that n_1 and n_2 are defined as the integers which satisfy

$$(M_1 N_2 n_1 + M_2 N_1 n_2) \bmod N = n \tag{3.5.13}$$

where M_1 and M_2 are defined as before. Comparing Eqs. 3.5.13 and 3.5.11 (substituting n for k) that n_1 and n_2 are simply given by

$$n_1 = n \bmod N_1, \quad \text{and} \quad n_2 = n \bmod N_2. \tag{3.5.14}$$

Consider the case where $N = 15$, $N_1 = 3$, and $N_2 = 5$. The parameters for the Chinese remainder theorem are

$$M_1 = (N_2)^{-1} \bmod N_1 = (5)^{-1} \bmod 3 = 2$$

and

$$M_2 = (N_1)^{-1} \bmod N_2 = (3)^{-1} \bmod 5 = 2.$$

The index mappings for the input index k are given by

$$k_1 = (M_1 k) \bmod N_1 = (2k) \bmod 3$$

and

$$k_2 = (M_2 k) \bmod N_2 = (2k) \bmod 3.$$

The index mappings for the harmonic index n are

$$n_1 = n \bmod 3$$

k_1 \ k_2	0	1	2	3	4
0	x(0)	x(3)	x(6)	x(9)	x(12)
1	x(5)	x(8)	x(11)	x(14)	x(2)
2	x(10)	x(13)	x(1)	x(4)	x(7)

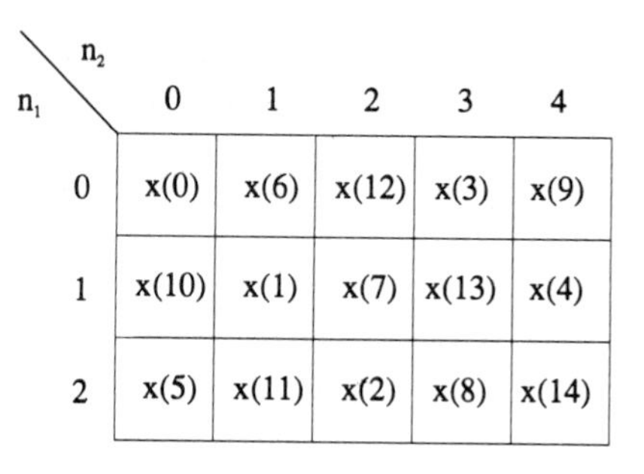

n_1 \ n_2	0	1	2	3	4
0	x(0)	x(6)	x(12)	x(3)	x(9)
1	x(10)	x(1)	x(7)	x(13)	x(4)
2	x(5)	x(11)	x(2)	x(8)	x(14)

Figure 3.5.11: Good-Thomas index mappings for $N_1 = 3$, $N_2 = 5$.

and

$$n_2 = n \bmod 5.$$

The index mappings may be viewed as mappings from a one-dimensional sequence to a two-dimensional sequence. Figure 3.5.11 shows the index mappings for this particular case.

At this point, the reader may be wondering why we have developed this somewhat confusing pair of index mappings. The reason becomes clear if we examine the resulting DFT. Beginning with the definition

$$X(n) = \sum_{k=0}^{N-1} x(k) W_N^{nk},$$

substitute Eqs. 3.5.11 and 3.5.13 for n and k, resulting in

$$X(< M_1 N_2 n_1 + M_2 N_1 n_2 >_N) = \sum_{k_1=0}^{N_1-1} \sum_{k_2=0}^{N_2-1} x(< N_2 k_1 + N_1 k_2 >_N)\ W_N^{<(M_1 N_2 n_1 + M_2 N_1 n_2)(N_2 k_1 + N_1 k_2)>_N} \tag{3.5.15}$$

where we have used the notation $< \cdot >_N$ to denote reduction modulo N. Examining the exponent to which W_N is raised in Eq. 3.5.15, we see that

$$(M_1 N_2 n_1 + M_2 N_1 n_2)(N_2 k_1 + N_1 k_2) = M_1 (N_2)^2 n_1 k_1 + M_2 (N_1)^2 n_2 k_2 + M_2 N_1 N_2 n_2 k_1 + M_1 N_2 N_1 n_1 k_2. \tag{3.5.16}$$

The last two terms on the right-hand side of Eq. 3.5.16 are multiples of N since $N = N_1 N_2$, and hence vanish when reduced modulo N. Therefore,

$$< (M_1 N_2 n_1 + M_2 N_1 n_2)(N_2 k_1 + N_1 k_2) >_N = < M_1 (N_2)^2 n_1 k_1 + M_2 (N_1)^2 n_2 k_2 >_N \quad (3.5.17)$$

Also, since $M_1 = (N_2)^{-1} \bmod N_1$ and $M_2 = (N_1)^{-1} \bmod N_2$, Eq. 3.5.17 simplifies to

$$< (M_1 N_2 n_1 + M_2 N_1 n_2)(N_2 k_1 + N_1 k_2) >_N = < N_2 n_1 k_1 + N_1 n_2 k_2 >_N . \quad (3.5.18)$$

Finally, if we make the identifications

$$x(k_1, k_2) = x(< N_2 k_1 + N_1 k_2 >_N)$$

and

$$X(n_1, n_2) = X(< M_1 N_2 n_1 + M_2 N_1 n_2 >_N)$$

and substitute Eq. 3.5.18 into Eq. 3.5.15, we get

$$X(n_1, n_2) = \sum_{k_1=0}^{N_1-1} \sum_{k_2=0}^{N_2-1} x(k_1, k_2) W_N^{N_2 n_1 k_1} W_N^{N_1 n_2 k_2}. \quad (3.5.19)$$

Notice that $W_N^{N_1} = W_{N_2}$ and $W_N^{N_2} = W_{N_1}$. Therefore, the DFT can be expressed as

$$X(n_1, n_2) = \sum_{k_1=0}^{N_1-1} \sum_{k_2=0}^{N_2-1} x(k_1, k_2) W_{N_1}^{n_1 k_1} W_{N_2}^{n_2 k_2}. \quad (3.5.20)$$

Equation 3.5.20 is similar to the Cooley-Tukey FFT with the crucial difference being the absence of the twiddle factors. The only additional expense is in the complicated index mappings.

In practice, the input sequence $\{x(k)\}$ is mapped to the two-dimensional sequence $\{x(k_1, k_2)\}$ where k_1 and k_2 are as defined in Eq. 3.5.12. Next, a DFT is performed on each row of $\{x(k_1, k_2)\}$, giving the intermediate sequence $\{G(k_1, n_2)\}$. DFTs are then performed on the columns of $\{G(k_1, n_2)\}$ giving the two-dimensional sequence $\{X(n_1, n_2)\}$. Finally, the elements $X(n)$ are extracted from the two-dimensional sequence $\{X(n_1, n_2)\}$ by way of the index mapping in Eq. 3.5.13. The saving in complexity over the Cooley-Tukey FFT is N less multiplications due to the disappearance of the twiddle factors. As with the Cooley-Tukey FFT, the Good-Thomas FFT can be nested several levels deep, provided that the blocklengths at each stage are relatively prime.

3.5.5 Final Notes on the FFT

The DFT in its general form is used to transform a complex time series in to a complex collection of harmonics. When the time series is real, significant savings in computation can be made. For instance, the DFTs of two real sequences can be obtained simultaneously using a single complex DFT. To show this, let $x(k)$ and $y(k)$ be real N-point sequences and form the complex sequence $z(k)$ as

$$z(k) = x(k) + jy(k).$$

It follows that

$$Z(n) = X(n) + jY(n),$$

but because both $X(n)$ and $Y(n)$ will be complex in general, it is difficult to determine from $Z(n)$ which part belongs to $X(n)$ and which belongs to $Y(n)$. Recall, however, that

$$z^*(k) \overset{DFT}{\longleftrightarrow} Z^*(-n \bmod N)$$

where

$$Z^*(-n \bmod N) = X^*(-n \bmod N) - jY^*(-n \bmod N).$$

Because $x(k)$ and $y(k)$ are real, we have $X^*(-n \bmod N) = X(n)$ and likewise for $Y(n)$ (from Table 3.3.1) so that

$$Z^*(-n \bmod N) = X(n) - jY(n).$$

Thus,

$$X(n) = \frac{Z(n) + Z^*(-n \bmod N)}{2}$$

and

$$Y(n) = \frac{Z(n) - Z^*(-n \bmod N)}{2j}$$

and we have found the DFTs of the real sequences $x(k)$ and $y(k)$.

Similarly, suppose $\{x(k)\}$ is a real sequence of length $2N$. From $\{x(k)\}$, form the two real length-N sequences $\{a(k)\}$ and $\{b(k)\}$ where

$$a(k) = x(2k) \quad \text{and} \quad b(k) = x(2k+1), \quad k = 0, 1, \ldots, N-1.$$

Now, form the complex time series $\{c(k)\}$ as

$$c(k) = a(k) + jb(k), \quad k = 0, 1, \ldots, N-1.$$

Next, the DFT of $\{c(k)\}$ gives $\{C(n)\}$ and the constituent DFTs $\{A(n)\}$ and $\{B(n)\}$ are found as above according to

$$A(n) = \frac{C(n) + C^*(-n \bmod N)}{2}$$

and

$$B(n) = \frac{C(n) - C^*(-n \bmod N)}{2j}.$$

Finally, it is simple to show that the $2N$-point DFT $\{X(n)\}$ can be obtained from $\{A(n)\}$ and $\{B(n)\}$ by

$$X(n) = A(n) + W_{2N}^{-n} B(n), \quad n = 0, 1, \ldots, N-1$$

and

$$X(n+N) = A(n) - W_{2N}^{-n} B(n), \quad n = 0, 1, \ldots, N-1.$$

Even with this additional stage of butterfly operations, a substantial reduction in complexity is achieved. Direct evaluation of the length-$2N$ DFT requires $2N \log_2(2N)$ multiplications, whereas this approach requires $N + N \log_2 N$ multiplications, which represents a 50% savings.

It should be mentioned that FFT algorithms can be used for computing both the DFT and the inverse DFT. Structurally, the equations are nearly identical. The DFT is given by

$$X(n) = \sum_{i=0}^{N-1} x(k) W_N^{nk}$$

and the IDFT is given by

$$x(k) = \frac{1}{N} X(n) W_N^{-nk}.$$

In matrix form, the DFT was represented as

$$\boldsymbol{X} = \boldsymbol{V}\boldsymbol{x}$$

and we have seen that the IDFT can be represented as

$$\boldsymbol{x} = \frac{1}{N} \boldsymbol{V}^H \boldsymbol{X}.$$

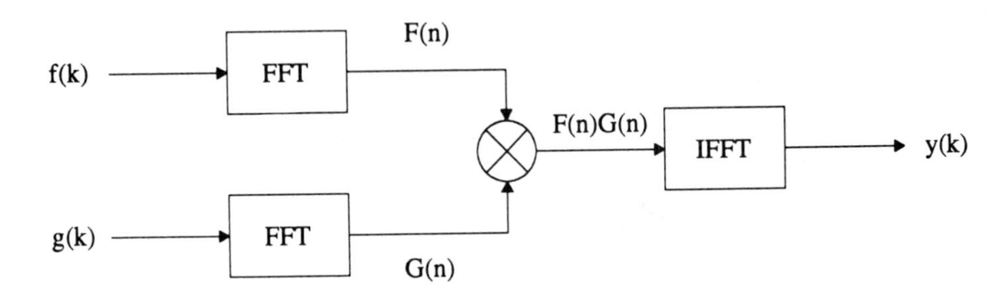

Figure 3.5.12: Using the FFT to compute linear convolution.

Thus, and algorithm for computing the DFT can be used to compute the IDFT by first replacing $\boldsymbol{V}$ by $\boldsymbol{V}^H$, using the DFT algorithm to compute $\boldsymbol{V}^H\boldsymbol{X}$, and then dividing by N. Since the i,l-th element of $\boldsymbol{V}$ is given by

$$[\boldsymbol{V}]_{i,l} = W_N^{il},$$

the i,l-th element of $\boldsymbol{V}^H$ is simply given by

$$[\boldsymbol{V}^H]_{i,l} = W_N^{-il},$$

which is just the complex conjugate of $[\boldsymbol{V}]_{il}$. Therefore, for an algorithm such as the radix-2 FFT, the IFFT can be computed by complex-conjugating the twiddle factors, performing the FFT, and dividing by N.

Finally, we earlier alluded to the idea that the FFT could be used for efficient linear convolution. To crystallize this notion, suppose $\boldsymbol{f}$ and $\boldsymbol{g}$ are sequences of length M and N, respectively. Since the product of the DFTs $F(n)G(n)$ is the DFT of the cyclic convolution $\boldsymbol{f} \otimes \boldsymbol{g}$ and we have linear convolution can be performed using cyclic convolution, we can use the FFT to compute linear convolution. This is done by zero-padding $\boldsymbol{f}$ and $\boldsymbol{g}$ to *at least* length $M + N - 1$. The minimum length is dictated by the blocklength necessary to use the FFT of choice. For example, to use the radix-2 FFT, the length needs to be taken as a power of two which is greater than or equal to $N + M - 1$. The product $F(n)G(n)$ is then computed, and the inverse FFT computed. This is shown in Fig. 3.5.12.

To assess the potential savings in complexity, assume that $\boldsymbol{f}$ and $\boldsymbol{g}$ are complex and of length N where N is already a power of 2. Then direct linear convolution requires $M_{conv} = N^2$ complex multiplications. Instead, zero-pad both sequences to length $2N$ and compute $F(n)$ and $G(n)$ using the radix-2 FFT. Each FFT will require $N\log_2(2N)$ complex multiplications for a total of $2N\log_2(2N)$. Multiplying $F(n)G(N)$ requires N complex multiplications, and the inverse FFT of $F(n)G(n)$ requires an additional $N\log_2(2N)$ complex multiplications. Therefore, the overall computation requires

$$M_{FFT} = 3N\log_2(2N) + N$$

complex multiplications. For large N, the ratio M_{FFT}/M_{conv} is approximately equal to

$$M_{FFT}/M_{conv} = \frac{3\log_2(2N)}{N}.$$

For even modest N, the savings can be substantial. For example, for $N = 1024$, the FFT method requires roughly three percent of the number of multiplications used by the direct method.

Chapter 4

DIGITAL FILTER DESIGN

4.1 Infinite Impulse Response Filters

There are several techniques for designing infinite impulse response (IIR) digital filters. The two basic design methodologies are frequency-domain methods and time-domain methods. Frequency-domain methods typically consist of specifying a magnitude frequency profile and then using polynomial approximation techniques to approximate the desired profile in the frequency domain. Time-domain methods are concerned with determining z-domain transfer functions which approximate a desired impulse response. The most popular IIR design techniques are the frequency-domain methods. Accordingly, we will devote most of our discussion to these techniques.

The first step in a discussion of frequency-domain IIR design is a review of analog filter design. The reason for this is that there are several methods for mapping an analog filter to a discrete-time IIR filter. Depending on the type of mapping, salient characteristics of the analog frequency response can be preserved in the discrete-time domain.

4.2 Classical Analog Filter Design

The first technique for IIR filter design we will study is based on the mapping of classical analog filters. The reason for this is simple. The field of analog filter design is very old and very well developed. Consequently, there exists a wide collection of analog filters which are capable of meeting a desired frequency response profile. The analog prototype mapping paradigm is explained as follows. Given a set of filter specifications, typically defined as a collection of break frequencies and a piecewise constant magnitude profile, a classical analog filter is first derived which meets these specifications. Next, a mapping is made from the analog filter to the desired digital filter. We will study both these classical analog filters and mapping techniques in detail.

Recall that the s-domain description of an analog filter is given by

$$H(s) = \frac{b_0 s^M + b_{M-1}s^{M-1} + \cdots + b_1 s + b_0}{s^N + a_{N-1}s^{N-1} + \cdots + a_1 s + a_0},$$

where $M \leq N$ to prevent poles at infinity. The magnitude of $H(s)$ along the $j\omega$-axis describes the magnitude frequency response of the analog filter, $|H(j\omega)|$.

The analog *lowpass* filter is the most important magnitude profile we will need to examine in detail. This is because other magnitude profiles can be derived by appropriate transformations of the lowpass filter. Thus, the problem which must be considered is the *approximation* of a desired lowpass magnitude profile by some appropriate approximation technique. This approximation consists of determining a rational function $H(s)$ which, when evaluated along the $j\omega$-axis, has a magnitude which approximates the desired magnitude response. These approximations are typically one of three types: Butterworth, Elliptic, or Chebyshev. Since analog filter design is well-documented and a detailed discussion of analog filter approximations would take us too far afield, we will only give an in-depth discussion of the Butterworth filter.

The desired magnitude profile of a lowpass filter consists of three frequency regions: the *passband*, the *transition band*, and the *stopband*. Ideally, the magnitude response should be unity in the passband and zero in the stopband. As the name implies, the magnitude makes the transition from unity to zero in the transition band. Since we will be approximating the desired magnitude profile, we need to bound the approximation error. That is, we need to specify a maximum acceptable deviation from unity in the passband and a maximum acceptable deviation from zero in the stopband. With the passband defined as the frequency range $0 \leq \omega \leq \omega_c$ and the stopband defined as the frequency range $\omega \geq \omega_r$, we have the set of conditions

$$1 - \delta_1 \leq |H(j\omega)| \leq 1, \quad 0 \leq \omega \leq \omega_c$$

and

$$|H(j\omega)| \leq \delta_2, \quad \omega_r \leq \omega.$$

The response is left unspecified in the transition band, which consists of the frequency range $[\omega_c, \omega_r]$. Fig. 4.2.1 gives a graphical depiction of the lowpass specifications. We can now describe each approximation in detail.

The prototypical analog filter we will consider is the lowpass filter. The lowpass filter is the starting point from which other magnitude characteristics can be derived. We will see that highpass, bandpass, and bandstop filters can be obtained very simply from the lowpass filter. For each approximation technique we will consider, it will be assumed that the cutoff frequency is normalized to $\omega_c = 1$. This is because there are frequency transformation

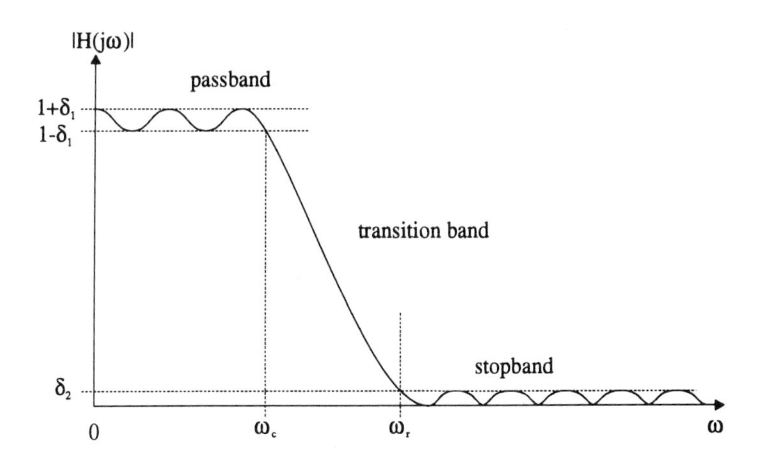

Figure 4.2.1: Analog lowpass filter magnitude specification.

techniques which allow a lowpass filter to be designed with a cutoff frequency of $\omega_c = 1$ and translated to the desired cutoff frequency. These frequency transformations are simple algebraic substitution rules.

4.2.1 Butterworth Approximation

The magnitude squared response of a Butterworth filter is given by

$$|H(j\omega)|^2 = \frac{1}{1+\omega^{2N}}. \tag{4.2.1}$$

Notice that $|H(0)|^2 = 1$ and that $|H(j1)|^2 = 0.5$. Thus, the gain at $\omega = 1$ is -3 dB. The dependence of the magnitude on N is shown in Fig 4.2.2. Notice that the gain at dc is independent of the order N as is the gain at $\omega = 1$. As N increases, the steepness of the transition band increases.

It is easily shown that the first $2N-1$ derivatives of the Butterworth magnitude response are equal to zero at dc. This is a property known as *maximal flatness.* The passband of a Butterworth is extremely flat and deviates very little from unity for low frequencies. Furthermore, the Butterworth magnitude response is monotonically decreasing and approaches zeros as ω approaches infinity.

In order to determine the poles and zeros of the Butterworth filter, the magnitude can be rewritten as

$$|H(j\omega)|^2 = H(j\omega)H^*(j\omega),$$

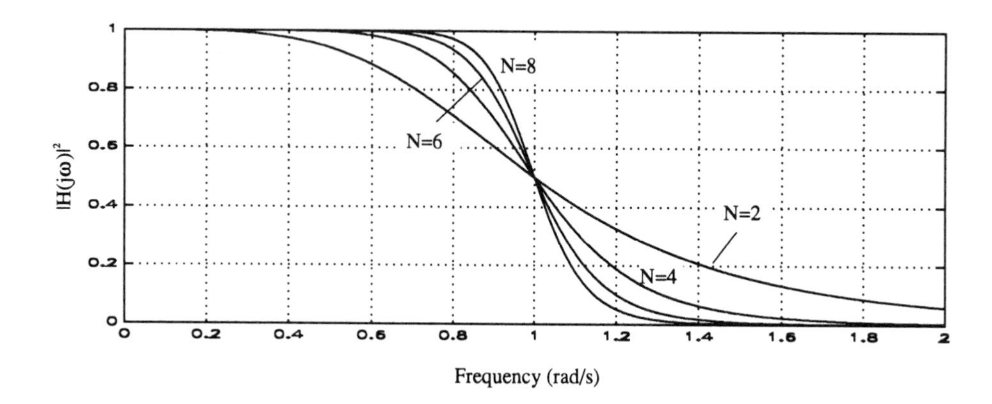

Figure 4.2.2: Magnitude squared Butterworth response for several values of N.

and since $h_c(t)$ is assumed to be real, it follows that

$$H^*(j\omega) = H(-j\omega).$$

Thus,

$$|H(j\omega)|^2 = H(s)H(-s)|_{s=j\omega} . \tag{4.2.2}$$

Therefore, the transfer function of the Butterworth filter must satisfy

$$H(s)H(-s) = \frac{1}{1 + (-js)^{2N}} \tag{4.2.3}$$

The analog Butterworth filter thus has no zeros. To obtain the poles, we must find the roots of the denominator above. These roots satisfy

$$1 + (-js)^{2N} = 0,$$

which can be rewritten as

$$1 + (-1)^N s^{2N} = 0.$$

For N odd, this reduces to

$$s^{2N} = 1,$$

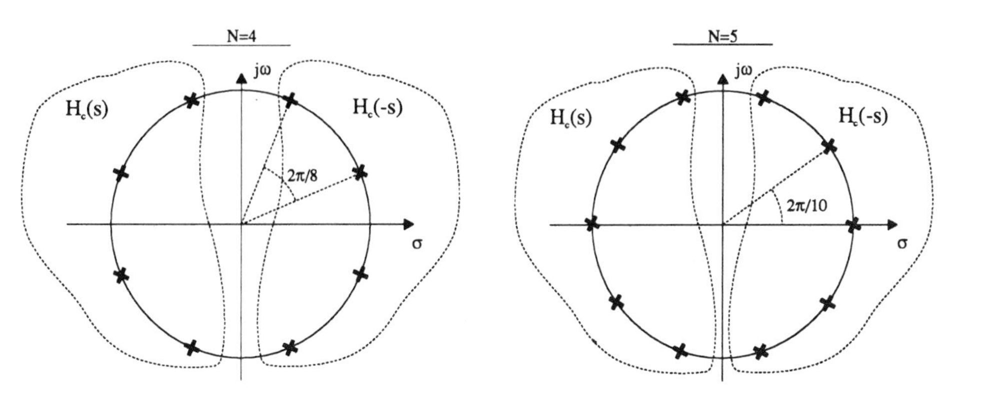

Figure 4.2.3: Pole locations of $H(s)H(-s)$ for a Butterworth filter.

which has roots

$$s_k = e^{jk\pi/N}, \quad k = 0, 1, \ldots, 2N-1. \tag{4.2.4}$$

For N even, the poles are given by the solutions to

$$s^{2N} = -1,$$

which gives

$$s_k = e^{j(2k+1)\pi/2N}, \quad k = 0, 1, \ldots, 2N-1. \tag{4.2.5}$$

It can be seen that the $2N$ poles are distributed along the periphery of the unit circle in the s-plane with an angular spacing of π/N between poles. For odd N, there will be poles on the real axis, but not for even N. It is also simple to show using Eqs. 4.2.4 and 4.2.5 that no poles will ever fall on the imaginary axis. The pole distributions for even and odd N are shown in Fig. 4.2.3.

The question now remains as to which poles belong to $H(s)$ and which belong to $H(-s)$. The solution is simple: because the filter is assumed to be stable, the poles in the left-half plane belong to $H(s)$ and the poles in the right-half plane belong to $H(-s)$.

Example 4.1

For $N = 2$, we find from Eq. 4.2.5 that the pole locations of $H(s)H(-s)$ are

$$e^{j\pi/4}, \quad e^{j3\pi/4}, \quad e^{j5\pi/4}, \quad e^{j7\pi/4}.$$

The left-half plane poles are located at $e^{j3\pi/4}$ and $e^{j5\pi/4}$ so that

$$H(s) = \frac{1}{(s - e^{j3\pi/4})(s - e^{j5\pi/4})} = \frac{1}{s^2 + \sqrt{2}s + 1}.$$

The next consideration in designing a lowpass Butterworth filter is determining the appropriate order, N. We wish to choose N so that the desired magnitude profile is met with the understanding that N should be the *minimum* such value. This is because filter order translates into complexity and throughput.

Assume that we require the magnitude-squared at ω_a to be smaller than δ_2^2. Then we seek the value of N such that

$$\delta_2^2 = \frac{1}{1 + \omega_a^{2N}}.$$

This means that

$$\frac{1}{\delta_2^2} - 1 = \omega_a^{2N}$$

so that

$$\log_{10}(1/\delta_2^2 - 1) = 2N \log_{10}(\omega_a).$$

Solving for N, we get

$$N = \frac{\log_{10}(1/\delta_2^2 - 1)}{2\log_{10}(\omega_a)}. \tag{4.2.6}$$

Eq. 4.2.6 gives the exact value of N for which the magnitude-squared response is equal to δ_2^2 at $\omega = \omega_a$. Typically, this value of N will not be an integer so that we will need to round to the next-highest integer. In this case, the filtering requirements will be slightly exceeded.

Example 4.2

Suppose it is required that a Butterworth filter have a cutoff frequency of $w_c = 1$ and we want to have the magnitude-squared equal to 0.01 or less when $w_a = 2$. It is thus seen that

$$\delta_2^2 = 0.01$$

so that using Eq. 4.2.6, we find

$$N = \frac{\log_{10}(100 - 1)}{2\log_{10} 2} = 3.31.$$

Thus, we choose $N = 4$, which gives a magnitude-squared at ω_a equal to

$$|H(j\omega_a)|^2 = \frac{1}{1 + 2^8} \approx .004,$$

or - 24 dB.

4.2.2 Chebyshev Approximation

The Butterworth filter had the characteristic that it was maximally flat in the passband and monotonically decreasing over all frequencies. One drawback of the Butterworth filter is the need for relatively high order, N, to meet a given transition band steepness. By relaxing the requirements of monotonicity and maximal flatness, lower order filters can result. One such filter is the *Chebyshev* filter, which is based on the use of Chebyshev polynomials to meet a desired magnitude profile.

The magnitude-squared of a Chebyshev filter is described by

$$|H(j\omega)|^2 = \frac{1}{1+\epsilon^2 C_N^2(\omega)} \tag{4.2.7}$$

where $C_N(\omega)$ is the N-th Chebyshev polynomial, given by

$$C_N(\omega) = \cos(N\cos^{-1}(\omega)).$$

Recall that the arc-cosine function will produce an imaginary value for arguments which are greater than unity in magnitude. Therefore, we can define $C_N(\omega)$ over two ranges as

$$C_N(\omega) = \begin{cases} \cos(N\cos^{-1}(\omega)), & 0 \le \omega \le 1 \\ \cosh(N\cosh^{-1}(\omega)), & \omega > 1. \end{cases} \tag{4.2.8}$$

The magnitude-squared of a Chebyshev filter is shown in Fig. 4.2.4. Notice that the response is equiripple present over the range $0 \le \omega \le 1$. This is known as the *ripple passband*, and the amount of ripple is controlled by the parameter ϵ. For frequencies greater than one, the response is monotonically decreasing.

The Chebyshev polynomials are defined recursively. It is simple to see that

$$C_0(\omega) = \cos(0 \cdot \cos^{-1}(\omega)) = 1$$

and

$$C_1(\omega) = \cos(1 \cdot \cos^{-1}(\omega)) = \omega.$$

The remaining Chebyshev polynomials are determined by the recursion relation

$$C_{N+1}(\omega) = 2\omega C_N(\omega) - C_{N-1}(\omega).$$

For instance, we can generate $C_2(\omega)$ as

$$C_2(\omega) = 2\omega C_1(\omega) - C_0(\omega) = 2\omega^2 - 1.$$

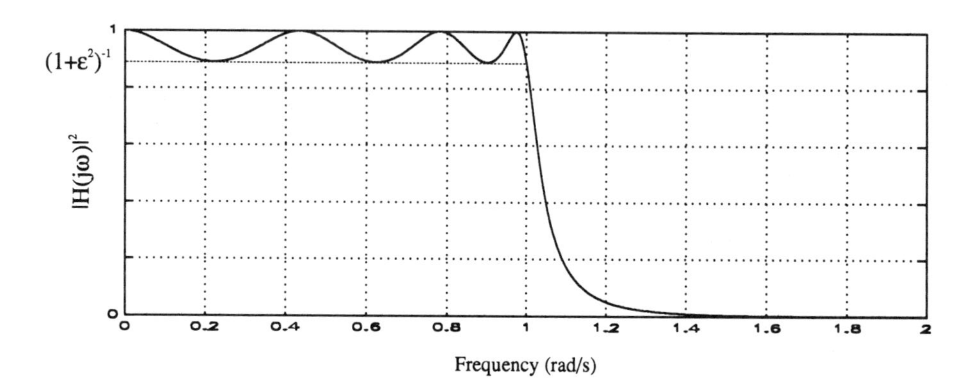

Figure 4.2.4: Chebyshev magnitude-squared response.

Because of the relation $C_N^2(\omega) = \cos^2(N\cos^{-1}(\omega))$, it follows that for N odd we have $C_N^2(0) = 0$ and that for N even we have $C_N^2(0) = 1$. Referring to Eq. 4.2.7, it then follows that

$$|H(j0)|^2 = 1, \quad N \text{ odd} \tag{4.2.9}$$

and

$$|H(j0)|^2 = \frac{1}{1+\epsilon^2}, \quad N \text{ even} . \tag{4.2.10}$$

Also, $C_N^2(1) = \cos^2(N\cos^{-1}(1)) = 1$ for all N which means that

$$|H(j1)|^2 = \frac{1}{1+\epsilon^2} \quad \text{for all } N. \tag{4.2.11}$$

Thus, ϵ can be related to the maximum allowable passband ripple δ_1. Referring to Fig. 4.2.4 and Eq. 4.2.11,

$$|H(j1)| = \frac{1}{\sqrt{1+\epsilon^2}} = 1 - \delta_1.$$

Epsilon is then chosen to meet or exceed

$$\epsilon^2 = \frac{1}{(1-\delta_1^2)} - 1. \tag{4.2.12}$$

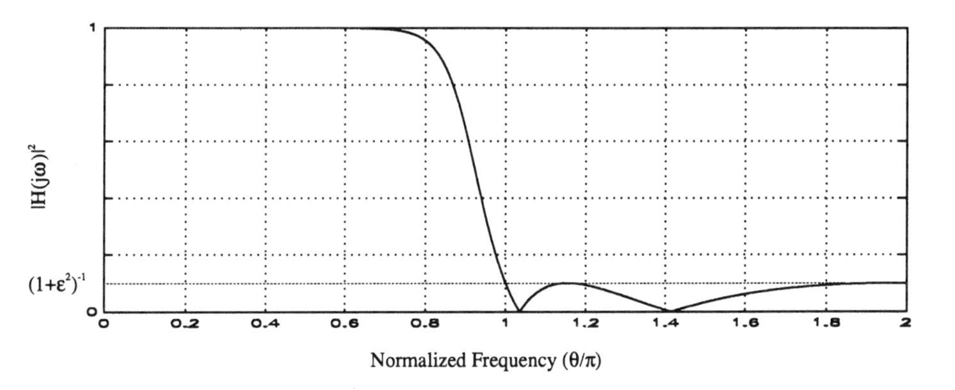

Figure 4.2.5: Magnitude-squared response of a Chebyshev-II lowpass filter.

It is simple to see from Eq. 4.2.7 that the Chebyshev filter has no zeros. In fact, it can be shown that the Chebyshev filter is capable of producing the steepest transition band among the class of filters which have rational transfer functions and *no* zeros.

A second type of Chebyshev filter is known as the *inverse Chebyshev filter*. The inverse Chebyshev filter differs from the Chebyshev filter in that it has a maximally flat passband and an equiripple stopband (see Fig. 4.2.5). It is common to refer to the Chebyshev filter as the *Chebyshev-I* filter and the inverse Chebyshev filter as the *Chebyshev II* filter; this is the convention we will adapt henceforth.

The magnitude-squared function for the Chebyshev-II lowpass filter with cutoff frequency equal to one is given by

$$|H(j\omega)|^2 = \frac{1}{1 + [\epsilon^2 C_N^2(\omega_a/\omega)]^{-1}} \tag{4.2.13}$$

where ω_a is the desired stopband frequency. Because of the term $[C_N^2(\omega_a/\omega)]^{-1}$ in the denominator of Eq. 4.2.13, the Chebyshev-II filter will have zeros as well as poles. At the stopband frequency ω_a, the magnitude-squared response is equal to $(1 + \epsilon^{-2})^{-1}$, which is equal to the magnitude of the stopband ripple. The Chebyshev-II filter is useful in applications where a flat passband is important, yet the order of the required Butterworth filter is too high.

4.2.3 Elliptic Approximation

We have seen that the Chebyshev I and II filters are capable of a steeper transition band than the Butterworth filter for a fixed order, N. The Butterworth filter is useful because it has a maximally flat passband and a monotonically decreasing stopband. The drawback of the Butterworth filter is the high order, N, which is needed to meet a given magnitude profile. The Chebyshev-I filter was optimal in the sense that it is capable of the steepest transition among the class of all-pole filters. The Chebyshev-II filter was seen to have a maximally flat passband and an equiripple stopband. If we are willing to allow ripple in both the passband and the stopband, it is possible to obtain an even steeper transition band. This is the idea behind the elliptic filter.

The elliptic filter possesses both poles and zeros and can be shown to be capable of realizing the steepest possible transition among the class of all rational transfer functions. The magnitude-squared function of the Elliptic lowpass filter with unity cutoff frequency is given by

$$|H(j\omega)|^2 = \frac{1}{1+\epsilon^2 U_N(\omega)}$$

where $U_N(x)$ is the N-th Jacobian elliptic function and ϵ is related to the passband ripple. The elliptic functions U_N have been extensively tabulated and there are many computer programs available to compute them.

Given maximum allowable passband and stopband ripples, δ_1 and δ_2, and stopband frequency ω_a, the order of the elliptic filter which meets these requirements is given by

$$N = \frac{K(1/\omega_a)K(\sqrt{1-\delta_2^2(1+\epsilon^2)}/\sqrt{1-\delta_2^2})}{K(\epsilon\delta_2/\sqrt{1-\delta_2^2})K(\sqrt{1-(1/\omega_a)^2})}$$

where the passband ripple is equal to $1+\epsilon^2$ and the function $K(x)$ is the complete elliptic integral of the first kind, given by

$$K(x) = \int_0^{\pi/2} \frac{d\theta}{\sqrt{1-x^2\sin^2\theta}}.$$

A detailed discussion of the elliptic filter is beyond the scope of this book, but suffice it to say that most commercially available filter design packages support elliptic filter design.

The magnitude response of an elliptic lowpass filter is shown in Fig. 4.2.6.

4.3 Analog Frequency Transformations

So far, we have only discussed how to design lowpass filters with unity cutoff frequency. We will now show how to design lowpass, highpass, bandpass, and bandstop filters with arbitrary

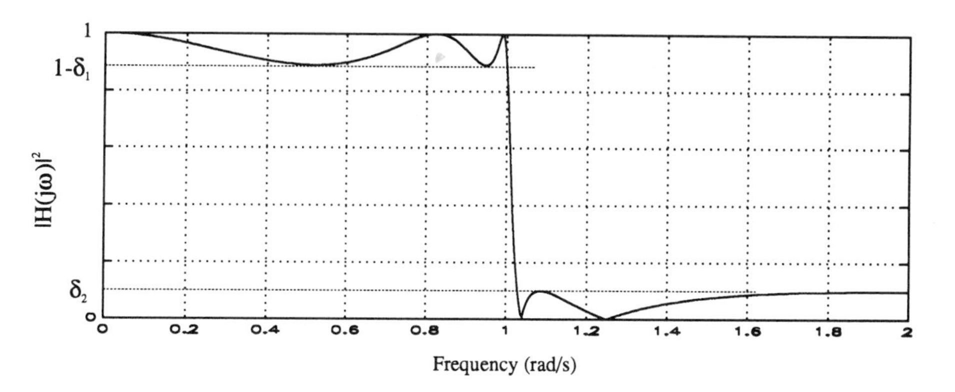

Figure 4.2.6: Elliptic lowpass filter magnitude-squared response.

band edges. It is assumed that we have an analog lowpass filter $H(s')$ with cutoff frequency $\omega_c' = 1$. This $H(s')$ is known as the *prototype lowpass filter.* The basic idea behind analog frequency transformations is to begin with this prototype lowpass filter $H(s')$. Assume we have some mapping f which maps the s plane to the s' plane, where

$$s' = f(s). \tag{4.3.1}$$

The mapping f must meet certain conditions, the most important of which is that the imaginary axis of the s plane must map to the imaginary axis of the s' plane. Thus, we have a relationship of the form

$$j\omega' = f(j\omega). \tag{4.3.2}$$

We take as our frequency-transformed filter $H(s)$ where

$$H_T(s) = H(s')|_{s'=f(s)} = H(f(s)). \tag{4.3.3}$$

Since it is the response of the filter along the $j\omega$ axis we are interested in, we can study the effect of the mapping f along the imaginary axis. Because of Eq. 4.3.3, it follows that

$$H_T(j\omega) = H(f(j\omega)). \tag{4.3.4}$$

Figure 4.3.1 gives a geometric interpretation of the mapping in Eq. 4.3.4. The magnitude response of the prototype lowpass filter $H(s')$ is shown on the left. To the right, we have shown a mapping $\omega' = f(\omega)$ which transforms the prototype lowpass filter into a lowpass filter with a different cutoff frequency. To find the new cutoff frequency, we follow a horizontal line from $\omega' = 1$ to the graph of $\omega' = f(\omega)$. We follow this point vertically down to the graph of $H_T(j\omega)$ to locate the new cutoff frequency for the frequency-transformed filter. This is performed for all points ω' to obtain the picture of $H_T(j\omega)$.

In order to transform an analog lowpass filter $H(s')$ with unity cutoff frequency to an analog lowpass filter $H(s)$ with cutoff frequency ω_c, we use the mapping

$$s = \omega_c s'. \tag{4.3.5}$$

This means that

$$s' = \frac{s}{\omega_c}.$$

In other words, we replace every occurrence of s' in $H(s')$ with s/ω_c.

Example 4.3

A first order Butterworth filter with unity cutoff frequency is given by

$$H(s') = \frac{1}{s'+1}.$$

Suppose we wish to place the new cutoff frequency at $\omega_c = 5$. We then replace s' by $s/5$ giving

$$H(s) = \frac{1}{\frac{s}{5}+1} = \frac{5}{s+5}.$$

It can be seen that this indeed produces a unity magnitude passband (because $H(j0) = 1$) and that the new cutoff frequency is located where we desired.

In order to convert a lowpass filter $H(s')$ with unity cutoff frequency to a highpass filter $H(s)$ with cutoff frequency ω_c, we use the substitution

$$s' = \frac{\omega_c}{s}. \tag{4.3.6}$$

Example 4.4

To design a first-order Butterworth highpass filter with cutoff frequency $\omega_c = 2$, we begin with

$$H(s') = \frac{1}{s'+1}$$

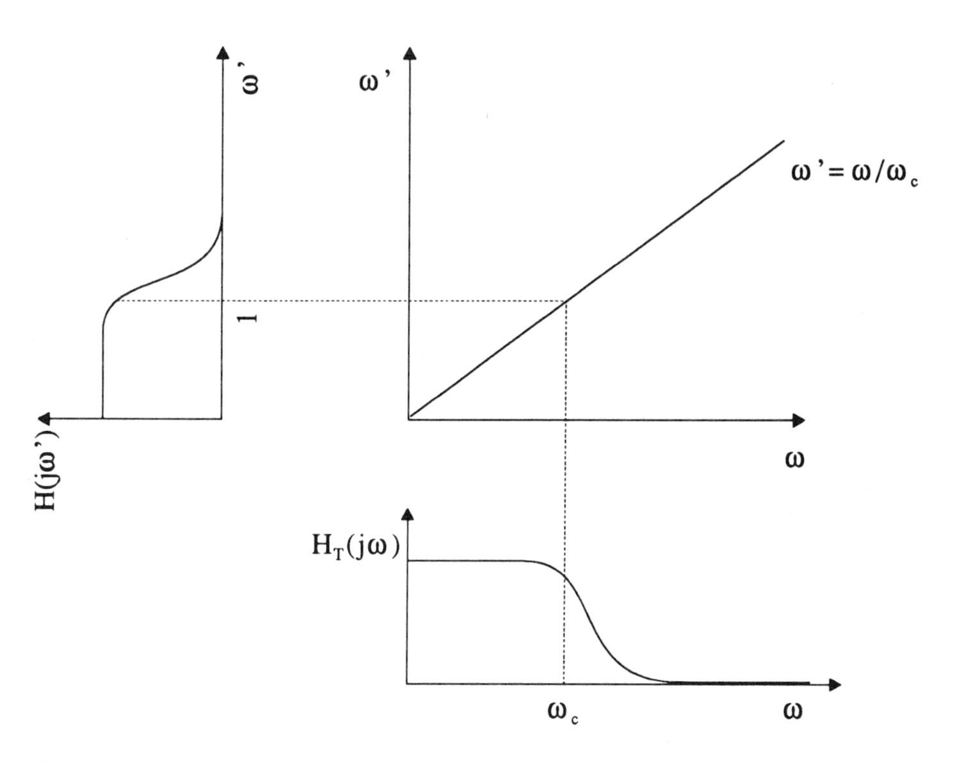

Figure 4.3.1: Converting a prototype lowpass filter to a lowpass filter with desired cutoff frequency using an analog frequency transformation.

and substitute

$$s' = \frac{2}{s},$$

giving

$$H(s) = \frac{1}{\frac{2}{s} + 1} = \frac{s}{s+2}.$$

Notice that the highpass filter contains zeros as well as poles.

To convert a lowpass filter $H(s')$ with unity cutoff frequency into a bandpass filter $H(s)$ with lower cutoff frequency ω_l and upper cutoff frequency ω_u, we make the substitution

$$s' = \frac{s^2 + \omega_l \omega_u}{s(\omega_u - \omega_l)}. \tag{4.3.7}$$

Similarly, to convert $H(s')$ to a bandstop filter with lower cutoff frequency ω_l and upper cutoff frequency ω_u, we make the substitution

$$s' = \frac{s(\omega_u - \omega_l)}{s^2 + \omega_l \omega_u}. \tag{4.3.8}$$

These transformations are summarized in Table 4.1.

Example 4.5

Suppose we wish to design a Butterworth bandpass filter with lower cutoff frequency $\omega_l = 10$ and upper cutoff frequency $\omega_u = 20$. Furthermore, we want an attenuation of at least 20 dB for frequencies in the range

$$0 \le |\omega| \le 5 \quad \text{and} \quad |\omega| \ge 50.$$

Referring to the Table 4.1, the appropriate transformation is

$$s' = f(s) = \frac{s^2 + 200}{10s}.$$

When evaluated at $s = j\omega$, we have

$$\omega' = \frac{\omega^2 - 200}{10\omega}.$$

As expected, we find that

$$\omega_l' = f(j\omega_l) = 1$$

and

$$\omega_u' = f(j\omega_u) = -1.$$

The frequency $\omega = 5$ corresponds to the prototype frequency

$$\omega'_{10} = f(j5) = -3.5$$

and $\omega = 50$ corresponds to

$$\omega_{50} = f(j50) = 4.6.$$

In order to insure that the stopband magnitude of -20 dB is met, it is necessary to make sure that the magnitude of the analog prototype at $\omega' = -3.5$ (and hence at $\omega' = 3.5$ because the response is symmetric) is less than -20 dB. For then, the monotonicity of the stopband of the lowpass prototype guarantees that the magnitude of the prototype at $\omega' = 4.6$ will be less than -20 dB. Using Eq. 4.2.6, we find that $N = 1.83$, so we round up to $N = 2$. Thus, the analog prototype is given by

$$H(s') = \frac{1}{s'^2 + \sqrt{2}s' + 1}.$$

Finally, the bandpass filter is given by

$$H_T(s) = H(f(s)) = \frac{1}{\left(\frac{s^2+200}{10s}\right)^2 + \sqrt{2}\left(\frac{s^2+200}{10s}\right) + 1},$$

which gives

$$H_T(s) = \frac{100s^2}{s^4 + 10\sqrt{2}s^3 + 500s^2 + 2000\sqrt{2}s + 40,000}.$$

4.4 Impulse Invariant IIR Design

A plausible way to map an analog filter to a discrete-time filter is to require that the discrete-time filter's impulse response match the analog filter's impulse response at the sampling instants kT. Heuristically, we expect that if the time-domain properties are preserved, the frequency-domain properties should then follow.

Suppose we have an analog filter

$$H_c(s) = \frac{n(s)}{d(s)} = \frac{a_M s^M + a_{M-1}s^{M-1} + \cdots + a_1 s + a_0}{s^N + b_{N-1}s^{N-1} + \cdots + a_1 s + a_0}, \quad M < N$$

with impulse response $h_c(t)$. The impulse invariant design method maps $H_c(s)$ to the discrete-time filter $H(z)$ which has impulse response

$$h(k) = Th_c(kT) \tag{4.4.1}$$

Type	*Transformation*	*New Cutoff(s)*
Lowpass	$s' = \dfrac{s}{\omega_c}$	ω_c
Highpass	$s' = \dfrac{\omega_c}{s}$	ω_c
Bandpass	$s' = \dfrac{s^2 + \omega_l \omega_u}{s(\omega_u - \omega_l)}$	ω_l, ω_u
Bandstop	$s' = \dfrac{s(\omega_u - \omega_l)}{s^2 + \omega_l \omega_u}$	ω_l, ω_u

Table 4.1: Analog frequency transformations for lowpass prototype with unity cutoff frequency.

where T is the sampling rate of the discrete-time filter. In order to determine $H(z)$, assume for now that $H_c(s)$ is of order N and has distinct poles. Then $H_c(s)$ has a partial fraction expansion of first-degree terms given by

$$H_c(s) = \sum_{i=1}^{N} \frac{\alpha_i}{s - p_i}$$

where the p_i are the roots of the denominator, *i.e.*,

$$d(s) = (s - p_1)(s - p_2) \cdots (s - p_n).$$

The impulse response is found by inverting the Laplace transform as given by the partial fraction expansion, giving

$$h_c(t) = \sum_{i=1}^{n} \alpha_i e^{p_i t}, \quad t \geq 0.$$

The impulse response of the digital filter, according to Eq. 4.4.1, is then

$$h(k) = T h_c(kT) = \sum_{i=1}^{N} \alpha_i T e^{p_i k T}$$

which we can also write as

$$h(k) = \sum_{i=1}^{N} \alpha_i (e^{p_i T})^k. \tag{4.4.2}$$

The $\mathcal{Z}$-transform of Eq. 4.4.2 is easily recognized as

$$H(z) = \sum_{i=1}^{N} \frac{\alpha_i T}{1 - e^{p_i T} z^{-1}}. \tag{4.4.3}$$

Equation 4.4.3 gives a closed-form expression for the discrete-time transfer function obtained by impulse invariance. It can be seen from this relationship that a pole of the analog filter at $s = p_i$ is mapped to a pole of the discrete-time filter located at

$$z_i = e^{p_i T}.$$

Suppose p_i is given by

$$p_i = \sigma_i + j\omega_i.$$

Then

$$z_i = e^{\sigma_i T} e^{j\omega_i T}.$$

Clearly, then, if the pole of the analog filter is in the left half-plane ($\sigma_i < 0$) the pole of the discrete-time filter will be inside the unit circle. Also, if the pole of the analog filter is on the imaginary axis ($\sigma_i = 0$), the pole of the discrete-time filter will lie on the unit circle. Hence, a stable analog filter will be mapped to a stable discrete-time filter. The impulse invariance technique is sometimes known as the *standard Z-transform.*

Example 4.6

Suppose $H_c(s)$ is given by

$$H_c(s) = \frac{1}{(s+1)(s+2)}$$

and we use impulse invariance to derive a discrete-time filter with sampling interval $T = 1$. The partial fraction expansion of $H_c(s)$ is

$$H_c(s) = \frac{1}{s+1} - \frac{1}{s+2}.$$

Therefore, we have the impulse response

$$h_c(t) = e^{-t} - e^{-2t}.$$

The impulse response of the discrete-time filter is given by

$$h(k) = Th_c(kT) = e^{-k} - e^{-2k}$$

which has the $\mathcal{Z}$-transform

$$H(z) = \frac{1}{1 - e^{-1}z^{-1}} - \frac{1}{1 - e^{-2}z^{-1}},$$

which we can write as

$$H(z) = \frac{(e^{-1} - e^{-2})z^{-1}}{1 - (e^{-1} + e^{-2})z^{-1} + e^{-3}z^{-2}}.$$

A logical question is how well the frequency domain properties of $H_c(s)$ are preserved by impulse invariance. Recall that if an analog signal $x_c(t)$ with Fourier transform $X_c(j\omega)$ is sampled with a sampling interval T, we have

$$X(e^{j\theta}) = \frac{1}{T} \sum_{r=-\infty}^{\infty} X_c\left(\frac{\theta}{T} + j\frac{2\pi r}{T}\right)$$

where the discrete-time signal $x(k)$ was obtained by

$$x(k) = T x_c(kT).$$

Therefore, since $h(k) = T h_c(kT)$, we have

$$H(e^{j\theta}) = \sum_{r=-\infty}^{\infty} H_c\left(\frac{\theta}{T} + j\frac{2\pi r}{T}\right). \tag{4.4.4}$$

Thus, the analog frequency response is scaled in frequency by the relationship

$$\theta = \omega T$$

and then copies of the scaled response are shifted and added. This is shown in Fig. 4.4.1. It can be seen that if the analog filter has substantial frequency content at frequencies greater than $\omega = \pi/T$, aliasing will result and the frequency response of the discrete-time filter will be distorted. Because π/T corresponds to half the sampling frequency, we require that the impulse response of the analog filter be sampled at twice its highest frequency component. This is merely a restatement of the Shannon sampling theorem. Impulse invariance results in a digital filter $H(e^{j\theta})$ which is an aliased version of $H_c(j\theta/T)$. If there is little frequency content in $H_c(j\omega)$ for frequencies greater than $\omega = \pi/T$, this aliasing will be minimal.

The distortion in the response of the discrete-time filter may be made small by sampling at a high enough rate T so that there is little frequency content in $H(s)$ beyond π/T. Clearly, this is possible if $H(s)$ is a lowpass filter or a bandpass filter where the passband is well below half the sampling frequency. For highpass and bandstop filters, impulse invariance will not work. We will have to develop other techniques whereby these filters can be transformed.

Example 4.7

Suppose we wish to design a Butterworth lowpass filter which has a sampling rate of $T = 5 \times 10^{-4}s$ rad/s, a cutoff frequency of 50 rad/s, and an attenuation of at least 20 dB for frequencies greater than 250 rad/s. We begin with the analog Butterworth filter. The analog prototype with unity cutoff frequency is given by

$$H_p(s') = \frac{1}{s'+1}.$$

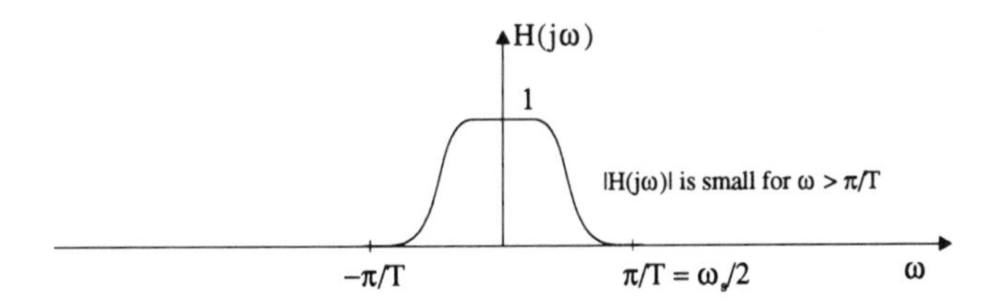

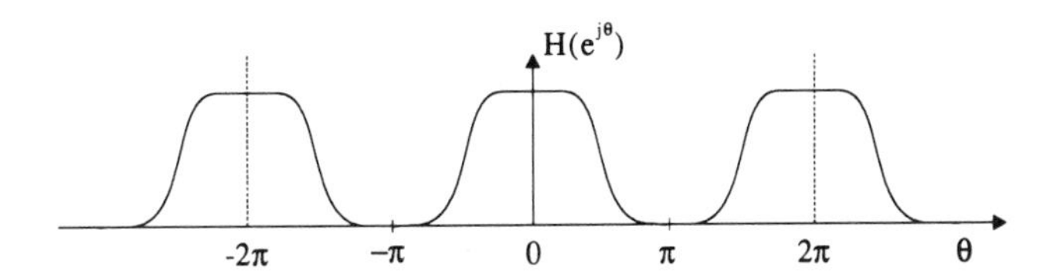

Figure 4.4.1: Obtaining the frequency response of a discrete-time filter by applying impulse invariance to an analog filter.

We apply the frequency transformation

$$s' = \frac{s}{\omega_c}$$

where ω_c is the new cutoff frequency, giving

$$H_c(s) = H_p(f(s)).$$

The frequency $s = 250$ corresponds to the prototype frequency

$$s' = \frac{250}{\omega_c} = 5.$$

Therefore, the specifications for the analog prototype are: cutoff frequency of one, and the attenuation must be at least 20 dB for frequencies greater than $\omega_a' = 5$. The attenuation of 20 dB translates to a magnitude of 0.1. Therefore, we determine the order to be equal to $N = 0.697$, which we round up to $N = 1$. The analog prototype is thus given by

$$H_p(s') = \frac{1}{s'+1}.$$

Applying $f(s)$, we have the frequency-transformed analog filter

$$H_c(s) = \frac{1}{\frac{250}{s}+1} = \frac{250}{s+250}.$$

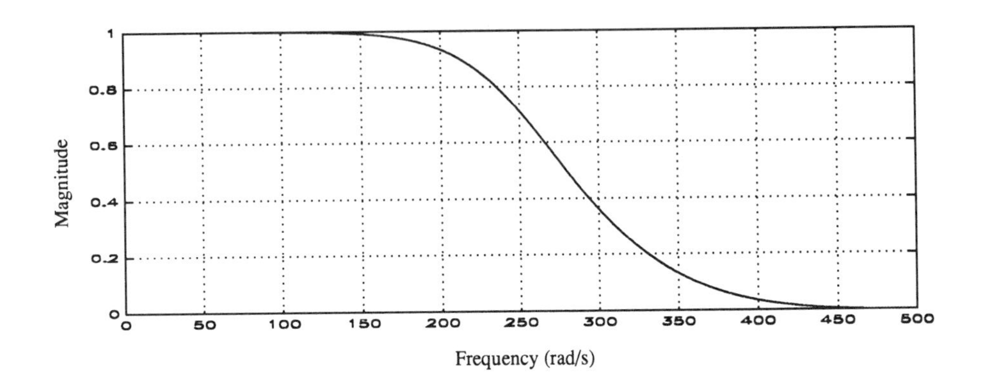

Figure 4.4.2: Analog and digital filter magnitude frequency responses for Example 4.7.

Applying impulse invariance, we get

$$H(z) = \frac{250T}{1 - e^{-250T}z^{-1}} = \frac{0.125}{1 - 0.8825z^{-1}}.$$

The frequency response of the analog and digital filters are shown in Fig. 4.4.2. Notice the distortion in the passband of the digital filter. The reason for this is simple: the analog filter is a first-order Butterworth filter, which has a very gradual rolloff. At half the sampling frequency, π/T, there is still substantial frequency content which will result in aliasing.

When designing digital filters, it is convenient to use the normalized frequency θ where

$$\theta = \omega T.$$

In this manner, frequencies pertaining to the digital filter are expressed relative to the sampling frequency. For instance, $\omega = \omega_s$ corresponds to $\theta = \omega_s T = 2\pi$, and half the sampling frequency corresponds to $\theta = \pi$.

Using this convention, we can study the effect of aliasing on the impulse invariant method very easily. Suppose we want to examine how well the impulse invariance method works for mapping first order analog Butterworth filters to discrete-time filters. We have seen that the transfer function of first-order Butterworth filter with cutoff frequency ω_c is given by

$$H_c(s) = \frac{\omega_c}{s + \omega_c}.$$

Therefore, for a sampling rate of T, we apply impulse invariance to get the discrete-time filter described by

$$H(z) = \frac{\omega_c T}{1 - e^{-\omega_c T} z^{-1}}.$$

The quantity $\omega_c T$, however, is simply the normalized cutoff frequency θ_c. Thus, $H(z)$ is given by

$$H(z) = \frac{\theta_c}{1 - e^{-\theta_c} z^{-1}}.$$

$H(z)$ has a zero at the origin and a pole at $z = e^{-\theta_c}$, as shown in Fig. 4.4.3. For θ_c small, the pole moves closer and closer to the unit circle. As θ_c approaches π, the pole moves toward the origin, causing a distortion in the lowpass magnitude characteristic. Thus, we should have θ_c small, which corresponds to a cutoff frequency which is small compared to the sampling frequency.

For this simple first order example, the maximal gain occurs at $z = 1$ and has a value of

$$G_{max} = \frac{1}{1 - e^{-\theta_c}}.$$

As θ_c approaches zero, we find that G_{max} approaches unity. The gain in the stopband, however, does not approach zero for any value of θ_c. In fact, the minimum gain occurs at $z = -1$ and can be seen to be equal to

$$G_{min} = \frac{1}{1 + e^{-\theta_c}}.$$

Thus, as θ_c approaches zero, G_{min} approaches 1/2. Hence, it is not possible to achieve any appreciable stopband attenuation, regardless of the sampling frequency or the bandwidth of the analog filter. The message we can derive from this example is that impulse invariance should be restricted to filters whose magnitude response dies off very rapidly compared to half the sampling frequency, which in turn implies that the denominator degree of the analog filter should be significantly greater than the numerator degree.

From now on, we will always use the normalized frequency when designing discrete-time filters. We should always be thinking in terms of normalized frequency. Thus, a discrete-time lowpass filter with a sampling rate of 100 Hz and a cutoff frequency of 25 Hz will have the same $\mathcal{Z}$-transform as a discrete-time lowpass filter with a sampling rate of 200 Hz and a cutoff frequency of 50 Hz. For both of these filters, we have

$$\theta_c = \frac{\pi}{2}.$$

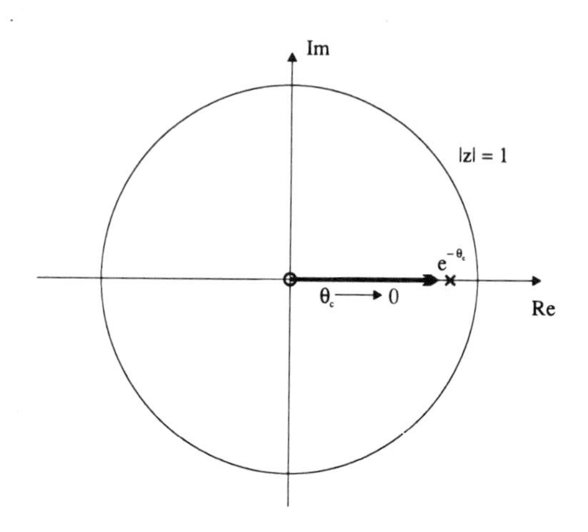

Figure 4.4.3: Pole-zero plot for first-order Butterworth digital filter obtained by impulse invariance.

To gain deeper insight into the mapping between the s plane and the z plane induced by impulse invariance, consider the mapping

$$z = e^{sT}$$

which is used to map the poles of the analog filter to the z-plane. Suppose we have two points s_1, s_2 in the complex plane given by

$$s_1 = \sigma + j\omega, \quad s_2 = \sigma + j(\omega + \frac{2\pi}{T}).$$

In other words, s_1 and s_2 have the same real part but their imaginary parts are separated by $2\pi/T$. Then s_1 is mapped to the point z_1 where

$$z_1 = e^{\sigma} e^{j\omega T}.$$

The point s_2 is mapped to z_2 where

$$z_2 = e^{\sigma} e^{j(\omega+2\pi/T)T} = e^{\sigma} e^{j\omega T}.$$

Therefore, $z_1 = z_2$ so that both points s_1 and s_2 map to the same location in the z-plane. To understand this visually, consider Fig. 4.4.4. We see that horizontal strips of width $2\pi/T$ in the s-plane are mapped to the z-plane. The left half of the strip maps to the interior of the unit circle and the right half of the strip maps to the exterior of the unit circle. The different strips map to the same location in the z-plane; this is the source of the aliasing.

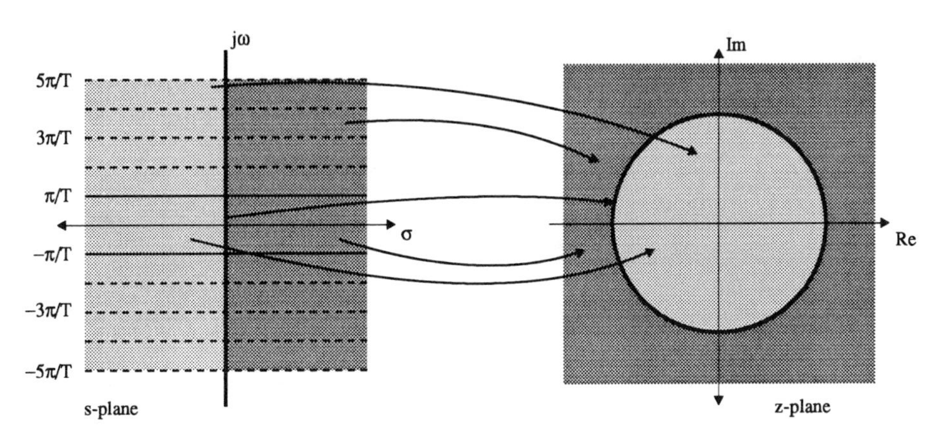

Figure 4.4.4: Mapping the s-plane to the z-plane by impulse invariance.

Example 4.8

An example where impulse invariance works slightly better than the previous example is provided by the following. A third-order analog Butterworth filter with cutoff frequency $\omega_c = 1$ is given by

$$H_c(s) = \frac{1}{s^3 + 2s^2 + 2s + 1}.$$

Suppose we wish to design a third-order discrete-time Butterworth filter with a sampling frequency equal to four times the cutoff frequency of the analog filter, namely

$$\omega_s = 4\omega_c = 4,$$

giving

$$T = \frac{2\pi}{\omega_s} = \frac{\pi}{2}.$$

We anticipate that this should produce acceptable results since the magnitude response of $H_c(s)$ dies off very quickly at $4\omega_c$. The partial fraction expansion of $H_c(s)$ is

$$H_c(s) = \frac{1}{s+1} + \frac{-0.5 - j0.2887}{s + 0.5 - j0.866} + \frac{-0.5 + j0.2887}{s + 0.5 + j0.866}.$$

Applying impulse invariance, we get

$$H(z) = \frac{1.5708}{1 - 0.2079z^{-1}} + \frac{0.0952 + j0.4459}{1 - (0.0952 + j0.4459)z^{-1}} + \frac{0.0952 - j0.4459}{1 - (0.0952 - j0.4459)z^{-1}}$$

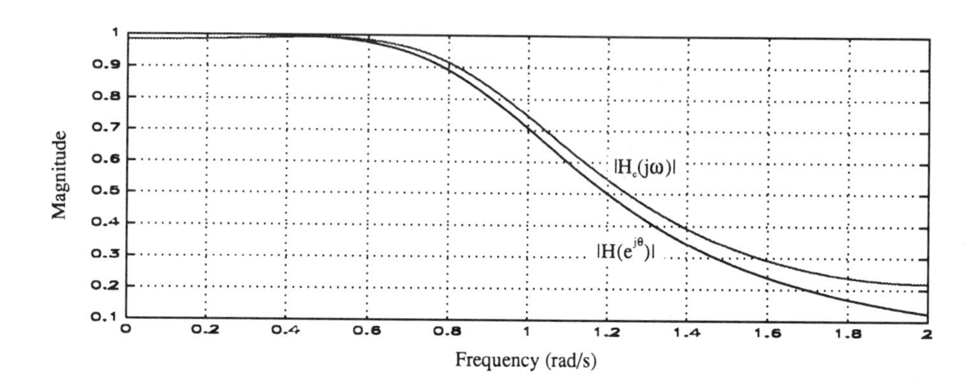

Figure 4.4.5: Frequency responses of third-order analog Butterworth lowpass filter and discrete-time filter obtained by impulse invariance for Example 4.8.

which simplifies to

$$H(z) = \frac{0.5813z^{-1} + 0.2114z^{-2}}{1 - 0.3984z^{-1} + 0.2475z^{-2} - 0.0432z^{-3}}.$$

The frequency range over which the discrete-time filter operates is from d.c. to half the sampling frequency, which corresponds to $\omega = 2$. The magnitude responses of $H_c(s)$ and $H(z)$ for $0 \leq \omega \leq 2$ are superimposed in Fig. 4.4.5. Notice the slight distortion in the passband, which is due to minor aliasing. We should expect that the response would improve if the sampling frequency were increased.

The impulse invariance technique is simply summarized as follows. We begin with a statement of the discrete-time filter specifications, including sampling frequency and critical frequencies. Next, a prototype analog filter $H_c(s)$ is designed which matches the discrete-time specifications using any of the classical prototypes. Impulse invariance is then applied, resulting in a discrete-time filter $H(z)$. We are assured that the time-domain property of impulse invariance is preserved. If, however, aliasing occurs, there is no guarantee that the desired frequency domain properties of the analog filter are preserved by $H(z)$.

4.5 The Bilinear Z-Transform

The motivation for impulse invariance was to match the time-domain properties of a discrete-time filter with an analog filter. We have seen that this leads to a discrete-time filter with a frequency response which is close to that of the analog filter if the amount of aliasing is minimal. If, however, the analog filter is not lowpass or bandpass with a narrow bandwidth which is centered at a low frequency, the effects of aliasing can introduce severe distortion into the derived discrete-time filter. Recall that the standard $\mathcal{Z}$-transform (impulse invariance) is a many-to-one mapping which maps strips of width $2\pi/T$ from the s-plane to the z-plane. It is precisely this many-to-one nature which is responsible for the aliasing. This suggests the need for another mapping of the s-plane to the z-plane.

The idea behind the bilinear $\mathcal{Z}$-transform is to use a mapping ϕ from the s-plane to the z-plane which is *one-to-one*. In particular, ϕ should map the imaginary axis of the s-plane in a one-to-one manner onto the unit circle of the z-plane. As usual, we would also like the left half-plane to map to the interior of the unit circle so that a stable analog filter will map to a stable discrete-time filter. One such mapping ϕ which meets these requirements is

$$z = \phi(s) = \frac{1+s}{1-s}. \tag{4.5.1}$$

This mapping is shown in Fig. 4.5.1. Clearly, $\phi(s)$ is invertible, with an inverse given by

$$s = \phi^{-1}(z) = \frac{z-1}{z+1}. \tag{4.5.2}$$

To verify that the imaginary axis maps to the unit circle, let $s = j\omega$ and apply Eq. 4.5.1, giving

$$|z| = \frac{|1+j\omega|}{|1-j\omega|} = 1.$$

Because the entire imaginary axis maps to the unit circle, there is a corresponding *frequency warping*. Given a point $e^{j\theta}$ on the unit circle, we can determine the analog frequency which maps to it by applying the inverse mapping in Eq. 4.5.2, which gives

$$\omega = \frac{e^{j\theta}-1}{e^{j\theta}+1} = j\frac{\sin(\theta/2)}{\cos(\theta/2)} = \tan(\theta/2), \tag{4.5.3}$$

which, as expected, is on the imaginary axis. Let's define the restriction of ϕ^{-1} to the unit circle as the function $\Omega(\theta)$ where

$$\Omega(\theta) = \phi^{-1}(z)\Big|_{z=e^{j\theta}}.$$

From Eq. 4.5.3, it follows that

$$\Omega(\theta) = \tan(\theta/2). \tag{4.5.4}$$

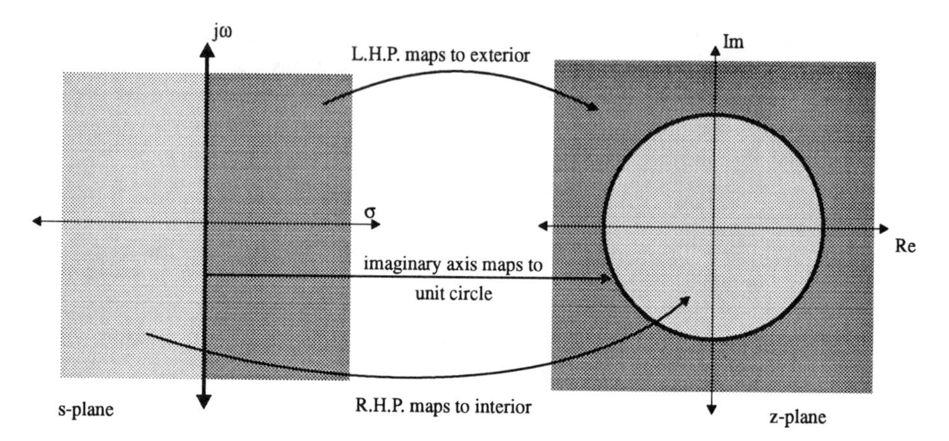

Figure 4.5.1: Mapping the s-plane to the z-plane using the bilinear $\mathcal{Z}$-transform.

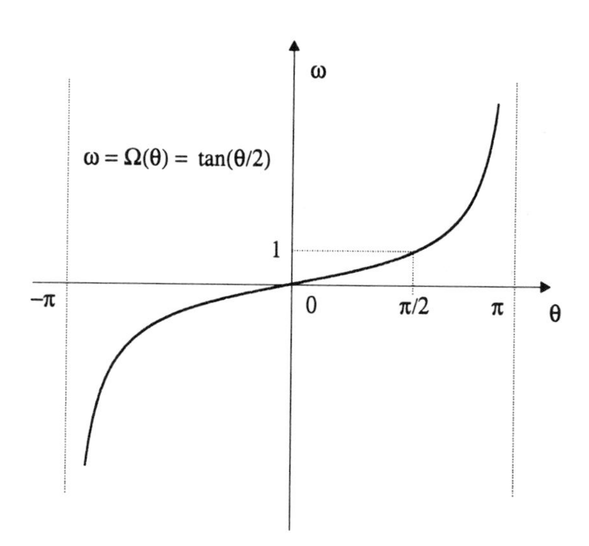

Figure 4.5.2: Frequency warping function for the bilinear $\mathcal{Z}$-transform .

Examining Eq. 4.5.4, we see that as θ goes from $-\pi$ to π, $\Omega(\theta)$ increases monotonically from $-\infty$ to ∞. Equation 4.5.4 is known as the *frequency warping* equation for the bilinear $\mathcal{Z}$-transform and is illustrated in Fig. 4.5.2.

Given an analog filter $H_c(s)$, we apply the bilinear $\mathcal{Z}$-transform by taking the discrete-time filter as

$$H(z) = H_c(\phi^{-1}(z)) \tag{4.5.5}$$

which gives the frequency response

$$H(e^{j\theta}) = H_c(j\Omega(\theta)). \tag{4.5.6}$$

Because of the bijectivity of the mapping ϕ, no aliasing will occur. The only distortion incurred by the discrete-time filter is due to the nonlinear frequency warping. Equation 4.5.6 is illustrated in Fig. 4.5.3. Examining the figure, to find the value of $H(e^{j\theta})$ at a frequency θ_0, we simply follow the vertical line from the point θ_0 to the intersection with the graph of $\Omega(\theta)$ and then follow the line from ω_0 which intersects the graph of $\Omega(\theta)$ horizontally. It then follows that $H(e^{j\theta_0}) = H_c(\omega_0)$.

Because of the nonlinear warping of the frequency axis, we need to be able to determine the critical frequencies of the analog filter so that they will map to the desired frequency for the discrete-time filter. For example, suppose we wish to design a discrete-time lowpass filter which has a cutoff frequency at $\theta_c = \omega_c T$. If we design the analog lowpass filter with a cutoff frequency of ω_c, the frequency warping will relocate the cutoff frequency of the discrete-time filter to a location other than $\omega_c T$. We know from Eq. 4.5.4, however, that the analog frequency $\Omega(\theta_c)$ is mapped by the bilinear $\mathcal{Z}$-transform to θ_c. Therefore, if we design the analog filter with a cutoff frequency of $\Omega(\theta_c)$, the discrete-time filter will have its cutoff frequency located at the proper frequency, θ_c. This is known as *prewarping.*

Using the bilinear $\mathcal{Z}$-transform consists of four steps. First we specify the discrete-time filter in terms of normalized frequency, θ. Next, the critical frequencies are prewarped using Eq. 4.5.4 to locate the analog critical frequencies. Then the analog filter $H_c(s)$ is designed using any of the techniques we have developed. Finally, the discrete-time filter $H(z)$ is obtained by replacing the variable s with $(z-1)/(z+1)$. There will be no aliasing, and this technique can be used for arbitrary magnitude characteristics.

Example 4.9

We wish to design a discrete-time Butterworth filter $H(z)$ which is lowpass with a sampling frequency of 1000 Hz and has a cutoff frequency of 250 Hz. We would like the magnitude at 375 Hz to be less than 0.1.

In terms of normalized frequencies, we find

$$\theta_c = 2\pi \frac{250}{1000} = \frac{\pi}{2}$$

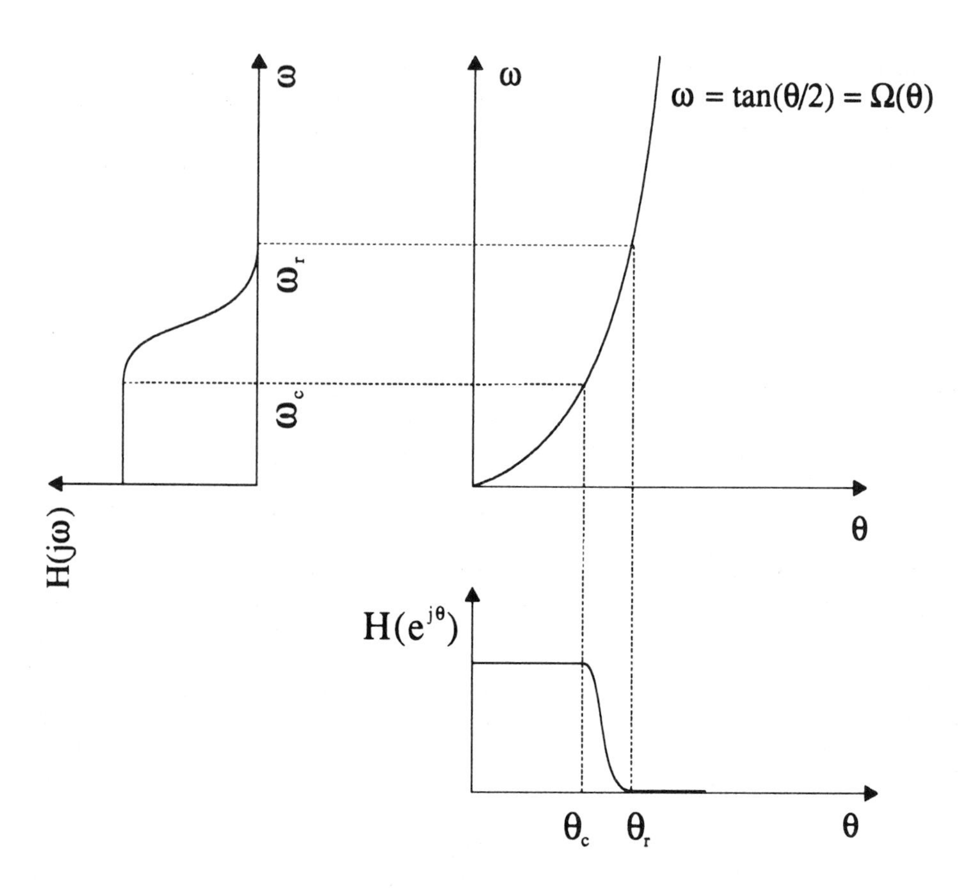

Figure 4.5.3: Illustration of the bilinear $\mathcal{Z}$-transform .

and

$$\theta_a = 2\pi\frac{375}{1000} = \frac{3\pi}{4}.$$

Applying prewarping, we get

$$\omega_c = \Omega(\theta_c) = \tan(\theta_c/2) = 1.0$$

and

$$\omega_a = \Omega(\theta_a) = \tan(\theta_a/2) = 3.077.$$

Therefore, we need to design an analog Butterworth lowpass filter which has a cutoff frequency of 1.0 rad/s and a gain of no more than 0.1 for frequencies greater than 3.077 rad/s. The order calculation for Butterworth filters gives an order $N = 3$. The transfer function of a third-order Butterworth filter with unity cutoff frequency is

$$H_c(s) = \frac{1}{s^3 + 2s^2 + 2s + 1}.$$

We make the substitution $s = (z-1)/(z+1)$, giving

$$H(z) = H_c\left(\frac{z-1}{z+1}\right)$$

which yields

$$H(z) = \frac{1}{\left(\frac{z-1}{z+1}\right)^3 + 2\left(\frac{z-1}{z+1}\right)^2 + 2\left(\frac{z-1}{z+1}\right) + 1},$$

or,

$$H(z) = \frac{z^3 + 3z^2 + 3z + 1}{6z^3 + 2z}.$$

The magnitude response of this filter is shown in Fig. 4.5.4.

4.6 Discrete-Time Frequency Transformations

The previous sections have suggested one possible technique for designing discrete-time filters with lowpass, highpass, bandpass, and bandstop filters. We begin with an analog lowpass filter and perform a frequency transformation on the *analog filter*, followed by a transformation from the s-plane to the z-plane. We saw that impulse invariance could be used for lowpass filters and for certain bandpass filters, but that the bilinear $\mathcal{Z}$-transform needed to be used for other filters to avoid aliasing. Another approach to designing discrete-time filters is to use *discrete-time frequency transformations*. These frequency transformations begin with a

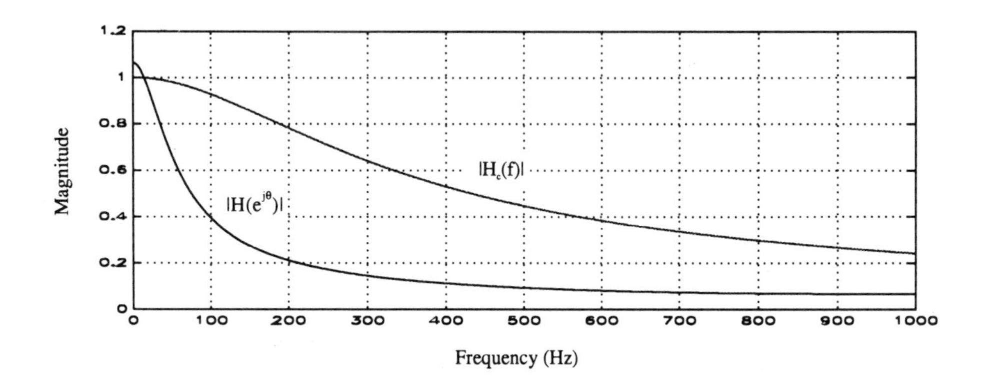

Figure 4.5.4: Magnitude response of third-order Butterworth lowpass filter for Example 4.9.

discrete-time lowpass filter and perform an algebraic transformation of the z-plane to obtain the desired frequency-selective filter.

Suppose we have a desired frequency response $H_d(z)$. We begin with a prototype lowpass filter $H(\tilde{z})$ and perform a mapping from the $\tilde{z}$-plane to the z-plane of the form

$$\tilde{z}^{-1} = g(z^{-1}) \tag{4.6.1}$$

such that

$$H_d(z) = H(\tilde{z})|_{\tilde{z}^{-1}=g(z^{-1})} \,. \tag{4.6.2}$$

We have expressed $\tilde{z}$ as a function of z in anticipation of the fact that our filters will be expressed as rational functions of z^{-1} rather than z. Thus, once we know the transformation g, the new filter $H_d(z)$ is obtained by replacing every occurrence of $\tilde{z}^{-1}$ in $H(\tilde{z})$ with $g(z^{-1})$.

The transformation g must satisfy certain constraints. First, we want rational functions to map to rational functions. Therefore, we require that $g(z^{-1})$ be a rational function of z^{-1}. Furthermore, a causal and stable filter should map to a causal and stable filter. This implies that the *interior* of the unit circle in the $\tilde{z}$-plane must map to the *interior* of the unit circle in the z-plane and that the contour $|\tilde{z}| = 1$ should map to the contour $|z| = 1$. From these requirements, it is relatively simple to infer a structural form for g. The most general form of the function g which satisfies all of these requirements is

$$\tilde{z}^{-1} = \pm \prod_{i=1}^{N} \frac{z^{-1} - \alpha_i}{1 - \alpha_i z^{-1}}, \quad |\alpha_i| < 1. \tag{4.6.3}$$

This mapping is seen to be a cascade of allpass factors. Rational functions of this form are known as *Blaschke products* [RM87].

To study the effects of these frequency transformations on the frequency response of a discrete-time filter, we can examine the behavior of $g(z^{-1})$ on the unit circle. A point $z = e^{j\theta}$ on the unit circle in the z-plane is related to a point $\tilde{z} = e^{j\tilde{\theta}}$ in the $\tilde{z}$-plane by

$$e^{-j\tilde{\theta}} = g(e^{-j\theta})$$

because $g(z)$ is a cascade of allpass factors. Consider the case where $N = 1$ and the positive sign is taken in Eq. 4.6.3. We then have

$$\tilde{z}^{-1} = \frac{z^{-1} - \alpha}{1 - \alpha z^{-1}}$$

and

$$e^{-j\tilde{\theta}} = \frac{e^{-j\theta} - \alpha}{1 - \alpha e^{-j\theta}}.$$

Solving for $\tilde{\theta}$ in terms of θ, we get

$$\tilde{\theta} = \tan^{-1}\left[\frac{(1 - \alpha^2)\sin(\theta)}{(1 + \alpha^2)\cos(\theta) - 2\alpha}\right]. \tag{4.6.4}$$

Eq. 4.6.4 expresses the frequency warping induced by the mapping g. Figure 4.6.1 shows this mapping for several values of α. For fixed θ and $\tilde{\theta}$, the proper value of α is found by solving Eq. 4.6.4 for α, giving

$$\alpha = \frac{\sin[(\tilde{\theta}_c - \theta_c)/2]}{\sin[(\tilde{\theta}_c + \theta_c)/2]}. \tag{4.6.5}$$

The mapping g transforms a lowpass filter with cutoff frequency $\tilde{\theta}_c$ to a lowpass filter with cutoff frequency θ_c in much the same manner as the bilinear $\mathcal{Z}$-transform. Given a filter $H(\tilde{z})$ with known cutoff frequency $\tilde{\theta}_c$ and a desired filter $H_d(z)$ with desired cutoff frequency θ_c, the value of α for the frequency transformation is given by Eq. 4.6.5 as

$$\alpha = \frac{\sin[(\tilde{\theta}_c - \theta_c)/2]}{\sin[(\tilde{\theta}_c + \theta_c)/2]}.$$

This ensures that θ_c will map to $\tilde{\theta}_c$ under the mapping g. Then, $H_d(z)$ is obtained simply as

$$H_d(z) = H(\tilde{z})|_{\tilde{z}^{-1}=g(z^{-1})}$$

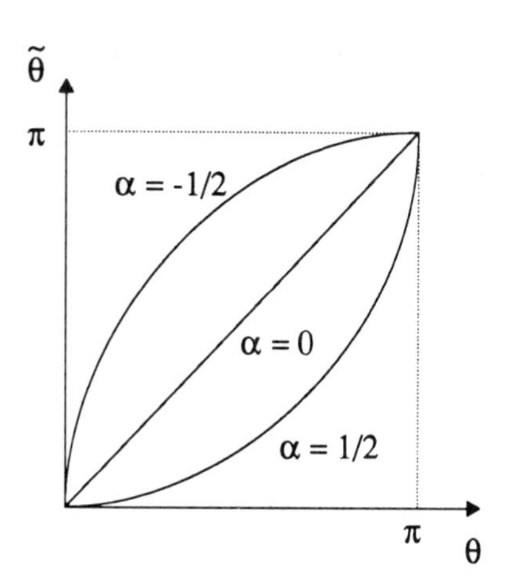

Figure 4.6.1: Lowpass to lowpass discrete-time frequency transformations for several values of α.

where, for the simple first-order case,

$$g(z^{-1}) = \frac{z^{-1} - \alpha}{1 - \alpha z^{-1}}.$$

The magnitude of $H_d(e^{j\theta})$ at $\theta = \theta_c$ then equals the magnitude of $H(e^{j\tilde{\theta}})$ at $\tilde{\theta} = \tilde{\theta}_c$.

Example 4.10

The transfer function of a second-order butterworth lowpass filter with cutoff frequency $\tilde{\theta}_c = \pi/2$ is given by

$$H(\tilde{z}) = \frac{0.2929(1 + 2\tilde{z}^{-1} + \tilde{z}^{-2})}{1 + 0.1715\tilde{z}^{-2}}.$$

Suppose we wish to transform this to a lowpass filter with cutoff frequency $\theta_c = 3\pi/4$. First, the value of α is found according to Eq. 4.6.5 as

$$\alpha = \frac{\sin[(\pi/2 - 3\pi/4))/2]}{\sin[(\pi/2 + 3\pi/4)/2]} = 0.4142.$$

Then, the frequency transformation is given by

$$\tilde{z}^{-1} = \frac{z^{-1} - 0.4142}{1 - 0.4142z^{-1}}.$$

If the above expression is substituted for $\tilde{z}^{-1}$ in $H(\tilde{z}^{-1}$, we obtain after some algebraic manipulation

$$H_d(z) = \frac{0.5691(1 + 2z^{-1} + z^{-2})}{1 + 0.9428z^{-1} + 0.3333z^{-2}}.$$

It is readily verified that $H_d(z)$ satisfies the design objective.

We will now summarize the four important discrete-time frequency transformations. For each one, it is assumed that we are starting with a lowpass filter with cutoff frequency $\tilde{\theta}_c$. Notice that there is no explicit reference to the sampling frequency. This is because we can perform all computations with the normalized frequency $\theta = \omega T$.

Lowpass to lowpass If the desired cutoff frequency is θ_c, use

$$\tilde{z}^{-1} = \frac{z^{-1} - \alpha}{1 - \alpha z^{-1}}$$

where

$$\alpha = \frac{\sin[(\tilde{\theta}_c - \theta_c)/2]}{\sin[(\tilde{\theta}_c + \theta_c)/2]}.$$

Lowpass to highpass To design a highpass filter with upper cutoff frequency θ_u, use

$$\tilde{z}^{-1} = -\frac{z^{-1} + \alpha}{1 + \alpha z^{-1}}$$

where

$$\alpha = \frac{\cos[(\tilde{\theta}_c - \theta_u)/2]}{\sin[(\tilde{\theta}_c + \theta_u)/2]}.$$

Lowpass to bandpass To design a bandpass filter with lower cutoff frequency θ_l and upper cutoff frequency θ_u, use

$$\tilde{z}^{-1} = -\frac{z^{-2} - \dfrac{2\alpha k}{k+1} z^{-1} + \dfrac{k-1}{k+1}}{\dfrac{k-1}{k+1} z^{-2} - \dfrac{2\alpha k}{k+1} z^{-1} + 1}$$

where

$$\alpha = \frac{\cos[(\theta_l + \theta_u)/2]}{\cos[(\theta_u - \theta_l)/2]}$$

and

$$k = \cot[(\theta_u - \theta_l)/2] \tan(\tilde{\theta}_c/2).$$

Lowpass to bandstop To design a bandstop filter with lower cutoff frequency and upper cutoff frequency θ_u, use

$$z^{-1} = \frac{z^{-2} - \frac{2\alpha k}{k+1}z^{-1} - \frac{k-1}{k+1}}{\frac{1-k}{k+1}z^{-2} - \frac{2\alpha k}{k+1}z^{-1} + 1}$$

where

$$\alpha = \frac{\cos[(\theta_l + \theta_u)/2]}{\cos[(\theta_u - \theta_l)/2]}$$

and

$$k = \tan[(\theta_u - \theta_l)/2]\tan(\tilde{\theta}_c/2).$$

4.7 FIR Filter Design

The next few sections will examine FIR filters in detail, including their design, analysis, and performance. We will see, in general, that the order required of an FIR to meet a desired magnitude profile will be considerably higher than an IIR. The power of the FIR, however, lies in its ease of implementation and the simplicity with which it can be analyzed.

Whereas IIR filter design bears a strong resemblance to analog filter design, FIR filters are unique to digital filtering. As a consequence, most of the FIR design techniques are not derived from classical analog methods. Rather, the majority of FIR design techniques come from polynomial approximation theory and are somewhat computationally complex. Once designed, however, FIR filters can possess attributes which are not possible for IIR filters. The most important of these are *linear phase* and *constant group delay.* This makes FIR filters extremely useful in applications which demand little phase distortion. Furthermore, the FIR is *a priori* stable, and its fixed-point effects are extremely easy to analyze. Consequently, FIR filters are well-suited to implementation by low-cost fixed-point processors.

An FIR filter is a purely feed-forward system. The transfer function of an N-th order FIR filter is given by

$$H(z) = \sum_{k=0}^{N-1} h_k z^{-k},$$

which means that the input/output relationship is expressed by

$$y(k) = \sum_{n=0}^{N-1} h_n x(k-n).$$

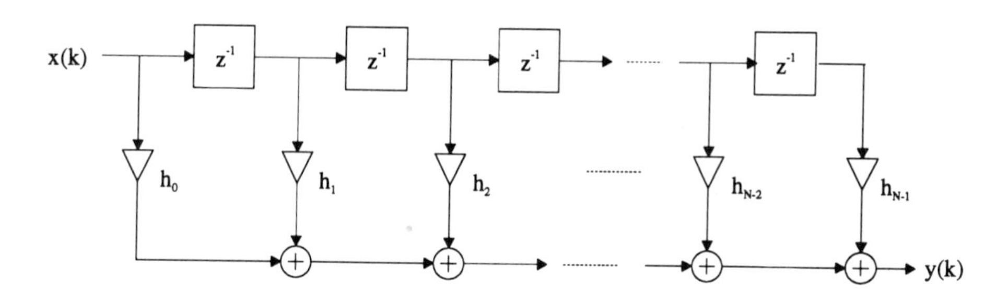

Figure 4.7.1: A direct-form FIR filter.

A block diagram which realizes the FIR transfer function is shown in Fig. 4.7.1. This implementation is known as a *direct-form FIR implementation.*

Referring to Fig. 4.7.1 or either of the above equations, it is immediately clear that the impulse response of the FIR is given by

$$\boldsymbol{h} = \{h_0, h_1, h_2, \ldots, h_{N-1}, 0, 0, \ldots\}.$$

Thus, the impulse response is of finite duration (hence the name). Because the numerator of the FIR transfer function is of degree $N-1$, there will be $N-1$ zeros in the complex plane. If we rewrite the transfer function of an FIR as a function of z, the denominator will be equal to z^{N-1} so that there are exactly $N-1$ poles at the origin.

Example 4.11

Suppose an FIR is described by

$$H(z) = \frac{1}{N}\sum_{k=0}^{N-1} z^{-k}.$$

This corresponds to the input/output relationship

$$y(k) = \frac{1}{N}(x(k) + x(k-1) + x(k-2) + \cdots + x(k-N-1),$$

which corresponds to an N-sample moving average. There will be $N-1$ poles at the origin. Because $H(z)$ can be rewritten as

$$H(z) = \frac{z^{N-1} + z^{N-2} + \cdots + z + 1}{z^{N-1}},$$

the filter zeros are the $N-1$ roots of the polynomial

$$p(z) = z^{N-1} + z^{N-2} + \cdots + z + 1.$$

To simplify, we can use the identity

$$z^N - 1 = (z^{N-1} + z^{N-2} + \cdots + z + 1)(z - 1)$$

so that

$$p(z) = \frac{z^N - 1}{z - 1}$$

and hence

$$H(z) = \frac{z^N - 1}{z^{N-1}(z - 1)}.$$

The polynomial $z^N - 1$ has N roots distributed uniformly along the unit circle with angular spacing $2\pi/N$. The root at $z = 1$ is canceled by the root of the denominator at $z = 1$. Thus, the FIR has $N - 1$ zeros given by

$$z_k = e^{j2\pi k/N}, \quad k = 1, 2, \ldots, N - 1$$

and $N - 1$ poles at the origin. The pole-zero distribution for this example is shown in Fig. 4.7.2a and the magnitude response is shown in Fig. 4.7.2b for the case $N = 8$. We can reconcile these results by using a little common sense. Assume we apply a sinusoidal input with frequency $2\pi k/N$ for some non-zero k. This means that the input is periodic with period N/k. A N-point moving average will simply compute the average of this sinusoid over precisely k periods, which obviously equals zero.

4.8 Linear Phase FIR Filters

One of the most important characteristics of FIR filters is the possibility of obtaining linear phase. The frequency response of a length N FIR is given by

$$H(e^{j\theta}) = \sum_{k=0}^{N-1} h(k) e^{-jk\theta}.$$

The FIR is said to be linear phase if

$$H(e^{j\theta}) = H_1(\theta) e^{-j(\alpha\theta + \beta)} \tag{4.8.1}$$

where α and β are constant and $H_1(\theta)$ is a real function of θ. To understand the importance of linear phase, consider the case where $\beta = 0$. Then

$$H(e^{j\theta}) = H_1(\theta) e^{-j\alpha\theta}.$$

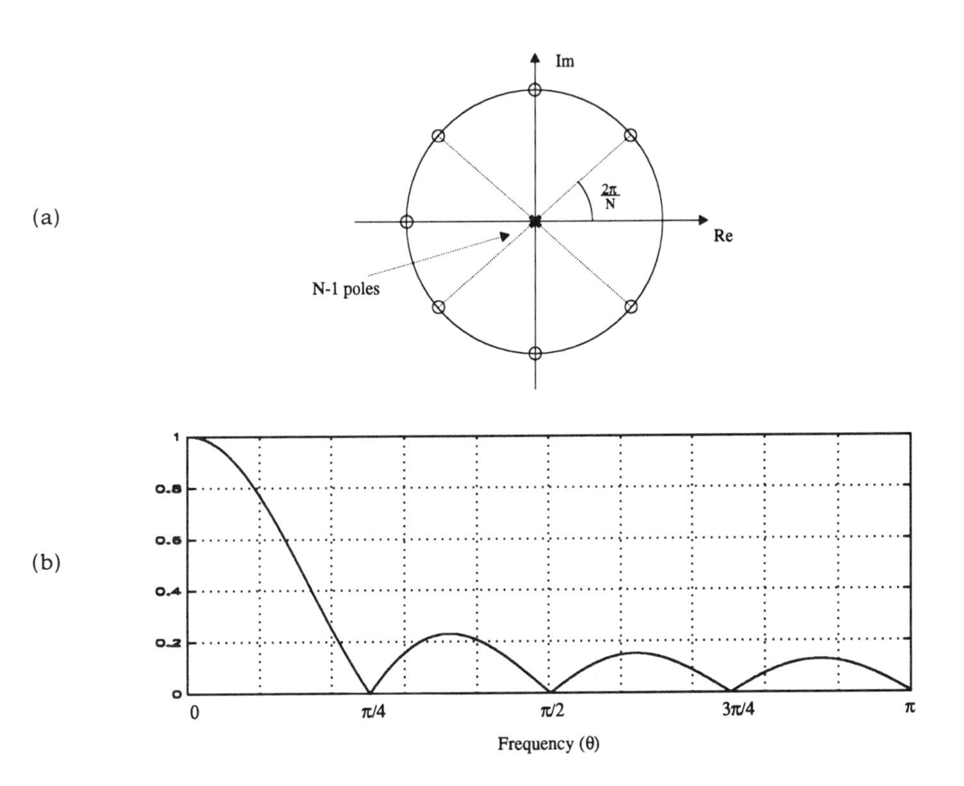

Figure 4.7.2: (a) Pole-zero distribution for Example 4.11; (b) magnitude response for Example 4.11.

Let the input to the FIR be a complex exponential $e^{jk\theta_0}$. By the definition of frequency response, the output will be

$$y(k) = H_1(\theta_0)e^{j\theta_0(k-\alpha)}.$$

Because the function $H(\theta)$ is real, the output will be scaled in magnitude by $H_1(\theta_0)$ and delayed in time by α samples. Furthermore, this time delay is *independent of* θ_0. Thus, the time delay between the input and output will be the same, regardless of frequency. This is important in applications such as data communication, where nonlinear phase can cause synchronization problems. Another area where linear phase is important is in audio signal processing. Consider the problem of designing a graphic equalizer. A graphic equalizer is typically used to alter the magnitude response of an audio system in order to compensate (*i.e.*, boost or attenuate) deviations from a flat response. If the phase response of the equalizer is not linear (as is typically the case), there can be an audible "dispersive" effect. This is due to the fact that certain frequencies are delayed more than others when passing through the equalizer.

With group delay defined by

$$grd(H(e^{j\theta})) = -\frac{d\angle H(e^{j\theta})}{d\theta},$$

it immediately follows that for a linear phase FIR, the group delay is equal to α. A linear phase FIR is said to possess *flat* group delay.

An FIR can be made linear phase if its coefficients are symmetric. There are four ways in which this can be achieved: the FIR can have either even or odd length and the coefficients can have either even or odd symmetry. For an FIR of length N, even symmetry is defined by the condition

$$h(k) = h(N-1-k) \tag{4.8.2}$$

and odd symmetry by

$$h(k) = -h(N-1-k). \tag{4.8.3}$$

To show how linear phase results from these conditions, assume N is odd and given by $N = 2M+1$. Also, let the coefficients have even symmetry. Then Eq. 4.8.2 implies that the coefficients are symmetric about the midpoint, M. This means that

$$h(M-k) = h(M+k), \quad k = 0, 1, \ldots, M. \tag{4.8.4}$$

Then

$$H(e^{j\theta}) = \sum_{k=0}^{2M} h(k)e^{-jk\theta} = \sum_{k=-M}^{M} h(M+k)e^{-j(k+M)\theta},$$

which can be rewritten as

$$H(e^{j\theta}) = h(M)e^{-jM\theta} + \sum_{k=1}^{M} h(M-k)e^{-j(M-k)\theta} + \sum_{k=1}^{M} h(M+k)e^{-j(k+M)\theta}.$$

Factoring out $e^{-jM\theta}$ and using Eq. 4.8.4,

$$H(e^{j\theta}) = e^{-jM\theta}[h(M) + 2\sum_{k=1}^{M} h(M+k)\cos(k\theta)].$$

This satisfies the conditions for linear phase expressed by Eq. 4.8.1 with

$$H_1(\theta) = h(M) + 2\sum_{k=1}^{M} h(M+k)\cos(k\theta)$$

and

$$\alpha = M, \quad \beta = 0.$$

The three other possibilities for linear phase are summarized as follows. If $N = 2M+1$ and the coefficients possess odd symmetry, then

$$H_1(\theta) = h(M) + 2\sum_{k=1}^{M} h(M+k)\sin(k\theta)$$

and

$$\alpha = M, \quad \beta = \pi/2.$$

If $N = 2M$ and the coefficients have even symmetry, there will be symmetry about the fictitious "midpoint" $M - 1/2$. In this case, we have

$$H_1(\theta) = 2\sum_{k=1}^{M} h(M-1+k)\cos((k-1/2)\theta)$$

and

$$\alpha = M - 1/2, \quad \beta = 0.$$

Finally, for $N = 2M$ with odd symmetry, we again have symmetry about $M - 1/2$ and

$$H_1(\theta) = 2\sum_{k=1}^{M} h(M-1+k)\sin((k-1/2)\theta)$$

and

$$\alpha = M - 1/2, \quad \beta = \pi/2.$$

Notice that for all of these linear phase FIR types, the group delay is equal to $(N-1)/2$.

Linear phase FIRs, in addition to exhibiting coefficient symmetry, also have symmetric zero locations. To see this, let $H(z)$ be a linear phase FIR given by

$$H(z) = h_0 + h_1 z^{-1} + h_2 z^{-2} + \cdots + h_N z^N.$$

Define the *reverse* of $H(z)$ by

$$H_{rev}(z) = h_N + h_{N-1} z^{-1} + \cdots + h_1 z^{N-1} + h_0 z^N.$$

Comparing $H(z)$ and $H_{rev}(z)$, it is clear that

$$H_{rev}(z) = z^{-N} H(1/z).$$

Because $H(z)$ is linear phase, the coefficients are either even- or odd-symmetric so that

$$H_{rev}(z) = \pm H(z).$$

Therefore, for a linear phase FIR we have

$$z^{-N} H(1/z) = \pm H(z).$$

Consider the zeros of $H(z)$. Assume that $H(z_0) = 0$. By the above,

$$z_0^{-N} H(1/z_0) = 0.$$

This implies that $H(1/z_0) = 0$. Hence, the zeros of a linear phase FIR occur in reciprocal pairs. If there are an odd number of zeros, it is fairly straightforward to show that one of the zeros must fall at $z = \pm 1$.

4.9 FIR Design by Windowing

The first FIR design technique we will discuss uses finite-duration windows applied to infinite-duration sequences. We already introduced this concept in Chapter 2. Basically, the idea is as follows. We begin with the impulse response of an IIR filter which has a desired magnitude response. Applying a data window to this impulse response will result in a "blurring" of the ideal spectrum due to the convolution effect of windowing in the time domain. We will have to deal with effects such as Gibbs phenomenon and weakened transition bands. These will be dealt with by choosing the appropriate window.

Suppose we wish to design an FIR which approximates an ideal lowpass filter with a cutoff frequency of $\theta_c = \pi/2$. We begin with an ideal lowpass filter. The ideal lowpass filter with cutoff frequency $\pi/2$ has impulse response

$$h(k) = \frac{\sin(\pi k/2)}{\pi k}.$$

Recall that the symmetric window of length N was defined by

$$v_N(k) = \begin{cases} 1, & |k| \le (N-1)/2 \\ 0, & \text{otherwise} \end{cases}$$

If we wish to approximate the ideal lowpass filter with an FIR of length N, we can apply the window $v_N(k)$ to the sequence $h(k)$ which generates the FIR $h_1(k) =$, where

$$h_1(k) = v_N(k)h(k) = \begin{cases} h(k), & |k| \le (N-1)/2 \\ 0, & \text{otherwise.} \end{cases}$$

This FIR, however, is non-causal because it has an impulse response which is non-zero before $k = 0$. To make the FIR causal, we can time-shift it to the right by $(N-1)/2$ samples (which has no effect on the magnitude spectrum), giving

$$h_1(k) = \frac{\sin(\frac{\pi}{2}(k - (N-1)/2))}{\pi(k - (N-1)/2)}, \quad k = 0, 1, 2, \ldots, N-1.$$

For example, if $N = 129$, we have

$$h_1(k) = \frac{\sin((k-64)\pi/2)}{\pi(k-64)}, \quad k = 0, 1, 2, \ldots, 128.$$

The magnitude spectrum for the rectangular window is shown for various choices of N in Fig. 4.9.1.

There is still the matter of how to choose N. Clearly, there is a tradeoff between ripple magnitude, stopband suppression, and computational complexity. This will be discussed later. The ripple in the passband and stopband is due to the window. Recall from our discussion in Chapter 2 that both the mainlobe width and the sidelobe amplitude of the window will have the effect of smoothing the windowed response because of the convolution in the frequency domain. Qualitatively, we can see that a narrower mainlobe will result in a steeper transition for the windowed filter (see Fig. 4.9.1). Because the mainlobe width varies inversely with the rectangular window length, N, larger N will result in a steeper transition. The sidelobes, however, will cause "ringing" at the transition edges. Furthermore, we saw

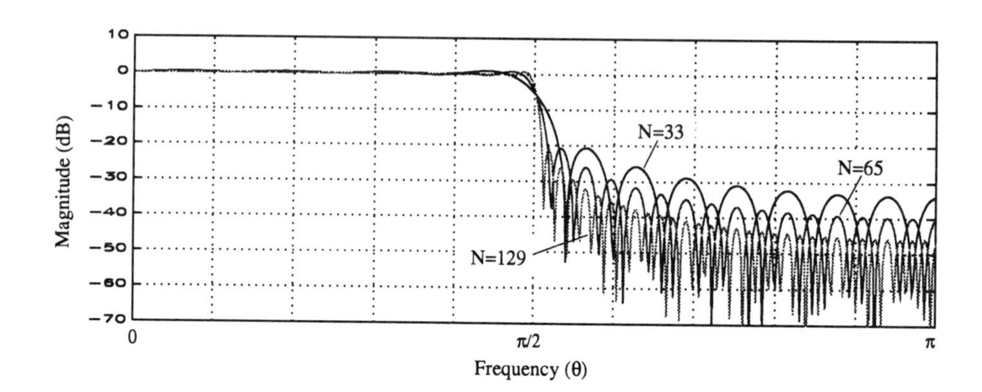

Figure 4.9.1: Lowpass FIR designed by symmetric rectangular windowing of ideal lowpass filter for $N = 33, 65, 129$.

that the sidelobe amplitude is essentially independent of N. The ringing is caused by the first and subsequent sidelobes being slid past the discontinuity in the ideal response in the convolution integral. Because the sidelobe amplitude ratio does not decrease with N, there will always be ripple at the transition band edges when using a rectangular window.

We should anticipate that it is possible to minimize these effects if there exist windows with narrower mainlobes and smaller sidelobe amplitudes. Indeed, there are. Unfortunately, the objectives of narrow mainlobes and small sidelobe amplitude are somewhat in conflict (again verifying the basic premise that nothing comes for free in nature). The study of these windows now follows.

Suppose the desired response of an FIR is $H_d(e^{j\theta})$. FIR design by rectangular windowing has the property of minimizing the mean-squared error between the desired and realized frequency responses of the FIR. To see this, define the mean-squared error ε by

$$\varepsilon = \int_{-\pi}^{\pi} |H_d(e^{j\theta}) - H_{FIR}(e^{j\theta})|^2 \, d\theta$$

subject to the FIR constraint

$$h_{FIR}(k) = 0, \quad k < 0, \quad \text{and} \quad k \geq N.$$

The mean-squared error provides a measure of the total deviation of the FIR frequency response from the desired frequency response. It is not immediately obvious how to minimize

ε subject to the FIR constraint. However, using Parseval's theorem, we have

$$\varepsilon = \sum_{k=-\infty}^{\infty} |h_d(k) - h_{FIR}(k)|^2.$$

Clearly, then, to minimize ε, we must choose

$$h_{FIR}(k) = h_d(k), \quad k = 0, 1, \ldots, N-1,$$

which is simply the rectangular-windowed ideal response. For this choice of $h_{FIR}(k)$, we have

$$\varepsilon = \sum_{k=-\infty}^{-1} |h_d(k)|^2 + \sum_{k=N}^{\infty} |h_d(k)|^2 = ||\boldsymbol{h}_d||_2^2 - ||\boldsymbol{h}_{FIR}||_2^2.$$

We have seen, however, that FIR design by rectangular windowing can lead to excessive ripple and overshoot at the transition edges. Thus, the concept of minimizing the mean-squared error is not always compatible with "good" FIR design. Rather, we would like an FIR with less ripple and overshoot. This is possible using other window types.

Recall that the rectangular window has a mainlobe width of $4\pi/N$ and a sidelobe amplitude of roughly -13.6 dB. The ripple in the rectangular window's frequency response is due to the fact that the time series drops abruptly from unity to zero. Smoother frequency responses are possible if we allow the window to taper gradually to zero at its endpoints. The Hamming window is one such window, and is derived from the rectangular window. We begin with the symmetric rectangular window $v_N(k)$, which we know has frequency response

$$V_N(e^{j\theta}) = \frac{\sin(N\theta/2)}{\sin(\theta/2)}.$$

This response is shown in Fig. 4.9.2. It is possible to attenuate the sidelobes of $V_N(e^{j\theta})$ by adding shifted copies of $V_N(e^{j\theta})$ at the points where the sidelobes occur. Thus, consider the frequency response given by

$$W_{Ham}(e^{j\theta}) = \frac{1}{2}V_N(e^{j\theta}) + \frac{1}{4}V_N(e^{j(\theta-2\pi/N)}) + \frac{1}{4}V_N(e^{j(\theta+2\pi/N)}).$$

This will result in a cancellation of sidelobes as shown in Fig. 4.9.2. Notice, however, that the mainlobe width has increased. The window coefficients are derived by taking the inverse DTFT of $W_{Ham}(e^{j\theta})$, which gives

$$w_{Ham}(k) = \frac{1}{2}v_N(k) + \frac{1}{2}\cos(2\pi k/N)v_N(k).$$

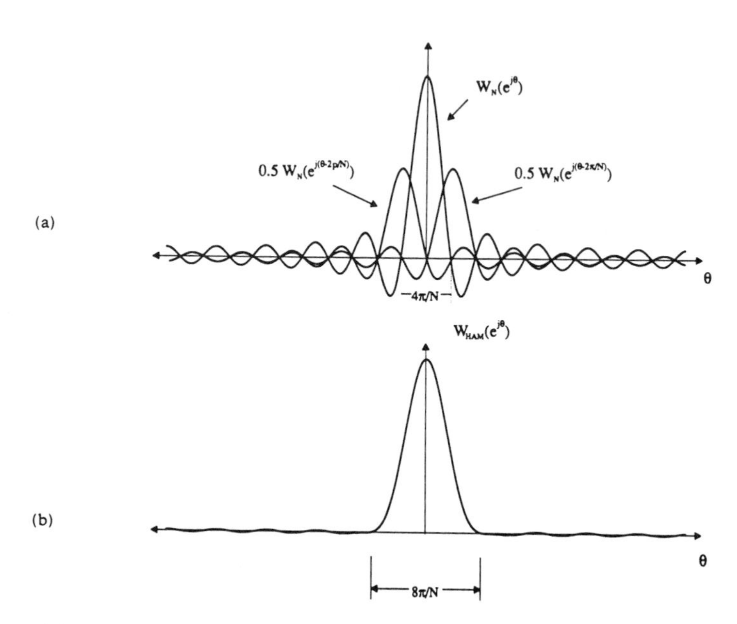

Figure 4.9.2: (a) Frequency response $V_N(e^{j\theta})$ of symmetric rectangular window; (b) summing shifted copies of $V_N(e^{j\theta})$ to attenuate sidelobes.

We will usually use an odd window length, N, so that $N = 2M + 1$. The window $w_{Ham}(k)$ is called a Hamming window, and is thus given by

$$w_{Ham}(k) = \begin{cases} 0.5 + 0.5\cos(2\pi k/N), & |k| \leq M \\ 0, & \text{otherwise} \end{cases}$$

The Hamming window has a mainlobe width of $8\pi/N$ and a peak sidelobe amplitude which is approximately -41 dB below the mainlobe. The frequency response of a 65-point Hamming window is shown in Fig. 4.9.3.

The *Hanning* window is obtained by a slight modification of the Hamming window, and is given by

$$w_{Han}(k) = \begin{cases} 0.54 + 0.46\cos(2\pi k/N), & |k| \leq M \\ 0, & \text{otherwise} \end{cases}$$

As with the Hamming window, the Hanning window also has a mainlobe width of $8\pi/N$ but has a peak sidelobe amplitude which is approximately -31 dB below the mainlobe.

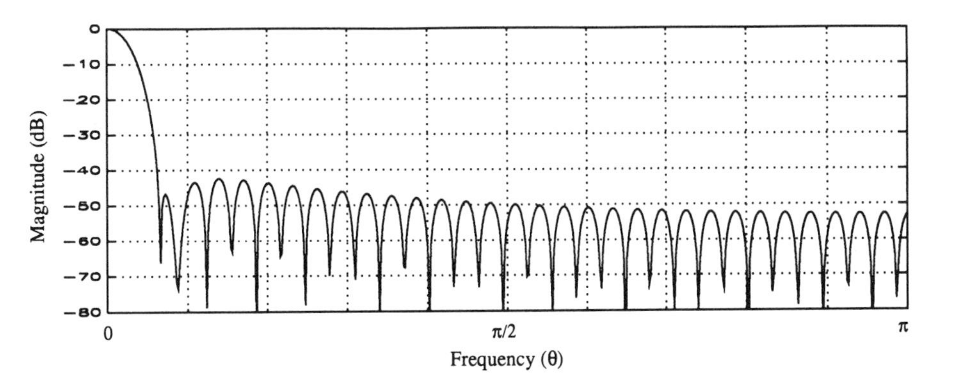

Figure 4.9.3: Frequency response of 65-point Hamming window.

The sidelobes of the rectangular window can be attenuated even more if we are willing to add more shifted copies of its frequency response than the Hamming or Hanning windows. The resulting window will have a larger mainlobe width but less ripple. This is the idea behind the *Blackman* window. The Blackman window is defined by

$$w_B(k) = \begin{cases} 0.42 - 0.5\cos(2\pi k/N) + 0.08\cos(4\pi k/N), & |k| \leq M \\ 0, & \text{otherwise} \end{cases}$$

The Blackman window has a mainlobe width of $12\pi/N$ and a peak sidelobe amplitude which is approximately -57 dB below the mainlobe.

The triangular, or *Bartlett* window is defined by

$$w_T(k) = \begin{cases} 1 - |k|/(M+1) & |k| \leq M \\ 0, & \text{otherwise} \end{cases}$$

The triangular window has a mainlobe width of $8\pi/N$, but a peak sidelobe amplitude which is -25 dB below the mainlobe, which is only slightly better than the rectangular window. The use of the triangular window is motivated primarily by positivity conditions for spectral estimation (which will be discussed later).

For the purposes of comparison, the magnitude responses of 33-point Hamming, Hanning, Bartlett, and Blackman windows are shown in Fig. 4.9.4.

There are many ways in which to formulate a performance index by which to measure the optimality of a given window function. The following criterion leads to another useful class of windows: given a cutoff frequency θ_c and an order N, minimize the energy in the frequency range $\theta_c \leq \theta \leq \pi$ over all unit-energy sequences $\{w(k)\}$ of length N. It was shown by Slepian [Sle78] that the solution to this optimization problem is a *prolate spheroidal* sequence. In

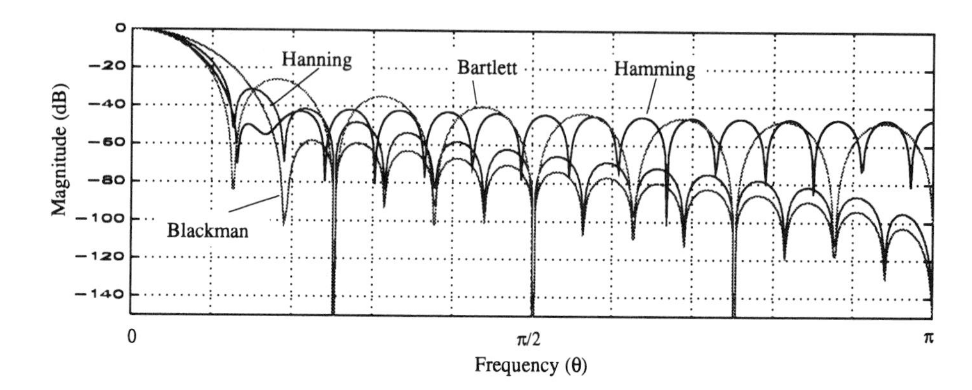

Figure 4.9.4: Magnitude response of 33-point Hamming, Hanning, Bartlett, and Blackman windows.

practice, computing the prolate spheroidal sequence is computationally difficult. However, Kaiser showed [Kai74b] that a good approximation to the optimal solution could be obtained using Bessel functions.

The windows we have discussed thus far have the characteristic that sidelobe amplitude is traded for mainlobe width. The Kaiser window technique is slightly more flexible in that there is more control over the mainlobe width and the sidelobe amplitude for a given order N. The Kaiser window of length $N = 2M + 1$ is given by

$$w_K(k) = \frac{I_0\left(\beta\sqrt{1 - \left(\frac{k}{M}\right)^2}\right)}{I_0(\beta)}, \quad |k| \leq M$$

where $I_0(\cdot)$ is the zeroth order modified Bessel function of the first kind, given by

$$I_0(x) = 1 + \sum_{k=1}^{\infty} \left[\left(\frac{1}{k!}\frac{x}{2}\right)^k\right]^2.$$

There are two parameters for the Kaiser window: the window length and the value of β. Qualitatively, increasing N while holding β constant decreases the mainlobe width but does

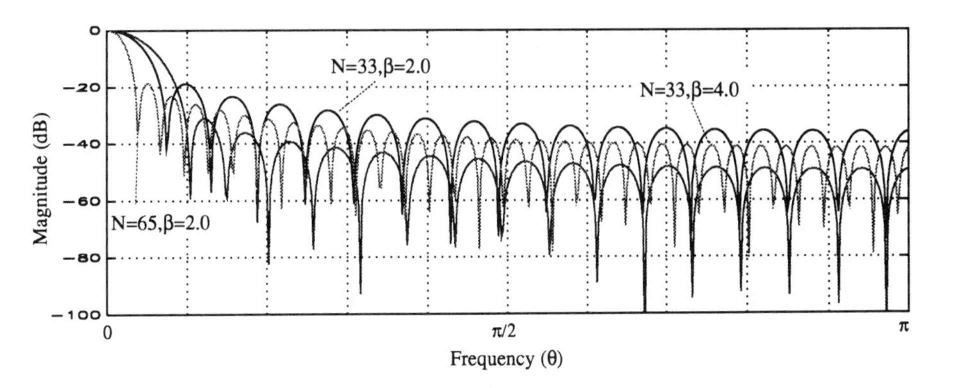

Figure 4.9.5: Kaiser window frequency responses.

not appreciably change the sidelobe amplitude. Similarly, the sidelobe level can be modified for fixed N by changing β.

Figure 4.9.5 shows the magnitude responses of three Kaiser windows. The first window has $N = 33$ and $\beta = 2.0$, the second window has $N = 33$ and $\beta = 4.0$ and the third window has $N = 65$ and $\beta = 2.0$. From this figure, the effects of different choices of N and β can be seen. Notice that for the two windows with $\beta = 2.0$, the maximum sidelobe amplitudes are roughly equal, while the larger order N decreases the mainlobe width. For the two windows with equal order, the mainlobe widths are approximately equal while the larger β gives smaller maximum sidelobe amplitude.

To apply a particular window to a filter design problem, recall that multiplication of two sequences in the time domain corresponds to convolution of Fourier transforms in the frequency domain. The reason ripple and overshoot occur when using a rectangular window to truncate an infinite sequence is because of the large ripple in the rectangular window's frequency response. This is due to the abrupt transition in the time domain from one to zero. It can be seen that the windows we have discussed above have a more gradual "taper" to zero in the time domain. Consequently, if the infinite sequence is windowed by one of these windows, less ripple can be expected at the expense of a wider transition region (due to the increased mainlobe width).

Let's consider a brief example. We begin with a length-33 approximation to an ideal

Window	Mainlobe Width	Sidelobe Amplitude (dB)
Rectangular	$4\pi/N$	-13.6 dB
Hamming	$8\pi/N$	-41
Hanning	$8\pi/N$	-31
Bartlett	$8\pi/N$	-25
Blackman	$12\pi/N$	-57
Kaiser	see text	see text

Table 4.2: Characteristics of some popular window functions

lowpass filter with cutoff frequency $\pi/2$. This gives the sequence

$$h(k) = \frac{\sin(k\pi/2)}{k\pi}, \quad |k| \leq 16.$$

Next, we window with a 33-point Hamming window, giving

$$h'(k) = w_{Ham}(k)h(k), \quad |k| \leq 16.$$

The sequence is then time-shifted for causality and has the frequency response shown in Fig. 4.9.6. Comparing with the rectangularly windowed filter, we can observe the effect of the window: the transition is not as steep, but the stopband attenuation is greater.

There are many other window functions we have not discussed here for the purposes of brevity. An excellent reference on the subject is given by [Har78]. There is no answer to the question "what is the ideal window?" The best that can be done is to have an understanding of the fundamentals so that an intelligent choice can be made depending on application-dependent needs. Table 4.2 provides a brief summary of the characteristics of some common windows.

4.10 FIR Design by Frequency Sampling

Another approach to FIR design is based directly on matching desired frequency response specifications rather than on truncated Fourier series. Specifically, suppose $H_d(e^{j\theta})$ is some desired frequency response. What we will attempt to do is find a sequence of length N whose DFT matches $H_d(e^{j\theta})$ at the N frequencies $2\pi n/N$, $n = 0, 1, \ldots, N-1$. To this end, define $H(n)$ by

$$H(n) = H_d(e^{j2\pi n/N}).$$

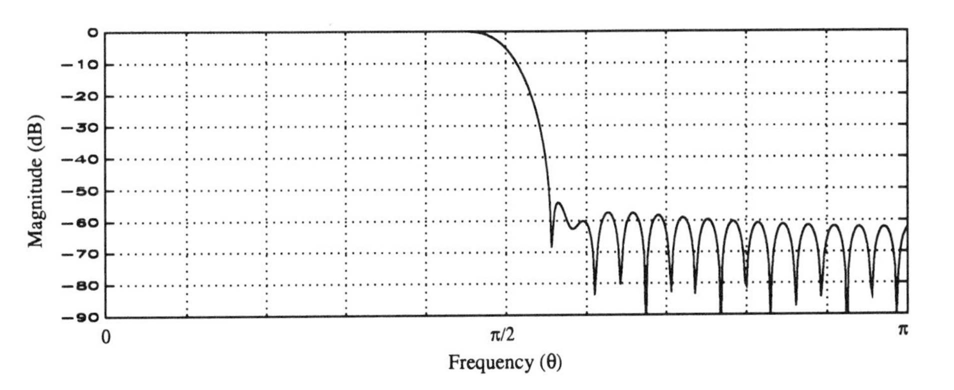

Figure 4.9.6: Hamming-windowed lowpass filter.

The corresponding FIR coefficients are given by the IDFT of $H(n)$, which gives

$$h(k) = \frac{1}{N} \sum_{n=0}^{N-1} H(n) e^{j2\pi nk/N}. \tag{4.10.1}$$

If the DTFT of $h(k)$ is given by $H(e^{j\theta})$, we will then have

$$H(e^{j\theta})\Big|_{\theta=2\pi n/N} = H_d(e^{j\theta})\Big|_{\theta=2\pi n/N}, \quad n = 0, 1, \ldots, N-1.$$

In other words, the frequency response of the FIR matches $H_d(e^{j\theta})$ at the N DFT points. The same can not be said, however, for the rest of the frequency response. This will be analyzed soon.

We can obtain an expression for the $\mathcal{Z}$-transform, and hence the DTFT of the derived FIR by interpolating through the frequency samples $H(n)$. The transfer function of the FIR is given by

$$H(z) = \sum_{k=0}^{N-1} h(k) z^{-k}.$$

Substituting Eq. 4.10.1 for $h(k)$ gives

$$H(z) = \frac{1}{N} \sum_{k=0}^{N-1} \left(\sum_{n=0}^{N-1} H(n) e^{j2\pi nk/N} \right) z^{-k}.$$

Interchanging the order of summation, we have

$$H(z) = \frac{1}{N} \sum_{n=0}^{N-1} H(n) \left(\sum_{k=0}^{N-1} (e^{j2\pi n/N} z^{-1})^k \right).$$

The inner summation is a geometric series which sums to

$$\sum_{k=0}^{N-1} (e^{j2\pi n/N} z^{-1})^k = \frac{1 - z^{-N}}{1 - e^{j2\pi n/N} z^{-1}}.$$

If we define $Q_n(z)$ by

$$Q_n(z) = \frac{1}{1 - e^{j2\pi n/N} z^{-1}}, \tag{4.10.2}$$

it follows that

$$H(z) = \frac{(1 - z^{-N})}{N} \sum_{n=0}^{N-1} H(n) Q_n(z) = (1 - z^{-N}) \sum_{n=0}^{N-1} \frac{H(n)}{1 - e^{j2\pi n/N} z^{-1}}. \tag{4.10.3}$$

Using Eq. 4.10.3, the FIR $H(z)$ can be implemented as the cascade of a comb filter and a parallel bank of filters $Q_n(z)$, each with gain given by $H(n)$, as shown in Fig. 4.10.1. The filter $Q_n(z)$ is a first-order system with a single zero at the origin and a single pole at $z = e^{j2\pi n/N}$. Each of the filters $Q_n(z)$ is highly frequency-selective around the frequency $\theta = 2\pi n/N$. Thus, the $Q_n(z)$ constitute an analysis bank where each analysis filter is a resonator centered about the frequency $\theta = 2\pi n/N$. The poles of the $Q_n(z)$ are exactly canceled by the zeros due to the comb filter, $(1 - z^{-N})/N$. All that will remain are the zeros of $H(z)$ which come from the summation in Eq. 4.10.3.

The decomposition of the frequency-sampling FIR into a cascade of a comb filter and a bank of resonators can simplify the implementation if the filter $H(z)$ is narrow-band. In this case, many of the $H(n)$ will be equal to zero and there will be no need to compute the response of the resonators corresponding to the $H(n)$ which are zero.

We are still left with the problem of needing to perform complex arithmetic since the $H(n)$ and the poles of the resonators are, in general, complex. Fortunately, we can exploit symmetry in the frequency samples, $H(n)$. In particular, we would like the FIR coefficients

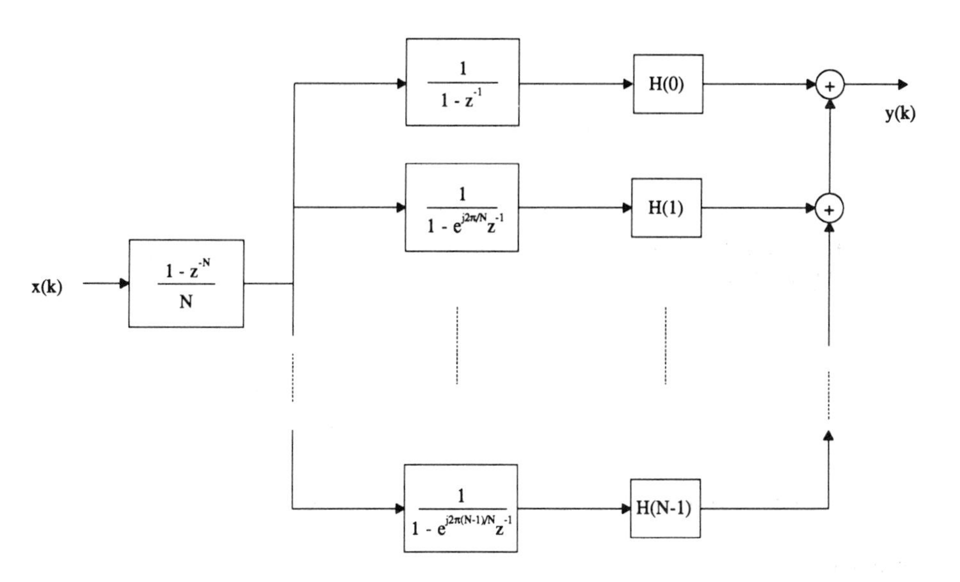

Figure 4.10.1: Decomposition of a frequency sampling FIR.

$h(k)$ to be real. There are several ways in which this can be accomplished. Consider the case where N is odd. The inverse DFT can be written as

$$h(k) = H(0) + \frac{1}{N} \sum_{n=1}^{N-1} H(n) e^{j2\pi nk/N}.$$

The frequencies at which $H_d(e^{j\theta})$ is sampled are

$$\theta_n = 0, \frac{2\pi}{N}, 2\frac{2\pi}{N}, \ldots, (N-1)\frac{2\pi}{N},$$

which are distributed about the unit circle as shown in Fig. 4.10.2. From the figure, it is clear that

$$e^{j\theta_n} = (e^{j\theta_{N-n}})^* = e^{-j\theta_{N-n}} \quad n = 1, 2, \ldots, (N-1)/2.$$

Therefore, if the frequency samples satisfy

$$H(N-n) = H^*(n), \quad n = 1, 2, \ldots, (N-1)/2, \tag{4.10.4}$$

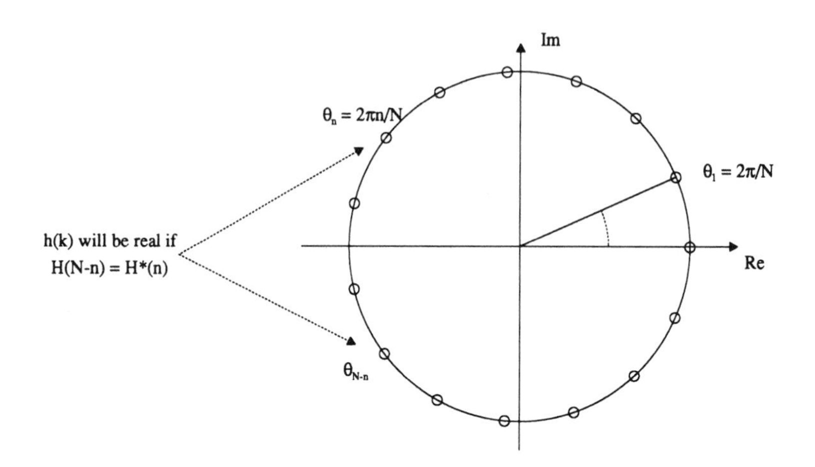

Figure 4.10.2: Distribution of frequency samples about the unit circle for N odd.

we can write

$$h(k) = H(0) + \sum_{n=1}^{(N-1)/2} H(n)e^{j2\pi nk/N} + \sum_{n=1}^{(N-1)/2} H^*(n)(e^{j2\pi nk/N})^*.$$

Combining both summations, we get

$$h(k) = H(0) + \sum_{n=1}^{(N-1)/2} 2\text{Re}(H(n)e^{j2\pi nk/N})$$

so that $h(k)$ will be real. Furthermore, if the frequency samples $H(n)$ are real and symmetric, we have

$$h(k) = H(0) + \sum_{n=1}^{(N-1)/2} 2H(n)\cos(2\pi nk/N).$$

The case where N is even requires a slight modification and will be omitted here.

With the symmetry conditions expressed in Eq. 4.10.4, Eq. 4.10.3 can be expressed as

$$H(z) = \frac{(1-z^{-N})}{N}\left(\frac{H(0)}{1-z^{-1}} + \sum_{n=1}^{(N-1)/2}\left(\frac{H(n)}{1-e^{j2\pi n/N}} + \frac{H^*(n)}{1-e^{-j2\pi n/N}}\right)\right)$$

which reduces to

$$H(z) = \frac{(1-z^{-N})}{N}\left(\frac{H(0)}{1-z^{-1}} + \sum_{n=1}^{(N-1)/2}\frac{2\text{Re}(H(n)) - 2\text{Re}(H(n)e^{j2\pi n/N})z^{-1}}{1-2\cos(\frac{2\pi n}{N})z^{-1}+z^{-2}}\right) \quad (4.10.5)$$

This is a decomposition of $H(z)$ into the cascade of a comb and an analysis bank where the analysis filters all have real coefficients. If the frequency samples are not only conjugate-symmetric, but real as well, we then have

$$H(z) = \frac{(1 - z^{-N})}{N} \left(\frac{H(0)}{1 - z^{-1}} + \sum_{n=1}^{(N-1)/2} \frac{2H(n) - 2H(n)\cos(2\pi n/N)z^{-1}}{1 - 2\cos(\frac{2\pi n}{N})z^{-1} + z^{-2}} \right) \tag{4.10.6}$$

Example 4.12

Suppose we wish to design a frequency-sampling FIR to approximate an ideal lowpass filter of order $N = 33$ with cutoff frequency $\theta_c = \pi/8$. The frequencies which are sampled occur at

$$\theta_n = \frac{2\pi n}{33}.$$

Therefore, we can choose

$$H(n) = \begin{cases} 1, & 0 \le n \le 4 \\ 0, & 5 \le n \le 16. \end{cases}$$

To meet the symmetry conditions expressed by Eq. 4.10.4, we can choose the rest of the $H(n)$ according to

$$H(n) = \begin{cases} 0, & 17 \le n \le 27 \\ 1, & 29 \le n \le 32. \end{cases}$$

The frequency samples of the ideal response are shown in Fig. 4.10.3. With the $H(n)$ given as above, the FIR coefficients $h(k)$ will be real and the FIR will have the frequency response shown in Fig. 4.10.3. Notice that the frequency response $H(e^{j\theta})$ matches the desired response at the discrete frequencies θ_n but there is ringing elsewhere. This ringing can be reduced by relaxing the transition band and choosing $H(4) = H(29) = 0.5$. Again, the FIR coefficients will be real, and the frequency response is also shown in Fig. 4.10.3. Notice that the ringing at the band edge has been reduced.

Direct implementation of the 33rd order FIR will require 33 multiplications and additions per output point. Suppose instead that we use the frequency-sampling decomposition as expressed in Eq. 4.10.6. The FIR transfer function $H(z)$ can then be written as

$$H(z) = \frac{(1 - z^{-33})}{33} \left(\frac{1}{1 - z^{-1}} + \sum_{n=1}^{4} \frac{2 - 2\cos(\frac{2\pi n}{33})z^{-1}}{1 - 2\cos(\frac{2\pi n}{33})z^{-1} + z^{-2}} \right).$$

Each of the second-order analysis filters can be implemented in a manner which requires three multiplications and three additions, as will be shown when we discuss state variables. The first-order filter requires no multiplication and one addition and the comb filter requires one multiplication and one addition. Therefore, the entire FIR can be implemented with a total of 13 multiplications and 14 additions, which is more efficient than the direct-form implementation.

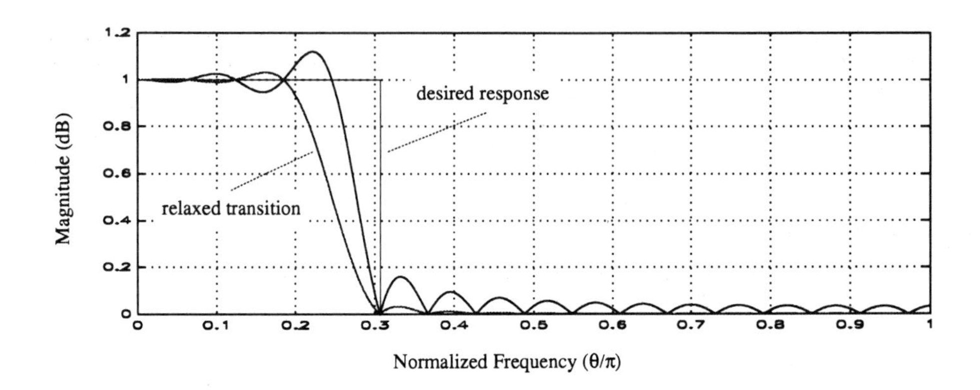

Figure 4.10.3: Ideal response and frequency samples for Example 4.12; frequency response of FIR designed by frequency sampling; and frequency response of FIR designed by frequency sampling with relaxed transition band.

4.11 Equiripple FIR Design

The frequency sampling and window design methods for FIR filters are fairly simple and frequently yield very good results. It was shown that the rectangular window corresponds to Fourier series truncation and gives a FIR which is optimal in the mean-squared error sense. Consider for a moment, however, the case of a simple lowpass filter designed by any of the windowing techniques. Notice that in order to meet a desired stopband attenuation criterion, we end up with a filter which meets the criterion at the very beginning of the stopband and then greatly exceeds the specifications in the remainder of the stopband. In a sense, this can be regarded as "overdesigning." That is to say, perhaps there exists an FIR of lower order which still meets the stopband criterion without exceeding it as drastically as the window method. From the standpoint of implementation, reduced filter order is important because it facilitates higher throughput and better fixed-point behavior.

FIR Filters which are designed using Fourier series have their approximation errors concentrated at the band edges. If the approximation error is allowed to be spread equally about the entire pass- and stopband, it is possible to obtain a filter which meets the design objectives with a lower order than that obtained from the Fourier series. This is the principle behind the *equiripple FIR* design method.

The equiripple FIR design is based on classical polynomial approximation theory and is optimal with respect to a performance metric which is different than the least-squares metric used by the Fourier series design methods. That is, we are concerned with minimizing the maximum error over a set of frequencies. As such, the equiripple design method is referred to as a *minimax* method. In an equiripple FIR, the local extrema in the passband are all equal and the local extrema in the stopband are all equal.

To design an equiripple lowpass filter, the passband and stopband edges θ_p and θ_s are specified along with the maximum passband ripple, δ_1 and the maximum stopband ripple, δ_2. The equiripple filter which meets these specifications will have the smallest possible order of any FIR. The solution to the equiripple FIR problem is based on the famous *alternation theorem* from polynomial approximation theory [Che66]. Based on this theorem, the *Parks-McClellan technique* makes use of an iterative algorithm called the *Remez exchange algorithm* to find the equiripple FIR. The details are rather complicated and are given in [MP73].

Most digital filter design packages incorporate the Parks-McClellan technique for equiripple FIR design. Using the Parks-McClellan technique, it is possible to design not only lowpass filters, but highpass, bandpass, arbitrary magnitude response, Hilbert transformer, and differentiator filters, as well.

Let's examine the design of an equiripple lowpass filter. Typically, the order of the filter, M, will not be known prior to the design. What is usually specified is $\theta_p, \theta_s, \delta_1$, and δ_2. There is no absolute rule for determining the required filter order, although a number of approximations have been derived. One such approximation is due to Kaiser, who obtained

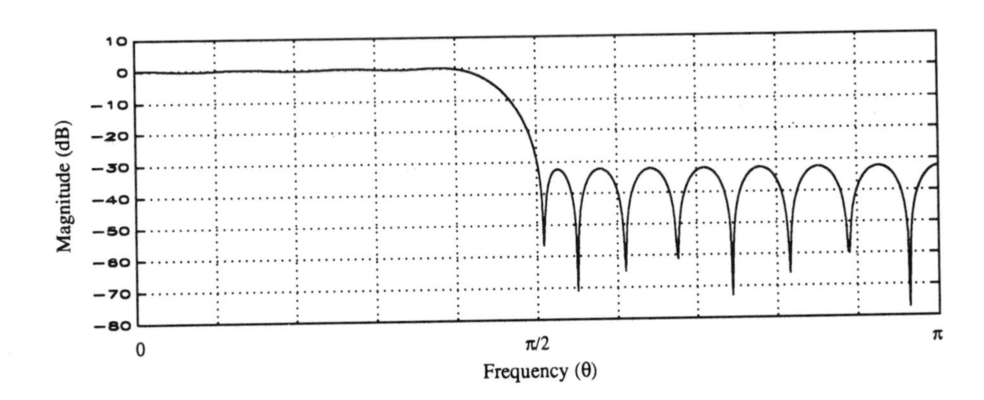

Figure 4.11.1: Frequency response for 30-th order equiripple FIR in example 4.13.

the formula

$$M \approx \frac{-20\log_{10}(\sqrt{\delta_1\delta_2}) - 13)}{14.6(\theta_s - \theta_p)/(2\pi)} + 1. \qquad (4.11.1)$$

Qualitatively, we can see the effect of the ripple size and the transition width on the filter order. As the ripple is allowed to grow, the filter order will decrease. Similarly, if the transition width increases, the filter order decreases.

Example 4.13

Suppose we wish to design an equiripple lowpass FIR with passband over the range $[0, 0.2\pi]$ and stopband over the range $[.25\pi, \pi]$. Furthermore, suppose the passband should have a magnitude within 0.02 of unity and the stopband within 0.02 of zero. Thus, $\delta_1 = \delta_2 = 0.02$. We thus have

$$H_d(e^{j\theta}) = \begin{cases} 1, & 0 \leq \theta \leq 0.2\pi \\ 0, & 0.25\pi \leq \theta \leq \pi \end{cases}$$

The approximate order M is determined by Eq. 4.11.1 to be equal to 30. The Parks-McClellan algorithm was used to generate the 30-th order equiripple FIR whose frequency response is shown in Fig. 4.11.1. Notice the equiripple behavior in the pass and stopbands. The objective was to allow a ripple of no more than 0.02 in the pass and stopbands. This corresponds to a magnitude of roughly -33 dB in the stopband and 0.17 dB in the passband, which is satisfied by the filter in Fig. 4.11.1.

Chapter 5

STOCHASTIC PROCESSES

5.1 Introduction

The purpose of this chapter is to provide a brief review of the theory of stationary stochastic processes and introduce some of the concepts we will need for Wiener filtering, adaptive filtering, fixed-point filter design, and spectral estimation. It is assumed that the reader is already familiar with the basic notions of probability theory. If the reader is unfamiliar with the basic theory, Appendix A may be consulted. For further background, the interested reader is referred to any standard reference on probability theory and stochastic processes, such as the comprehensive treatments by Papoulis [Pap65] or Parzen [Par62].

Recall that a wide-sense stationary (WSS) stochastic process is a stochastic process whose first and second order moments are invariant to shifts in time. That is,

$$\mathcal{E}[x(k+m)] = \mathcal{E}[x(k)] \quad \text{for all } k$$

and

$$\mathcal{E}[x(k+m)x(k+n)] = \mathcal{E}[x(m)x(n)] \quad \text{for all } k.$$

If $\{x(k)\}$ is WSS, the mean is a constant

$$\mathcal{E}[x(k)] = \mu.$$

Because the second-order moments are invariant to time shifts, they can be characterized by a one-dimensional autocorrelation sequence $r_{xx}(k)$, where

$$r_{xx}(n) = \mathcal{E}[x(k)x(k+n)].$$

If the mean, μ is equal to zero, then the autocorrelation sequence is equal to the autocovariance sequence. For a real stochastic process $x(k)$, the autocorrelation sequence satisfies

$$r_{xx}(k) = r_{xx}(-k) \tag{5.1.1}$$

so that the autocorrelation sequence is real and even. For a WSS process, we define the function $P_{xx}(z)$ by

$$P_{xx}(z) = \sum_{k=-\infty}^{\infty} r_{xx}(k) z^{-k}. \tag{5.1.2}$$

The function $P_{xx}(z)$ is seen to be the $\mathcal{Z}$-transform of the autocorrelation sequence. Because $\{r_{xx}(k)\}$ is real and even, it immediately follows that

$$P_{xx}(z) = P_{xx}(z^{-1}). \tag{5.1.3}$$

For an arbitrary real and even autocorrelation sequence $\{r_{xx}(k)\}$, there is no guarantee that $P_{xx}(z)$ will be a rational function. Most of the stochastic processes we will study, however, result from uncorrelated noise being passed through linear time-invariant systems which are described by rational transfer functions. Consequently, as we will see, the resulting power spectral densities will be rational. Therefore, we will primarily deal with functions $P_{xx}(z)$ which are rational functions of z.

An immediate consequence of Eq. 5.1.3 is that the poles and zeros of $P_{xx}(z)$ occur in *reciprocal pairs*. That is, if $z = p_0$ is a pole of $P_{xx}(z)$ then so is p_0^{-1}. The same is true for the zeros. This will provide a convenient *factorization* of $P_{xx}(z)$. Because $P_{xx}(z)$ is the $\mathcal{Z}$-transform of the autocorrelation sequence, the autocorrelation sequence may be recovered from the PSD by $\mathcal{Z}$-transform inversion. In general,

$$r_{xx}(k) = \frac{1}{2\pi j} \oint P_{xx}(z) z^{k-1}\, dz. \tag{5.1.4}$$

In particular, the power, $r_{xx}(0)$, can be computed as

$$\sigma_x^2 = r_{xx}(0) = \frac{1}{2\pi j} \oint P_{xx}(z) z^{-1}\, dz.$$

The *power spectrum*, $P_{xx}(\theta)$ of a WSS stochastic process $\{x(k)\}$ is defined as the Fourier transform of the autocorrelation sequence,

$$P_{xx}(\theta) = \sum_{k=-\infty}^{\infty} r_{xx}(k) e^{-jk\theta}. \tag{5.1.5}$$

Again, because the autocorrelation sequence $\{r_{xx}(k)\}$ is real and even, the power spectrum $P_{xx}(\theta)$ is a real and even function of θ. Because $P_{xx}(\theta)$ is the Fourier transform of $\{r_{xx}(k)\}$, the autocorrelation sequence can be recovered from the power spectrum by

$$r_{xx}(k) = \frac{1}{2\pi} \int_{-\pi}^{\pi} P_{xx}(\theta) e^{jk\theta}\, d\theta. \tag{5.1.6}$$

The signal power, $r_{xx}(0)$ is thus computed by

$$r_{xx}(0) = \frac{1}{2\pi} \int_{-\pi}^{\pi} P_{xx}(\theta)\, d\theta. \tag{5.1.7}$$

According to Eq. 5.1.7, the signal power is determined by the integral of the power spectrum over the range $-\pi \leq \theta \leq \pi$. As such, we can regard the power spectrum as a distribution of the signal power in the frequency domain. The function $P_{xx}(\theta)\, d\theta$ can be interpreted as the contribution to the total signal power due to frequencies between θ and $\theta + d\theta$.

Example 5.1

Let $x(k)$ be a zero-mean white noise process. We then have

$$r_{xx}(k) = \sigma^2 \delta(k).$$

From the definition,

$$P_{xx}(z) = \sum_{k=-\infty}^{\infty} \sigma^2 \delta(k) z^{-k} = \sigma^2.$$

Similarly, we find that $P_{xx}(\theta) = \sigma^2$. Thus, the zero-mean white noise process has a power spectrum which is "flat" and equal to σ^2 for all θ. This means that the signal power of the white noise process is distributed uniformly among all frequencies.

5.2 WSS Signals and Linear Systems

Suppose a WSS signal is passed through a linear system $H(z)$. For the time being, no assumption is made about the causality of the input: it is allowed to start at $-\infty$. What can we say about the output? If the input is $x(k)$, we have

$$y(k) = \sum_{m=-\infty}^{\infty} h(m) x(k-m)$$

so that

$$\mathcal{E}[y(k)] = \mathcal{E}\left[\sum_{m=-\infty}^{\infty} h(m) x(k-m) \right].$$

Because $x(k)$ is WSS, it has mean μ. Using the linearity of the expectation operator,

$$\mathcal{E}[y(k)] = \mu \sum_{m=-\infty}^{\infty} h(m).$$

Clearly, if $h(k)$ is absolutely summable, the mean of the output will be bounded and given by

$$\mathcal{E}[y(k)] = \mu H(e^{j0}). \tag{5.2.1}$$

If the input is zero-mean, the output will also be zero-mean. Thus, we have shown that the mean of the output is constant.

What about the correlation sequence? To show that the correlation sequence is invariant to a shift in time, assume the contrary. We compute

$$r_{yy}(k, k+m) = \mathcal{E}[y(k)y(k+m)].$$

Where

$$\mathcal{E}[y(k)y(k+m)] = \mathcal{E}\left[\sum_{r=-\infty}^{\infty} h(r)x(k-r) \sum_{s=-\infty}^{\infty} h(s)x(k+m-s)\right]$$

which becomes

$$\mathcal{E}[y(k)y(k+m)] = \sum_{r=-\infty}^{\infty} \sum_{s=-\infty}^{\infty} h(r)h(s)\mathcal{E}[x(k-r)x(k+m-s)].$$

Because $x(k)$ is WSS,

$$\mathcal{E}[x(k-r)x(k+m-s)] = r_{xx}(m+r-s)$$

so that

$$\mathcal{E}[y(k)y(k+m)] = \sum_{r=-\infty}^{\infty} h(r) \sum_{s=-\infty}^{\infty} h(s)r_{xx}(m+r-s). \tag{5.2.2}$$

Thus, the output correlation is also invariant to shift in time and is a function only of the lag m, which means that the output is also WSS. Henceforth, we can refer to the output autocorrelation as $r_{yy}(m)$. To obtain a simplified expression for $r_{yy}(m)$, we make the substitution $l = s - r$ in Eq. 5.2.2, which gives

$$r_{yy}(m) = \sum_{r=-\infty}^{\infty} h(r) \sum_{l=-\infty}^{\infty} h(l+r)r_{xx}(m-l).$$

Reversing the order of summation,

$$r_{yy}(m) = \sum_{l=-\infty}^{\infty} r_{xx}(m-l)\left[\sum_{r=-\infty}^{\infty} h(r)h(r+l)\right].$$

The inner summation is recognized as the deterministic autocorrelation sequence of the impulse response, $h(k)$ (denoted by $r_{hh}(k)$). Therefore,

$$r_{yy}(m) = \sum_{l=-\infty}^{\infty} r_{hh}(l) r_{xx}(m-l). \tag{5.2.3}$$

so that the output autocorrelation sequence is given by the convolution of the filter's autocorrelation sequence and the input autocorrelation sequence. Taking the $\mathcal{Z}$-transform of Eq. 5.2.3, we have

$$P_{yy}(z) = P_{hh}(z) P_{xx}(z).$$

We previously showed that the deterministic autocorrelation sequence has $\mathcal{Z}$-transform

$$P_{hh}(z) = H(z) H(z^{-1}).$$

Therefore,

$$P_{yy}(z) = H(z) H(z^{-1}) P_{xx}(z). \tag{5.2.4}$$

Also,

$$P_{yy}(\theta) = H(e^{j\theta}) H(e^{-j\theta}).$$

Because the impulse response was assumed to be real, it follows that

$$H(e^{-j\theta}) = H^*(e^{j\theta})$$

and therefore,

$$P_{yy}(\theta) = |H(e^{j\theta})|^2 P_{xx}(\theta). \tag{5.2.5}$$

Equations 5.2.4 and 5.2.5 are sometimes referred to as the *Wiener-Khinchine theorem*. Consider the case where $H(z)$ is a very narrow bandpass filter satisfying

$$H(e^{j\theta}) = \begin{cases} 1, & |\theta - \theta_c| \leq B/2 \\ 0, & \text{otherwise} \end{cases}$$

Then the output power is due to frequency components about the center frequency θ_c and from Eq. 5.2.5, it follows that

$$P_{yy}(\theta) = \begin{cases} P_{xx}(\theta), & |\theta - \theta_c| \leq B/2 \\ 0, & \text{otherwise} \end{cases}$$

Therefore, the output power $r_{yy}(0)$ is obtained by integrating $P_{xx}(\theta)$ over the region $\theta_c - B/2 \leq |\theta| \leq \theta_c + B/2$, and in this manner it is seen that the PSD gives a measure of the contribution to the signal power as a function of frequency.

Finally, we wish to compute the crosscorrelation between the input and the output when a linear system is fed with a WSS input. Again, we assume that the output is not WSS, giving

$$r_{xy}(k, k+m) = \mathcal{E}[x(k)y(k+m)] = \sum_{r=-\infty}^{\infty} \mathcal{E}[x(k)h(r)x(k+m-r)].$$

Rearranging, we have

$$r_{xy}(k, k+m) = \sum_{r=-\infty}^{\infty} h(r)\mathcal{E}[x(k)x(k+m-r)] = \sum_{r=-\infty}^{\infty} h(r)r_{xx}(m-r)$$

so that the crosscorrelation depends only on the lag index, m. Thus, the crosscorrelation between the input and the output is given by the convolution of the filter's input response and the input's autocorrelation sequence, *i.e.*,

$$r_{xy}(k) = h(k) * r_{xx}(k).$$

The corresponding $\mathcal{Z}$-transform relationship gives the *cross spectral density* (CSD) $P_{xy}(z)$ as

$$P_{xy}(z) = H(z)P_{xx}(z) \tag{5.2.6}$$

and we also have

$$P_{xy}(\theta) = H(e^{j\theta})P_{xx}(\theta). \tag{5.2.7}$$

If the roles of $x(k)$ and $y(k)$ are reversed, we obtain the crosscorrelation $r_{yx}(k)$ where

$$r_{yx}(k) = \mathcal{E}[y(n)x(n+k)].$$

It is obvious that $r_{xy}(k)$ and $r_{yx}(k)$ are related by

$$r_{yx}(k) = r_{xy}(-k).$$

Because $r_{yx}(k)$ is obtained by time-reversing $r_{xy}(k)$, it follows that

$$P_{yx}(z) = P_{xy}(z^{-1}). \tag{5.2.8}$$

Therefore,

$$P_{yx}(z) = P_{xx}(z^{-1})H(z^{-1})$$

and because $P_{xx}(z) = P_{xx}(z^{-1})$,

$$P_{yx}(z) = P_{xx}(z)H(z^{-1}). \tag{5.2.9}$$

Finally, assume that $d(k)$ and $x(k)$ are jointly WSS stationary and that $P_{xd}(z)$ is known. If $x(k)$ is passed through a stable filter $H(z)$, we have shown that the output $y(k)$ is also WSS. We know how to compute $P_{xy}(z)$ and $P_{yy}(z)$. We need to be able to express the CSD $P_{yd}(z)$ in terms of $P_{xd}(z)$. We begin with the crosscorrelation sequence $r_{yd}(k)$,

$$r_{dy}(k) = \mathcal{E}[d(n)y(n+k)] = \mathcal{E}\left[\sum_{i=-\infty}^{\infty} h_i d(n)x(n+k-i)\right]$$

which becomes

$$r_{dy}(k) = \sum_{i=-\infty}^{\infty} h_i r_{dx}(k-i).$$

We immediately recognize this as a convolution of $\{h_i\}$ and $\{r_{dx}(i)\}$ so that

$$P_{dy}(z) = H(z)P_{dx}(z).$$

Replacing z with z^{-1},

$$P_{dy}(z^{-1}) = H(z^{-1})P_{dx}(z^{-1})$$

which, by Eq. 5.2.8, means that

$$P_{yd}(z) = H(z^{-1})P_{xd}(z).$$

The PSD and CSD relationships established in this chapter are summarized in Table 5.1.

Asymptotic Stationarity

The derivation of the transform relationships in the previous section implicitly assumed that the input stochastic process $\boldsymbol{x}$ which was applied to the linear system $H(z)$ exists for *all time*. This is a theoretical constraint which must be satisfied to guarantee that the output stochastic process will be truly wide-sense stationary. In practice, however, the input must begin at some starting time in the finite past. It follows that the output cannot be precisely WSS, for there is some particular significance to the starting time. If the linear system $H(z)$ is stable, the statistics of the output will undergo a transient phase after which the output eventually takes on the characteristics of a WSS stochastic process. The duration of this transient phase is determined by the time constant of $H(z)$. This phenomenon is known as *asymptotic stationarity*. For our purposes, we will not be concerned with the transient behavior of asymptotically stationary stochastic processes. Rather, we can safely assume that the input was applied sufficiently far in the past so that the output is for all intents and purposes WSS.

Given $\boldsymbol{x}, \boldsymbol{y}, \boldsymbol{d}, \boldsymbol{h}$ where $\boldsymbol{y} = \boldsymbol{h} * \boldsymbol{x}$:
$P_{yy}(z) = H(z)H(z^{-1})P_{xx}(z)$
$P_{xy}(z) = H(z)P_{xx}(z)$
$P_{yx}(z) = H(z^{-1})P_{xx}(z)$
$P_{dy}(z) = H(z)P_{dx}(z)$
$P_{yd}(z) = H(z^{-1})P_{xd}(z)$

Table 5.1: Power and cross spectral density relationships.

5.3 Spectral Factorization

Let $w(k)$ be a WSS signal with PSD $P_{ww}(\theta)$. We are interested in determining if $w(k)$ can be modeled as the output of a linear system $H(z)$ which is fed with white noise $u(k)$. If this is possible, we know from the Wiener-Khinchine theorem that

$$P_{ww}(z) = H(z)H(z^{-1})P_{uu}(z)$$

and

$$P_{ww}(\theta) = |H(e^{j\theta})|^2 P_{uu}(\theta).$$

If $u(k)$ is white with unit variance, then a trivial solution to our problem is

$$H(e^{j\theta}) = \sqrt{P_{ww}(\theta)}.$$

This, however, can lead to a noncausal solution and if minimum-phase is not required, the solution is nonunique. This is because if $F(z)$ is allpass, then $F(z)H(z)$ will also solve our problem. If we require that $H(z)$ be causal, however, the situation is more interesting. The existence of a solution is given by the following theorem [GS58].

Theorem 4 (Kolmogorov-Szego) *Let $P_{ww}(\theta)$ be real, even, and nonnegative. If $P_{ww}(\theta)$ satisfies the conditions*

$$\int_{-\pi}^{\pi} P_{ww}(\theta)\, d\theta < \infty$$

and

$$\exp\left(\frac{1}{2\pi}\int_{-\pi}^{\pi}\ln(P_{ww}(\theta))\,d\theta\right) > 0$$

then there exists a causal, finite-energy sequence $\boldsymbol{h}$ *such that*

$$P_{ww}(\theta) = |H(e^{j\theta})|^2.$$

Obtaining such a sequence $\boldsymbol{h}$ given $P_{ww}(\theta)$ is known as *spectral factorization.* This theorem makes no mention of *rationality.* In general, it is difficult to infer a form for $P_{ww}(z)$ directly from an expression for $P_{ww}(\theta)$. If $P_{ww}(\theta)$ is a rational function of $\cos(\theta)$, we can determine a rational $P_{ww}(z)$ for which

$$P_{ww}(\theta) = P_{ww}(z)\big|_{z=e^{j\theta}}$$

by choosing

$$P_{ww}(z) = P_{ww}(\theta)\big|_{\cos(\theta)=\frac{1}{2}(z-z^{-1})}\,.$$

In the special case where $P_{ww}(z)$ is a rational function of z, the Kolmogorov-Szego theorem implies that it is possible to find a *rational* function $H(z)$ such that

$$P_{ww}(z) = H(z)H(z^{-1})$$

where $H(z)$ is minimum phase. This $H(z)$ is fairly simple to compute. We have already seen that for rational $P_{ww}(z)$, the poles and the zeros must occur in reciprocal pairs. Assuming a rational $P_{ww}(z)$ of the form

$$P_{ww}(z) = \frac{B(z)}{A(z)},$$

the numerator can be factored as

$$B(z) = N(z)N(z^{-1})$$

where $N(z)$ is built up from the zeros inside the unit circle. The denominator can be factored as

$$A(z) = D(z)D(z^{-1})$$

where $D(z)$ is built up from the poles inside the unit circle. Thus,

$$P_{ww}(z) = \frac{N(z)N(z^{-1})}{D(z)D(z^{-1})}$$

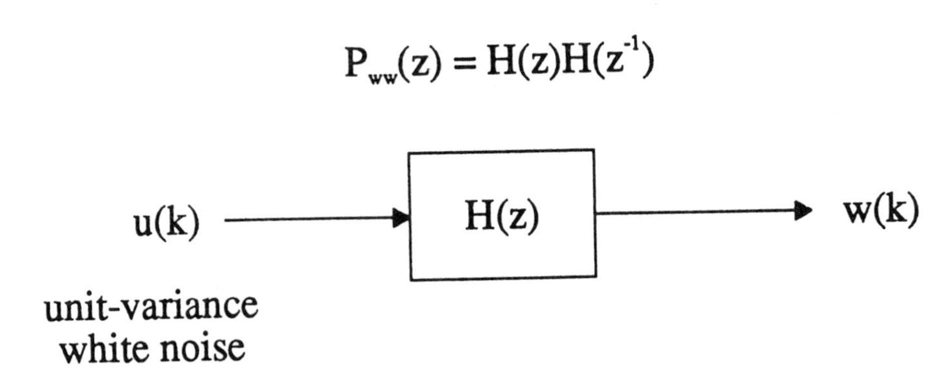

Figure 5.3.1: Using spectral factorization to synthesize a stochastic process $w(k)$ as the output of a causal, minimum-phase filter when driven with white noise.

and we take as $H(z)$ the causal, minimum phase function $H(z)$ where

$$H(z) = \frac{N(z)}{D(z)}.$$

With $H(z)$ thus constructed, we have a causal, minimum-phase filter which can be used to synthesize the stochastic process $\{w(k)\}$. If the input to $H(z)$ is zero-mean, unit-variance white noise $\{u(k)\}$, the PSD of the output is equal to

$$H(z)H(z^{-1})P_{uu}(z) = H(z)H(z^{-1}),$$

which equals $P_{ww}(z)$. This procedure is known as *spectral factorization* and is illustrated in Fig. 5.3.1.

Example 5.2

Suppose the stochastic process $\{w(k)\}$ has the autocorrelation sequence

$$r_{ww}(k) = 0.5^{|k|}.$$

The PSD is given by

$$P_{ww}(z) = \sum_{k=0}^{\infty} 0.5^k z^{-k} + \sum_{k=-\infty}^{-1} 0.5^{-k} z^{-k}$$

which can be simplified to

$$P_{ww}(z) = \frac{0.75}{(1-0.5z^{-1})(1-0.5z)}.$$

If we identify $H(z)$ with

$$H(z) = \frac{\sqrt{0.75}}{1-0.5z^{-1}},$$

it follows that

$$P_{ww}(z) = H(z)H(z^{-1}).$$

Thus, the causal, finite-energy sequence $\boldsymbol{h}$ is given by

$$h(k) = \sqrt{0.75}(0.5)^k, \quad k \geq 0.$$

Alternatively, $w(k)$ can be regarded as the output of the filter $H(z)$ when driven with unit-variance white noise.

The Wold decomposition

The Wold decomposition [Pap65] shows that a stationary stochastic process can be represented as the output of a causal MA system of possibly infinite order when driven with white noise. Suppose $\{x(k)\}$ is WSS with autocorrelation sequence $\{r_{xx}(k)\}$ and

$$P_{xx}(z) = \sum_{k=-\infty}^{\infty} r_{xx}(k)z^{-k}.$$

If $\{r_{xx}(k)\}$ is a valid autocorrelation sequence, then $\log P_{xx}(z)$ will be analytic in an annular region which includes the unit circle. This allows $\log P_{xx}(z)$ to be expanded in a Laurent series as

$$\log P_{xx}(z) = \sum_{k=-\infty}^{\infty} c_{xx}(k)z^{-k} \tag{5.3.1}$$

where the $c_{xx}(k)$ are called the *cepstral coefficients*. Clearly, the sequence $\{c_{xx}(k)\}$ has $\mathcal{Z}$-transform $\log P_{xx}(z)$. When evaluated on the unit circle, we have

$$\log P_{xx}(\theta) = \sum_{k=-\infty}^{\infty} c_{xx}(k)e^{-jk\theta}.$$

Because $P_{xx}(\theta)$ is real and even (it is a power spectrum), $\log P_{xx}(\theta)$ is also real and even. This means that the cepstral coefficients form an even sequence since

$$c_{xx}(k) = \frac{1}{2\pi}\int_{-\pi}^{\pi}(\log P_{xx}(\theta))e^{jk\theta}\,d\theta.$$

Using Eq. 5.3.1, it immediately follows that

$$P_{xx}(z) = \exp\left[\sum_{k=-\infty}^{\infty} c_{xx}(k)z^{-k}\right]. \tag{5.3.2}$$

Because $\{c_{xx}(k)\}$ is even, we have

$$\sum_{k=-\infty}^{\infty} c_{xx}(k)z^{-k} = c_{xx}(0) + \sum_{k=1}^{\infty} c_{xx}(k)z^{-k} + \sum_{k=1}^{\infty} c_{xx}(k)(z^{-1})^{-k}. \tag{5.3.3}$$

Thus, Eq. 5.3.2 becomes

$$P_{xx}(z) = \sigma_v^2 H(z)H(z^{-1}) \tag{5.3.4}$$

where

$$\sigma_v^2 = \exp[c_{xx}(0)]$$

and

$$H(z) = \exp\left[\sum_{k=1}^{\infty} c_{xx}(k)z^{-k}\right]. \tag{5.3.5}$$

Equation 5.3.4 evaluated on the unit circle gives the relationship

$$P_{xx}(\theta) = \sigma_v^2|H(e^{j\theta})|^2. \tag{5.3.6}$$

Clearly, the causal part of the cepstral sequence is associated with $H(z)$ and the anticausal part with $H(z^{-1})$. The filter $H(z)$ can be used to synthesize the stochastic process $\{x(k)\}$. With $H(z)$ expanded in a Laurent series as

$$H(z) = \sum_{k=0}^{\infty} h(k)z^{-k},$$

suppose $H(z)$ is driven by white noise $\{v(k)\}$ with power σ_v^2. Then the output $\{x(k)\}$ will be stationary with power spectral density

$$P_{xx}(\theta) = \sigma_v^2|H(e^{j\theta})|^2.$$

This representation of $\{x(k)\}$ as the output of a (possibly infinite order) MA filter $H(z)$ when driven with white noise is known as the *Wold decomposition.* Equivalently, the process $\{x(k)\}$ with PSD $P_{xx}(\theta)$ may be *whitened* by applying it to the filter $1/H(z)$. The output, $\{v(k)\}$, is known as the *innovations sequence* associated with the stochastic process $\{x(k)\}$.

5.4 Models of Stochastic Processes

An important class of stochastic processes can be represented by a rational transfer function model. These stochastic processes occur frequently in practice, and the rational transfer function model is often used as an approximate representation method for other stochastic processes, as well. A stochastic process which is represented by a rational transfer function model can be generated by driving a system which has a rational transfer function with a white noise input. The input and output are related by

$$x(k) = -\sum_{n=1}^{p} a_n x(k-n) + \sum_{n=0}^{q} b_n v(k-n) \tag{5.4.1}$$

where $\{v(k)\}$ is white with zero mean and power σ_v^2. Such as stochastic process is called *autoregressive moving average* (ARMA). The a_i are known as the *autoregressive parameters* and the b_i are called the *moving average parameters.* To explicitly indicate the numerator and denominator orders, we refer to the process as an ARMA(q,p) process. The transfer function of the system is

$$H(z) = \frac{B(z)}{A(z)} = \frac{b_0 + b_1 z^{-1} + \cdots + b_q z^{-q}}{1 + a_1 z^{-1} + a_2 z^{-2} + \cdots + a_p z^{-p}}$$

where it is assumed that the roots of $A(z)$ are inside the unit circle to guarantee that $H(z)$ is stable and causal. This assumption is necessary to insure that the output sequence $\{x(k)\}$ is WSS. The PSD is then given by the Wiener-Khinchine theorem as

$$P_{xx}(z) = H(z)H(z^{-1})P_{vv}(z),$$

and since $P_{vv}(z) = \sigma_v^2$, we have

$$P_{xx}(z) = \sigma_v^2 \frac{B(z)B(z^{-1})}{A(z)A(z^{-1})}. \tag{5.4.2}$$

Similarly, the power spectrum is given by

$$P_{xx}(\theta) = \sigma_v^2 \frac{|B(e^{j\theta})|^2}{|A(e^{j\theta})|^2}. \tag{5.4.3}$$

We can assume that the numerator and denominator polynomials are monic without loss of generality since an arbitrary filter gain can be "absorbed" by the noise power σ_v^2. Figure 5.4.1 shows how an ARMA process is generated from a white noise input.

The system $H(z)$ which is used to generate the ARMA process is called the ARMA *synthesis filter.* It is interesting to note that we may recover the driving noise $\{v(k)\}$ if the

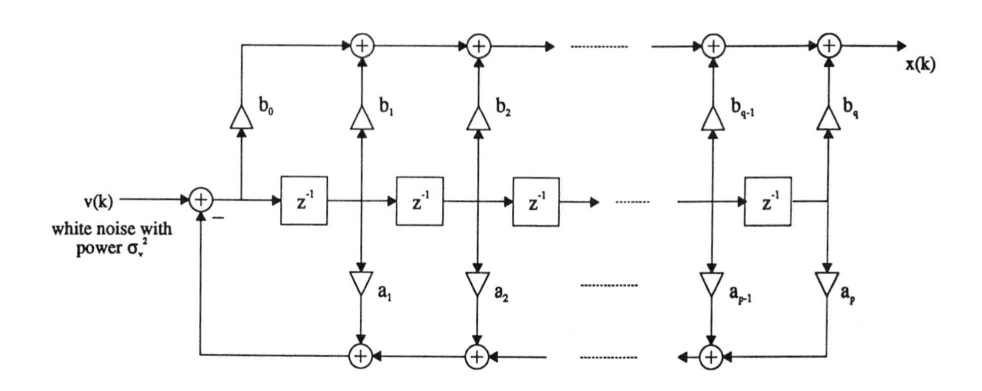

Figure 5.4.1: ARMA(q, p) stochastic process model (shown with $p = q$).

ARMA process $\{x(k)\}$ is applied as the input to the filter $H^{-1}(z)$. This inverse filter is known as the ARMA *analysis filter*.

If we remove the autoregressive part of the filter, which means that all of the a_i equal zero except $a_0 = 1$ and assume that $b_0 = 1$ we have an input-output relationship given by

$$x(k) = 1 + \sum_{n=1}^{q} b_n x(k-n). \tag{5.4.4}$$

This is called a *moving average* model and denoted by MA(q). The transfer function of the system which generates the MA(q) process is

$$H(z) = B(z) = 1 + \sum_{n=1}^{q} b_n z^{-n}$$

so that the PSD is given by

$$P_{xx}(z) = \sigma_v^2 B(z) B(z^{-1}).$$

This means that the power spectrum is simply

$$P_{xx}(\theta) = \sigma_v^2 |B(e^{j\theta})|^2.$$

The transfer function $B(z)$ is known as the MA process synthesis filter and is seen to be an all-zero filter of order q. Fig. 5.4.2 illustrates the MA process model. The driving noise can

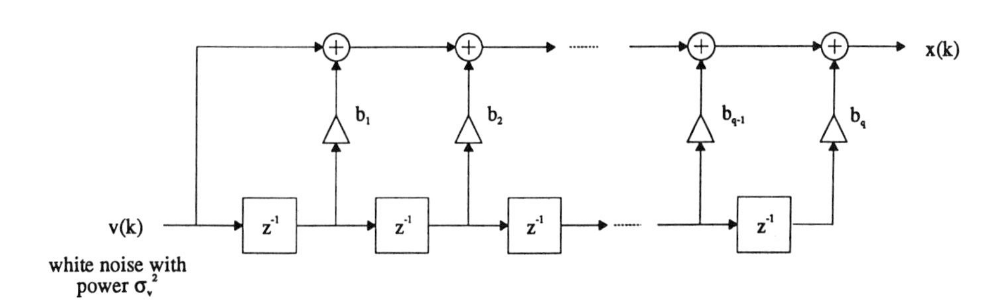

Figure 5.4.2: MA(q) stochastic process model.

be recovered by applying the time series $\{x(k)\}$ to the all-pole filter $B^{-1}(z)$, which is called the analysis filter.

Finally, if we remove the moving average part of an ARMA model, which means that all b_i are zero except $b_0 = 1$, we are left with an *autoregressive process* denoted by AR(p). For the AR(p) process, we have

$$x(k) = -\sum_{n=1}^{p} a_n x(k-n) + v(k). \tag{5.4.5}$$

The transfer function of the system which generates the AR(p) process is

$$H(z) = \frac{1}{A(z)} = \frac{1}{1 + a_1 z^{-1} + \cdots + a_p z^{-p}}$$

so that the PSD is given by

$$P_{xx}(z) = \frac{\sigma_v^2}{A(z)A(z^{-1})}.$$

This means that the power spectrum is simply

$$P_{xx}(\theta) = \frac{\sigma_v^2}{|A(e^{j\theta})|^2}.$$

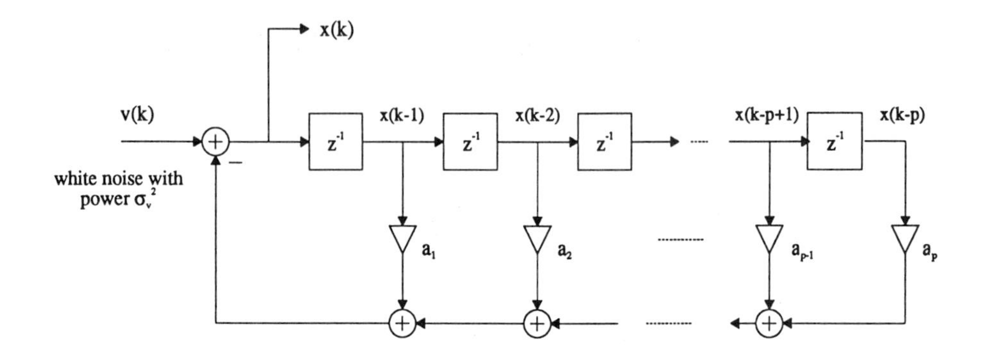

Figure 5.4.3: AR(p) stochastic process model.

The transfer function $A(z)$ is known as the AR process synthesis filter and is seen to be an all-pole filter of order p. Fig. 5.4.3 illustrates the AR process model. The driving noise can be recovered by applying the time series $\{x(k)\}$ to the all-zero filter $A^{-1}(z)$, which is called the analysis filter.

We can make qualitative statements about the power spectra of ARMA, AR, and MA models. Because the MA model is produced by an all-zero filter, MA spectra are capable of achieving sharp nulls when there are zeros near the unit circle. Similarly, AR models can achieve sharp peaks at frequencies corresponding to poles near the unit circle. ARMA spectra can have deep nulls and sharp peaks. A comparison of these spectra is shown in Fig. 5.4.4

In practice, we will frequently be concerned with the problem of spectral *estimation*, which is covered in detail later in the book. The problem of spectral estimation is estimating the power spectrum of a stochastic process given a finite set of measurements from a *single realization* of the process. There are two important classes of spectral estimation techniques: nonparametric techniques and parametric techniques. The nonparametric techniques make no assumptions about a model for the process and instead base a spectral estimate on the measurements alone. These techniques tend to perform poorly compared to the parametric techniques, which *do* assume a model (MA, AR, or ARMA) for the process and base a spectral estimate on the derived model parameters. One of the basic problems is determining which model is appropriate: MA, AR, or ARMA.

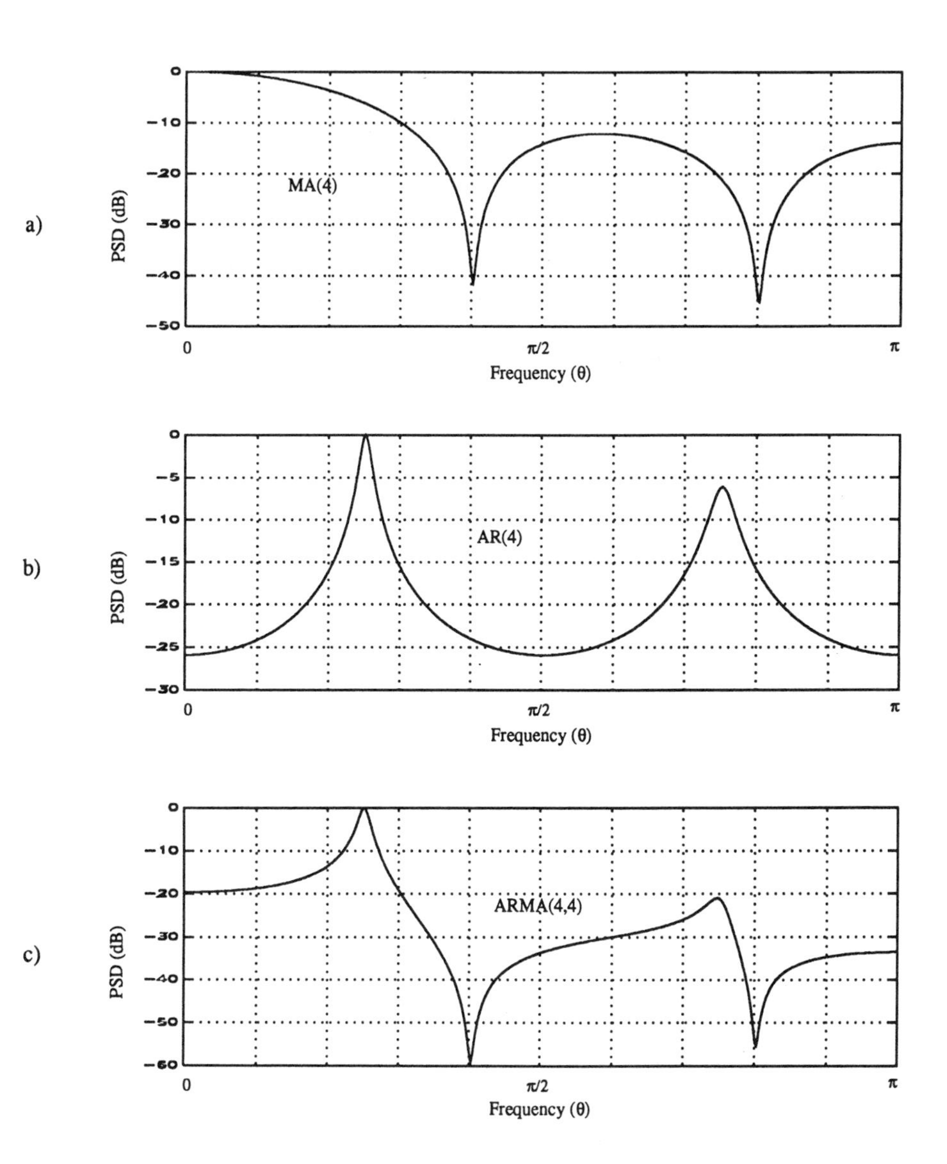

Figure 5.4.4: (a) MA(4) spectrum (b) AR(4) spectrum (c) ARMA(4,4) spectrum.

Both the Wold decomposition theorem and the Kolmogorov-Szego theorem provide important connections between the different rational transfer function models. The Wold decomposition states that an AR or an ARMA process can be represented by a MA model of possibly infinite order. The Kolmogorov-Szego theorem implies that a MA or an ARMA process may be represented by an AR model of possibly infinite order. These results are significant because they allow us to obtain a good approximation even if the wrong model is chosen. For instance, if we are trying to model an AR(p, q) process with an AR model, the results can still be acceptable if a large enough order is chosen for the AR model.

To show the relationship between the coefficients of an ARMA(p, q) model and an AR(∞) model, let $G(z)$ be the denominator polynomial of the AR(∞) model so that

$$\frac{1}{G(z)} = \frac{B(z)}{A(z)}$$

which means that

$$G(z)B(z) = A(z).$$

Taking the inverse $\mathcal{Z}$-transform, we have

$$\sum_{n=0}^{q} g(k-n)b_n = a_k$$

because $b_n = 0$ for $n < 0$ and $n > q$. Therefore,

$$g(k) = -\sum_{n=1}^{q} g(k-n)b_n + a_k.$$

Finally, since $a_k = 0$ for $k > p$, we get

$$g(k) = \begin{cases} 1, & k = 0 \\ -\sum_{n=1}^{q} g(k-n)b_n + a_k, & 1 \le k \le p \\ -\sum_{n=1}^{q} g(k-n)b_n, & k \ge p \end{cases} \tag{5.4.6}$$

The recursion is initialized with $g(-1), g(-2), \ldots, g(-q) = 0$. Working in the other direction, suppose we are given the parameters of an AR(∞) model and would like to compute the equivalent ARMA(p, q) model. In general, this is a highly nontrivial problem. [1] If we know

[1]This is a classic problem in mathematical system theory known as the *realization problem*.

p and q *a priori*, however, the problem is simplified greatly. Using Eq. 5.4.6, we have the relationship for $k > p$

$$g(k) = -\sum_{n=1}^{q} b_n g(k-n).$$

Using this for $k = p+1$ through $k = p+q$ gives q equations which can be solved for the q unknown MA parameters b_i. In matrix form, we have

$$\begin{bmatrix} g(p) & g(p-1) & \cdots & g(p-q+1) \\ g(p+1) & g(p) & \cdots & g(p-q+2) \\ \vdots & \vdots & \ddots & \vdots \\ g(p+q-1) & g(p+q-2) & \cdots & g(p) \end{bmatrix} \begin{bmatrix} b_1 \\ b_2 \\ \vdots \\ b_q \end{bmatrix} = - \begin{bmatrix} g(p+1) \\ g(p+2) \\ \vdots \\ g(p+q) \end{bmatrix}.$$

Next, we use Eq. 5.4.6 again for $k = 1, \ldots, p$, giving

$$g(k) = -\sum_{n=1}^{q} g(k-n) b_n + a_k, \quad 1 \le k \le p$$

which can be rearranged to give the AR parameters as

$$a_k = g(k) + \sum_{n=1}^{p} b_n g(k-n), \quad 1 \le k \le p.$$

In matrix form, we have

$$\begin{bmatrix} a_1 \\ a_2 \\ \cdots \\ a_p \end{bmatrix} = \begin{bmatrix} g(1) & 1 & 0 & \cdots & 0 \\ g(2) & g(1) & 1 & \cdots & 0 \\ \vdots & \vdots & \vdots & \ddots & \vdots \\ g(p) & g(p-1) & g(p-2) & \cdots & g(p-q) \end{bmatrix} \begin{bmatrix} 1 \\ b_1 \\ \vdots \\ b_q \end{bmatrix}.$$

Thus, only the first $p+q$ coefficients of the AR(∞) polynomial $G(z)$ are necessary to compute both $A(z)$ and $B(z)$. If, however, $G(z)$ did not actually arise from an ARMA(p,q) model, $G(z)$ and $A(z)/B(z)$ will only agree up to the first $p+q$ terms.

If we reverse the roles of $A(z)$ and $B(z)$ in the preceding discussion, it is possible to relate the parameters of a MA(∞) model $L(z)$ to an AR(p,q) model through

$$l(k) = \begin{cases} 1, & k = 0 \\ -\sum_{n=1}^{p} l(k-n) a_n + b_k, & 1 \le k \le q \\ -\sum_{n=1}^{q} l(k-n) a_n, & k \ge q \end{cases} \tag{5.4.7}$$

Relating the model to the autocorrelation sequence

For the AR, MA, and AR models, it is possible to derive relationships between the model parameters and the autocorrelation sequences. We begin with the ARMA model. Since

$$P_{xx}(z) = \sigma_v^2 \frac{B(z)B(z^{-1})}{A(z)A(z^{-1})}, \tag{5.4.8}$$

it follows that

$$P_{xx}(z)A(z) = \sigma_v^2 \frac{B(z)B(z^{-1})}{A(z^{-1})} = \sigma_v^2 B(z)H(z^{-1}). \tag{5.4.9}$$

Now, recall that $P_{xx}(z)$ is the $\mathcal{Z}$-transform of $\{r_{xx}(k)\}$ and $H(z^{-1})$ is the $\mathcal{Z}$-transform of $\{h(-k)\}$. Thus, if we take the inverse $\mathcal{Z}$-transform of both sides of Eq. 5.4.9, we get

$$\sum_{n=0}^{p} a_n r_{xx}(k-n) = \sigma_v^2 \sum_{n=0}^{q} b_n h(n-k). \tag{5.4.10}$$

Using the fact that $a_0 = 1$, Eq. 5.4.10 becomes

$$r_{xx}(k) = -\sum_{n=1}^{p} a_n r_{xx}(k-n) + \sigma_v^2 \sum_{n=0}^{q} b_n h(n-k). \tag{5.4.11}$$

Because the second summation in Eq. 5.4.11 is expanded as

$$\sum_{n=0}^{q} b_n h(n-k) = b_0 h(-k) + b_1 h(1-k) + \cdots + b_q h(q-k),$$

it is clear that the second summation has no contribution to $r_{xx}(k)$ if $k > q$ since $H(z)$ is assumed causal. We can rewrite this summation as

$$\sum_{n=0}^{q} b_n h(n-k) = \sum_{n=0}^{q-k} h(n) b_{k+n}.$$

Thus, we have

$$r_{xx}(k) = \begin{cases} -\sum_{n=1}^{p} a_n r_{xx}(k-n) + \sigma_v^2 \sum_{n=0}^{q-k} h(n) b_{k+n}, & k = 0, 1, \ldots, q \\ -\sum_{n=1}^{p} a_n r_{xx}(k-n) & k \geq q+1. \end{cases} \tag{5.4.12}$$

The p AR parameters of the ARMA model can be computed from the second equation above. For $k \geq q+1$, we have

$$r_{xx}(k) = -\sum_{n=1}^{p} a_n r_{xx}(k-n).$$

The p equations in p unknowns for $k = q+1, q+2, \ldots, q+p$ can be written in matrix form as

$$\begin{bmatrix} r_{xx}(q) & r_{xx}(q-1) & \cdots & r_{xx}(q-p+1) \\ r_{xx}(q+1) & r_{xx}(q) & \cdots & r_{xx}(q-p+2) \\ \vdots & \vdots & \ddots & \vdots \\ r_{xx}(q+p-1) & r_{xx}(q+p-2) & \cdots & r_{xx}(q) \end{bmatrix} \begin{bmatrix} a_1 \\ a_2 \\ \vdots \\ a_p \end{bmatrix} = - \begin{bmatrix} r_{xx}(q+1) \\ r_{xx}(q+2) \\ \vdots \\ r_{xx}(q+p) \end{bmatrix}. \quad (5.4.13)$$

Equation 5.4.13 is known as the *extended Yule-Walker* equation for the ARMA process and allows us to compute the AR parameters from the autocorrelation sequence. The relationship for the MA parameters is more difficult to compute because of the convolution between the MA parameters and the ARMA impulse response in Eq. 5.4.6.

For a purely autoregressive process, it is simple to determine the relationship between the autocorrelation sequence and the AR parameters. Since $b_i = \delta(i)$, we have

$$r_{xx}(k) = \begin{cases} -\sum_{n=1}^{p} a_n r_{xx}(k-n) + \sigma_v^2 \sum_{n=0}^{q-k} h(n)\delta(k+n), & k = 0, 1, \ldots, q \\ -\sum_{n=1}^{p} a_n r_{xx}(k-n), & k \geq q+1. \end{cases} \quad (5.4.14)$$

The top equation becomes

$$r_{xx}(k) = -\sum_{n=1}^{p} a_n r_{xx}(k-n) + \sigma_v^2 h(-k), \quad k = 0, 1, \ldots, q \quad (5.4.15)$$

and since $h(-k) = 0$ for $k > 0$,

$$r_{xx}(k) = \begin{cases} -\sum_{n=1}^{p} a_n r_{xx}(-n) + \sigma_v^2 & k = 0 \\ -\sum_{n=1}^{p} a_n r_{xx}(k-n) & k \geq 1 \end{cases} \quad (5.4.16)$$

and we have as usual $r_{xx}(-k) = r_{xx}(k)$ for real stochastic processes. The second line of Eq. 5.4.16 can be used to solve for the AR parameters from the first $p+1$ elements of the autocorrelation sequence. In matrix form, we have

$$\begin{bmatrix} r_{xx}(0) & r_{xx}(1) & \cdots & r_{xx}(p-1) \\ r_{xx}(1) & r_{xx}(0) & \cdots & r_{xx}(p-2) \\ \vdots & \vdots & \ddots & \vdots \\ r_{xx}(p-1) & r_{xx}(p-2) & \cdots & r_{xx}(0) \end{bmatrix} \begin{bmatrix} a_1 \\ a_2 \\ \vdots \\ a_p \end{bmatrix} = - \begin{bmatrix} r_{xx}(1) \\ r_{xx}(2) \\ \vdots \\ r_{xx}(p) \end{bmatrix}. \tag{5.4.17}$$

Equation 5.4.17 is known as the *Yule-Walker equation* for the AR process. Notice that the matrix formed from the autocorrelation is Toeplitz and symmetric. There exists an efficient algorithm for inverting this set of equations which is known as the Levinson-Durbin algorithm. The solution can be computed in $O(p^2)$ operations and is discussed later when we study linear prediction.

Both lines of Eq. 5.4.16 can be incorporated into a single system of equations which will be important in subsequent discussions. This is called the *augmented normal equation* for reasons which will become apparent later. Specifically, we have

$$\begin{bmatrix} r_{xx}(0) & r_{xx}(1) & \cdots & r_{xx}(p) \\ r_{xx}(1) & r_{xx}(0) & \cdots & r_{xx}(p-1) \\ \vdots & \vdots & \ddots & \cdots \\ r_{xx}(p) & r_{xx}(p-1) & \cdots & r_{xx}(0) \end{bmatrix} \begin{bmatrix} 1 \\ a_1 \\ \vdots \\ a_p \end{bmatrix} = \begin{bmatrix} \sigma_v^2 \\ 0 \\ \vdots \\ 0 \end{bmatrix}. \tag{5.4.18}$$

It is important to note that the first $p+1$ elements of the autocorrelation sequence completely determine the power spectrum of an AR process. This is because

$$P_{xx}(\theta) = \sum_{k=-\infty}^{\infty} r_{xx}(k)e^{-jk\theta}$$

and any $r_{xx}(k)$ for $|k| > p$ can be computed recursively as

$$r_{xx}(k) = -\sum_{n=1}^{p} a_n r_{xx}(k-n)$$

once the a_i have been computed from $r_{xx}(0)$ through $r_{xx}(p)$ via Eq. 5.4.17. Also, the first row of Eq. 5.4.18 shows that the power of the driving white noise may be expressed as

$$\sigma_v^2 = \sum_{i=0}^{p} a_i r_x(i) \tag{5.4.19}$$

where $a_0 = 1$.

Example 5.3

Suppose $\{x(k)\}$ is an AR(1) process which is modeled by

$$x(k) = -\alpha x(k-1) + v(k)$$

where $\{v(k)\}$ is zero-mean white noise with power σ_v^2. In this case, $a_1 = \alpha$ and $\{r_{xx}(k)\}$ satisfies the recursion

$$r_{xx}(k) = -\alpha r_{xx}(k-1).$$

Therefore,

$$r_{xx}(k) = (-\alpha)^k r_{xx}(0), \quad k > 0,$$

and, of course, $r_{xx}(-k) = r_{xx}(k)$. To determine $r_{xx}(0)$, we use Eq. 5.4.19, which says that

$$r_{xx}(0) + \alpha r_{xx}(1) = \sigma_v^2$$

Thus,

$$r_{xx}(0) + \alpha(-\alpha) r_{xx}(0) = \sigma_v^2$$

which means that

$$r_{xx}(0) = \frac{\sigma_v^2}{1-\alpha^2}.$$

Therefore, the autocorrelation sequence is given by

$$r_{xx}(k) = \frac{\sigma_v^2}{1-\alpha^2}(-\alpha^k), \quad k > 0.$$

Therefore, the AR(1) autocorrelation sequence is either damped or oscillatory, depending on the sign of α. Figure 5.4.5 shows the AR(1) power spectrum for several values of α. Notice that the power spectrum is either lowpass or highpass, depending on the sign of α. This is to be expected since

$$P_{xx}(\theta) = \frac{1}{|A(e^{j\theta})|^2} = \frac{1}{|1+\alpha e^{j\theta}|^2}.$$

Consequently, the magnitude of $P_{xx}(\theta)$ grows as α moves closer to the unit circle. It should be clear that the AR(1) process will be either highpass or lowpass, and that at least an AR(2) model is necessary in order to have a bandpass power spectrum.

Finally, we can derive the relationship between the autocorrelation sequence and the MA parameters of a MA model. Using Eq. 5.4.6 and remembering that $a_i = \delta(i)$ and $h(i) = b_i$ for a MA model, we have

$$r_{xx}(k) = \begin{cases} \sigma_v^2 \sum_{n=0}^{q-k} b_n b_{k+n} & k = 0, 1, \ldots, q \\ 0 & k \geq q+1. \end{cases} \tag{5.4.20}$$

and, as usual, $r_{xx}(-k) = r_{xx}(k)$ for real stochastic processes. Clearly, the relationship between $r_{xx}(k)$ and the MA parameters is nonlinear.

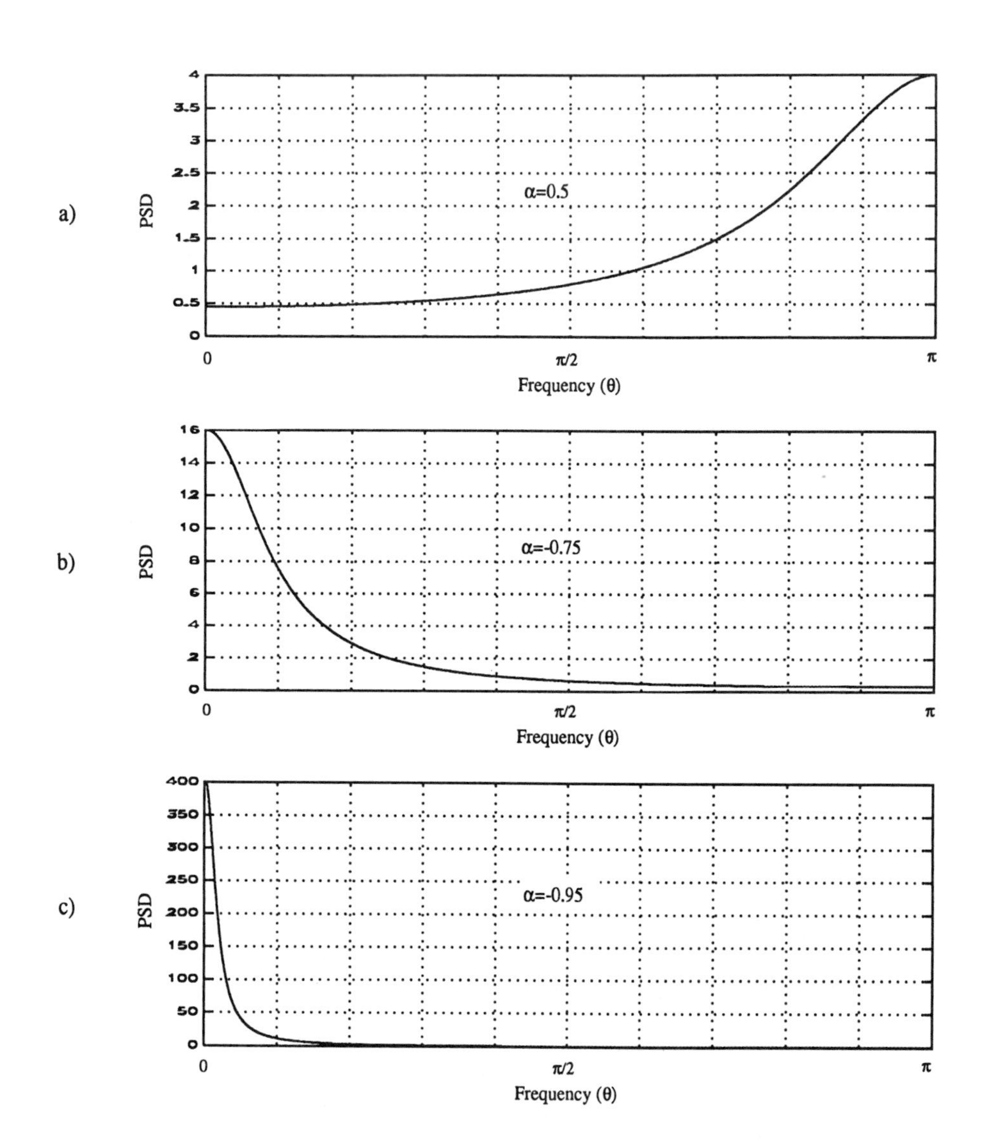

Figure 5.4.5: Power spectrum of AR(1) process with a) $\alpha = 0.5$; (b) $\alpha = -0.75$; (c) $\alpha = -0.95$.

5.5 Vector Processes

We will frequently be interested in describing the statistics of a vector of observations of a WSS stochastic process. This ability is critical for an understanding of optimal and adaptive FIR filtering. Let us denote by $\boldsymbol{x}(k)$ the vector of the N most recent samples of the WSS stochastic process $\{x(k)\}$,

$$\boldsymbol{x}(k) = [x(k), x(k-1), \ldots, x(k-N+1)]^T.$$

If we assume that the process is zero-mean, then

$$\mathcal{E}[\boldsymbol{x}(k)] = \mathbf{0}.$$

The *correlation matrix*, $\boldsymbol{R}_N$ is defined by

$$\boldsymbol{R}_N = \mathcal{E}[\boldsymbol{x}(k)\boldsymbol{x}^T(k)]$$

with i, j-th element

$$[\boldsymbol{R}_N]_{i,j} = \mathcal{E}[x(k-i)x(k-j)] = r_{xx}(i-j).$$

Because $r_{xx}(k)$ is an even sequence, $\boldsymbol{R}_N$ will be a symmetric matrix given by

$$\boldsymbol{R}_N = \begin{bmatrix} r_{xx}(0) & r_{xx}(1) & \cdots & r_{xx}(N-1) \\ r_{xx}(1) & r_{xx}(0) & \cdots & r_{xx}(N-2) \\ \vdots & \vdots & \ddots & \vdots \\ r_{xx}(N-1) & r_{xx}(N-2) & \cdots & r_{xx}(0) \end{bmatrix}.$$

In addition to being symmetric, $\boldsymbol{R}_N$ is also *Toeplitz.*

Because $\boldsymbol{R}_N$ is symmetric, its eigenvalues are all real. We can also show that $\boldsymbol{R}_N$ is positive semidefinite: let $\boldsymbol{q}$ be an arbitrary vector and define the random variable z by

$$z = \boldsymbol{q}^T\boldsymbol{x}(k).$$

Then $\mathcal{E}[z^2] \geq 0$ by definition. But

$$\mathcal{E}[z^2] = \mathcal{E}[\boldsymbol{q}^T\boldsymbol{x}(k)\boldsymbol{x}^T(k)\boldsymbol{q}] = \boldsymbol{q}^T\boldsymbol{R}_N\boldsymbol{q} \geq 0.$$

Since $\boldsymbol{q}$ was arbitrary, this is equivalent to $\boldsymbol{R}_N$ being positive semidefinite. Therefore, not only are the eigenvalues of $\boldsymbol{R}_N$ real, they are also non-negative. Furthermore, since $\boldsymbol{R}_N$ is symmetric, we know that we can find a set of orthonormal eigenvectors. Thus, there exists a unitary matrix $\boldsymbol{Q}$ such that

$$\boldsymbol{R}_N = \boldsymbol{Q}\boldsymbol{\Lambda}\boldsymbol{Q}^H$$

where

$$\boldsymbol{Q}\boldsymbol{Q}^H = \boldsymbol{Q}^H\boldsymbol{Q} = \boldsymbol{I}$$

and

$$\boldsymbol{\Lambda} = \text{diag}(\lambda_1, \lambda_2, \ldots, \lambda_N)$$

where the λ_i are the eigenvalues of $\boldsymbol{R}_N$.

Define the *reversed* vector $\boldsymbol{x}^B(k)$ by

$$\boldsymbol{x}^B(k) = [x(k-N+1), x(k-N+2), \ldots, x(k)]^T.$$

It is simple to show that the correlation matrix of the reversed vector is the same as that of $\boldsymbol{x}(k)$, *i.e.*,

$$\mathcal{E}[\boldsymbol{x}^B(k)\boldsymbol{x}^{BT}(k)] = \boldsymbol{R}_N.$$

If we increase the size of the observation vector from N to $N+1$, we need an expression for the new correlation matrix $\boldsymbol{R}_{N+1}$. The matrix $\boldsymbol{R}_{N+1}$ can be put in a useful form if we first note that

$$\boldsymbol{x}_{N+1}(k) = \begin{bmatrix} x(k) \\ \boldsymbol{x}_N(k-1) \end{bmatrix} = \begin{bmatrix} \boldsymbol{x}_N(k) \\ x(k-N) \end{bmatrix} \tag{5.5.1}$$

where the subscripts N and $N+1$ are used for clarity to indicate dimensions N and $N+1$, respectively. Let's use the first expression in Eq. 5.5.1. We have

$$\boldsymbol{R}_{N+1} = \mathcal{E}[\boldsymbol{x}_{N+1}(k)\boldsymbol{x}_{N+1}^T(k)] = \begin{bmatrix} \mathcal{E}[\boldsymbol{x}_N(k)\boldsymbol{x}_N^T(k)] & \mathcal{E}[x(k)\boldsymbol{x}_N^T(k)] \\ \mathcal{E}[x(k)\boldsymbol{x}_N(k-1)] & \mathcal{E}[\boldsymbol{x}_N(k-1)\boldsymbol{x}_N^T(k-1)] \end{bmatrix}. \tag{5.5.2}$$

Define the vector $\boldsymbol{r}$ by

$$\boldsymbol{r} = \mathcal{E}[x(k)\boldsymbol{x}_N(k-1)] = \begin{bmatrix} r_{xx}(1) \\ r_{xx}(2) \\ \vdots \\ r_{xx}(N) \end{bmatrix}. \tag{5.5.3}$$

Because of stationarity, $\mathcal{E}[\boldsymbol{x}_N(k-1)\boldsymbol{x}_N^T(k-1)] = \boldsymbol{R}_N$. Therefore, R_{N+1} can be expressed by

$$\boldsymbol{R}_{N+1} = \begin{bmatrix} r_{xx}(0) & \boldsymbol{r}^T \\ \boldsymbol{r} & \boldsymbol{R}_N \end{bmatrix}. \tag{5.5.4}$$

Similarly, if we use the second expression for $\boldsymbol{x}_{N+1}(k)$ in Eq. 5.5.1, we find that

$$\boldsymbol{R}_{N+1} = \begin{bmatrix} \boldsymbol{R}_N & \boldsymbol{r}^B \\ \boldsymbol{r}^{BT} & r_{xx}(0) \end{bmatrix} \tag{5.5.5}$$

where $\boldsymbol{r}^B$ is the reverse of $\boldsymbol{r}$,

$$\boldsymbol{r}^B = \begin{bmatrix} r_{xx}(M) \\ r_{xx}(M-1) \\ \vdots \\ r_{xx}(1) \end{bmatrix}.$$

Equations 5.5.4 and 5.5.5 will be very useful when we discuss forward and backward linear prediction.

There is an important connection between the eigenvalues of the correlation matrix and the power spectral density of the stochastic process. It can be shown [Hay86] that

$$\min_\theta P_{xx}(\theta) \leq \lambda_i \leq \max_\theta P_{xx}(\theta).$$

That is, the eigenvalues are bounded by the minimum and maximum values of the power spectral density. This further implies that

$$\frac{\lambda_{max}}{\lambda_{min}} \leq \frac{\max_\theta P_{xx}(\theta)}{\min_\theta P_{xx}(\theta)}.$$

As the dimension of the correlation matrix goes to infinity, the ratio of the maximum to the minimum eigenvalues actually approaches the ratio of the maximum to the minimum power spectral density. As we will see, the eigenvalue spread is an important quantity in the analysis of adaptive algorithms. Qualitatively, we can see that the eigenvalue spread will be very small for white noise processes since they have *flat* power spectral densities. Conversely, a large eigenvalue spread corresponds to highly correlated data.

Example 5.4

Suppose $x(k)$ is a complex exponential of the form

$$x(k) = Ae^{j(k\theta_0+\phi)}.$$

If the amplitude A and the phase ϕ are assumed to be constants, then this process cannot be WSS since the mean and autocorrelation will depend on k. Instead, assume the amplitude is constant and the phase is random and uniformly distributed over the interval $[0, 2\pi)$. Then it is simple to show that

$$\mathcal{E}[x(k)] = 0$$

and

$$r_{xx}(k) = A^2 e^{j(\theta_0 k + \phi)}$$

so that $x(k)$ is WSS. Next, consider the stochastic process which consists of a sum of complex exponentials where the phases of the exponentials are uncorrelated with one another. That is,

$$x(k) = \sum_{i=1}^{M} A_i e^{j(\theta_i k + \phi_i)}.$$

Because the phases are uncorrelated, it follows that the exponentials are uncorrelated with one another and the autocorrelation sequence for $x(k)$ is given by

$$r_{xx}(k) = \sum_{i=1}^{M} A_i^2 e^{j\theta_i k}.$$

It is simple to verify that the $N \times N$ autocorrelation matrix $\boldsymbol{R}$ for the process $x(k)$ is given by

$$\boldsymbol{R} = \boldsymbol{S}\boldsymbol{D}\boldsymbol{S}^H$$

where

$$\boldsymbol{D} = diag(A_1^2, A_2^2, \ldots, A_M^2)$$

and

$$\boldsymbol{S} = \begin{pmatrix} 1 & 1 & \cdots & 1 \\ e^{j\theta_1} & e^{j\theta_2} & \cdots & e^{j\theta_M} \\ \vdots & \vdots & \ddots & \vdots \\ e^{j(N-1)\theta_1} & e^{j(N-1)\theta_2} & \cdots & e^{j(N-1)\theta_M} \end{pmatrix}.$$

If $x(k)$ also contains an additive white noise component $v(k)$ which is uncorrelated with the complex exponentials, that is,

$$x(k) = \sum_{i=1}^{M} A_i e^{j(\theta_i k + \phi_i)} + v(k),$$

then the autocorrelation sequence is given by

$$r_{xx}(k) = \sum_{i=1}^{M} A_i^2 e^{j\theta_i k} + \sigma_v^2 \delta(k)$$

where σ_v^2 is the power of the white noise. The correlation matrix for $x(k)$ is then given by

$$\boldsymbol{R} = \boldsymbol{S}\boldsymbol{D}\boldsymbol{S}^H + \sigma_v^2 \boldsymbol{I}.$$

Chapter 6

STATE VARIABLE ANALYSIS

6.1 Introduction

Up to this point, we have only given basic input/output descriptions of digital filters. We have seen that the impulse response, $\boldsymbol{h}$, characterizes the input/output behavior, and that knowledge of $\boldsymbol{h}$ is equivalent to knowledge of the transfer function, $H(z)$. The problem we have considered thus far is how to find $H(z)$ in order to meet a desired set of filtering characteristics.

In reality, this is only half of the problem. The second half of the problem is to obtain an algorithm which describes how to perform the series of arithmetic operations related to $H(z)$. For an IIR or FIR digital filter, there are three primitive operations which must be performed: addition, multiplication, and data moves.

We refer to the problem of implementing the digital filter as the *realization* problem. Realization refers to the actual manner in which a given transfer function is implemented. By *implementation*, we are only concerned with the specification of the order in which data moves, additions, and multiplications are performed. The realization problem does not have a unique solution. In fact, we will see that there are an infinite number of solutions to it. The question remains as to which solution is preferable. There are two aspects of a filter's behavior which are affected by the realization: the speed and the fixed-point behavior. While allocating more hardware (*i.e.*, more than one multiplier and adder) will change the throughput, the fixed-point behavior is more or less independent of the amount of hardware. Thus, for most of our discussions, we make no distinction as to how much hardware is used for the filter's construction. In the case of a microprocessor implementation, realization simply refers to the order in which operations are performed.

The natural language for internal description of digital filters is linear algebra. We will be using the *state variable approach* which uses matrix difference equations and was developed and refined by control theorists during the 1960s. Where DSP differs from linear control theory, however, is in its concern with issues such as finite precision effects and nonlinear phenomena such as zero-input limit cycling. These issues are not typically treated in most introductory texts on DSP or control theory. We will see, however, that a simple and elegant treatment of these topics can be provided using the state variable approach.

6.2 The Direct-II Realization

Before giving a thorough development of the state variable method for the analysis of linear systems, we will first examine a simple realization problem. That is, given a transfer function of order N, we wish to construct a realization of the transfer function using shift registers, adders, and multipliers. This example will give the motivation for the state variable method.

Perhaps the simplest of all possible realizations for an IIR digital filter is the *direct-II* realization. Let $H(z)$ be a given by

$$H(z) = \frac{b_0 + b_1 z^{-1} + b_2 z^{-2} + \cdots + b_N z^{-N}}{1 + a_1 z^{-1} + a_2 z^{-2} + \cdots + a_N z^{-N}} = \frac{Y(z)}{U(z)}.$$

Introduce the intermediate quantity $X(z)$ according to

$$H(z) = \frac{Y(z)}{X(z)} \frac{X(z)}{U(z)}$$

where

$$\frac{X(z)}{U(z)} = \frac{1}{1 + a_1 z^{-1} + a_2 z^{-2} + \cdots + a_N z^{-N}} \tag{6.2.1}$$

and

$$\frac{Y(z)}{X(z)} = b_0 + b_1 z^{-1} + b_2 z^{-2} + \cdots + b_N z^{-N}. \tag{6.2.2}$$

Simple manipulation of Eq. 6.2.1 yields

$$X(z) = U(z) - a_1 z^{-1} X(z) - a_2 z^{-2} X(z) - \cdots - a_N z^{-N} X(z),$$

which, in the time domain, corresponds to the difference equation

$$x(k) = u(k) - a_1 x(k-1) - a_2 x(k-2) - \cdots - a_N x(k-N). \tag{6.2.3}$$

This difference equation can be realized with a chain of N delays which is "tapped" with multipliers, as shown in Fig. 6.2.1. Notice that the input to the first delay is $x(k)$.

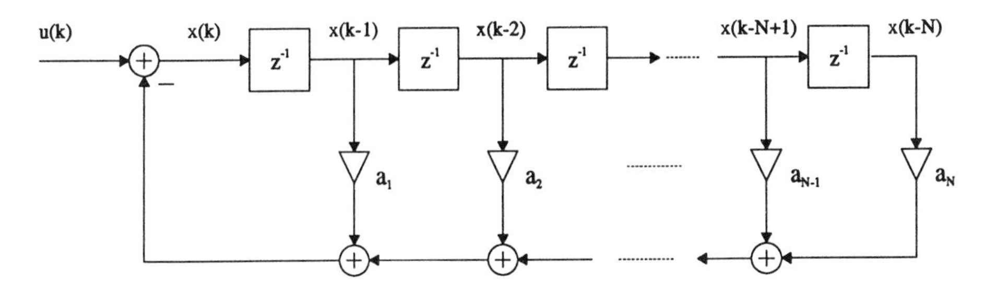

Figure 6.2.1: Realization of equation relating $x(k)$ to $u(k)$.

Now, consider Eq. 6.2.2. Simple manipulation gives

$$Y(z) = b_0X(z) + b_1z^{-1}X(z) + b_2z^{-2}X(z) + \cdots + b_Nz^{-N}X(z),$$

which corresponds to the difference equation

$$y(k) = b_0x(k) + b_1x(k-1) + b_2x(k-2) + \cdots + b_Nx(k-N). \qquad (6.2.4)$$

Equation 6.2.4 can be realized by summing the delayed copies of $x(k)$, weighted by the coefficients b_i, as shown in Fig. 6.2.2. The collection of shift registers, adders, and multipliers as configured in Fig. 6.2.2 is known as the *direct-II* realization of $H(z)$. This realization is canonical in the sense that an N-th order transfer function can be realized with precisely N delays.

We now proceed to show that the direct-II model can be described in terms of a pair of matrix difference equations. This method of representation will give a description of all of the internal signals in the direct-II model.

Denote the output of the right-most shift register in Fig. 6.2.2 by $x_1(k)$, so that

$$x_1(k) = x(k-N).$$

Moving from right to left, let the output of the next shift-register be called $x_2(k)$, giving

$$x_2(k) = x(k-N+1).$$

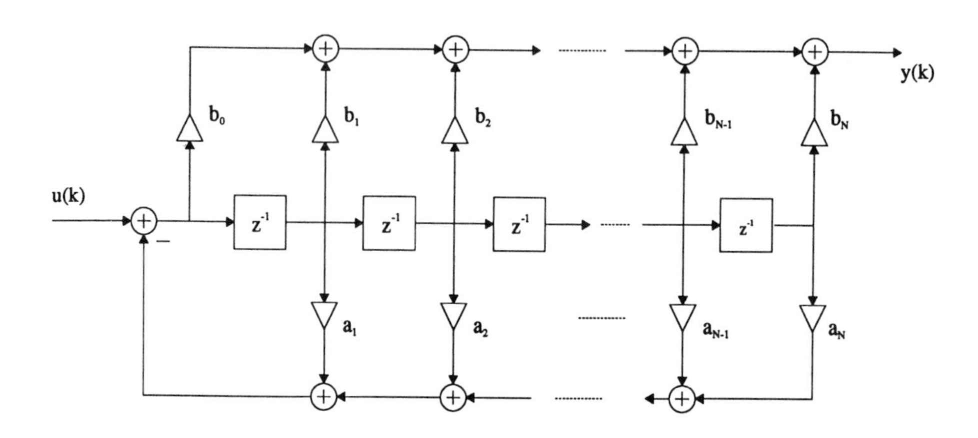

Figure 6.2.2: Direct-II realization of $H(z)$.

Continuing in this manner, the outputs of each shift register are labeled, terminating with the left-most shift register, $x_N(k)$, where

$$x_N(k) = x(k).$$

For any shift register other than the left-most one, its contents at time $k+1$ are the same as the contents of the shift register to its left at time k. Therefore,

$$x_i(k+1) = x_{i+1}(k), \quad i = 1, 2, \ldots, N-1.$$

More explicitly, we have

$$\begin{aligned} x_1(k+1) &= x_2(k) \\ x_2(k+1) &= x_3(k) \\ \vdots \quad & \quad \vdots \quad \vdots \\ x_{N-1}(k+1) &= x_N(k) \end{aligned} \tag{6.2.5}$$

These equations describe the evolution of the shift register contents in time. We are missing an equation for the evolution of the left-most shift register, however. This equation is simple to derive. The output of x_N at time $k+1$ is given by the sum of the input at time k and the contents of the other shift registers at time k, weighted by the coefficients a_i. That is,

$$x_N(k+1) = u(k) - a_N x_1(k) - a_{N-1} x_2(k) - \cdots - a_1 x_N(k). \tag{6.2.6}$$

The shift register contents, in a manner to be made precise later, can be regarded as the *state* of the system. We also call the $x_i(k)$ the *state variables* for the system. Define the *state vector*, $\boldsymbol{x}(k)$, by

$$\boldsymbol{x}(k) = \begin{bmatrix} x_1(k) \\ x_2(k) \\ x_3(k) \\ \vdots \\ x_N(k) \end{bmatrix}.$$

Equations 6.2.5 and 6.2.6 can be put in the matrix-vector form

$$\boldsymbol{x}(k+1) = \begin{bmatrix} 0 & 1 & 0 & \cdots & 0 \\ 0 & 0 & 1 & \cdots & 0 \\ \vdots & \vdots & \vdots & \ddots & \vdots \\ 0 & 0 & 0 & \cdots & 1 \\ -a_N & -a_{N-1} & -a_{N-2} & \cdots & -a_1 \end{bmatrix} \boldsymbol{x}(k) + \begin{bmatrix} 0 \\ 0 \\ 0 \\ \vdots \\ 1 \end{bmatrix} u(k) \tag{6.2.7}$$

Equation 6.2.7 is known as the *state equation* for the system and describes the evolution of the state in time. Notice that the *next state* is given as a function of the *present* state and the *present* input. Define the matrix $\boldsymbol{A}$ by

$$\boldsymbol{A} = \begin{bmatrix} 0 & 1 & 0 & \cdots & 0 \\ 0 & 0 & 1 & \cdots & 0 \\ \vdots & \vdots & \vdots & \ddots & \vdots \\ 0 & 0 & 0 & \cdots & 1 \\ -a_N & -a_{N-1} & -a_{N-2} & \cdots & -a_1 \end{bmatrix}$$

and the vector $\boldsymbol{b}$ by

$$\boldsymbol{b} = \begin{bmatrix} 0 \\ 0 \\ 0 \\ \vdots \\ 1 \end{bmatrix}.$$

The state equations can then be written in the compact form

$$\boldsymbol{x}(k+1) = \boldsymbol{A}\boldsymbol{x}(k) + \boldsymbol{b}u(k). \tag{6.2.8}$$

The state variable representation is not yet complete. We now need to describe how the output is generated from the state and the input. Notice that each state variable has two paths to the output. The first path is directly from the state variable through the multiplier above it. The second path is an undelayed feedback path through the first adder and up through the b_0 multiplier. Also, the input has an undelayed path to the output through b_0, as well. In this manner, we have

$$y(k) = (b_N - a_N b_0)x_1(k) + \cdots + (b_1 - a_1 b_0)x_N(k) + b_0 u(k). \tag{6.2.9}$$

We can rewrite Eq. 6.2.9 in vector form as

$$y(k) = \begin{bmatrix} b_N - a_N b_0, & b_{N-1} - a_{N-1} b_0, & \cdots, & b_1 - a_1 b_0 \end{bmatrix} \boldsymbol{x}(k) + b_0 u(k). \tag{6.2.10}$$

This equation is known as the *output equation* for the state variable model. Examining Eq. 6.2.10, we see that the *present* output is given as a function of the *present* state and the *present* input. Define the vector $\boldsymbol{c}$ by

$$\boldsymbol{c} = \begin{bmatrix} b_N - a_N b_0 & b_{N-1} - a_{N-1} b_0 & \cdots & b_1 - a_1 b_0 \end{bmatrix},$$

and the scalar d by

$$d = b_0.$$

Equation 6.2.9 can then be written in the concise form

$$y(k) = \boldsymbol{c}\boldsymbol{x}(k) + du(k). \tag{6.2.11}$$

This completes the state variable model for the direct-II realization. The system is completely described by the state and output equations (Eqs. 6.2.8 and 6.2.11)

$$\begin{aligned} \boldsymbol{x}(k+1) &= \boldsymbol{A}\boldsymbol{x}(k) + \boldsymbol{b}u(k) \\ y(k) &= \boldsymbol{c}\boldsymbol{x}(k) + du(k) \end{aligned} \tag{6.2.12}$$

Figure 6.2.2 corresponds in an obvious way to the transfer function $H(z)$: the branch gains correspond directly to the coefficients of the transfer function. This clarity is not preserved by the state variable equations, however. The elements of the $\boldsymbol{A}$ matrix correspond in an obvious way, as well, but the elements of the $\boldsymbol{c}$ vector are somewhat less obvious. This is because of the presence of the coefficient b_0 in the feedforward path. We can make a slight modification to the direct-II architecture which eliminates this problem. There are two paths from each state to the output: one from the state x_i through the branch with gain b_i and one through the feedback path with loop gain $-a_i b_0$. In order to eliminate this second path, we move the branch with gain b_0 to the left of the summing node. Now, replace each branch with gain b_i with a branch of gain $b_i - a_i b_0$. This is shown in Fig. 6.2.3. The original direct-II architecture was canonical with respect to the transfer function in that the gains of each branch could written down directly from looking at the transfer function. The modified

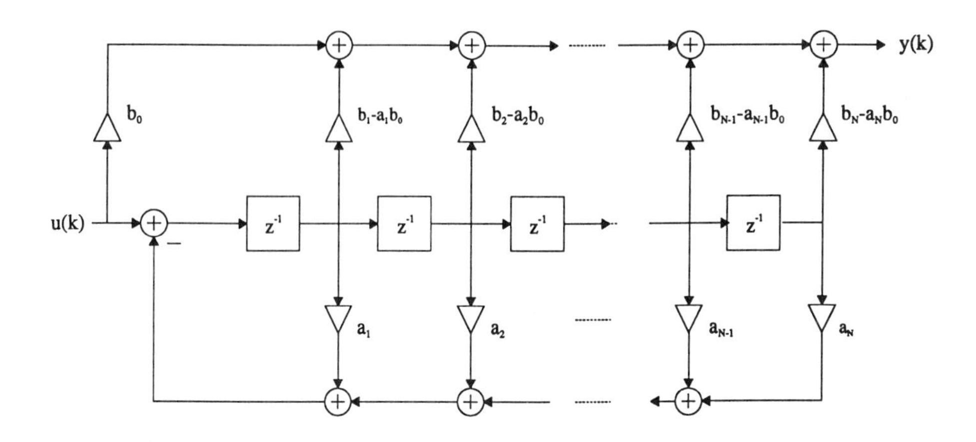

Figure 6.2.3: Modified direct-II architecture.

direct-II architecture is canonical with respect to the state variable representation in that its branch gains correspond identically to the elements of the matrices.

It is interesting to note that the modified direct-II architecture can be obtained by writing $H(z)$ as a *proper* ratio of polynomials. That is, forcing the numerator to have degree one less than the denominator, we have

$$H(z) = b_0 + \frac{(b_1 - a_1 b_0) + (b_2 - a_2 b_0)z^{-1} + \cdots + (b_N - a_N b_0)z^{-(N-1)}}{a_0 + a_1 z^{-1} + \ldots + a_N z^{-N}}. \tag{6.2.13}$$

Notice that the coefficients of the modified direct-II architecture correspond to the state variable model in an obvious way.

6.3 The State Variable Model

The previous section showed how a transfer function could be realized with a collection of shift registers, adders, and multipliers. It will be seen that the solution to the realization problem is not unique; there are many different realizations which have the same transfer function. It is important to classify these realizations and determine the mathematical rules which relate them to one another. This is the essence of the state variable approach.

What is significant about the state variable representation is that it gives an explicit "recipe" for computing the system's behavior. That is, we have equations for updating each internal variable in the system and an equation for computing the output from these internal variables and the input. This "recipe" is not available directly from the input/output SDE for the system. An obvious question is why we should care about having such a detailed description. There are two principal reasons. First, we will often implement digital filters with microprocessors, and hence must have a way to manage information internally. Secondly, and perhaps more important, certain computational recipes may lead to better behavior than others, especially when fixed-point hardware is used. A state variable model explicitly indicates the order in which computations are performed, and some structures will behave better than others.

In the previous section, we introduced the notion of state and gave equations for the evolutions of the state and the output for a particular system. In this section, we will generalize these ideas for arbitrary linear time-invariant systems.

The *state* of a system is loosely defined as a minimal collection of information, the knowledge of which, along with the input, allows us to compute the output of the system for all time. The number of state variables is called the *dimension* of the system. All of the systems we will consider are *finite dimensional*, with state variables

$$x_1(k), x_2(k), \ldots, x_N(k).$$

The *state vector*, $\boldsymbol{x}(k)$, is defined by

$$\boldsymbol{x}(k) = \begin{bmatrix} x_1(k) \\ x_2(k) \\ \vdots \\ x_N(k) \end{bmatrix}.$$

Taking a cue from the previous section, the dynamics (*i.e.*, the time-evolution) of the filter can be described by a pair of equations: one describes the next state as a function of the present state and the present input, the other describes the present output as a function of the present state and the present input. These equations are given by

$$\boldsymbol{x}(k+1) = \boldsymbol{f}(\boldsymbol{x}(k), u(k)) \tag{6.3.1}$$

and

$$y(k) = g(\boldsymbol{x}(k), u(k)). \tag{6.3.2}$$

The function $\boldsymbol{f}$ is a vector-valued function and g is a scalar function. For the special case of a linear system, the mappings $\boldsymbol{f}$ and g will be linear.

For a *linear* system, the function $\boldsymbol{f}$ produces the next state $\boldsymbol{x}(k+1)$ as a linear time-invariant function of the present state $\boldsymbol{x}(k)$ and the present input $u(k)$. Namely, each state variable's next value is a linear combination of each state variable's present value and the present input so that

$$\begin{array}{lcl} x_1(k+1) & = & a_{11}x_1(k) + a_{12}x_2(k) + \cdots + a_{1N}x_N(k) + b_1u(k) \\ x_2(k+1) & = & a_{21}x_1(k) + a_{22}x_2(k) + \cdots + a_{2N}x_N(k) + b_2u(k) \\ \cdots & \cdots & \cdots \\ x_N(k+1) & = & a_{N1}x_1(k) + a_{N2}x_2(k) + \cdots + a_{NN}x_N(k) + b_Nu(k) \end{array} \tag{6.3.3}$$

A more compact description of this relationship is the matrix difference equation

$$\boldsymbol{x}(k+1) = \boldsymbol{A}\boldsymbol{x}(k) + \boldsymbol{b}u(k) \tag{6.3.4}$$

where

$$\boldsymbol{A} = \begin{bmatrix} a_{11} & a_{12} & \cdots & a_{1N} \\ a_{21} & a_{22} & \cdots & a_{2N} \\ \vdots & \vdots & \vdots & \vdots \\ a_{N1} & a_{N2} & \cdots & a_{NN} \end{bmatrix} \quad \text{and} \quad \boldsymbol{b} = \begin{bmatrix} b_1 \\ b_2 \\ \vdots \\ b_N \end{bmatrix}. \tag{6.3.5}$$

For the direct-II model, we have already seen what values the coefficients a_{ij} and b_i assume.

Now that we have described the evolution of the state, we need a description of the output as a function of the state and the input. Whereas the state evolution equation describes the *next state* as a function of the present state and the present input, the output can be computed as a linear function of the present state and the present input. Specifically,

$$y(k) = c_1x_1(k) + c_2x_2(k) + \cdots + c_Nx_N(k) + du(k). \tag{6.3.6}$$

This can be represented compactly by the matrix equation

$$y(k) = \boldsymbol{c}\boldsymbol{x}(k) + \boldsymbol{d}u(k) \tag{6.3.7}$$

where

$$\boldsymbol{c} = \begin{bmatrix} c_1 & c_2 & c_3 & \cdots & c_N \end{bmatrix}, \quad \text{and} \quad d = d.$$

Again, we have seen how $\boldsymbol{c}$ and d are determined for the particular case of the direct-II model.

Thus, a linear time-invariant system can be described by the pair of equations

$$\begin{array}{rcll} \boldsymbol{x}(k+1) & = & \boldsymbol{A}\boldsymbol{x}(k) & + \ \boldsymbol{b}u(k) \\ y(k) & = & \boldsymbol{c}\boldsymbol{x}(k) & + \ du(k) \end{array}. \tag{6.3.8}$$

The matrix $\boldsymbol{A}$ describes the interactions or "coupling" between states. The matrix $\boldsymbol{b}$ describes the connection of each state to the input. The matrix $\boldsymbol{c}$ describes the connection of each

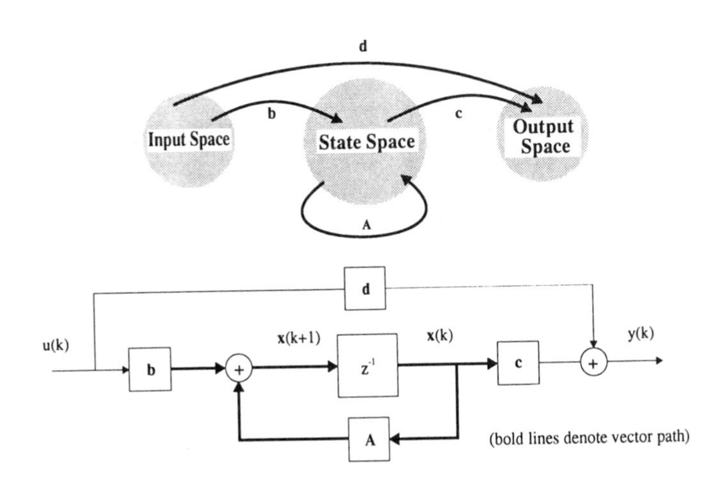

Figure 6.3.1: Geometric interpretation of a linear system.

state to the output, and the matrix $\boldsymbol{d}$ describes the direct coupling from the input to the output.

The state vector is an N-dimensional vector, and when the system has real coefficients and is driven by a real input, the state vector can be regarded as an element of the vector space R^N, which in turn is called the *state space*. The time-evolution of the state vector in the state space is often referred to as a *state trajectory*. The trajectory is influenced by both the input and the coupling between the state variables, as expressed by the $\boldsymbol{A}$ matrix. A useful geometric interpretation of a system is given by regarding the system matrices as mappings. That is, the matrix $\boldsymbol{A}$ maps the state space to itself, $\boldsymbol{b}$ maps inputs to the state space, $\boldsymbol{c}$ maps the state space to outputs, and d maps inputs directly to outputs with no interaction through the state space. This geometric interpretation is depicted in Fig. 6.3.1.

6.4 Solution of the State Equations

It has been established that a fundamental description of linear time-invariant systems is given by the state variable equations

$$\begin{aligned} \boldsymbol{x}(k+1) &= \boldsymbol{A}\boldsymbol{x}(k) + \boldsymbol{b}u(k) \\ y(k) &= \boldsymbol{c}\boldsymbol{x}(k) + du(k) \end{aligned} . \tag{6.4.1}$$

Given an initial value of the state vector at time k_0, we would like to be able to determine both the state and the output at an arbitrary time k. This is simple if we begin with the state equation,

$$\boldsymbol{x}(k+1) = \boldsymbol{A}\boldsymbol{x}(k) + \boldsymbol{b}u(k). \tag{6.4.2}$$

Given $\boldsymbol{x}(k_0)$, it follows from Eq. 6.4.2 that

$$\boldsymbol{x}(k_0+1) = \boldsymbol{A}\boldsymbol{x}(k_0) + \boldsymbol{b}u(k_0).$$

At time $k_0 + 2$,

$$\boldsymbol{x}(k_0+2) = \boldsymbol{A}\boldsymbol{x}(k_0+1) + \boldsymbol{b}u(k_0+1) = \boldsymbol{A}^2\boldsymbol{x}(k_0) + \boldsymbol{A}\boldsymbol{b}u(k_0) + \boldsymbol{b}u(k_0+1).$$

Continuing the recursion, we find that at time $k_0 + n$,

$$\begin{aligned} \boldsymbol{x}(k_0+n) &= \boldsymbol{A}^n\boldsymbol{x}(k_0) + \boldsymbol{A}^{n-1}\boldsymbol{b}u(k_0) + \boldsymbol{A}^{n-2}\boldsymbol{b}u(k_0+1) + \cdots \\ &\quad + \boldsymbol{A}\boldsymbol{b}u(k_0+n-2) + \boldsymbol{b}u(k_0+n-1) \end{aligned} \tag{6.4.3}$$

Now, let $k = k_0 + n$ so that Eq. 6.4.3 becomes

$$\begin{aligned} \boldsymbol{x}(k) &= \boldsymbol{A}^{k-k_0}\boldsymbol{x}(k_0) + \boldsymbol{A}^{k-k_0-1}\boldsymbol{b}u(k_0) + \boldsymbol{A}^{k-k_0-2}\boldsymbol{b}u(k_0+1) + \cdots \\ &\quad + \boldsymbol{A}\boldsymbol{b}u(k-2) + \boldsymbol{b}u(k-1) \end{aligned} \tag{6.4.4}$$

In closed-form, Eq. 6.4.4 becomes

$$\boldsymbol{x}(k) = \boldsymbol{A}^{k-k_0}\boldsymbol{x}(k_0) + \sum_{i=k_0}^{k-1} \boldsymbol{A}^{k-i-1}\boldsymbol{b}u(i). \tag{6.4.5}$$

The output of the system is now easily obtained. Recall that

$$y(k) = \boldsymbol{c}\boldsymbol{x}(k) + du(k). \tag{6.4.6}$$

Therefore, using Eq. 6.4.5, it follows that

$$y(k) = \boldsymbol{c}\boldsymbol{A}^{k-k_0}\boldsymbol{x}(k_0) + \boldsymbol{c}\sum_{i=k_0}^{k-1} \boldsymbol{A}^{k-i-1}\boldsymbol{b}u(i) + du(k). \tag{6.4.7}$$

Equation 6.4.7 consists of two parts: the response due to the initial state, and the response due to the input. If the initial state is set to to zero, we get the zero-state response, $y_{zs}(k)$, where

$$y_{zs}(k) = \boldsymbol{c}\sum_{i=k_0}^{k-1} \boldsymbol{A}^{k-i-1}\boldsymbol{b}u(i) + du(k). \tag{6.4.8}$$

If the input is set to zero, we get the zero-input response, $y_{zi}(k)$, where

$$y_{zi}(k) = \boldsymbol{c}\boldsymbol{A}^{k-k_0}\boldsymbol{x}(k_0). \tag{6.4.9}$$

It immediately follows that

$$y(k) = y_{zs}(k) + y_{zi}(k). \tag{6.4.10}$$

Because we are studying linear time-invariant systems, there is no loss of generality if the starting time is taken to be $k_0 = 0$. In this case, Eq. 6.4.5 becomes

$$\boldsymbol{x}(k) = \boldsymbol{A}^k\boldsymbol{x}(0) + \sum_{i=0}^{k-1} \boldsymbol{A}^{k-i-1}\boldsymbol{b}u(i) \tag{6.4.11}$$

and the Eq. 6.4.7 becomes

$$y(k) = \boldsymbol{c}\boldsymbol{A}^k\boldsymbol{x}(0) + \boldsymbol{c}\sum_{i=0}^{k-1} \boldsymbol{A}^{k-i-1}\boldsymbol{b}u(i) + du(k). \tag{6.4.12}$$

In order to obtain a closed-form expression for the state or the output as in Eqs. 6.4.11 and 6.4.12, the matrix power $\boldsymbol{A}^k$ needs to be computed. For the present, assume that the eigenvalues of $\boldsymbol{A}$ are distinct (we will see that this corresponds to a filter with no repeated poles). Then there exists an invertible matrix $\boldsymbol{T}$ such that

$$\boldsymbol{T}^{-1}\boldsymbol{A}\boldsymbol{T} = \boldsymbol{\Lambda} = \begin{bmatrix} \lambda_1 & 0 & 0 & \cdots & 0 \\ 0 & \lambda_2 & 0 & \cdots & 0 \\ \vdots & \ddots & \vdots & \vdots & \vdots \\ 0 & 0 & 0 & \cdots & \lambda_N \end{bmatrix}. \tag{6.4.13}$$

The matrix $\boldsymbol{T}$ has columns which are eigenvectors of $\boldsymbol{A}$ and the diagonal elements of $\boldsymbol{\Lambda}$ are the eigenvalues corresponding to the eigenvectors. Consequently, Eq. 6.4.13 implies that

$$\boldsymbol{A} = \boldsymbol{T}\boldsymbol{\Lambda}\boldsymbol{T}^{-1} \tag{6.4.14}$$

so that

$$\boldsymbol{A}^2 = \boldsymbol{T}\boldsymbol{\Lambda}\boldsymbol{T}^{-1}\boldsymbol{T}\boldsymbol{\Lambda}\boldsymbol{T}^{-1} = \boldsymbol{T}\boldsymbol{\Lambda}^2\boldsymbol{T}^{-1}. \tag{6.4.15}$$

It is simple to see that in general,

$$\boldsymbol{A}^k = \boldsymbol{T}\boldsymbol{\Lambda}^k\boldsymbol{T}^{-1}. \tag{6.4.16}$$

Therefore, if $\boldsymbol{\Lambda}^k$ can be computed, it is simple to compute $\boldsymbol{A}^K$ using Eq. 6.4.15. Because $\boldsymbol{\Lambda}$ is diagonal, $\boldsymbol{\Lambda}^k$ is given by

$$\boldsymbol{\Lambda}^k = \begin{bmatrix} \lambda_1^k & 0 & 0 & \cdots & 0 \\ 0 & \lambda_2^k & 0 & \cdots & 0 \\ \vdots & \vdots & \vdots & \ddots & \vdots \\ 0 & 0 & 0 & \cdots & \lambda_N^k \end{bmatrix}. \tag{6.4.17}$$

Thus, Eq. 6.4.15 becomes

$$\boldsymbol{A}^k = \boldsymbol{T} \begin{bmatrix} \lambda_1^k & 0 & 0 & \cdots & 0 \\ 0 & \lambda_2^k & 0 & \cdots & 0 \\ \vdots & \vdots & \vdots & \ddots & \vdots \\ 0 & 0 & 0 & \cdots & \lambda_N^k \end{bmatrix} \boldsymbol{T}^{-1}.$$

Internal stability

In Chapter 1, bounded-input bounded-output (BIBO) stability was presented. A similar idea for systems described by state variables is that of *bounded-input bounded-state* (BIBS) stability. Namely, a system is BIBS stable if for all bounded inputs, the state remains bounded. This is fairly simple to characterize. It can be shown that a system is BIBS stable if and only if the zero-state response $\boldsymbol{x}_{zs}(k)$ of the *state* converges to zero for *all* initial states $\boldsymbol{x}(0)$. Because

$$\boldsymbol{x}_{zs}(k) = \boldsymbol{A}^k \boldsymbol{x}(0),$$

BIBS stability is completely determined by the $\boldsymbol{A}$ matrix. Recalling that

$$\boldsymbol{A}^k = \boldsymbol{T} \begin{bmatrix} \lambda_1^k & 0 & 0 & \cdots & 0 \\ 0 & \lambda_2^k & 0 & \cdots & 0 \\ \vdots & \vdots & \vdots & \ddots & \vdots \\ 0 & 0 & 0 & \cdots & \lambda_N^k \end{bmatrix} \boldsymbol{T}^{-1},$$

we see that $\boldsymbol{A}^k$ is a linear combination of the *modes*, λ^k. Therefore, $\boldsymbol{A}^k \boldsymbol{x}(0)$ converges to zero for all $\boldsymbol{x}(0)$ if and only if the modes λ^k themselves are stable. This means that the system is BIBS stable if and only if

$$|\lambda_i| < 1, \quad i = 1, 2, \ldots, N.$$

From the standpoint of filter implementation, BIBS stability is important. Clearly, we would like the shift register contents of the filter to remain bounded if the output is to have any meaning. BIBO stability is not sufficient to ensure this, for consider the system governed by the state equation

$$\begin{bmatrix} x_1(k+1) \\ x_2(k+1) \end{bmatrix} = \begin{bmatrix} 0.5 & 0 \\ 0 & 2 \end{bmatrix} \begin{bmatrix} x_1(k) \\ x_2(k) \end{bmatrix} + \begin{bmatrix} 1 \\ 1 \end{bmatrix} u(k)$$

and the output equation

$$y(k) = x_1(k).$$

If $x_2(0)$ is non-zero, the state $x_2(k)$ will diverge to infinity, while the output remains bounded. In other words, the output remains bounded even though the magnitude of the state diverges. This is because $x_2(k)$ is not observable at the output.[1] If BIBS stability is required, not only will the state remain bounded, but so will the output, since it is a linear function of the state.

6.5 Impulse Response

The solution the the state variable equations can be put in a form which explicitly displays the impulse response. Given the state-variable model

$$\begin{aligned} \boldsymbol{x}(k+1) &= \boldsymbol{A}\boldsymbol{x}(k) + \boldsymbol{b}u(k) \\ y(k) &= \boldsymbol{c}\boldsymbol{x}(k) + du(k) \end{aligned},$$

assume the filter is started from zero initial condition. Then

$$\boldsymbol{x}(1) = \boldsymbol{A}\boldsymbol{x}(0) + \boldsymbol{b}\delta(0) = \boldsymbol{b}$$

and

$$y(0) = \boldsymbol{c}\boldsymbol{x}(0) + d\delta(0) = d.$$

Next,

$$\boldsymbol{x}(2) = \boldsymbol{A}\boldsymbol{x}(1) + \boldsymbol{b}\delta(1) = \boldsymbol{A}\boldsymbol{b}$$

and

$$y(1) = \boldsymbol{c}\boldsymbol{x}(1) + d\delta(1) = \boldsymbol{c}\boldsymbol{b} = \boldsymbol{c}\boldsymbol{A}^0\boldsymbol{b}.$$

[1]For a precise definition of observability, the reader is referred to any standard reference on linear system theory (*e.g.*, [Kai80]).

Continuing, for $k > 0$, it is simple to see that

$$\boldsymbol{x}(k) = \boldsymbol{A}^{k-1}\boldsymbol{b} \tag{6.5.1}$$

and

$$y(k) = \boldsymbol{c}\boldsymbol{A}^{k-1}\boldsymbol{b} + d\delta(k). \tag{6.5.2}$$

Therefore, the impulse response is given by

$$h(k) = \begin{cases} \boldsymbol{d}, & k = 0 \\ \boldsymbol{c}\boldsymbol{A}^{k-1}\boldsymbol{b}, & k > 0. \end{cases} \tag{6.5.3}$$

6.6 $\mathcal{Z}$-Transform Solution of the State Variable Equations

Given the state variable equations

$$\begin{array}{rcl} \boldsymbol{x}(k+1) & = & \boldsymbol{A}\boldsymbol{x}(k) + \boldsymbol{b}u(k) \\ y(k) & = & \boldsymbol{c}\boldsymbol{x}(k) + du(k) \end{array},$$

another useful method of solution of the state equations is given by taking $\mathcal{Z}$-transforms. This leads to the pair of equations

$$\begin{array}{rcl} z\boldsymbol{X}(z) - z\boldsymbol{x}(0) & = & \boldsymbol{A}\boldsymbol{X}(z) + \boldsymbol{b}U(z) \\ Y(z) & = & \boldsymbol{c}\boldsymbol{X}(z) + \boldsymbol{d}U(z). \end{array} \tag{6.6.1}$$

The first equation of Eq. 6.6.1 can be solved for $\boldsymbol{X}(z)$ as

$$\boldsymbol{X}(z) = (z\boldsymbol{I} - \boldsymbol{A})^{-1}\boldsymbol{b}U(z) + z(z\boldsymbol{I} - \boldsymbol{A})^{-1}\boldsymbol{x}(0)$$

so that

$$Y(z) = \boldsymbol{c}(z\boldsymbol{I} - \boldsymbol{A})^{-1}\boldsymbol{b}U(z) + \boldsymbol{d}U(z) + \boldsymbol{c}z(z\boldsymbol{I} - \boldsymbol{A})^{-1}\boldsymbol{x}(0).$$

Again, the output response is seen to consist of the zero-input response and the zero-state response, where

$$Y_{zi}(z) = \boldsymbol{c}z(z\boldsymbol{I} - \boldsymbol{A})^{-1}\boldsymbol{x}(0) \tag{6.6.2}$$

and

$$Y_{zs}(z) = (\boldsymbol{c}(z\boldsymbol{I} - \boldsymbol{A})^{-1}\boldsymbol{b} + d)U(z). \tag{6.6.3}$$

The transfer function is defined as the ratio of the $\mathcal{Z}$-transform of the zero-state response to the $\mathcal{Z}$-transform of the input so that

$$H(z) = \mathbf{c}(z\boldsymbol{I} - A)^{-1}\boldsymbol{b} + d. \tag{6.6.4}$$

It is worth showing that the same result can be obtained by taking the $\mathcal{Z}$-transform of the impulse response, as given by Eq. 6.5.3 directly, giving

$$H(z) = \sum_{k=0}^{\infty} h(k)z^{-k} = \boldsymbol{d}z^0 + \sum_{k=1}^{\infty} \mathbf{c}\boldsymbol{A}^{k-1}\boldsymbol{b}z^{-k}. \tag{6.6.5}$$

Equation 6.6.5 can be rewritten as

$$H(z) = \boldsymbol{d} + z^{-1}\sum_{k=1}^{\infty} \mathbf{c}(\boldsymbol{A}/z)^{k-1}\boldsymbol{b},$$

and upon shifting the index of summation,

$$H(z) = \boldsymbol{d} + z^{-1}\mathbf{c}\left[\sum_{k=0}^{\infty}(\boldsymbol{A}/z)^k\right]\boldsymbol{b}. \tag{6.6.6}$$

It can be shown that the matrix power series above converges if the magnitude of z is larger than the magnitude of the maximum eigenvalue of $\boldsymbol{A}$. The value to which the series converges is

$$\sum_{k=0}^{\infty}(\boldsymbol{A}/z)^k = (\boldsymbol{I} - z^{-1}\boldsymbol{A})^{-1} \tag{6.6.7}$$

(notice the analogy with scalar geometric series). Thus, Eq. 6.6.6 becomes

$$H(z) = \boldsymbol{d} + z^{-1}\mathbf{c}(\boldsymbol{I} - z^{-1}\boldsymbol{A})^{-1}B = \mathbf{c}(z\boldsymbol{I} - \boldsymbol{A})^{-1}\boldsymbol{b} + \boldsymbol{d},$$

as expected.

In order to obtain $H(z)$ as given by Eq. 6.6.4, we need to be able to compute $(z\boldsymbol{I} - \boldsymbol{A})^{-1}$. One useful method is to use the formula

$$(z\boldsymbol{I} - \boldsymbol{A})^{-1} = \frac{\operatorname{adj}(z\boldsymbol{I} - \boldsymbol{A})}{|z\boldsymbol{I} - \boldsymbol{A}|}. \tag{6.6.8}$$

If $\boldsymbol{A}$ is $n \times n$, then $\operatorname{adj}(z\boldsymbol{I} - \boldsymbol{A})$ will be a polynomial matrix with entries of degree at most $n-1$. Also, $|z\boldsymbol{I} - \boldsymbol{A}|$ will be a polynomial of degree n, so that $(z\boldsymbol{I} - \boldsymbol{A})^{-1}$ is a matrix of *proper* rational functions in z.

Example 6.1

Suppose

$$A = \begin{bmatrix} 0.5 & 1 \\ 0 & 0.25 \end{bmatrix}.$$

Then

$$(zI - A) = \begin{bmatrix} z - 0.5 & -1 \\ 0 & z - 0.25 \end{bmatrix}.$$

From the definition of adjoint,

$$\text{adj}(zI - A) = \begin{bmatrix} z - 0.25 & 1 \\ 0 & z - 0.5 \end{bmatrix}.$$

Also,

$$|zI - A| = (z - 0.25)(z - 0.5).$$

Finally, since

$$(zI - A)^{-1} = \frac{\text{adj}(zI - A)}{|zI - A|},$$

we have

$$(zI - A)^{-1} = \begin{bmatrix} \frac{1}{z-0.5} & \frac{1}{(z-0.25)(z-0.5)} \\ 0 & \frac{1}{z-0.25} \end{bmatrix},$$

which can be verified by pre- and post-multiplying. Another useful check is to invert the $\mathcal{Z}$-transform . We can perform partial-fraction expansion on the elements of the matrix, which gives

$$(zI - A)^{-1} = \begin{bmatrix} \frac{1}{z-0.5} & \frac{4}{z-0.5} - \frac{4}{z-0.25} \\ 0 & \frac{1}{z-0.25} \end{bmatrix},$$

and leads to the inverse $\mathcal{Z}$-transform

$$\begin{bmatrix} (0.5)^{k-1}u(k-1) & (4(0.5)^{k-1} - 4(0.25)^{k-1})u(k-1) \\ 0 & (0.25)^{k-1}u(k-1) \end{bmatrix}. \tag{6.6.9}$$

We already showed that the $\mathcal{Z}$-transform of the matrix sequence

$$\{A^k \mid k = 0, 1, 2, \ldots\}$$

is

$$(I - z^{-1}A)^{-1}.$$

Also,

$$(z\boldsymbol{I} - \boldsymbol{A})^{-1} = z^{-1}(\boldsymbol{I} - z^{-1}\boldsymbol{A})^{-1}.$$

Applying the time-shifting property of the $\mathcal{Z}$-transform , the matrix $(z\boldsymbol{I} - \boldsymbol{A})^{-1}$ is thus the $\mathcal{Z}$-transform of the matrix sequence

$$\{\boldsymbol{A}^{k-1} \mid k = 1, 2, \ldots\}.$$

We can check our result in this manner. For instance, Eq. 6.6.9 evaluated at time $k = 1$ yields the identity matrix, which agrees with the sequence. At $k = 2$, we have

$$\begin{bmatrix} 0.5 & 1 \\ 0 & 0.25 \end{bmatrix} = \boldsymbol{A},$$

which also agrees with the sequence.

If Eq. 6.6.8 is substituted into Eq. 6.6.4, we get

$$H(z) = \boldsymbol{c}\frac{\operatorname{adj}(z\boldsymbol{I} - \boldsymbol{A})}{|z\boldsymbol{I} - \boldsymbol{A}|}\boldsymbol{b} + d \tag{6.6.10}$$

so that

$$H(z) = \frac{\boldsymbol{c}\operatorname{adj}(z\boldsymbol{I} - \boldsymbol{A})\boldsymbol{b} + d|z\boldsymbol{I} - \boldsymbol{A}|}{|z\boldsymbol{I} - \boldsymbol{A}|}. \tag{6.6.11}$$

Clearly, the numerator of this expression is a polynomial of degree at most N. Therefore, the poles of $H(z)$ are precisely the roots of the determinant,

$$|z\boldsymbol{I} - \boldsymbol{A}| = 0, \tag{6.6.12}$$

which are the eigenvalues of $\boldsymbol{A}$[2].

Now that we know how to evaluate $(z\boldsymbol{I} - \boldsymbol{A})^{-1}$, we are in a position to examine a complete example. We will begin with a simple second-order transfer function description of a digital filter and obtain a direct-II state-variable model for the filter. Next, we will compute a closed-form expression for the internal state of the system. Finally, we will show that the transfer function obtained from the state-variable representation is the same as what we started with.

[2]This, of course, assumes there is no cancellation of terms between the numerator and the denominator. For our purposes, this is of no concern. In general, however, this is related to the concepts of *controllability* and *observability*, which can be found in any standard reference on control theory (again, [Kai80] is recommended).

Example 6.2

Suppose

$$H(z) = \frac{1 + 2z^{-1} + z^{-2}}{1 - 0.75z^{-1} + 0.125z^{-2}}.$$

Making the identification

$$b_0 = 1, b_1 = 2, b_2 = 1$$

and

$$a_0 = 1, a_1 = -0.75, a_2 = 0.125,$$

it then follows from Eqs. 6.2.7 and 6.2.10 that

$$\boldsymbol{A} = \begin{bmatrix} 0 & 1 \\ -0.125 & 0.75 \end{bmatrix}, \quad \boldsymbol{b} = \begin{bmatrix} 0 \\ 1 \end{bmatrix}, \quad \boldsymbol{c} = \begin{bmatrix} 0.875 & 2.75 \end{bmatrix}, \quad \boldsymbol{d} = 1.$$

We find that

$$(z\boldsymbol{I} - \boldsymbol{A}) = \begin{bmatrix} z & -1 \\ 0.125 & z - 0.75 \end{bmatrix},$$

and hence

$$\mathrm{adj}(z\boldsymbol{I} - \boldsymbol{A}) = \begin{bmatrix} z - 0.75 & 1 \\ -0.125 & z \end{bmatrix}.$$

Furthermore, $|z\boldsymbol{I} - \boldsymbol{A}| = (z - 0.5)(z - 0.25)$ so that

$$(z\boldsymbol{I} - \boldsymbol{A})^{-1} = \begin{bmatrix} \frac{z-0.75}{(z-0.5)(z-0.25)} & \frac{1}{(z-0.5)(z-0.25)} \\ \frac{-0.125}{(z-0.5)(z-0.25)} & \frac{z}{(z-0.5)(z-0.25)} \end{bmatrix}.$$

Observe that the eigenvalues of $\boldsymbol{A}$ are the poles of $H(z)$, as expected. Next,

$$(z\boldsymbol{I} - \boldsymbol{A})^{-1}\boldsymbol{b} = (z\boldsymbol{I} - \boldsymbol{A})^{-1}\begin{bmatrix} 0 \\ 1 \end{bmatrix} = \begin{bmatrix} \frac{1}{(z-0.5)(z-0.25)} \\ \frac{z}{(z-0.5)(z-0.25)} \end{bmatrix}.$$

Finally,

$$H(z) = \boldsymbol{c}(z\boldsymbol{I} - \boldsymbol{A})^{-1}\boldsymbol{b} + \boldsymbol{d}$$

which gives

$$H(z) = \begin{bmatrix} 0.875 & 2.75 \end{bmatrix}(z\boldsymbol{I} - \boldsymbol{A})^{-1}\boldsymbol{b} + 1 = \frac{1 + 2z^{-1} + z^{-2}}{1 - 0.75z^{-1} + 0.125z^{-2}}.$$

Thus, $\boldsymbol{c}(z\boldsymbol{I} - \boldsymbol{A})^{-1}\boldsymbol{b} + \boldsymbol{d} = H(z)$, as expected.

The state-variable representation is useful because it allows us to determine the impulse response from the input to each state variable. This is important because it will enable us to gain quantitative information about the internal shift register contents of the filter. We will need this information when we have to deal with issues such as finite wordlength effects and overflow. Because the relation from the input to the state is given by

$$\boldsymbol{X}(z) = (z\boldsymbol{I} - \boldsymbol{A})^{-1}\boldsymbol{b}U(z),$$

we find that the impulse response from the input to the state is obtained by inverting the transform $(z\boldsymbol{I} - \boldsymbol{A})^{-1}\boldsymbol{b}$, which yields

$$\begin{bmatrix} x_1(k) \\ x_2(k) \end{bmatrix} = \begin{bmatrix} 4\left[\left(\frac{1}{2}\right)^{k-1} - \left(\frac{1}{4}\right)^{k-1}\right] u(k-1) \\ 4\left[\left(\frac{1}{2}\right)^{k} - \left(\frac{1}{4}\right)^{k}\right] u(k-1) \end{bmatrix}.$$

This result makes sense intuitively, since the contents of state 2 (the second leftmost shift register) are the same as those of state 1, delayed by one sample.

While this example is rather simple, the techniques are valid for higher order systems, as well. While the computations are rather tedious to perform by hand, there is a wide assortment of numerical techniques for computer computation. We will discuss some of these techniques shortly.

While this example is rather simple, the techniques are valid for higher order systems, as well. While the computations are rather tedious to perform by hand, there is a wide assortment of numerical techniques to make the job simple for a computer. We will discuss some of these techniques shortly.

Example 6.3

For thoroughness, we will show how the impulse response from the input to the state could have been obtained using diagonalization of the $\boldsymbol{A}$ matrix in the previous example. Recall that the transfer function $H_s(z)$ from the input to the state is

$$H_s(z) = (z\boldsymbol{I} - \boldsymbol{A})^{-1}\boldsymbol{b},$$

which implies that the impulse response from the input to the state is

$$h_s(k) = \boldsymbol{A}^{k-1}\boldsymbol{b}.$$

We can decompose the $\boldsymbol{A}$ matrix as

$$\boldsymbol{A} = \boldsymbol{T}\boldsymbol{\Lambda}\boldsymbol{T}^{-1}$$

where $\boldsymbol{T}$ is the matrix of eigenvectors of $\boldsymbol{A}$ and $\boldsymbol{\Lambda}$ is a diagonal matrix of corresponding eigenvalues. It then follows that

$$h_s(k) = \boldsymbol{T}\boldsymbol{\Lambda}^{k-1}\boldsymbol{T}^{-1}\boldsymbol{b}.$$

We find that

$$\boldsymbol{T} = \begin{bmatrix} 1 & 1 \\ 0.25 & 0.5 \end{bmatrix}, \quad \boldsymbol{T}^{-1} = \begin{bmatrix} 2 & -4 \\ -1 & 4 \end{bmatrix},$$

and

$$\boldsymbol{\Lambda} = \begin{bmatrix} 0.25 & 0 \\ 0 & 0.5 \end{bmatrix}$$

so that

$$\boldsymbol{A}^{k-1} = \begin{bmatrix} 1 & 1 \\ 0.25 & 0.5 \end{bmatrix} \begin{bmatrix} (0.25)^{k-1} & 0 \\ 0 & (0.5)^{k-1} \end{bmatrix} \begin{bmatrix} 2 & -4 \\ -1 & 4 \end{bmatrix}.$$

Multiplying the matrices, we find that

$$\begin{bmatrix} x_1(k) \\ x_2(k) \end{bmatrix} = \begin{bmatrix} 4\left[\left(\frac{1}{2}\right)^{k-1} - \left(\frac{1}{4}\right)^{k-1}\right] \\ 4\left[\left(\frac{1}{2}\right)^{k} - \left(\frac{1}{4}\right)^{k}\right] \end{bmatrix},$$

which is the same result we obtained before.

Computational techniques

The methods we have presented for computing $(z\boldsymbol{I} - \boldsymbol{A})^{-1}$ are not well suited to implementation on a general-purpose digital computer. A method which is frequently used is *Leverrier's method*, which provides a simple and elegant solution to a difficult problem in symbolic computation.

To begin, recall that

$$(z\boldsymbol{I} - \boldsymbol{A})^{-1} = \frac{\operatorname{adj}(z\boldsymbol{I} - \boldsymbol{A})}{|z\boldsymbol{I} - \boldsymbol{A}|}. \tag{6.6.13}$$

If both sides of Eq. 6.6.13 are multiplied by $(z\boldsymbol{I} - \boldsymbol{A})$, we get

$$\boldsymbol{I} = \frac{\operatorname{adj}(z\boldsymbol{I} - \boldsymbol{A})}{|z\boldsymbol{I} - \boldsymbol{A}|}(z\boldsymbol{I} - \boldsymbol{A}). \tag{6.6.14}$$

Multiplying both sides of Eq. 6.6.14 by $|z\boldsymbol{I} - \boldsymbol{A}|$ gives

$$|z\boldsymbol{I} - \boldsymbol{A}|\boldsymbol{I} = \operatorname{adj}(z\boldsymbol{I} - \boldsymbol{A})(z\boldsymbol{I} - \boldsymbol{A}). \tag{6.6.15}$$

Now, recall that $|z\boldsymbol{I} - \boldsymbol{A}|$ is a polynomial of degree n in z (specifically, it is the characteristic polynomial for the matrix $\boldsymbol{A}$) and can be written as

$$|z\boldsymbol{I} - \boldsymbol{A}| = z^n + a_{n-1}z^{n-1} + a_{n-2}z^{n-2} + \cdots + a_1 z + a_0. \tag{6.6.16}$$

Furthermore, $\text{adj}(z\boldsymbol{I} - \boldsymbol{A})$ is a matrix of polynomials of degree $n-1$ and hence can be decomposed as a polynomial of degree $n-1$ with matrix coefficients, such as

$$\text{adj}(z\boldsymbol{I} - \boldsymbol{A}) = \boldsymbol{Q}_{n-1}z^{n-1} + \boldsymbol{Q}_{n-2}z^{n-2} + \cdots + \boldsymbol{Q}_1 z + \boldsymbol{Q}_0. \tag{6.6.17}$$

Substituting Eqs. 6.6.17 and 6.6.18 into Eq. 6.6.15, it follows that

$$\begin{aligned} z^n\boldsymbol{I} \;+\; & a_{n-1}z^{n-1}\boldsymbol{I} + a_{n-2}z^{n-2}\boldsymbol{I} + \cdots + a_1 z\boldsymbol{I} + a_0\boldsymbol{I} \\ & = (\boldsymbol{Q}_{n-1}z^{n-1} + \boldsymbol{Q}_{n-2}z^{n-2} + \cdots + \boldsymbol{Q}_1 z + \boldsymbol{Q}_0)(z\boldsymbol{I} - \boldsymbol{A}). \end{aligned} \tag{6.6.18}$$

If we multiply out the expression on the right of Eq. 6.6.18 and equate similar powers of z, the following relationships hold:

$$\begin{array}{lcc} \boldsymbol{Q}_{n-1} & = & \boldsymbol{I} \\ \boldsymbol{Q}_{n-2} & = & \boldsymbol{Q}_{n-1}\boldsymbol{A} + a_{n-1}\boldsymbol{I} \\ \boldsymbol{Q}_{n-3} & = & \boldsymbol{Q}_{n-2}\boldsymbol{A} + a_{n-2}\boldsymbol{I} \\ \cdots & \cdots & \cdots \\ \boldsymbol{Q}_{n-k} & = & \boldsymbol{Q}_{n-k-1}\boldsymbol{A} + a_{n-k-1}\boldsymbol{I} \\ \cdots & \cdots & \cdots \\ \boldsymbol{Q}_0 & = & \boldsymbol{Q}_1\boldsymbol{A} + a_1\boldsymbol{I} \\ -\boldsymbol{Q}_0\boldsymbol{A} & = & a_0\boldsymbol{I}. \end{array} \tag{6.6.19}$$

Equation 6.6.19 gives a recursive method for computing the matrices $\boldsymbol{Q}_i$. We start from $\boldsymbol{Q}_{n-1}$ and work the recursion backwards. The final recursion is simply a check. The only unknown parameters are the a_i which can either be obtained by computing the characteristic polynomial, or, more simply, using the rule

$$a_i = -\frac{1}{n-i}\,trace(\boldsymbol{Q}_i\boldsymbol{A}). \tag{6.6.20}$$

Once the a_i and the $\boldsymbol{Q}_i$ have been computed, Eqs. 6.6.16 and 6.6.17 are substituted into Eq. 6.6.13 to obtain

$$(z\boldsymbol{I} - \boldsymbol{A})^{-1} = \frac{\boldsymbol{Q}_{n-1}z^{n-1} + \boldsymbol{Q}_{n-2}z^{n-2} + \cdots + \boldsymbol{Q}_1 z + \boldsymbol{Q}_0}{z^n + a_{n-1}z^{n-1} + a_{n-2}z^{n-2} + \cdots + a_1 z + a_0}. \tag{6.6.21}$$

Example 6.4

Suppose

$$\boldsymbol{A} = \begin{bmatrix} 0 & 1 \\ -0.125 & 0.75 \end{bmatrix}.$$

In this case, $n = 2$. We begin with

$$\boldsymbol{Q}_1 = \begin{bmatrix} 1 & 0 \\ 0 & 1 \end{bmatrix}$$

and

$$a_1 = -\frac{1}{1} trace(\boldsymbol{Q}_1 \boldsymbol{A}) = -trace(\boldsymbol{A}) = -0.75.$$

Next,

$$\boldsymbol{Q}_0 = \boldsymbol{Q}_1 \boldsymbol{A} + a_1 \boldsymbol{I} = \begin{bmatrix} 0 & 1 \\ -0.125 & 0 \end{bmatrix} - \frac{3}{4} \begin{bmatrix} 1 & 0 \\ 0 & 1 \end{bmatrix},$$

so that

$$\boldsymbol{Q}_0 = \begin{bmatrix} -0.75 & 1 \\ -0.125 & 0 \end{bmatrix}$$

and

$$a_0 = -\frac{1}{2} trace(\boldsymbol{Q}_0 \boldsymbol{A}) = -\frac{1}{2} trace \left[\begin{bmatrix} -0.125 & 0 \\ 0 & -0.125 \end{bmatrix} \right] = 0.125.$$

As a check, it can be seen that $-\boldsymbol{Q}_0 \boldsymbol{A} = a_0 \boldsymbol{I}$. Finally,

$$(z\boldsymbol{I} - \boldsymbol{A})^{-1} = \frac{\boldsymbol{Q}_1 z + \boldsymbol{Q}_0}{z^2 + a_1 z + a_2}$$

which gives

$$(z\boldsymbol{I} - \boldsymbol{A})^{-1} = \frac{1}{z^2 - 0.75z + 0.125} \begin{bmatrix} z - 0.75 & 1 \\ -0.125 & z \end{bmatrix}.$$

In practice, Leverrier's algorithm tends to suffer from roundoff error problems for large filter orders. There are other computational solutions to the problem of converting a state-variable representation to a transfer function. One method is based on eigenvalue computations. There are many numerically stable "canned" routines available for eigenvalue computation. These routines can be used as the basis for a reliable procedure for transfer function computation. Given the state variable description $\{\boldsymbol{A}, \boldsymbol{b}, \boldsymbol{c}, \boldsymbol{d}\}$, the transfer function is given by

$$H(z) = \boldsymbol{c}(z\boldsymbol{I} - \boldsymbol{A})^{-1}\boldsymbol{b} + \boldsymbol{d}.$$

For a column vector $\boldsymbol{b}$ and a row vector $\boldsymbol{c}$, it can be shown that

$$\boldsymbol{c}(z\boldsymbol{I} - \boldsymbol{A})^{-1}\boldsymbol{b} = \frac{det(z\boldsymbol{I} - (\boldsymbol{A} - \boldsymbol{bc})) - det(z\boldsymbol{I} - \boldsymbol{A})}{det(z\boldsymbol{I} - \boldsymbol{A})}$$

so that

$$H(z) = \frac{det(z\boldsymbol{I} - (\boldsymbol{A} - \boldsymbol{bc})) - (\boldsymbol{d} - 1)det(z\boldsymbol{I} - \boldsymbol{A})}{det(z\boldsymbol{I} - \boldsymbol{A})}. \tag{6.6.22}$$

Given a square matrix $\boldsymbol{X}$, the characteristic polynomial $det(z\boldsymbol{I} - \boldsymbol{X})$ can be computed by first finding the eigenvalues $\lambda_1, \lambda_2, \ldots, \lambda_N$ of $\boldsymbol{X}$ using a standard eigenvalue routine and then forming the characteristic polynomial using the eigenvalues according to

$$det(z\boldsymbol{I} - \boldsymbol{X}) = (z - \lambda_1)(z - \lambda_2) \cdots (z - \lambda_N). \tag{6.6.23}$$

6.7 Filter Architectures

By now, it should be clear that there is a one-to-one correspondence between a state variable representation and a filter architecture. That is, the collection of matrices

$$\{\boldsymbol{A}, \boldsymbol{b}, \boldsymbol{c}, \boldsymbol{d}\}$$

uniquely specifies how to construct the filter from shift registers, adders, and multipliers. A worthwhile question is "What modifications can be made to the internal construction of the filter without modifying the input-output behavior?" What this question is really asking is how we can generate other filter architectures (and hence state variable descriptions) without altering the transfer function of the filter. This is an important question, since, as we will see, different architectures have different properties. While the theoretical transfer function from the input to the output may be the same for two different architectures, when implemented in hardware their behavior may be drastically different. This is usually a very difficult problem to analyze, but the state variable method makes the analysis extremely simple.

To this end, assume we have a state variable description

$$\begin{array}{rcll} \boldsymbol{x}(k+1) & = & \boldsymbol{A}\boldsymbol{x}(k) & + \ \boldsymbol{b}u(k) \\ y(k) & = & \boldsymbol{c}\boldsymbol{x}(k) & + \ \boldsymbol{d}u(k) \end{array} . \tag{6.7.1}$$

Let $\boldsymbol{T}$ be an invertible matrix and define the *new state* $\boldsymbol{q}(k)$ by

$$\boldsymbol{x}(k) = \boldsymbol{T}\boldsymbol{q}(k). \tag{6.7.2}$$

It then follows that

$$\boldsymbol{x}(k+1) = \boldsymbol{T}\boldsymbol{q}(k+1) \tag{6.7.3}$$

and substituting Eq. 6.7.3 into Eq. 6.7.1,

$$\begin{array}{rcll} \boldsymbol{T}\boldsymbol{q}(k+1) & = & \boldsymbol{A}\boldsymbol{T}\boldsymbol{q}(k) & + \ \boldsymbol{b}u(k) \\ y(k) & = & \boldsymbol{c}\boldsymbol{T}\boldsymbol{q}(k) & + \ \boldsymbol{d}u(k) \end{array} . \tag{6.7.4}$$

Multiplying the top equation of Eq. 6.7.4 by $\boldsymbol{T}^{-1}$ (which is possible since $\boldsymbol{T}$ is assumed invertible), we get the new state variable equations

$$\begin{array}{rcll} \boldsymbol{q}(k+1) & = & \boldsymbol{T}^{-1}\boldsymbol{A}\boldsymbol{T}\boldsymbol{q}(k) & + \ \boldsymbol{T}^{-1}\boldsymbol{b}u(k) \\ y(k) & = & \boldsymbol{c}\boldsymbol{T}^{-1}\boldsymbol{q}(k) & + \ \boldsymbol{d}u(k) \end{array} . \tag{6.7.5}$$

Thus, the system with state $\boldsymbol{q}(k)$ is described by the new state variable description

$$\{\boldsymbol{A}', \boldsymbol{b}', \boldsymbol{c}', \boldsymbol{d}'\} = \{\boldsymbol{T}^{-1}\boldsymbol{A}\boldsymbol{T}, \boldsymbol{T}^{-1}\boldsymbol{b}, \boldsymbol{c}\boldsymbol{T}, \boldsymbol{d}\}. \tag{6.7.6}$$

The original system has transfer function

$$H(z) = \boldsymbol{c}(z\boldsymbol{I} - \boldsymbol{A})^{-1}\boldsymbol{b} + \boldsymbol{d}.$$

To study the effect of the change of state on the transfer function, write the new transfer function $H'(z)$ as

$$H'(z) = \boldsymbol{c}'(z\boldsymbol{I} - \boldsymbol{A}')^{-1}\boldsymbol{b}' + \boldsymbol{d}'.$$

Substituting the relations for $\boldsymbol{A}', \boldsymbol{b}', \boldsymbol{c}'$, and $\boldsymbol{d}'$, from Eq. 6.7.6, it follows that

$$H'(z) = \boldsymbol{c}\boldsymbol{T}(z\boldsymbol{I} - \boldsymbol{T}^{-1}\boldsymbol{A}\boldsymbol{T})^{-1}\boldsymbol{T}^{-1}\boldsymbol{b} + \boldsymbol{d}. \tag{6.7.7}$$

Equation 6.7.7 can be rewritten as

$$H'(z) = \boldsymbol{c}(\boldsymbol{T}^{-1})^{-1}(z\boldsymbol{I} - \boldsymbol{T}^{-1}\boldsymbol{A}\boldsymbol{T})^{-1}(\boldsymbol{T})^{-1}\boldsymbol{b} + \boldsymbol{d}. \tag{6.7.8}$$

Recall that the inverse of the product of matrices is equal to the reversed product of the inverses. That is,

$$(\boldsymbol{X}\boldsymbol{Y}\boldsymbol{Z})^{-1} = \boldsymbol{Z}^{-1}\boldsymbol{Y}^{-1}\boldsymbol{X}^{-1}.$$

Therefore, Eq. 6.7.8 becomes

$$H'(z) = \boldsymbol{c}(\boldsymbol{T}(z\boldsymbol{I} - \boldsymbol{T}^{-1}\boldsymbol{A}\boldsymbol{T})\boldsymbol{T}^{-1})^{-1}\boldsymbol{b} + \boldsymbol{d}, \tag{6.7.9}$$

which upon simplification reduces to

$$H'(z) = \boldsymbol{c}(z\boldsymbol{I} - \boldsymbol{A})^{-1}\boldsymbol{b} + \boldsymbol{d} = H(z). \tag{6.7.10}$$

Thus, the new filter has the same transfer function as the original filter.

The critical result is that nonsingular transformations of the state have no effect on the transfer function of the filter. Equally important, *these are the only transformations of the filter which will leave the transfer function unmodified.* In other words, we have a complete description of the allowable modifications to a filter which will leave the input/output behavior unmodified: they must be representable as an invertible matrix multiplication of the state. It will be seen that nonsingular transformations of the state corresponding to a "re-wiring" of the system's block diagram without changing the transfer function.

6.8 Interconnection of Systems

6.8.1 The Cascade Architecture

We begin with the cascade architecture, shown in Fig. 6.8.1. The cascade architecture, in its most general form, consists of an interconnection of L filters described by the transfer functions

$$H_1(z), H_2(z), \ldots, H_L(z).$$

The overall transfer function of the cascade system is

$$H_c(z) = H_1(z)H_2(z)\cdots H_L(z).$$

In a cascade interconnection, the output of the i-th filter is fed to the input of the $i+1$-th filter. There is an external input supplied to the first filter and the overall output is the output of the $\boldsymbol{L}$-th filter.

We are interested in obtaining an overall state variable description for the cascade system. Suppose each filter has state $\boldsymbol{x}_i(k)$ and is described by the state-variable equations

$$\begin{array}{rcl} \boldsymbol{x}_i(k+1) &=& \boldsymbol{A}_i\boldsymbol{x}_i(k) + \boldsymbol{b}_i u_i(k) \\ y_i(k) &=& \boldsymbol{c}_i\boldsymbol{x}_i(k) + \boldsymbol{d}_i u_i(k) \end{array}, \quad i = 1, 2, \ldots, L.$$

The transfer function of the i-th system is given by

$$H_i(z) = \boldsymbol{c}_i(z\boldsymbol{I} - \boldsymbol{A}_i)^1\boldsymbol{b}_i + \boldsymbol{d}_i.$$

The overall state for the cascade is the aggregate of the states of the subfilters, denoted by $\boldsymbol{X}(k)$, where

$$\boldsymbol{X}(k) := \begin{bmatrix} \boldsymbol{x}_1(k) \\ \boldsymbol{x}_2(k) \\ \vdots \\ \boldsymbol{x}_L(k) \end{bmatrix}.$$

The problem is to determine the system matrices $\{\boldsymbol{A}_c, \boldsymbol{b}_c, \boldsymbol{c}_c, \boldsymbol{d}_c\}$ for the cascade state-variable model

$$\begin{array}{rcl} \boldsymbol{X}(k+1) &=& \boldsymbol{A}_c\boldsymbol{X}(k) + \boldsymbol{b}_c u(k) \\ y(k) &=& \boldsymbol{c}_c\boldsymbol{X}(k) + \boldsymbol{d}_c u(k) \end{array}.$$

The key to developing the overall state-variable model is *recursion*; the overall state-variable description is built up one section at a time.

Consider first the problem of determining the system matrices for a cascade of two filters with states $\boldsymbol{x}_1(k)$ and $\boldsymbol{x}_2(k)$, respectively. For the overall cascade system, the input is $u_1(k)$ and the output is $y_2(k)$. The first system is described by

$$\begin{aligned} \boldsymbol{x}_1(k+1) &= \boldsymbol{A}_1\boldsymbol{x}_1(k) + \boldsymbol{b}_1 u_1(k) \\ y_1(k) &= \boldsymbol{c}_1\boldsymbol{x}_1(k) + \boldsymbol{d}_1 u_1(k) \end{aligned} \tag{6.8.1}$$

and the second system is described by

$$\begin{aligned} \boldsymbol{x}_2(k+1) &= \boldsymbol{A}_2\boldsymbol{x}_2(k) + \boldsymbol{b}_2 u_2(k) \\ y_2(k) &= \boldsymbol{c}_2\boldsymbol{x}_2(k) + \boldsymbol{d}_2 u_2(k) \end{aligned}$$

Suppose the output of the first system, $y_1(k)$, is supplied as the input to the second system, $u_2(k)$. Then the state equation for the second system becomes

$$\boldsymbol{x}_2(k+1) = \boldsymbol{A}_2\boldsymbol{x}_2(k) + \boldsymbol{b}_2(\boldsymbol{c}_1\boldsymbol{x}_1(k) + \boldsymbol{d}_1 u_1(k))$$

which can be rewritten as

$$\boldsymbol{x}_2(k+1) = \boldsymbol{A}_2\boldsymbol{x}_2(k) + \boldsymbol{b}_2\boldsymbol{c}_1\boldsymbol{x}_1(k) + \boldsymbol{b}_2\boldsymbol{d}_1\boldsymbol{u}_1(k). \tag{6.8.2}$$

The output equation for the second system becomes

$$y_2(k) = \boldsymbol{c}_2\boldsymbol{x}_2(k) + \boldsymbol{d}_2(\boldsymbol{c}_1\boldsymbol{x}_1(k) + d_1\boldsymbol{u}_1(k))$$

which can be rewritten as

$$y_2(k) = \boldsymbol{c}_2\boldsymbol{x}_2(k) + \boldsymbol{d}_2\boldsymbol{c}_1\boldsymbol{x}_1(k) + \boldsymbol{d}_2\boldsymbol{d}_1\boldsymbol{u}_1(k). \tag{6.8.3}$$

Now, define the aggregate state by

$$\boldsymbol{X}(k) = \begin{bmatrix} \boldsymbol{x}_1(k) \\ \boldsymbol{x}_2(k) \end{bmatrix}.$$

Combining Eqs. 6.8.1 and 6.8.2, the evolution of the aggregate state is given by

$$\begin{bmatrix} \boldsymbol{x}_1(k+1) \\ \boldsymbol{x}_2(k+1) \end{bmatrix} = \begin{bmatrix} \boldsymbol{A}_1 & \boldsymbol{O} \\ \boldsymbol{b}_2\boldsymbol{c}_1 & \boldsymbol{A}_2 \end{bmatrix} \begin{bmatrix} \boldsymbol{x}_1(k) \\ \boldsymbol{x}_2(k) \end{bmatrix} + \begin{bmatrix} \boldsymbol{b}_1 \\ \boldsymbol{b}_2\boldsymbol{d}_1 \end{bmatrix} u_1(k). \tag{6.8.4}$$

Similarly, Eq. 6.8.3 is then used to write the output equation as

$$y_2(k) = \begin{bmatrix} \boldsymbol{d}_2\boldsymbol{c}_1 & \boldsymbol{c}_2 \end{bmatrix} \begin{bmatrix} \boldsymbol{x}_1(k) \\ \boldsymbol{x}_2(k) \end{bmatrix} + \boldsymbol{d}_2\boldsymbol{d}_1\boldsymbol{u}_1(k). \tag{6.8.5}$$

This completes the model for the cascade of two filters. For the more general case of L cascaded filters, the overall model is built up successively a stage at a time as above, until the final cascaded section.

For a cascade of L filters, it can be shown using the above technique that the overall state variable model from the input $u_1(k) = u(k)$ to the output $y(k) = y_L(k)$ is given by the matrices

$$\boldsymbol{A}_c = \begin{bmatrix} \boldsymbol{A}_1 & \boldsymbol{O} & \boldsymbol{O} & \cdots & \boldsymbol{O} \\ \boldsymbol{b}_2\boldsymbol{c}_1 & \boldsymbol{A}_2 & \boldsymbol{O} & \cdots & \boldsymbol{O} \\ \boldsymbol{b}_3\boldsymbol{d}_2\boldsymbol{c}_1 & \boldsymbol{b}_3\boldsymbol{c}_2 & \boldsymbol{A}_3 & \cdots & \boldsymbol{O} \\ \vdots & \vdots & \vdots & \ddots & \vdots \\ \boldsymbol{b}_L\boldsymbol{d}_{L-1}\cdots\boldsymbol{d}_2\boldsymbol{c}_1 & \boldsymbol{b}_L\boldsymbol{d}_{L-1}\cdots\boldsymbol{d}_3\boldsymbol{c}_2 & \boldsymbol{b}_L\boldsymbol{d}_{L-1}\cdots\boldsymbol{d}_4\boldsymbol{c}_3 & \cdots & \boldsymbol{A}_L \end{bmatrix}, \tag{6.8.6}$$

$$\boldsymbol{b}_c = \begin{bmatrix} \boldsymbol{b}_1 \\ \boldsymbol{b}_2\boldsymbol{d}_1 \\ \boldsymbol{b}_3\boldsymbol{d}_2\boldsymbol{d}_1 \\ \vdots \\ \boldsymbol{b}_L\boldsymbol{d}_{L-1}\boldsymbol{d}_{L-2}\cdots\boldsymbol{d}_1 \end{bmatrix} \tag{6.8.7}$$

$$\boldsymbol{c}_c = \begin{bmatrix} \boldsymbol{d}_L\boldsymbol{d}_{L-1}\cdots\boldsymbol{d}_2\boldsymbol{c}_1 & \boldsymbol{d}_L\boldsymbol{d}_{L-1}\cdots\boldsymbol{d}_3\boldsymbol{c}_2 & \boldsymbol{d}_L\boldsymbol{d}_{L-1}\cdots\boldsymbol{d}_4\boldsymbol{c}_3 & \cdots & \boldsymbol{c}_L \end{bmatrix}, \tag{6.8.8}$$

and

$$\boldsymbol{d}_c = \boldsymbol{d}_L\boldsymbol{d}_{L-1}\cdots\boldsymbol{d}_1. \tag{6.8.9}$$

The transfer function for the cascade system will then be given by

$$H_c(z) = \boldsymbol{c}_c(z\boldsymbol{I} - \boldsymbol{A}_c)^{-1}\boldsymbol{b}_c + \boldsymbol{d}_c.$$

The reason we have developed the cascade architecture is as follows. The fixed-point behavior of the direct-II architecture is quite poor. Although the direct-II architecture requires the fewest multiply/accumulates per filter cycle (which translates into higher peak throughput), the effects of roundoff noise and coefficient error are quite pronounced. The reason for this is that the poles of the direct-II system are sensitive to all of the coefficients a_i simultaneously. That is, any perturbation to any coefficient a_i will bring about changes in all of the poles. Physically, this is due to the fact that there is feedback from each state to the input. The cascade architecture, however, is capable of *isolating* small groups of poles and using "less" feedback.

As an example, consider an eighth-order transfer function,

$$H(z) = \frac{b_0 + b_1 z^{-1} + \cdots + b_8 z^{-8}}{1 + a_1 z^{-1} + \cdots + a_8 z^{-8}} = \frac{b(z)}{a(z)}.$$

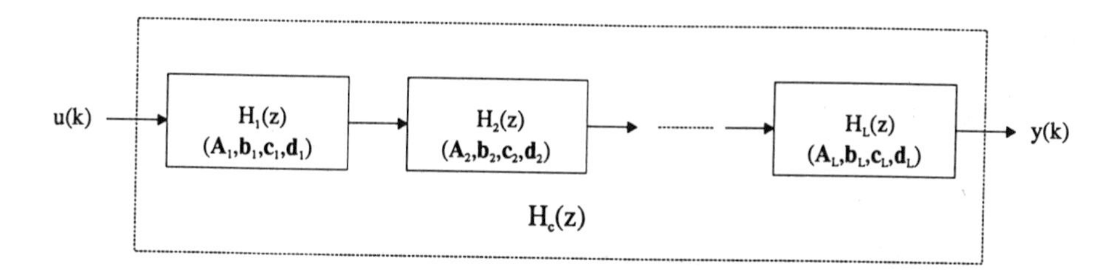

Figure 6.8.1: Cascade architecture.

The poles of the direct-II realization are the roots of $a(z)$, and any error in the coefficients will translate into errors in *all* eight root locations. Furthermore, the higher the degree of $a(z)$, the more severe the errors. It can also be shown that for tightly clustered roots, the situation is worse than for roots spread throughout the interior of the unit circle.

If, however, $H(z)$ is factorized as

$$H(z) = H_1(z)H_2(z)H_3(z)H_4(z)$$

where $H_i(z)$ is a second-order transfer function with real coefficients, we can generate a cascade architecture for $H(z)$. The formation of the poles is now done *by section* so that any coefficient error translates into a pole location error *for that section only.* Furthermore, the pole locations of a second order section are much less sensitive to coefficient errors than higher-order sections. The same is true for the zeros. Hence, the cascade architecture tends to allow fairly accurate pole and zero placement, even in the presence of coefficients. The poles and zeros of the cascade filter are simply the aggregate of the poles and zeros of the subfilters. The issue of pole and zero sensitivity to coefficient perturbations is studied in detail later in the chapter.

Now that we know how to write the state variable equations for a cascade of smaller subfilters, we can concern ourselves with the inverse problem. That is, given a transfer function $H(z)$, what is an appropriate decomposition of $H(z)$ into a cascade of smaller order subfilters? In other words, we seek a decomposition of the form

$$H(z) = H_1(z)H_2(z)\cdots H_L(z)$$

where

$$\sum_{i=1}^{L} \deg(H_i(z)) = \deg(H(z)).$$

We have two basic criteria for the subfilters:

1. The orders of the subfilters should be small to allow effective isolation of the coefficient errors from pole errors.

2. The coefficients of the subfilters should be real. This is because of the increased difficulty of complex multiplication. A single complex multiply requires *four* real multiplies.

A rule of thumb which follows these guidelines is that each real pole is used to generate a first order section, whereas complex conjugate pole pairs are used to generate a second order section. The first step in performing a cascade decomposition of a transfer function $H(z)$ is to factor the numerator and denominator to obtain their respective roots. Next, separate the numerator and denominator roots into collections of complex conjugate pairs and real roots. We are left with the decision of which zeros to pair with which poles. A reasonable rule is to group the poles with the zeros which are closest in the complex plane. Geometrically, it can be seen that this has the effect of minimizing the gain within each section, which is important if fixed-point arithmetic is used and overflow needs to be avoided. An example will illustrate.

Example 6.5

Suppose

$$H(z) = \frac{(1 - 0.5z^{-1} + 0.25z^{-2})(1 + 0.7z^{-1} + 0.49z^{-2})(1 - 0.2z^{-1})}{(1 + 0.8z^{-1} + 0.64z^{-2})(1 - 0.4z^{-1} + 0.16z^{-2})(1 - 0.25z^{-1})}.$$

The zeros of $H(z)$ are

$$z_1, z_1^* = 0.5e^{j\pi/3}, 0.5e^{-j\pi/3}, \quad z_2, z_2^* = 0.7e^{j4\pi/3}, 0.7e^{-j4\pi/3}, \quad z_3 = 0.2.$$

The poles of $H(z)$ are

$$p_1, p_1^* = 0.8e^{j4\pi/3}, 0.8e^{-j4\pi/3}, \quad p_2, p_2^* = 0.4e^{j\pi/3}, 0.4e^{-j\pi/3}, \quad p_3 = 0.25.$$

The cascade filter will consist of a cascade of two second order subfilters and one first order subfilter. The pole-zero grouping is performed by proximity. The pair z_1, z_1^* should be grouped with the pair p_2, p_2^*, the pair z_2, z_2^* should be grouped with the pair p_1, p_1^*, and we group z_3 with p_3. Thus, we have

$$H(z) = H_1(z)H_2(z)H_3(z)$$

where

$$H_1(z) = \frac{1 - 0.5z^{-1} + 0.25z^{-2}}{1 - 0.4z^{-1} + 0.16z^{-2}},$$

$$H_2(z) = \frac{1 + 0.7z^{-1} + 0.49z^{-2}}{1 + 0.8z^{-1} + 0.64z^{-2}},$$

and

$$H_3(z) = \frac{1 - 0.2z^{-1}}{1 - 0.25z^{-1}}.$$

Which choice of architecture to use for the first and second order subfilters can now be made. For now, we will assume a direct-II architecture. Later, we will consider other architectures for the subfilters. If a second order subfilter has transfer function

$$H_i(z) = \frac{b_{i0} + b_{i1}z^{-1} + b_{i2}z^{-2}}{1 + a_{i1}z^{-1} + a_{12}z^{-2}},$$

the state variable representation is

$$\boldsymbol{A}_i = \begin{bmatrix} 0 & 1 \\ -a_{i2} & -a_{i1} \end{bmatrix}, \quad \boldsymbol{b}_i = \begin{bmatrix} 0 \\ 1 \end{bmatrix}, \quad \boldsymbol{c}_i = \begin{bmatrix} b_{i2} - a_{i2}b_{i0} & b_{i1} - a_{i1}b_{i0} \end{bmatrix}, \quad \boldsymbol{d}_i = b_{i0}.$$

The direct-II realization of the first order subfilter $H_i(z)$ with transfer function

$$H_i(z) = \frac{b_{i0} + b_{i1}z^{-1}}{1 + a_{i1}z^{-1}}$$

is

$$\boldsymbol{A}_i = -a_{i1}, \quad \boldsymbol{b}_i = 1, \quad \boldsymbol{c}_i = b_{i1} - a_{i1}b_{i0}, \quad \boldsymbol{d}_i = b_{i0}.$$

Example 6.6

Referring to the previous example, we have

$$\boldsymbol{A}_1 = \begin{bmatrix} 0 & 1 \\ -0.16 & 0.4 \end{bmatrix}, \quad \boldsymbol{b}_1 = \begin{bmatrix} 0 \\ 1 \end{bmatrix}, \quad \boldsymbol{c}_1 = \begin{bmatrix} 0.09 & -0.1 \end{bmatrix}, \quad \boldsymbol{d}_1 = 1,$$

$$\boldsymbol{A}_2 = \begin{bmatrix} 0 & 1 \\ -0.64 & -0.8 \end{bmatrix}, \quad \boldsymbol{b}_2 = \begin{bmatrix} 0 \\ 1 \end{bmatrix}, \quad \boldsymbol{c}_2 = \begin{bmatrix} -0.15 & -0.1 \end{bmatrix}, \quad \boldsymbol{d}_2 = 1,$$

and

$$\boldsymbol{A}_3 = .25, \quad \boldsymbol{b}_3 = 1, \quad \boldsymbol{c}_3 = 0.05, \quad \boldsymbol{d}_3 = 1.$$

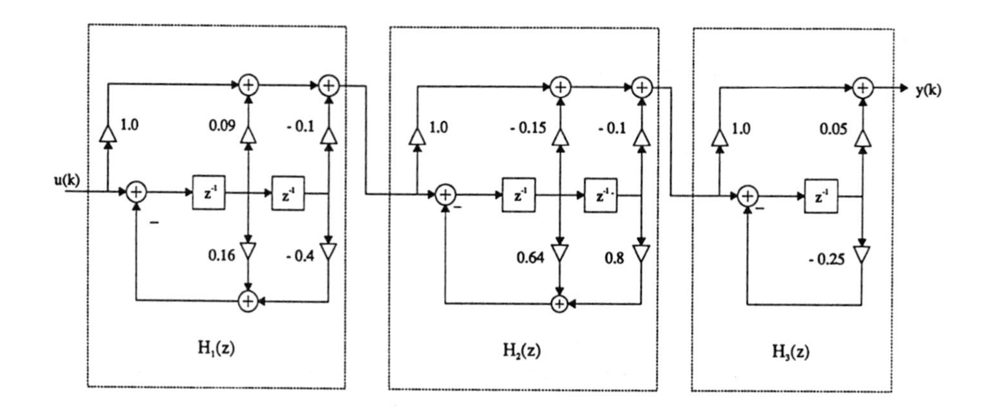

Figure 6.8.2: Cascade architecture for Example 6.6.

The cascade architecture is shown in Fig. 6.8.2 (recall the right-to-left convention we used for numbering the shift registers within individual direct-II sections). The overall state variable representation is given by

$$\boldsymbol{A}_c = \begin{bmatrix} 0 & 1 & 0 & 0 & 0 \\ -0.16 & 0.4 & 0 & 0 & 0 \\ 0 & 0 & 0 & 1 & 0 \\ 0.09 & -0.1 & -0.64 & -0.8 & 0 \\ 0.09 & -0.1 & -0.15 & -0.1 & 0.25 \end{bmatrix}, \quad \boldsymbol{b}_c = \begin{bmatrix} 0 \\ 1 \\ 0 \\ 1 \\ 1 \end{bmatrix},$$

and

$$\boldsymbol{c}_c = \begin{bmatrix} 0.09 & -0.1 & -0.15 & -0.1 & 0.05 \end{bmatrix}, \quad \boldsymbol{d}_c = 1.$$

6.8.2 The Parallel Architecture

Whereas the previous section was concerned with the cascade interconnection of subfilters, we are now interested in the *parallel* connection of subfilters. We will follow the same basic approach as the previous section in our discussion of the parallel architecture.

As before, assume that we have a collection of L filters

$$H_1(z), H_2(z), \ldots, H_L(z).$$

Again, the i-th filter is described by the state variable equations

$$\begin{aligned} \boldsymbol{x}_i(k+1) &= \boldsymbol{A}_i \boldsymbol{x}_i(k) + \boldsymbol{b}_i u_i(k) \\ y_i(k) &= \boldsymbol{c}_i \boldsymbol{x}_i(k) + \boldsymbol{d}_i u_i(k), \quad i = 1, \ldots, L. \end{aligned}$$

and the transfer function of the i-th system is given by

$$H_i(z) = \boldsymbol{c}_i (z\boldsymbol{I} - \boldsymbol{A}_i)^1 \boldsymbol{b}_i + \boldsymbol{d}_i.$$

This time, as in Fig. 6.8.3, all of the filters will be supplied with the same external input, $u(k)$, and we will sum the outputs to form the final output, $y(k)$. That is,

$$y(k) = \sum_{i=1}^{L} y_i(k).$$

It then follows that the transfer function of the parallel interconnection is

$$H_p(z) = \sum_{i=1}^{L} H_i(z).$$

The development of the state variable equations for the parallel interconnection is relatively since there is no coupling between the states of the subfilters. For the parallel filter, define the state $\boldsymbol{X}(k)$ by the concatenation of the states of the subfilters:

$$\boldsymbol{X}(k) = \begin{bmatrix} \boldsymbol{x}_1(k) \\ \boldsymbol{x}_2(k) \\ \vdots \\ \boldsymbol{x}_L(k) \end{bmatrix}.$$

It immediately follows that

$$\begin{aligned} \boldsymbol{X}(k+1) &= \boldsymbol{A}_p \boldsymbol{X}(k) + \boldsymbol{b}_p u(k) \\ y_p(k) &= \boldsymbol{c}_p \boldsymbol{X}(k) + \boldsymbol{d}_p u(k), \end{aligned} \tag{6.8.10}$$

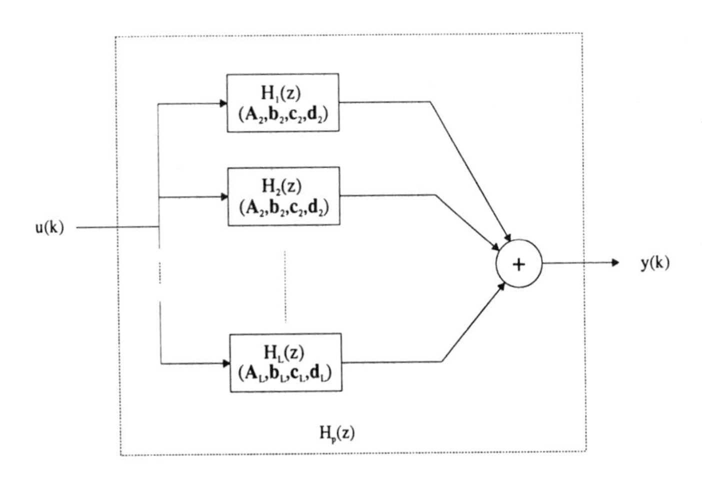

Figure 6.8.3: Parallel interconnection of subfilters.

where

$$\boldsymbol{A}_p = \begin{bmatrix} \boldsymbol{A}_1 & \boldsymbol{O} & \boldsymbol{O} & \cdots & \boldsymbol{O} \\ \boldsymbol{O} & \boldsymbol{A}_2 & \boldsymbol{O} & \cdots & \boldsymbol{O} \\ \boldsymbol{O} & \boldsymbol{O} & \boldsymbol{A}_3 & \cdots & \boldsymbol{O} \\ \vdots & \vdots & \vdots & \ddots & \vdots \\ \boldsymbol{O} & \boldsymbol{O} & \boldsymbol{O} & \cdots & \boldsymbol{A}_L \end{bmatrix}, \quad \boldsymbol{b}_p = \begin{bmatrix} \boldsymbol{b}_1 \\ \boldsymbol{b}_2 \\ \boldsymbol{b}_3 \\ \vdots \\ \boldsymbol{b}_L \end{bmatrix}, \tag{6.8.11}$$

and

$$\boldsymbol{c}_p = \begin{bmatrix} \boldsymbol{c}_1 & \boldsymbol{c}_2 & \boldsymbol{c}_3 & \cdots & \boldsymbol{c}_L \end{bmatrix}, \quad \boldsymbol{d}_p = \boldsymbol{d}_1 + \boldsymbol{d}_2 + \cdots + \boldsymbol{d}_L. \tag{6.8.12}$$

It then follows that

$$H_p(z) = \boldsymbol{c}_p(z\boldsymbol{I} - \boldsymbol{A}_p)^{-1}\boldsymbol{b}_p + \boldsymbol{d}_p. \tag{6.8.13}$$

Again, we are left with the question as to why one might find the parallel architecture useful. It can be seen from the definition of $H_p(z)$ as

$$H_p(z) = H_1(z) + H_2(z) + \cdots + H_L(z)$$

that the poles of $H_p(z)$ are simply the aggregate of the poles of the individual subfilters, $H_i(z)$. The same can not be said of the zeros. The zeros are obtained as the roots of a numerator which is formed by a collection of cross-multiplications of subfilter numerators and denominators. Thus, error in the coefficients will tend to have a pronounced effect on the zero locations. The pole locations are still relatively insensitive to coefficient errors since they are isolated in the smaller subfilters.

As before, we are interested in the same inverse problem. Specifically, given a transfer function $H(z)$, how can we decompose $H(z)$ into a parallel combination of L subfilters such that

$$H(z) = H_1(z) + H_2(z) + \cdots + H_L(z)$$

and

$$\sum_{i=1}^{L} \deg(H_i(z)) = \deg(H(z)).$$

This time, the solution is based on partial fraction expansion of $H(z)$. We find the poles of $H(z)$ and then decompose $H(z)$ into a sum of first and second order subfilters. We have the same constraint as before, namely, that the sections must consist of real coefficients only. Thus, the second order sections will consist of complex conjugate pole pairs and the first order sections will correspond to real poles.

Again, the first and second order sections can have arbitrary architecture, but we will use direct-II in what follows. An example will clarify

Example 6.7

Suppose that

$$H(z) = \frac{(1 - 0.5z^{-1} + 0.25z^{-2})(1 - 0.2z^{-1})}{(1 + 0.8z^{-1} + 0.64z^{-2})(1 - 0.25z^{-1})}.$$

In order to perform partial fraction expansion, we must first perform long division to yield a numerator which is of lower degree in z^{-1} than the denominator. We find that

$$H(z) = 1 + \frac{0.25 - 0.425z^{-1} + 0.0655z^{-2}}{(1 - 0.8z^{-1} + 0.64z^{-2})(1 - 0.2z^{-1})}.$$

Because real coefficients are required for practical implementation, the partial fraction expansion will be of the form

$$H(z) = 1 + \frac{A}{1 - 0.2z^{-1}} + \frac{B + Cz^{-1}}{1 - 0.8z^{-1} + 0.64z^{-2}},$$

and we find that

$$H(z) = 1 - \frac{0.0113}{1 - 0.2z^{-1}} - \frac{1.3387 + 0.3637z^{-1}}{1 - 0.8z^{-1} + 0.64z^{-2}}.$$

The parallel architecture for this example is shown in Fig. 6.8.4

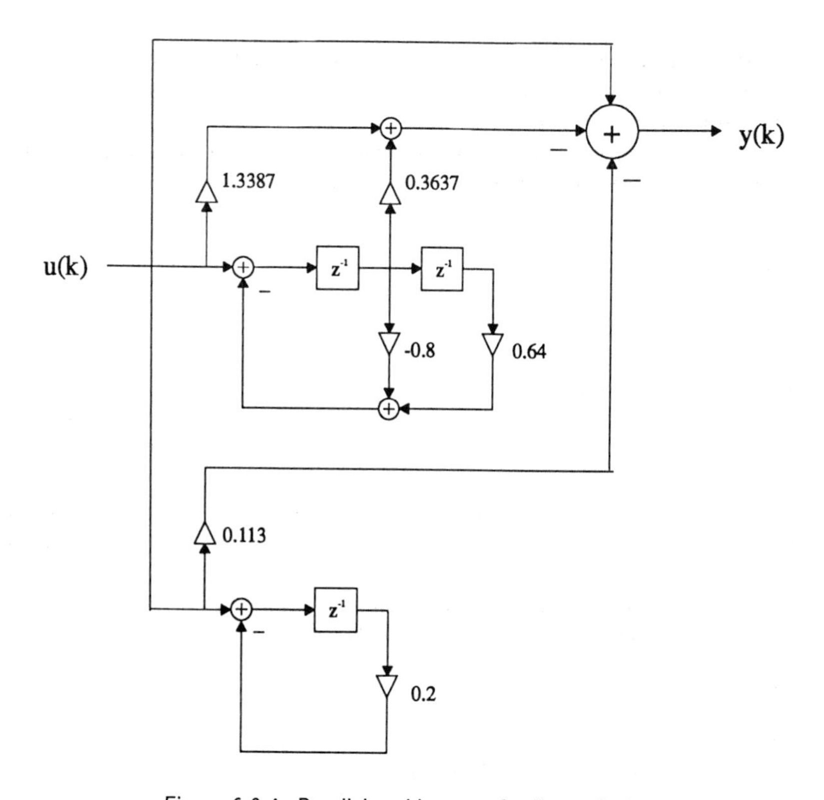

Figure 6.8.4: Parallel architecture for Example 6.7.

We have not yet made the connection between the direct-II architecture and either the cascade or parallel architecture in terms of state transformation. Recall that we mentioned that any two realizations of a transfer function must be related by a similarity transformation. That is, if $H(z)$ can be modeled by the state variable models

$$\{\boldsymbol{A}, \boldsymbol{b}, \boldsymbol{c}, \boldsymbol{d}\}$$

and

$$\{\boldsymbol{A}', \boldsymbol{b}', \boldsymbol{c}', \boldsymbol{d}'\},$$

there must exist an invertible matrix $\boldsymbol{T}$ such that

$$\boldsymbol{A}' = \boldsymbol{T}^{-1}\boldsymbol{A}\boldsymbol{T}, \quad \boldsymbol{b}' = \boldsymbol{T}^{-1}\boldsymbol{b}, \quad \boldsymbol{c}' = \boldsymbol{c}\boldsymbol{T}, \quad \boldsymbol{d}' = \boldsymbol{d}.$$

We begin with the parallel architecture. The case where $H(z)$ has distinct, real poles is simplest. In this case, we have shown that the eigenvalues of $\boldsymbol{A}$ are the poles of $H(z)$. Thus, there exists a real matrix, $\boldsymbol{T}$, such that

$$\boldsymbol{T}^{-1}\boldsymbol{A}\boldsymbol{T} = \boldsymbol{\Lambda}$$

where

$$\boldsymbol{\Lambda} = \begin{bmatrix} \lambda_1 & 0 & \cdots & 0 \\ 0 & \lambda_2 & \cdots & 0 \\ \vdots & \vdots & \ddots & \vdots \\ 0 & 0 & \cdots & \lambda_N \end{bmatrix}$$

where the λ_i are the eigenvalues of $\boldsymbol{A}$. The columns of $\boldsymbol{T}$ are the eigenvectors corresponding to λ_i. Then according to Eq. 6.7.2, if we make the change of state

$$\boldsymbol{x}(k) = \boldsymbol{T}\boldsymbol{q}(k),$$

or

$$\boldsymbol{q}(k) = \boldsymbol{T}^{-1}\boldsymbol{x}(k),$$

the new system will be described by the state variable equations

$$\begin{aligned} \boldsymbol{q}(k+1) &= \boldsymbol{T}^{-1}\boldsymbol{A}\boldsymbol{T}\boldsymbol{q}(k) + \boldsymbol{T}^{-1}\boldsymbol{b}u(k) \\ y(k) &= \boldsymbol{c}\boldsymbol{T}^{-1}\boldsymbol{q}(k) + \boldsymbol{d}u(k) \end{aligned} \qquad (6.8.14)$$

But because $\boldsymbol{T}^{-1}\boldsymbol{A}\boldsymbol{T} = \boldsymbol{\Lambda}$, Eq. 6.8.14 becomes

$$\begin{aligned} \boldsymbol{q}(k+1) &= \boldsymbol{\Lambda}\boldsymbol{q}(k) + \boldsymbol{T}^{-1}\boldsymbol{b}u(k) \\ y(k) &= \boldsymbol{c}\boldsymbol{T}^{-1}\boldsymbol{q}(k) + \boldsymbol{d}u(k) \end{aligned} . \qquad (6.8.15)$$

Thus, the new system is described by the state variable matrices

$$\{\boldsymbol{A}', \boldsymbol{b}', \boldsymbol{c}', \boldsymbol{d}'\} = \{\boldsymbol{\Lambda}, \boldsymbol{T}^{-1}\boldsymbol{b}, \boldsymbol{c}\boldsymbol{T}^{-1}, \boldsymbol{d}\}.$$

Notice that because $\boldsymbol{\Lambda}$ is diagonal, there is no coupling between the states of the new architecture. Hence, *the diagonalizing transformation, $\boldsymbol{T}$, yields a parallel architecture.*

Example 6.8

Consider again the filter

$$H(z) = \frac{1 + 2z^{-1} + z^{-2}}{1 - 0.75z^{-1} + 0.125z^{-2}}.$$

We found in example 2 that the direct-II architecture is described by the state variable matrices

$$A = \begin{bmatrix} 0 & 1 \\ -0.125 & 0.75 \end{bmatrix}, \quad b = \begin{bmatrix} 0 \\ 1 \end{bmatrix}, \quad c = \begin{bmatrix} 0.875 & 2.75 \end{bmatrix}, \quad d = 1.$$

The eigenvalues of A are

$$\lambda_1 = 0.25, \lambda_2 = 0.5$$

with corresponding eigenvectors

$$x_1 = \begin{bmatrix} 1 \\ 0.25 \end{bmatrix}, \quad x_2 = \begin{bmatrix} 1 \\ 0.5 \end{bmatrix}.$$

We define the transformation matrix T by

$$T = \begin{bmatrix} x_1 & x_2 \end{bmatrix}.$$

Then the new state variable matrices given by

$$A' = T^{-1}AT, \quad b' = T^{-1}b, \quad c' = cT, \quad d' = d.$$

If follows that

$$A' = \begin{bmatrix} 0.25 & 0 \\ 0 & 0.5 \end{bmatrix}, \quad b' = \begin{bmatrix} -4 \\ 4 \end{bmatrix}, \quad c' = \begin{bmatrix} 1.5625 & 2.25 \end{bmatrix}, \quad d' = 1.$$

These new state variable matrices correspond to the system

$$\begin{aligned} x_1(k+1) &= 0.25x_1(k) - 4u(k) \\ x_2(k+1) &= 0.5x_2(k) + 4u(k) \end{aligned}$$

and

$$y(k) = 1.5625x_1(k) + 2.25x_2(k) + u(k).$$

Notice that the new state variable description is "decoupled" in that there is no cross-dependence between the states x_1 and x_2.

We now consider the more complicated problem when the poles of $H(z)$ are complex. This time, we will have to settle for a "block-diagonal" A matrix. We first need the following result. Let A be a real $n \times n$ matrix with r real eigenvalues, λ_i, and $k = (n-r)/2$ complex eigenvalue pairs, $\sigma_i \pm j\omega_i$. Then there exists a real invertible T such that

$$A = T^{-1}AT = \begin{bmatrix} \lambda_1 & 0 & \cdots & 0 & 0 & 0 & \cdots & 0 & 0 \\ 0 & \lambda_2 & \cdots & 0 & 0 & 0 & \cdots & 0 & 0 \\ \vdots & \vdots & \ddots & \vdots & \vdots & \vdots & \ddots & \vdots & \vdots \\ 0 & 0 & \cdots & \lambda_r & 0 & 0 & \cdots & 0 & 0 \\ 0 & 0 & \cdots & 0 & \sigma_1 & \omega_1 & \cdots & 0 & 0 \\ 0 & 0 & \cdots & 0 & -\omega_1 & \sigma_1 & \cdots & 0 & 0 \\ \vdots & \vdots & \ddots & \vdots & \vdots & \vdots & \ddots & \vdots & \vdots \\ 0 & 0 & \cdots & 0 & 0 & 0 & \cdots & \sigma_k & \omega_k \\ 0 & 0 & \cdots & 0 & 0 & 0 & \cdots & -\omega_k & \sigma_k \end{bmatrix}.$$

To grasp the meaning of this result, because $\boldsymbol{A}$ is real with distinct eigenvalues, there exists a complete set of eigenvectors. Let the matrix $\boldsymbol{T}$ have columns consisting of the real eigenvectors of $\boldsymbol{A}$ and the real and imaginary part of each pair of complex eigenvectors. For the complex eigenvalues $\sigma \pm j\omega$ and the corresponding eigenvectors $\boldsymbol{u} + j\boldsymbol{v}$, it follows that

$$\boldsymbol{A}\boldsymbol{u} \pm j\boldsymbol{A}\boldsymbol{v} = \sigma\boldsymbol{u} - \omega\boldsymbol{v} \pm j(\sigma\boldsymbol{v} + \omega\boldsymbol{u}),$$

or

$$\boldsymbol{A}\boldsymbol{u} = \sigma\boldsymbol{u} - \omega\boldsymbol{v}, \quad \text{and} \quad \boldsymbol{A}\boldsymbol{v} = \omega\boldsymbol{u} + \sigma\boldsymbol{v}.$$

This implies the structure of the matrix $\boldsymbol{T}^{-1}\boldsymbol{A}\boldsymbol{T}$.

For the change of state induced by the relation

$$\boldsymbol{q}(k) = \boldsymbol{T}^{-1}\boldsymbol{x}(k),$$

the new state variable model

$$\{\boldsymbol{A}', \boldsymbol{b}', \boldsymbol{c}', \boldsymbol{d}'\} = \{\boldsymbol{\Lambda}, \boldsymbol{T}^{-1}\boldsymbol{b}, \boldsymbol{c}\boldsymbol{T}^{-1}, \boldsymbol{d}\}$$

only has coupling between the states corresponding to complex pairs of poles. The new system matrix $\boldsymbol{A}'$ is block diagonal, with 1×1 blocks corresponding to real poles and 2×2 blocks corresponding to complex pole pairs.

Example 6.9

Let's convert the cascade architecture from example 5 to a parallel architecture. Recall that the cascade architecture was described by the state variable matrices

$$\boldsymbol{A} = \begin{bmatrix} 0 & 1 & 0 & 0 & 0 \\ -0.16 & 0.4 & 0 & 0 & 0 \\ 0 & 0 & 0 & 1 & 0 \\ 0.09 & -0.1 & -0.64 & -0.8 & 0 \\ 0.09 & -0.1 & -0.15 & -0.1 & 0.25 \end{bmatrix}, \quad \boldsymbol{b} = \begin{bmatrix} 0 \\ 1 \\ 0 \\ 1 \\ 1 \end{bmatrix},$$

and

$$\boldsymbol{c} = \begin{bmatrix} 0.09 & -0.1 & -0.15 & -0.1 & 0.05 \end{bmatrix}, \quad \boldsymbol{d} = 1.$$

The eigenvalues of $\boldsymbol{A}$ are

$$\lambda_1 = 0.25, \quad \lambda_2, \lambda_2^* = 0.2 \pm j0.3464, \quad \lambda_3, \lambda_3^* = -0.4 \pm j0.6928$$

with associated eigenvectors

$$\boldsymbol{x}_1 = \begin{bmatrix} 0 \\ 0 \\ 0 \\ 0 \\ 1 \end{bmatrix}, \quad \boldsymbol{x}_2, \boldsymbol{x}_2^* = \begin{bmatrix} 1.0000 \\ 0.2000 \\ 0.0521 \\ 0.0375 \\ -0.0893 \end{bmatrix} \pm j \begin{bmatrix} 0.0000 \\ 0.3464 \\ -0.0782 \\ 0.0024 \\ -0.1558 \end{bmatrix},$$

$$\boldsymbol{x}_3, \boldsymbol{x}_3^* = \begin{bmatrix} 0.0000 \\ 0.0000 \\ 1.0000 \\ -0.4000 \\ 0.0260 \end{bmatrix} \pm j \begin{bmatrix} 0.0000 \\ 0.0000 \\ 0.0000 \\ 0.6928 \\ 0.1343 \end{bmatrix}.$$

We form the matrix $\boldsymbol{T}$ by

$$\boldsymbol{T} = \begin{bmatrix} \boldsymbol{x}_1 & \mathrm{Re}(\boldsymbol{x}_2) & \mathrm{Im}(\boldsymbol{x}_2) & \mathrm{Re}(\boldsymbol{x}_3) & \mathrm{Im}(\boldsymbol{x}_3) \end{bmatrix},$$

and compute $\boldsymbol{A}', \boldsymbol{b}', \boldsymbol{c}', \boldsymbol{d}'$ according to

$$\boldsymbol{A}' = \boldsymbol{T}^{-1}\boldsymbol{A}\boldsymbol{T}, \quad \boldsymbol{b} = \boldsymbol{T}^{-1}\boldsymbol{b}, \quad \boldsymbol{c}' = \boldsymbol{c}\boldsymbol{T}, \quad \boldsymbol{d}' = \boldsymbol{d},$$

which gives

$$\boldsymbol{A}' = \begin{bmatrix} 0.25 & 0 & 0 & 0 & 0 \\ 0 & 0.2 & 0.3464 & 0 & 0 \\ 0 & -0.3464 & .2 & 0 & 0 \\ 0 & 0 & 0 & -0.4 & 0.6928 \\ 0 & 0 & 0 & -0.6928 & -0.4 \end{bmatrix}, \quad \boldsymbol{b}' = \begin{bmatrix} 1.2338 \\ 0.0000 \\ 2.8868 \\ 0.2257 \\ 1.5637 \end{bmatrix},$$

$$\boldsymbol{c}' = \begin{bmatrix} 0.05 & 0.054 & -0.0309 & -0.1087 & -0.0626 \end{bmatrix}, \quad \boldsymbol{d}' = 1.$$

Notice the block-diagonal structure of the matrix $\boldsymbol{A}'$. These new matrices correspond to the system of equations

$$\begin{aligned} x_1(k+1) &= 0.25x_1(k) + 1.2338u(k) \\ x_2(k+1) &= 0.2x_2(k) + 0.3464x_3(k) \\ x_3(k+1) &= -0.3464x_2(k) + 0.2x_3(k) + 2.8868u(k) \\ x_4(k+1) &= -0.4x_4(k) + 0.6928x_5(k) + 0.2257u(k) \\ x_5(k+1) &= -0.6928x_4(k) - 0.4x_5(k) + 1.5637u(k) \end{aligned}$$

and

$$\begin{aligned} y(k) = {} & 0.05x_1(k) + 0.054x_2(k) - 0.0309x_3(k) - 0.1087x_4(k) \\ & - 0.0626x_5(k) + u(k). \end{aligned}$$

From the structure of the, it can be seen that the matrix $\boldsymbol{A}'$, it can be seen that the system is naturally decoupled into three non-interacting systems. The state x_1 belongs to a first-order filter. The states x_2 and x_3 belong to a second-order filter, and the states x_3 and x_4 belong to another second-order filter. Because $\boldsymbol{A}'$ is block-diagonal, there is no coupling between the subfilters.

6.9 Lattice Structures

Most of the architectures we have studied so far ar either canonical in that they are either related to the system's transfer function in a transparent manner or are easily derived be partial fraction expansion or factorization. There is a class of structures known as *lattice filters* which do not fall into this class of architectures. Lattice structures are fundamental in analysis and syntheses of speech as well as in adaptive applications such as linear prediction.

6.9.1 FIR Lattice Filters

We will first study the FIR lattice structure. The basic building block of the FIR lattice is shown in Fig. 6.9.1. This block is a two-input, two-output system with inputs $f^{(m-1)}(k)$ and $g^{(m-1)}(k)$ and outputs $f^{(m)}(k)$ and $g^{(m)}(k)$. The basic lattice elements are connected as shown in Fig. 6.9.1, with the first element being fed with the input $x(k)$ such that $f^{(0)}(k) = g^{(0)}(k) = x(k)$. The output of the last stage is $f^{(M)}(k) = y(k)$. The lattice is completely parameterized by the coefficients $k_1, k_2, \ldots, k_M$. The parameters k_i are known by several names, including *reflection coefficients* and *PARCOR coefficients.* These are names which come from the theory of signal modeling.

The FIR lattice structure can be seen to require $2N$ multiplications, although the direct form implementation only requires N multiplications. In this sense, the FIR lattice is not canonical and is not usually used for implementation of constant-coefficient FIRs. The lattice FIR has properties which make it very attractive for use in applications such as linear prediction and autoregressive signal modeling, which we will examine later.

The output of the lattice filter can be computed inductively. Referring to Fig. 6.9.1, the lattice equations are seen to be given by

$$\begin{aligned} f^{(0)}(k) &= g^{(0)}(k) = x(k) \\ f^{(m)}(k) &= f^{(m-1)}(k) + k_m g^{(m-1)}(k-1) \quad m = 1, 2, \ldots, M \\ g_m(k) &= k_m f^{(m-1)}(k) + g^{(m-1)}(k-1) \quad m = 1, 2, \ldots, M \\ y(k) &= f^{(M)}(k) \end{aligned} \tag{6.9.1}$$

Consider a three-stage lattice. For the first lattice stage, the outputs are given by

$$f^{(1)}(k) = x(k) + k_1 x(k-1) \tag{6.9.2}$$

and

$$g^{(1)}(k) = k_1 x(k) + x(k-1). \tag{6.9.3}$$

Moving on to the second stage,

$$f^{(2)}(k) = f^{(1)}(k) + k_2 g^{(1)}(k-1), \tag{6.9.4}$$

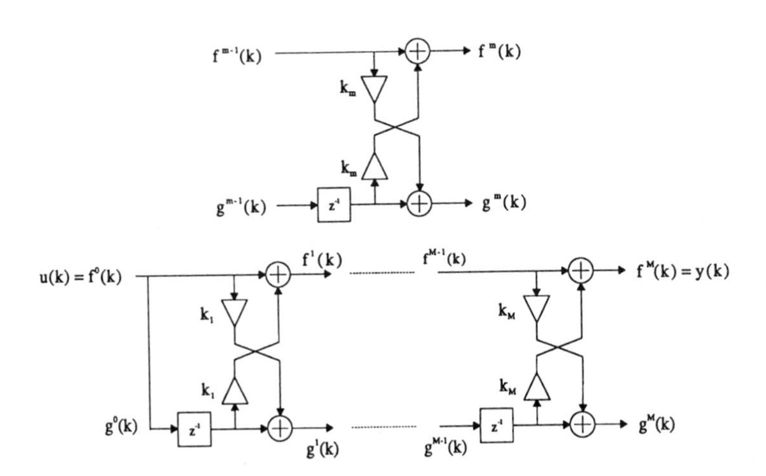

Figure 6.9.1: FIR lattice structure.

and upon substituting Eq. 6.9.2 for $f^{(1)}(k)$ into Eq. 6.9.4,

$$\begin{aligned} f^{(2)}(k) &= x(k) + k_1 x(k-1) + k_2[k_1 x(k-1) + x(k-2)] \\ &= x(k) + (k_1 + k_1 k_2)x(k-1) + k_2 x(k-2) \end{aligned} \tag{6.9.5}$$

and a similar computation for $g^{(2)}(k)$ gives

$$g^{(2)}(k) = k_2 x(k) + (k_1 + k_1 k_2)x(k-1) + x(k-2). \tag{6.9.6}$$

Finally, for the third stage, it is simple to show that

$$\begin{aligned} f^{(3)}(k) = x(k) &+ (k_1 + k_1 k_2 + k_2 k_3)x(k-1) \\ &+ (k_2 + k_1 k_3 + k_1 k_2 k_3)x(k-2) + k_3 x(k-3) \end{aligned}$$

and

$$\begin{aligned} g^{(3)}(k) = k_3 x(k) &+ (k_2 + k_1 k_3 + k_1 k_2 k_3)x(k-1) \\ &+ (k_1 + k_1 k_2 + k_2 k_3)x(k-2) + x(k-3). \end{aligned}$$

Notice that the coefficients for $g^{(m)}$ and $f^{(m)}$ are the reverse of one another.

In general, at the m-th stage, the lattice acts as an m-th order FIR from the input to $f^{(m)}(k)$. The relationship from the input to $f^{(m)}(k)$ is thus given by

$$f^{(m)}(k) = \sum_{n=0}^{m} a_n^{(m)} x(k-n) \tag{6.9.7}$$

Taking the $\mathcal{Z}$-transform of Eq. 6.9.7,

$$F^{(m)}(z) = A^{(m)}(z)X(z),$$

and because $F^{(0)}(z) = X(z)$,

$$A^{(m)}(z) = \frac{F^{(m)}(z)}{X(z)} = \frac{F^{(m)}(z)}{F^{(0)}(z)}. \tag{6.9.8}$$

Similarly, the lattice also as an m-th order FIR from the input to $g^{(m)}(k)$. The relationship from the input to $g^{(m)}(k)$ is given by

$$g^{(m)}(k) = \sum_{n=0}^{m} b_n^{(m)} x(k-n)$$

and can be described by the $\mathcal{Z}$-transform

$$G^{(m)}(z) = B^{(m)}(z)X(z).$$

Again, because $G^{(0)}(z) = X(z)$,

$$B^{(m)}(z) = \frac{G^{(m)}(z)}{X(z)} = \frac{G^{(m)}(z)}{G^{(0)}(z)}. \tag{6.9.9}$$

By definition, we have

$$A^{(0)}(z) = B^{(0)}(z) = 1$$

and the FIRs $A^{(m)}(z)$ and $B^{(m)}(z)$ are described by

$$A^{(m)}(z) = \sum_{i=0}^{m} a_i^{(m)} z^{-i}$$

and

$$B^{(m)}(z) = \sum_{i=0}^{m} b_i^{(m)} z^{-i}.$$

Additionally, the coefficients of $B^{(m)}(z)$ are the reverse of the coefficients of $A^{(m)}(z)$ which means that

$$b_i^{(m)} = a_{m-i}^{(m)}$$

which, in terms of polynomials, means that

$$B^{(m)}(z) = z^{-m} A^{(m)}(z^{-1}). \tag{6.9.10}$$

Taking the $\mathcal{Z}$-transform of Eq. 6.9.1, we have

$$\begin{aligned}
F^{(0)}(z) &= G^{(0)}(z) = X(z) \\
F^{(m)}(z) &= F^{(m-1)}(z) + k_m z^{-1} G^{(m-1)}(z) \quad m = 1, 2, \ldots, M \\
G^{(m)}(z) &= k_m F^{(m-1)}(z) + z^{-1} G^{(m-1)}(z) \quad m = 1, 2, \ldots, M \\
Y(z) &= F^{(M)}(z)
\end{aligned} \tag{6.9.11}$$

Using Eqs. 6.9.8 and 6.9.9 for $A^{(m)}(z)$ and $B^{(m)}(z)$, if the equations in Eq. 6.9.11 are divided by $X(z)$, we have

$$\begin{aligned}
A^{(0)}(z) &= B^{(0)}(z) = 1 \\
A^{(m)}(z) &= A^{(m-1)}(z) + k_m z^{-1} B^{(m-1)}(z) \quad m = 1, 2, \ldots, M \\
B^{(m)}(z) &= k_m A^{(m-1)}(z) + z^{-1} B^{(m-1)}(z) \quad m = 1, 2, \ldots, M \\
H(z) &= A^{(M-1)}(z)
\end{aligned} \tag{6.9.12}$$

The recursions expressed by the second and third rows of Eq. 6.9.12 can be put in the compact matrix form

$$\begin{bmatrix} A^{(m)}(z) \\ B^{(m)}(z) \end{bmatrix} = \begin{bmatrix} 1 & k_m \\ k_m & 1 \end{bmatrix} \begin{bmatrix} A^{(m-1)}(z) \\ z^{-1} B^{(m-1)}(z) \end{bmatrix}. \tag{6.9.13}$$

Consider now the problem of finding the FIR transfer function of an M-stage lattice given the coefficients $k_1, k_2, \ldots k_M$. We can use the recursion in Eq. 6.9.12 directly and exploit the symmetry between $A^{(m)}(z)$ and $B^{(m)}(z)$ as expressed by Eq. 6.9.10, giving the recursion

$$\begin{aligned}
A^{(0)}(z) &= B^{(0)}(z) = 1 \\
A^{(m)}(z) &= A^{(m-1)}(z) + k_m z^{-1} B^{(m-1)}(z) \quad m = 1, 2, \ldots, M \\
B^{(m)}(z) &= z^{-m} A^{(m)}(z^{-1}) \quad m = 1, 2, \ldots, M \\
H(z) &= A^{(M)}(z)
\end{aligned} \tag{6.9.14}$$

We start with the initial conditions $A^{(0)}(z) = B^{(0)}(z) = 1$ and iterate over the intermediate FIRs until the final stage $m = M$, which gives $H(z)$.

An expression for the intermediate FIR coefficients can be obtained by expanding the recursion in Eq. 6.9.14, giving

$$\sum_{i=0}^{m} a_i^{(m)} z^{-i} = \sum_{i=0}^{m-1} a_i^{(m-1)} z^{-i} + k_m z^{-1} \sum_{k=0}^{m-1} b_i^{(m-1)} z^{-i}.$$

Using the fact that $b_i^{(m-1)} = a_{m-1-i}^{(m-1)}$ gives

$$\sum_{i=0}^{m} a_i^{(m)} z^{-i} = \sum_{i=0}^{m-1} a_i^{(m-1)} z^{-i} + k_m \sum_{k=0}^{m-1} a_i^{(m-1-i)} z^{-i-1}. \tag{6.9.15}$$

If like powers of z^{-1} are equated in Eq. 6.9.15, we have

$$\begin{aligned} a_0^{(m)} &= 1 \\ a_m^{(m)} &= k_m \\ a_i^{(m)} &= a_i^{(m-1)} + k_m a_{m-i}^{(m-1)} \quad i = 1, 2, \ldots, m \end{aligned} \tag{6.9.16}$$

Example 6.10

Suppose we have a three-stage lattice FIR with $k_1 = 1/2, k_2 = 1/4, k_3 = 1/8$ and we wish to determine the transfer function $H(z)$. We use the recursion in Eq. 6.9.14, beginning with $A^{(0)}(z) = B^{(0)}(z) = 1$. Next,

$$A^{(1)}(z) = A^{(0)}(z) + k_1 z^{-1} B^{(0)}(z) = 1 + \frac{1}{2} z^{-1}.$$

Because $B^{(1)}(z)$ is the reverse of $A^{(1)}(z)$,

$$B^{(1)}(z) = \frac{1}{2} + z^{-1}.$$

Adding the second stage,

$$A^{(2)}(z) = A^{(1)}(z) + k_2 z^{-1} B^{(1)}(z)$$

which gives

$$A^{(2)}(z) = 1 + \frac{5}{8} z^{-1} + \frac{1}{4} z^{-2}$$

and

$$B^{(2)}(z) = \frac{1}{4} + \frac{5}{8} z^{-1} + z^{-2}.$$

Finally,

$$A^{(3)}(z) = A^{(2)}(z) + k_3 z^{-1} B^{(2)}(z),$$

giving

$$A^{(3)}(z) = 1 + \frac{21}{32} z^{-1} + \frac{21}{64} z^{-2} + \frac{1}{8} z^{-3}.$$

Thus, the lattice FIR has the impulse response coefficients

$$\{h_0, h_1, h_2, h_3\} = \{1, 21/32, 21/64, 1/8\}.$$

Now that we know how to obtain the direct FIR coefficients $\{h_i\}$ from the lattice parameters $\{k_i\}$, we consider the *inverse* problem, that of computing the $\{k_i\}$ from the $\{h_i\}$. The solution is to start with the FIR transfer function and work the recursions in Eq. 6.9.14 backwards. The recursions for $A^{(m)}(z)$ and $B^{(m)}(z)$ in Eq. 6.9.14 can be manipulated to obtain

$$A^{(m)}(z) = A^{(m-1)}(z) + k_m(B^{(m)}(z) - k_m A^{(m-1)}(z)).$$

Solving for $A^{(m-1)}(z)$, we have

$$A^{(m-1)}(z) = \frac{A^{(m)}(z) - k_m B^{(m)}(z)}{1 - k_m^2}, \quad m = M, M-1, \ldots, 1 \tag{6.9.17}$$

This recursion is begun with the initial condition

$$A^{(M)}(z) = H(z).$$

From Eq. 6.9.16, we found that

$$k_m = a_m^{(m)}.$$

Thus, Eq. 6.9.14 generates the successively lower-order FIRs, and we extract k_m from the final coefficient of each FIR $A^{(m)}(z)$.

Again, we can give an recursion for the k_m based on the intermediate FIR coefficients by substituting the expressions for $A^{(m)}(z)$ and $B^{(m)}(z)$ into Eq. 6.9.17 and collecting like powers of z^{-1}. This gives

$$k_m = a_m^{(m)}, \quad a_0^{(m-1)} = 1, \tag{6.9.18}$$

and

$$a_i^{(m-1)} = \frac{a_i^{(m)} - k_m a_{m-i}^{(m)}}{1 - k_m^2}, \quad 1 \le i \le m-1. \tag{6.9.19}$$

This recursion is started with $k_M = a_M^{(M)} = h_M$.

Example 6.11

This example illustrates how the lattice parameters are computed from an FIR transfer function. We will use with the FIR from the previous example,

$$H(z) = 1 + \frac{21}{32}z^{-1} + \frac{21}{64}z^{-2} + \frac{1}{8}z^{-3}.$$

Using Eq. 6.9.17, we start with

$$A^{(3)}(z) = H(z)$$

and $B^{(3)}(z)$ equal to the reverse of $A^{(3)}(z)$:

$$B^{(3)}(z) = \frac{1}{8} + \frac{21}{64}z^{-1} + \frac{21}{32}z^{-2} + z^{-3}.$$

The value of k_3 is given by

$$k_3 = a_3^{(3)} = \frac{1}{8}.$$

Then,

$$A^{(2)}(z) = \frac{A^{(3)}(z) - k_3 B^{(3)}(z)}{1 - k_3^2}$$

which gives

$$A^{(2)}(z) = 1 + \frac{5}{8}z^{-1} + \frac{1}{4}z^{-2}$$

and

$$B^{(2)}(z) = \frac{1}{4} + \frac{5}{8}z^{-1} + z^{-2}$$

and

$$k_2 = a_2^{(2)} = \frac{1}{4}.$$

Next,

$$A^{(1)}(z) = \frac{A^{(2)}(z) - k_2 B^{(2)}(z)}{1 - k_2^2} = 1 + \frac{1}{2}z^{-1}$$

so that

$$k_1 = a_1^{(1)} = \frac{1}{2}$$

and we are done. Notice that we have recovered the lattice parameters from the previous example, which is what we expected.

6.9.2 IIR Lattice Filters

Suppose an FIR described by $H(z)$ is fed with the input $x(k)$ to produce the output $y(k)$. The original signal $x(k)$ can be recovered from $y(k)$ by passing $y(k)$ through the all pole filter $1/H(z)$. This simple observation will allow us to develop an all-pole lattice filter based on our FIR lattice filter. That is, given an FIR lattice with input $x(k)$ and output $y(k)$, we wish to design a lattice which has input $y(k)$ and produces the original input, $x(k)$. This can be done simply by exchanging the roles of the input and the output. Consider an N-stage lattice and let the input be

$$x(k) = f^{(N)}(k)$$

and let the output be

$$y(k) = f^{(0)}(k).$$

This time, we will compute the $f^{(m)}$ in reverse order using Eq. 6.9.1. This gives

$$f^{(m-1)}(k) = f^{(m)}(k) - k_m g^{(m-1)}(k-1).$$

Because of the dependence of $f^{(m-1)}(k)$ on $g^{(m-1)}$ at time $k-1$, the recursion for $g^{(m)}(k)$ in Eq 6.9.1 can remain unchanged. Thus,

$$\begin{array}{lcll} f^{(N)}(k) & = & x(k) & \\ f^{(m-1)}(k) & = & f^{(m)}(k) - k_m g^{(m-1)}(k-1) & m = N, N-1, \ldots, 1 \\ g^{(m)}(k) & = & k_m f^{(m-1)}(k) + g^{(m-1)}(k-1) & m = N, N-1, \ldots, 1 \\ y(k) & = & f^{(0)}(k) = g^{(0)}(k) & \end{array} \tag{6.9.20}$$

The architecture implied by these equations is shown in Fig. 6.9.2.

Now that we know how to build FIR lattices and all-pole IIR lattices, a natural question is whether it is possible to build a lattice which has both poles and zeros. The answer is in the affirmative, but we need to modify the all-pole lattice architecture slightly by including a ladder network as shown in Fig. 6.9.3. In this case, the output is given by

$$y(k) = \sum_{i=0}^{N} \nu_i g^{(i)}(k). \tag{6.9.21}$$

Then

$$H(z) = \frac{Y(z)}{X(z)} = \sum_{i=0}^{N} \nu_i \frac{G^{(i)}(z)}{X(z)}. \tag{6.9.22}$$

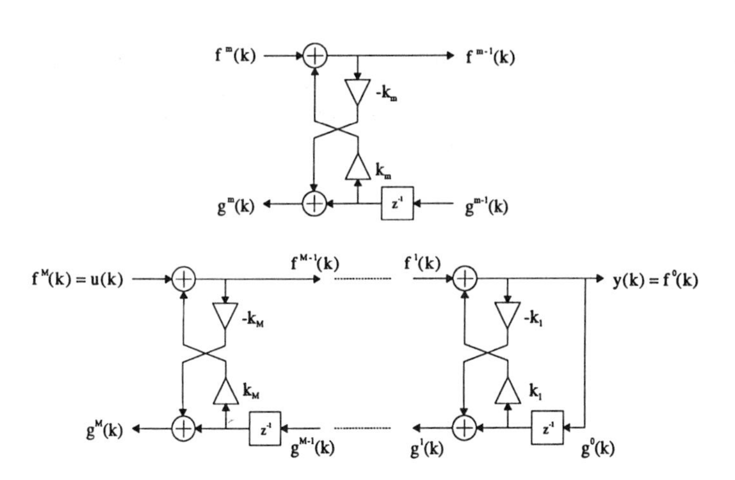

Figure 6.9.2: All-pole IIR lattice filter.

Recall from Eq. 6.9.20, however, that

$$f^{(N)}(k) = x(k) \quad \text{and} \quad f^{(0)}(k) = g^{(0)}(k) = y(k)$$

so that

$$H(z) = \sum_{i=0}^{N} \nu_i \frac{G^{(i)}(z)}{G^{(0)}(z)} \frac{F^{(0)}(z)}{F^{(N)}(z)}. \tag{6.9.23}$$

The ratio $G^{(i)}(z)/G^{(0)}(z)$ is simply $B^{(i)}(z)$ and the ratio $F^{(0)}(z)/F^{(N)}(z)$ is, by definition, the transfer function $1/A^{(N)}(z)$ of the all-pole lattice so that Eq. 6.9.23 becomes

$$H(z) = \sum_{i=0}^{N} \nu_i \frac{B^{(i)}(z)}{A^{(N)}(z)}. \tag{6.9.24}$$

Therefore, the transfer function of the lattice-ladder filter is

$$H(z) = \frac{\sum_{i=0}^{N} \nu_i B^{(i)}(z)}{A^{(N)}(z)}. \tag{6.9.25}$$

The poles of the lattice-ladder filter are determined by the all-pole lattice and the zeros are the roots of the polynomial

$$C(z) = \sum_{i=0}^{N} \nu_i B^{(i)}(z). \tag{6.9.26}$$

To build a lattice-ladder filter which realizes a given transfer function, the denominator is first realized as an all-pole lattice, which we already know how to do. The only problem remaining is how to determine the ladder coefficients ν_i given a desired numerator polynomial $C(z)$. To do this we begin with the relation

$$C^{(N)}(z) = C(z).$$

Define $C^{(m)}(z)$ by

$$C^{(m)}(z) = \sum_{i=0}^{m} \nu_i B^{(i)}(z).$$

It then follows that

$$C^{(m)}(z) = C^{(m-1)}(z) + \nu_m B^{(m)}(z). \tag{6.9.27}$$

Notice that $C^{(m-1)}(z)$ will be of degree $m-1$ and $B^{(m)}(z)$ will be of degree m. We have seen that $b_m^{(m)}$ is always equal to one. Therefore, from Eq. 6.9.27, it must be true that

$$\nu_m = c_m^{(m)}. \tag{6.9.28}$$

Therefore, we start with

$$\nu_N = C_N^{(N)}$$

and work backwards from eq. 6.9.27, using

$$C^{(m-1)}(z) = C^{(m)}(z) - \nu_m B^{(m)}(z) \tag{6.9.29}$$

and recognizing at each stage that

$$c_{m-1}^{(m-1)} = \nu_{m-1}. \tag{6.9.30}$$

Example 6.12

Suppose $H(z)$ is given by

$$H(z) = \frac{1 + 2z^{-1} + 3z^{-2} + 4z^{-3}}{1 + \frac{21}{32}z^{-1} + \frac{21}{64}z^{-2} + \frac{1}{8}z^{-3}}.$$

With $A^{(3)}(z)$ given by

$$A^{(3)}(z) = 1 + \frac{21}{32}z^{-1} + \frac{21}{64}z^{-2} + \frac{1}{8}z^{-3},$$

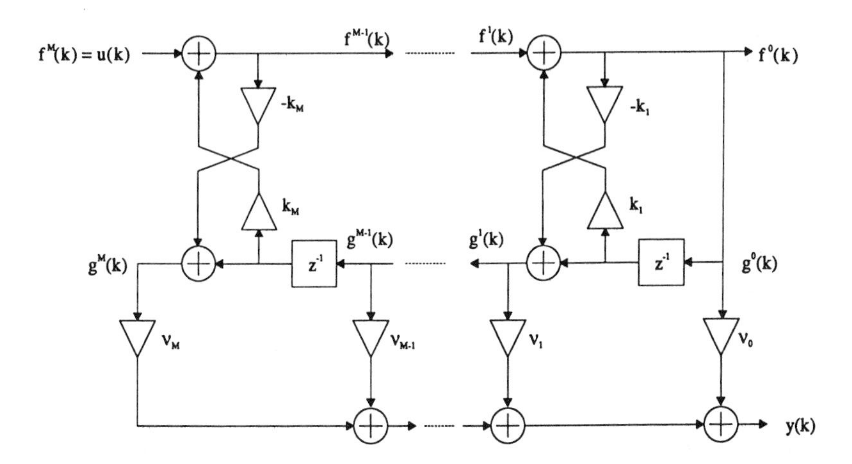

Figure 6.9.3: Lattice-ladder filter.

we have already seen how to realize $1/A^{(3)}(z)$ with an all-pole lattice. Also, we have already computed the intermediate quantities $A^{(2)}, B^{(2)}, A^{(1)}, B^{(1)}$ in the previous examples. All we must do now is utilize the recursion in Eq. 6.9.27 to generate $\nu_3, \nu_2, \nu_1, \nu_0$. We begin with

$$C^{(3)}(z) = 1 + 2z^{-1} + 3z^{-2} + 4z^{-3}$$

and recognize immediately that

$$\nu_3 = c_3^{(3)} = 4.$$

Next,

$$C^{(2)}(z) = C^{(3)}(z) - \nu_3 B^{(3)}(z),$$

which gives

$$C^{(2)}(z) = \frac{1}{2} + \frac{11}{16}z^{-1} + \frac{3}{8}z^{-2}$$

so that

$$\nu_2 = c_2^{(2)} = \frac{3}{8}.$$

Continuing for $m = 1$, we have

$$C^{(1)}(z) = C^{(2)}(z) - \nu_2 B^{(2)}(z) = \frac{13}{32} + \frac{29}{64}z^{-1}$$

giving

$$\nu_1 = \frac{29}{64}.$$

Finally,

$$C^{(0)}(z) = C^{(1)}(z) - \nu_1 B^{(1)}(z) = \frac{23}{128}$$

so that

$$\nu_0 = \frac{23}{128}$$

and we are finished.

6.10 State Variables and Asymptotic Stationarity

We have seen how a linear time-invariant system responds to a WSS input. If the input is zero-mean, so is the output. If the PSD of the input is $P_{uu}(\theta)$, then the PSD of the output is

$$P_{yy}(\theta) = |H(e^{j\theta})|^2 P_{uu}(\theta).$$

We have not, however, examined the *internal* response of the system. This will require the use of our state variable methods for the analysis of linear systems. Another problem we have not yet considered in detail is what happens when the stochastic process excites a linear system at a particular starting time $k = 0$. We will show in this section that if certain conditions are met, the internal states and the output of the system will eventually become stationary.

Assume we have a system described by the state variable model

$$\boldsymbol{x}(k+1) = \boldsymbol{A}\boldsymbol{x}(k) + \boldsymbol{b}u(k).$$

We will need some results from linear control theory. For now, we are only concerned with the state equation

$$\boldsymbol{x}(k+1) = \boldsymbol{A}\boldsymbol{x}(k) + \boldsymbol{b}u(k).$$

This system will subsequently be referred to by the pair

$$(\boldsymbol{A}, \boldsymbol{b}).$$

Recall that this system is BIBO stable if and only if all of the eigenvalues of $\boldsymbol{A}$ satisfy

$$\lambda_i(\boldsymbol{A}) < 1, \quad i = 1, 2, \ldots, n.$$

Henceforth, we will refer to such a matrix as a *stable matrix*. We begin with an important lemma.

Lemma 1 *Let $\boldsymbol{A}$ be an $n \times n$ matrix with all eigenvalues bounded by unity modulus. Then for any $n \times n$ matrix $\boldsymbol{W}$, the matrix series*

$$\sum_{k=0}^{\infty} \boldsymbol{A}^k \boldsymbol{W} (\boldsymbol{A}^T)^k$$

converges.

This result is not difficult to prove if one first considers the case where $n = 1$ and then showing it is true for diagonal matrices, as well. This lemma can be used to prove the following important theorem.

Theorem 5 *Let $(\boldsymbol{A}, \boldsymbol{b})$ describe a linear system and suppose that $\boldsymbol{Q}$ is positive semidefinite. Then there is a unique positive semidefinite matrix $\boldsymbol{K}$ satisfying*

$$\boldsymbol{K} - \boldsymbol{A}\boldsymbol{K}\boldsymbol{A}^T = \boldsymbol{b}\boldsymbol{Q}\boldsymbol{b}^T \tag{6.10.1}$$

if and only if $\boldsymbol{A}$ is stable.

To prove this, assume that $\boldsymbol{A}$ is stable. Denote the matrix $\boldsymbol{K}$ by

$$\boldsymbol{K} = \sum_{k=0}^{\infty} \boldsymbol{A}^k \boldsymbol{b}\boldsymbol{Q}\boldsymbol{b}^T (\boldsymbol{A}^T)^k. \tag{6.10.2}$$

By the first lemma, this matrix series converges because of the stability of $\boldsymbol{A}$. Also, $\boldsymbol{K}$ is positive semidefinite because $\boldsymbol{b}\boldsymbol{Q}\boldsymbol{b}^T$ is positive semidefinite. The matrix $\boldsymbol{b}\boldsymbol{b}^T$ is positive semidefinite because

$$\boldsymbol{z}^T \boldsymbol{b}\boldsymbol{Q}\boldsymbol{b}^T \boldsymbol{z} = (\boldsymbol{b}^T \boldsymbol{z})^T \boldsymbol{Q} (\boldsymbol{b}^T \boldsymbol{z}) \geq 0$$

for all vectors $\boldsymbol{z}$ due to the assumed positive semidefiniteness of $\boldsymbol{Q}$. Next, consider the matrix $\boldsymbol{A}^k \boldsymbol{b}\boldsymbol{Q}\boldsymbol{b}^T (\boldsymbol{A}^k)^T$. Then

$$\boldsymbol{z}^T \boldsymbol{A}^k \boldsymbol{b}\boldsymbol{Q}\boldsymbol{b}^T (\boldsymbol{A}^k)^T \boldsymbol{z} = (\boldsymbol{A}^{k^T} \boldsymbol{z})^T \boldsymbol{b}\boldsymbol{Q}\boldsymbol{b}^T (\boldsymbol{A}^{k^T} \boldsymbol{z}),$$

and because $\boldsymbol{b}\boldsymbol{Q}\boldsymbol{b}^T$ is positive semidefinite, the above is nonnegative for any k. Hence, the matrix

$$\boldsymbol{A}^k \boldsymbol{b}\boldsymbol{Q}\boldsymbol{b}^T (\boldsymbol{A}^T)^k$$

is positive semidefinite for any k. Finally, it is easy to see that the sum of positive semidefinite matrices is positive semidefinite, for if $\boldsymbol{A}$ and $\boldsymbol{B}$ are positive semidefinite, then

$$\boldsymbol{z}^T (\boldsymbol{A} + \boldsymbol{B}) \boldsymbol{z} = \boldsymbol{z}^T \boldsymbol{A} \boldsymbol{z} + \boldsymbol{z}^T \boldsymbol{B} \boldsymbol{z} \geq 0$$

because of the positive semidefiniteness of $\boldsymbol{A}$ and $\boldsymbol{B}$. Thus, we have seen that $\boldsymbol{K}$ as defined by Eq. 6.10.2 is positive semidefinite. We omit the proof that $\boldsymbol{K}$ is unique. The proof of the converse (that the existence of $\boldsymbol{K}$ implies stability of $\boldsymbol{A}$) is more involved, and can be found in any standard reference on linear system theory [Kai80].

To show that $\boldsymbol{K}$ as defined by Eq. 6.10.2 satisfies Eq. 6.10.1, we have

$$\boldsymbol{K} - \boldsymbol{AKA}^T = \sum_{k=0}^{\infty} \boldsymbol{A}^k \boldsymbol{bQb}^T (\boldsymbol{A}^T)^k - \boldsymbol{A} \left(\sum_{k=0}^{\infty} \boldsymbol{A}^k \boldsymbol{bQb}^T (\boldsymbol{A}^T)^k \right) \boldsymbol{A}^T$$

which equals

$$\sum_{k=0}^{\infty} \boldsymbol{A}^k \boldsymbol{bQb}^T (\boldsymbol{A}^T)^k - \boldsymbol{A} \sum_{k=1}^{\infty} \boldsymbol{A}^k \boldsymbol{bQb}^T (\boldsymbol{A}^T)^k = \boldsymbol{A}^0 \boldsymbol{bQb}^T (\boldsymbol{A}^T)^0$$

so that

$$\boldsymbol{K} - \boldsymbol{AKA}^T = \boldsymbol{bQb}^T.$$

This equation is easily solved for $\boldsymbol{K}$ by decomposing it into a set of n^2 equations in n^2 unknowns.

Example 6.13

Suppose

$$\boldsymbol{A} = \begin{pmatrix} 0 & 1 \\ -1/8 & -3/4 \end{pmatrix}, \quad \boldsymbol{b} = \begin{pmatrix} 0 \\ 1 \end{pmatrix}$$

and

$$\boldsymbol{Q} = \begin{bmatrix} 1 & 0 \\ 0 & 1 \end{bmatrix}.$$

Furthermore, $\boldsymbol{A}$ is stable and $\boldsymbol{K}$ as defined by Eq. 6.10.2 is symmetric so that

$$\boldsymbol{K} = \begin{pmatrix} k_1 & k_2 \\ k_2 & k_3 \end{pmatrix}.$$

The equation $\boldsymbol{K} - \boldsymbol{AKA}^T = \boldsymbol{bQb}^T$ yields the set of equations

$$\begin{aligned} k_1 &= k_3 \\ k_2 &= -\tfrac{1}{8}k_2 - \tfrac{3}{4}k_3 \\ k_3 &= \tfrac{1}{64}k_1 + \tfrac{3}{16}k_2 + \tfrac{9}{16}k_3 + 1 \end{aligned}$$

which are easily solved for k_1, k_2 and k_3.

We are now in a position to make use of the results we have just presented. Assume we have the system

$$\boldsymbol{x}(k+1) = \boldsymbol{A}\boldsymbol{x}(k) + \boldsymbol{b}u(k)$$

where $\boldsymbol{A}$ is stable and $u(k)$ is zero-mean white noise with variance σ^2. We would like to compute the correlation of the state,

$$\boldsymbol{K} = \mathcal{E}[\boldsymbol{x}(k)\boldsymbol{x}^T(k)].$$

The i, j-th element of $\boldsymbol{K}$ is given by

$$[\boldsymbol{K}]_{i,j} = \mathcal{E}[x_i(j)x_j(k)]$$

and in particular, the diagonal elements of $\boldsymbol{K}$ are given by

$$[\boldsymbol{K}]_{i,i} = \mathcal{E}[x_i^2(k)].$$

Notice that we have not ascribed a time index to $\boldsymbol{K}$. This is because $\boldsymbol{A}$ is assumed to be stable and hence each of the states will be asymptotically stationary.

From our earlier discussion, it is clear that since $u(k)$ is zero-mean, so is the state, $\boldsymbol{x}(k)$. To compute the correlation, $\boldsymbol{K}$, assume that the system is started from the initial state $\boldsymbol{x}(0)$. Then

$$\mathcal{E}[\boldsymbol{x}(k+1)\boldsymbol{x}^T(k+1)] = \mathcal{E}[(\boldsymbol{A}\boldsymbol{x}(k) + \boldsymbol{b}u(k))(\boldsymbol{A}\boldsymbol{x}(k) + \boldsymbol{b}u(k))^T]. \tag{6.10.3}$$

Because

$$\boldsymbol{x}(k) = \boldsymbol{A}^k\boldsymbol{x}(0) + \sum_{m=0}^{k-1} \boldsymbol{A}^{k-m-1}\boldsymbol{b}u(m),$$

the state at time k depends only on the input up to time $k-1$, the cross-terms in Eq. 6.10.3 vanish so that

$$\mathcal{E}[\boldsymbol{x}(k+1)\boldsymbol{x}^T(k+1)] = \boldsymbol{A}\mathcal{E}[\boldsymbol{x}(k)\boldsymbol{x}^T(k)]\boldsymbol{A}^T + \sigma^2\boldsymbol{b}\boldsymbol{b}^T.$$

Because of asymptotic stationarity,

$$\mathcal{E}[\boldsymbol{x}(k+1)\boldsymbol{x}^T(k+1)] = \mathcal{E}[\boldsymbol{x}(k)\boldsymbol{x}^T(k)] = \boldsymbol{K}.$$

We then have

$$\boldsymbol{K} = \boldsymbol{A}\boldsymbol{K}\boldsymbol{A}^T + \sigma^2\boldsymbol{b}\boldsymbol{b}^T.$$

This equation has a solution according to the theorem, because $\boldsymbol{A}$ is assumed to be stable and we have $\boldsymbol{Q} = \sigma^2\boldsymbol{I}$.

6.11 Fixed-Point Digital Filter Design

For most digital filtering applications, the signal to be processed is an analog signal which must be converted to digital by an analog-to-digital (A/D) converter. Converting an analog signal to a digital signal consists of two parts: sampling and quantization. Sampling refers to the process of capturing instantaneous "snapshots" of the continuous-time signal, and quantization is the process of converting these samples into finite-length binary numbers.

There are many methods used for the representation of fixed-point binary numbers, such as signed magnitude, ones complement, and twos complement. By far, the most popular is the twos complement representation representation due to the simplicity with which it can be implemented.

Given a real number $|x| \leq 1$, x can be represented as

$$x = -b_0 + \sum_{i=1}^{\infty} b_i 2^{-i}$$

where the b_i (called *bits*) can assume the value of either one or zero. The bit b_0 is equal to zero if x is positive and is equal to one if x is negative. More generally, real numbers x in the range $|x| < \Delta$ can be represented by

$$x = \left[-b_0 + \sum_{i=1}^{\infty} b_i 2^{-i} \right] \Delta$$

where the same rules hold for b_0.

In practice, we only have a finite-length register in which to store the number x. For a register of length $B+1$, x is approximated by $[x]_Q$ (the Q indicates *quantized*) where

$$[x]_Q = \left[-b_0 + \sum_{i=1}^{B} b_i 2^{-i} \right] \Delta.$$

With $B+1$ bits, it is possible to represent 2^{B+1} different numbers between $-\Delta$ and Δ. These numbers are all uniformly spaced with a distance of

$$q = \frac{\Delta - (-\Delta)}{2^{B+1}} = 2^{-B} \Delta$$

between numbers. In other words, all of the representable numbers are integer multiples of q. The number q is called the *quantization step size.*

In generating $[x]_Q$ from x, we will assume that x is rounded to the nearest multiple of q. The quantization characteristic for twos complement is shown in Fig. 6.11.1. The *quantization error,*

$$e = x - [x]_Q$$

seen to be bounded in magnitude by $q/2$. With a fixed number of bits, the quantization error can be made smaller by making the value of Δ smaller. However, this limits the allowable

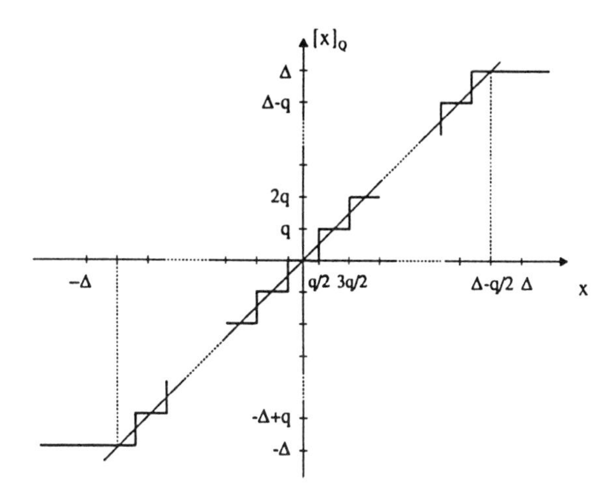

Figure 6.11.1: Two's complement quantization characteristic.

range of x and can introduce overflows. Instead, if Δ is increased while holding B constant, there will be an increase in quantization error.

There twos complement representation uses *wraparound* to cope with overflow. With wraparound overflow, a value of x which has magnitude greater than Δ is mapped to $[x]_Q$ as though the quantization characteristic were periodically extended. One desirable property of the wraparound characteristic is that if a series of quantized numbers is added together, no overflow will occur if the sum is in-range, even though intermediate overflows may have occurred.

For analysis purposes, it is useful to have a statistical characterization of the quantization error. It has been shown for broadband signals $x(k)$ that the quantization error sequence $e(k)$ is approximately white noise which is uncorrelated with $x(k)$. Each error $e(k)$ can reasonably be modeled as being uniformly distributed over the range $[-q/2, q/2]$. Thus, each error has a probability function given by

$$p(e) = \begin{cases} \frac{1}{q}, & e \in [-q/2, q/2] \\ 0, & \text{otherwise} \end{cases}$$

The error sequence is zero-mean, with variance given by

$$\sigma_e^2 = \int -q/2^{q/2} e^2 p(e)\, de = \int_{-q/2}^{q/2} \frac{e^2}{q}\, de = \frac{q^2}{12}.$$

In practice, we can model a quantizer as an additive noise source with zero mean and power $q^2/12$. Schematically, this is shown in Fig. 6.11.2. This model for quantization accounts only for roundoff error and does not take into account the phenomenon of overflow. For analysis purposes, we will need to ensure that overflow does not occur, which will be discussed soon.

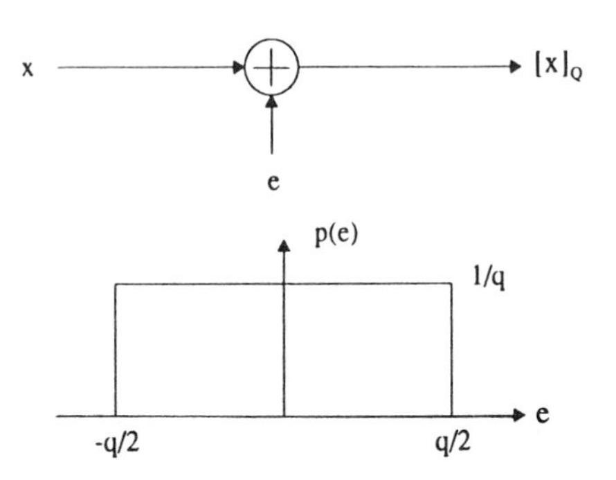

Figure 6.11.2: Representing quantization as an additive noise source.

One potentially troubling problem with the wraparound overflow characteristic is the existence of *zero-input overflow oscillations.* These are also known as *zero-input limit cycles.* As the name implies, there may exist initial filter states which do not decay to zero when no input is applied, even though the filter is stable. The state-variable representation allows us to study this phenomenon in detail.

Recall that a digital filter can be represented by the pair of equations

$$\begin{array}{rcl} \boldsymbol{x}(k+1) & = & \boldsymbol{A}\boldsymbol{x}(k) + \boldsymbol{b}u(k) \\ y(k) & = & \boldsymbol{c}\boldsymbol{x}(k) + du(k) \end{array}.$$

Only the state equation will be of interest in this discussion, and it is furthermore assumed that the input is identically zero. Therefore, we are interested in the equation

$$\boldsymbol{x}(k+1) = \boldsymbol{A}\boldsymbol{x}(k)$$

started from the initial state $\boldsymbol{x}(0)$. The solution to this equation is

$$\boldsymbol{x}(k) = \boldsymbol{A}^k\boldsymbol{x}(0)$$

and if the system is stable, any initial state will decay to zero. Let's represent the overflow characteristic by the function $O(\cdot)$ where

$$O(x) = \begin{cases} x, & |x| < \Delta \\ < \Delta & |x| > \Delta \end{cases}$$

What is important about the function $O(\cdot)$ is that

$$|x| \geq O(x)$$

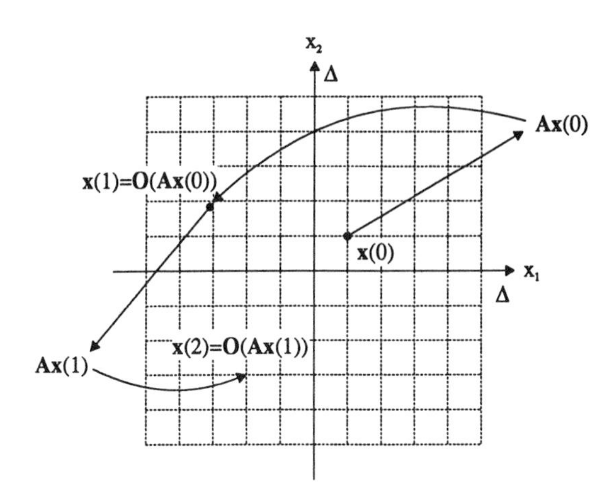

Figure 6.11.3: Illustration of overflow oscillations in a second-order fixed-point system.

for all x. Then the state actually evolves according to

$$\boldsymbol{x}(k+1) = O[\boldsymbol{A}\boldsymbol{x}(k)]$$

where O acts on each component of $\boldsymbol{x}(k)$ as

$$[O[\boldsymbol{x}(k)]]_i = O[x_i(k)].$$

If each state is represented as a B-bit number, the states which can be represented can be visualized as points inside an N-dimensional hypercube centered at the origin.

If floating-point arithmetic is used and the system is stable, the initial state $\boldsymbol{x}(0)$ will converge to the origin. The situation for fixed-point arithmetic is more complicated. Here is how an overflow oscillation may occur. Suppose the initial state $\boldsymbol{x}(0)$ is a point inside the hypercube of representable states. The next state is given by $\boldsymbol{x}(1) = O[\boldsymbol{A}\boldsymbol{x}(0)]$. If $\boldsymbol{A}\boldsymbol{x}(0)$ lies outside the hypercube, it will be mapped back inside the hypercube by the overflow function $O[\cdot]$ (this ignores the quantization error, which is negligible compared to the overflow error if overflow error has occurred). It is still possible that $\boldsymbol{x}(1)$ is such that $\boldsymbol{x}(2) = \boldsymbol{A}\boldsymbol{x}(1)$ will lie outside the hypercube, in which case $O[\boldsymbol{A}\boldsymbol{x}(1)]$ again maps back inside the hypercube. This pattern of $\boldsymbol{A}$ mapping a vector outside the hypercube and $O[\cdot]$ mapping back into the hypercube can repeat over and over depending on the matrix $\boldsymbol{A}$. The state can oscillate between fixed points, or converge to a single nonzero fixed point. This is illustrated in Fig. 6.11.3.

The key to eliminating these zero-input limit cycles is to ensure that overflows do not happen in the first place. This can be accomplished through scaling and the proper choice of filter architecture. The reason overflow occurred in the previous example is that the matrix $\boldsymbol{A}$ maps vectors $\boldsymbol{x}$ to vectors $\boldsymbol{Ax}$ which have a length greater than that of $\boldsymbol{x}$. This is the only way a vector inside the state-space grid could get mapped to a vector outside the grid. Let the matrix norm $||\boldsymbol{A}||$ be defined by

$$||\boldsymbol{A}|| = \max_{||\boldsymbol{x}|| \neq 0} \frac{||\boldsymbol{Ax}||}{||x||} = \max_{||\boldsymbol{x}|| \neq 0} \left[\frac{\boldsymbol{x}^T \boldsymbol{A}^T \boldsymbol{Ax}}{\boldsymbol{x}^T \boldsymbol{x}} \right]^{1/2}.$$

In other words, the norm of $\boldsymbol{A}$ is equal to the maximum ratio of $||\boldsymbol{Ax}||$ to $||\boldsymbol{x}||$ over all vectors $\boldsymbol{x}$. Therefore, a sufficient condition [MMR81] to ensure that zero-input limit cycles can not occur is

$$||\boldsymbol{A}|| < 1.$$

Consider the direct-II realization of the transfer function

$$H(z) = 1 + \frac{b_1 z^{-1} + b_2 z^{-2}}{1 + a_1 z^{-1} + a_2 z^{-2}}.$$

Assume that the denominator has complex poles

$$p_1, p_2 = \alpha \pm j\beta.$$

It is fairly simple to show that the poles are related to the denominator coefficients by

$$a_1 = -2\alpha, \quad a_2 = \alpha^2 + \beta^2.$$

The $\boldsymbol{A}$ matrix for this system is given by

$$\boldsymbol{A} = \begin{bmatrix} 0 & 1 \\ -a_2 & -a_1 \end{bmatrix} = \begin{bmatrix} 0 & 1 \\ -\alpha^2 - \beta^2 & 2\alpha \end{bmatrix}.$$

Suppose we apply the change of state defined by

$$\boldsymbol{x} = \boldsymbol{Tz}$$

where

$$\boldsymbol{T} = \begin{bmatrix} -1/\beta & 0 \\ -\alpha/\beta & 1 \end{bmatrix}.$$

Then the $\boldsymbol{A}$ matrix for the new system with state $\boldsymbol{z}$ is given by

$$\bar{\boldsymbol{A}} = \boldsymbol{T}^{-1} \boldsymbol{AT},$$

which we can show is equal to

$$\bar{A} = \begin{bmatrix} \alpha & -\beta \\ \beta & \alpha \end{bmatrix}.$$

The matrix $\bar{A}$ satisfies

$$\bar{A}^T \bar{A} = \bar{A}\bar{A}^T$$

and is known as a *normal* matrix. Let's look at the norm of $\bar{A}$. We have

$$\bar{A}^T \bar{A} = \begin{bmatrix} \alpha^2 + \beta^2 & 0 \\ 0 & \alpha^2 + \beta^2 \end{bmatrix}$$

so that

$$||\bar{A}|| = \max_{||x|| \neq 0} \left[\frac{x^T A^T A x}{x^T x} \right]^{1/2} = \sqrt{\alpha^2 + \beta^2}.$$

Because $\sqrt{\alpha^2 + \beta^2}$ is equal to the magnitude of the complex poles of $H(z)$, which was assumed to be stable, it follows that

$$||\bar{A}|| < 1.$$

Thus, the second-order system described by the normal matrix is incapable of producing zero-input limit cycles.

6.12 Scaling Fixed-Point Digital Filters

The analysis of roundoff noise can only be performed once it is ensured that the filter is free from overflow. Namely, we must make sure that all of the internal states have not exceeded the maximum bound which is representable in the fixed-point format.

Suppose the filter has state variables $x_1(k), x_2(k), \ldots, x_N(k)$ and that the maximum magnitude which can be represented is Δ. Then to avoid overflow, we must have

$$|x_i(k)| \leq \Delta, \quad i = 1, 2, \ldots, N$$

for all k. If this constraint is not met, the filter architecture must be modified by a process known as *scaling*. The state variable method provides an ideal framework for the study of scaling. Recall that the state variable representation provides a natural decomposition of the filter's input-output function into two mappings. The first mapping is from the input to the internal states and the second mapping is from the internal states to the output. Intuitively, we would expect that the transfer function from the input to the output can be left intact by reducing the gain from the input to the states and correspondingly increasing the gain from the states to the output. Indeed, this is the idea behind scaling.

There are several different scaling paradigms, each related to a different class of inputs. Suppose the impulse response from the input to the i-th state is given by $\boldsymbol{f}_i$. We have seen that the transfer function from the input to the state is given by

$$F(z) = \frac{\boldsymbol{X}(z)}{U(z)} = (z\boldsymbol{I} - \boldsymbol{A})^{-1}\boldsymbol{b}.$$

Thus, $F_i(z)$ is the i-th element of $F(z)$. The state $x_i(k)$ can be computed as

$$x_i(k) = \sum_{n=0}^{\infty} f_i(n)u(k-n).$$

Consider first the case where the input $u(k)$ is bounded by unity, *i.e.*,

$$|u(k)| \leq 1.$$

Then

$$|x_i(k)| = \left| \sum_{n=0}^{\infty} f_i(n)u(k-n) \right|.$$

Using the Cauchy-Schwartz inequality, we then have

$$|x_i(k)| \leq \sum_{n=0}^{\infty} |f_i(n)||u(k-n)| = \sum_{n=0}^{\infty} |f_i(n)|.$$

Therefore, the magnitude of the state is bounded by

$$|\boldsymbol{x}_i(k)| \leq ||\boldsymbol{f}_i||_1,$$

the l^1 norm of the impulse response from the input to the i-th state. Therefore, if we can find a nonsingular transformation of the state which gives $||f_i||_1 \leq \Delta$, we can be sure that $x_i(k)$ will be bounded by Δ for all inputs which are bounded by unity magnitude. The logical extension for larger magnitude inputs is obvious.

Similarly, suppose the input is a complex exponential,

$$u(k) = e^{jk\theta}.$$

Then

$$x_i(k) = \sum_{n=0}^{\infty} f_i(n)e^{j(k-n)\theta} = e^{jk\theta} \sum_{n=0}^{\infty} f_i(n)e^{-jn\theta}.$$

Thus,

$$|x_i(k)| \leq |F_i(e^{j\theta})|$$

and in particular,

$$|x_i(k)| \leq \max_{\theta} |F_i(e^{j\theta})|.$$

Therefore, for unit-magnitude complex exponential inputs, the magnitude of state $x_i(k)$ is bounded by the maximum magnitude of the frequency response from the input to $x_i(k)$. It is simple to show that the same is true for real sinusoidal inputs.

The most popular scaling criterion is based on the l^2 norm. Suppose the input signal $\{u(k)\}$ has finite energy. Without loss of generality, we can assume that

$$||\boldsymbol{u}||_2 = \sum_{k=-\infty}^{\infty} u^2(k) \leq 1.$$

Then it is simple to show that

$$|x_i(k)| \leq\leq \left[\sum_{k=0}^{\infty} f_i^2(k)\right]^{1/2} = ||\boldsymbol{f}_i||_2$$

where $\boldsymbol{f}_i$ is the impulse response from the input to the i-th state. The reason that the l^2 magnitude bound is popular is because it can be computed easily. It is difficult to obtain analytic expressions for the l^1 and maximum frequency response bounds. However, as we will soon see, the l^2 norm of a rational system is easily computed as the solution to a matrix equation.

The l^2, l^1, and frequency response criteria provide increasingly conservative bounds for the state variables. We have already seen that for a signal $\boldsymbol{f}$,

$$||\boldsymbol{f}||_2 \leq ||\boldsymbol{f}||_1.$$

The frequency response bound lies in between the l^2 and l^1 bounds, giving the relationship

$$||\boldsymbol{f}||_2 \leq \max_{\theta} |F(e^{j\theta})| \leq ||\boldsymbol{f}_1||.$$

These criteria can be used to provide bounds on the magnitude of the state variables of the filter for deterministic input signals. For random signals, we instead choose to bound the mean-squared value of the state variables. Suppose $\{u(k\}$ is a white noise input with zero mean and unit variance. We have

$$\mathcal{E}[x^2(k)] = \mathcal{E}\left[\sum_{n=-\infty}^{\infty} \sum_{m=-\infty}^{\infty} f(n)f(m)u(k-n)u(k-m)\right].$$

Therefore,

$$\mathcal{E}[x^2(k)] = \sum_{n=-\infty}^{\infty} \sum_{m=-\infty}^{\infty} f(n)f(m)\mathcal{E}[\boldsymbol{u}(k-n)u(k-m)].$$

Because $\{u(k)\}$ is white with unit variance,

$$\mathcal{E}[u(k-n)u(k-m)] = \delta(n-m)$$

so that

$$\mathcal{E}[x^2(k)] = \sum_{n=-\infty}^{\infty} f^2(n).$$

Therefore, the mean-squared value of the state is given by

$$\mathcal{E}[x^2(k)] = ||\boldsymbol{f}||_2^2.$$

If the input is WSS but not white, then

$$\mathcal{E}[x^2(k)] = r_{xx}(0)$$

and we use the Wiener-Khinchine theorem which yields

$$\mathcal{E}[x^2(k)] = \frac{1}{2\pi}\int_{-\pi}^{\pi} |F(e^{j\theta})|^2 P_{uu}(\theta)\, d\theta.$$

Once a magnitude bound in chosen, the scaling operation is performed in the following manner. Suppose we wish to bound the magnitude of the i-th state by Δ. Given the impulse response $\boldsymbol{f}_i$ from the input to $x_i(k)$, we compute $||\boldsymbol{f}_i||$ where the norm corresponds to the input class of interest. The state variable representation is transformed in a manner which leaves the transfer function intact but changes the norm of the impulse response from the input to the i-th state to Δ (assuming that $||u|| = 1$). We are then assured that the magnitude of $x_i(k)$ can never exceed Δ (in what follows, we will usually assume $\Delta = 1$).

6.13 l^2 Scaling

The l^2 scaling paradigm is important both because of its computational simplicity and its applicability to both deterministic and random inputs. We have seen that if the input $\boldsymbol{u}$ is finite energy with $||\boldsymbol{u}||_2 = 1$, then

$$|x_i(k)| \leq ||\boldsymbol{f}_i||_2.$$

Or, if the input is white noise with unit power, then

$$\mathcal{E}[x_i^2(k)] = ||\boldsymbol{f}_i||_2^2$$

which means that

$$\sqrt{\mathcal{E}[x_i^2(k)]} = ||\boldsymbol{f}_i||_2.$$

The l^2 scaling method begins with choosing some value s such that

$$s||\boldsymbol{f}_i||_2 = 1. \tag{6.13.1}$$

In other words, we would like the l^2 norm of the impulse response from the input to the i-th state to be equal to s^{-1} where s is equal to some "safety" factor.

For deterministic unit-energy inputs, if the scaling policy expressed by Eq. 6.13.1 is met, we are guaranteed that the i-th state will never exceed s^{-1}. For unit-variance white noise inputs, we instead interpret the scaling policy to mean that

$$\sqrt{\mathcal{E}[x_i^2(k)]} = s^{-1}.$$

This gives a measure of the spread of the state about its mean, which will be zero if the input is zero-mean. For example, if it is desired to bound the state by unity, a choice of $s = 1$ will allow approximately one standard deviation to be represented without overflow. This still leaves a fairly high probability of overflow. If we wish to bound the state by unity with a lower probability of overflow, a larger value of s should be chosen.

Let's see how $||\boldsymbol{f}_i||_2$ can be computed without summing any geometric series or using Parseval's theorem. In Eq. 6.4.5, we saw that the state response was given by

$$\boldsymbol{x}(k) = \sum_{n=0}^{\infty} \boldsymbol{A}^n \boldsymbol{b} u(k+1-n).$$

Assuming a zero-mean white noise input, the covariance $\boldsymbol{K}$ of the state is given by

$$\boldsymbol{K} = \mathcal{E}[\boldsymbol{x}(k)\boldsymbol{x}^T(k)] = \sum_{n=0}^{\infty}\sum_{m=0}^{\infty} \boldsymbol{A}^n \boldsymbol{b} \mathcal{E}[u(k+1-n)u(k+1-m)]\boldsymbol{b}^T(\boldsymbol{A}^T)^m. \tag{6.13.2}$$

Because $\{u(k)\}$ is white noise,

$$\mathcal{E}[u(k+1-n)u(k+1-m)] = \delta(n-m)$$

and Eq. 6.13.2 becomes

$$\boldsymbol{K} = \sum_{n=0}^{\infty} \boldsymbol{A}^n \boldsymbol{b}\boldsymbol{b}^T(\boldsymbol{A}^T)^n. \tag{6.13.3}$$

Now, recall that the impulse response from the input to the state is given by

$$\boldsymbol{f}(k) = \boldsymbol{A}^{k-1}\boldsymbol{b}, \quad k > 0. \tag{6.13.4}$$

Therefore, we can see that Eq. 6.13.3 is equivalent to

$$\boldsymbol{K} = \sum_{n=0}^{\infty} \boldsymbol{f}(k)\boldsymbol{f}^T(k). \tag{6.13.5}$$

In particular,

$$K_{ii} = \sum_{n=0}^{\infty} \boldsymbol{f}_i^2(k) = ||\boldsymbol{f}_i||_2^2.$$

Therefore, the l^2 norm of $\boldsymbol{f}_i$ can be extracted as the i-th diagonal element of $\boldsymbol{K}$, and we have

$$||\boldsymbol{f}_i||_2 = \sqrt{K_{ii}}. \tag{6.13.6}$$

The l^2 scaling requirement then becomes

$$s\sqrt{K_{ii}} = 1. \tag{6.13.7}$$

All we need to do is find a simple way to compute the state covariance, $\boldsymbol{K}$. To this end, recall that if white noise is applied to a LTI system, the output is WSS. We have seen that the response from the input to the i-th state is expressible as a rational LTI system, namely

$$X(z) = (z\boldsymbol{I} - \boldsymbol{A})^{-1}\boldsymbol{b}U(z)$$

so that

$$X_i(z) = [(z\boldsymbol{I} - \boldsymbol{A})^{-1}\boldsymbol{b}U(z)]_i.$$

Thus, $x_i(k)$ will be WSS for white noise inputs. Next, we use the relationship

$$\boldsymbol{x}(k+1) = \boldsymbol{A}\boldsymbol{x}(k) + \boldsymbol{b}u(k)$$

to obtain

$$\begin{aligned}\mathcal{E}[\boldsymbol{x}(k+1)\boldsymbol{x}^T(k+1)] &= \boldsymbol{A}\mathcal{E}[\boldsymbol{x}(k)\boldsymbol{x}^T(k)]\boldsymbol{A}^T + \boldsymbol{b}\mathcal{E}[u^2(k)]\boldsymbol{b}^T \\ &\quad + \boldsymbol{A}\mathcal{E}[\boldsymbol{x}(k)u(k)]\boldsymbol{b}^T + \boldsymbol{b}\mathcal{E}[\boldsymbol{x}(k)u(k)]\boldsymbol{A}^T.\end{aligned} \tag{6.13.8}$$

Because $\boldsymbol{x}(k)$ is WSS, it follows that

$$\mathcal{E}[\boldsymbol{x}(k+1)\boldsymbol{x}^T(k+1)] = \mathcal{E}[\boldsymbol{x}(k)\boldsymbol{x}^T(k)] = \boldsymbol{K}. \tag{6.13.9}$$

Furthermore, because $\boldsymbol{x}(k)$ depends on $u(n)$ only for $n = 0, 1, \ldots, k-1$, it follows that $\boldsymbol{x}(k)$ and $u(k)$ are *independent*. Therefore,

$$\mathcal{E}[\boldsymbol{x}(k)u(k)] = \boldsymbol{0}. \tag{6.13.10}$$

Substituting Eqs. 6.13.10 and 6.13.9 into Eq. 6.13.8, we then have

$$\boldsymbol{K} = \boldsymbol{A}\boldsymbol{K}\boldsymbol{A}^T + \boldsymbol{b}\boldsymbol{b}^T. \tag{6.13.11}$$

Equation 6.13.11 is known as a *matrix Lyapunov equation* and gives the state covariance as the solution to a simple quadratic matrix equation. The expression is quadratic in $\boldsymbol{A}$ and $\boldsymbol{b}$, but linear in $\boldsymbol{K}$. It is simple to expand Eq. 6.13.11 to solve for the individual elements of $\boldsymbol{K}$.

Once the matrix $\boldsymbol{K}$ is found, the l^2 scaling procedure is straightforward. We need to find a nonsingular transformation $\boldsymbol{T}$ of the state which forces the requirement of Eq. 6.13.1 to be met. Recall that the transformation

$$\boldsymbol{z} = \boldsymbol{T}\boldsymbol{x}$$

transforms the system

$$\begin{aligned} \boldsymbol{x}(k+1) &= \boldsymbol{A}\boldsymbol{x}(k) + \boldsymbol{b}u(k) \\ y(k) &= \boldsymbol{c}\boldsymbol{x}(k) + du(k) \end{aligned}$$

into the system

$$\begin{aligned} \boldsymbol{z}(k+1) &= \bar{\boldsymbol{A}}\boldsymbol{z}(k) + \bar{\boldsymbol{b}}u(k) \\ y(k) &= \bar{\boldsymbol{c}}\boldsymbol{z}(k) + \bar{d}u(k) \end{aligned}$$

without altering the transfer function from the input to the output. The new system matrices are given by

$$\bar{\boldsymbol{A}} = \boldsymbol{T}^{-1}\boldsymbol{A}\boldsymbol{T}, \quad \bar{\boldsymbol{b}} = \boldsymbol{T}^{-1}\boldsymbol{b}, \quad \bar{\boldsymbol{c}} = \boldsymbol{c}\boldsymbol{T}, \quad \bar{d} = d.$$

Let's examine the effect of the transformation $\boldsymbol{T}$ on the matrix $\boldsymbol{K}$. Using the fact that

$$\boldsymbol{A} = \boldsymbol{T}\bar{\boldsymbol{A}}\boldsymbol{T}^{-1}$$

and

$$\boldsymbol{b} = \boldsymbol{T}\bar{\boldsymbol{b}},$$

Eq. 6.13.11 becomes

$$\boldsymbol{K} = \boldsymbol{T}\bar{\boldsymbol{A}}\boldsymbol{T}^{-1}\boldsymbol{K}(\boldsymbol{T}^T)^{-1}\bar{\boldsymbol{A}}^T\boldsymbol{T}^T + \boldsymbol{T}\bar{\boldsymbol{b}}\bar{\boldsymbol{b}}^T\boldsymbol{T}^T. \tag{6.13.12}$$

Multiplying both sides of Eq. 6.13.12 on the left by $\boldsymbol{T}^{-1}$ and on the right by $(\boldsymbol{T}^T)^{-1}$, we then have

$$\boldsymbol{T}^{-1}\boldsymbol{K}(\boldsymbol{T}^T)^{-1} = \bar{\boldsymbol{A}}\boldsymbol{T}^{-1}\boldsymbol{K}(\boldsymbol{T}^T)^{-1}\bar{\boldsymbol{A}}^T + \bar{\boldsymbol{b}}\bar{\boldsymbol{b}}^T. \tag{6.13.13}$$

Equation 6.13.13 is immediately recognized as the matrix Lyapunov equation for the system described by $(\bar{\boldsymbol{A}}, \bar{\boldsymbol{b}})$. Therefore, the covariance for the transformed system is given by

$$\bar{\boldsymbol{K}} = \boldsymbol{T}^{-1}\boldsymbol{K}(\boldsymbol{T}^T)^{-1}. \tag{6.13.14}$$

The l^2 scaling problem then can be solved by finding a transformation $\boldsymbol{T}$ which gives

$$s\sqrt{\bar{K}_{ii}} = 1. \tag{6.13.15}$$

Suppose $\boldsymbol{T}$ is a diagonal matrix with diagonal entries T_{ii}. Then according to Eq. 6.13.14, the diagonal element of $\bar{\boldsymbol{K}}$ are given by

$$\bar{K}_{ii} = \frac{K_{ii}}{T_{ii}^2}. \tag{6.13.16}$$

Thus, the l^2 scaling constraint can be met by choosing T_{ii} to satisfy

$$s\sqrt{\frac{K_{ii}}{T_{ii}^2}} = 1$$

which means that

$$T_{ii} = s\sqrt{K_{ii}}. \tag{6.13.17}$$

Therefore, the nonsingular state transformation defined by

$$\boldsymbol{T} = \begin{bmatrix} T_{11} & 0 & \cdots & 0 \\ 0 & T_{22} & \cdots & 0 \\ \vdots & \vdots & \ddots & \vdots \\ 0 & 0 & \cdots & T_{NN} \end{bmatrix} \tag{6.13.18}$$

will yield a new system with the same transfer function, but the state variables will all satisfy the l^2 scaling constraint. The transformation may be simplified somewhat if we choose

$$\boldsymbol{T} = s\sqrt{\max_i(K_{ii})}\boldsymbol{I},$$

but will result in some of the state variables being "overscaled," which can impact the quantization error behavior of the filter. This will be discussed later.

In practice, the matrix $\boldsymbol{K}$ can be found either by solving a system of linear equations for the elements of $\boldsymbol{K}$ or by iterative methods. We have seen that the equation

$$\boldsymbol{K} = \boldsymbol{A}\boldsymbol{K}\boldsymbol{A}^T + \boldsymbol{b}\boldsymbol{b}^T \tag{6.13.19}$$

has a solution $\boldsymbol{K}$ which is symmetric and positive definite whenever the eigenvalues of $\boldsymbol{A}$ are inside the unit circle (corresponding to a stable system). In particular, $\boldsymbol{K}$ can be expressed in closed form as

$$\boldsymbol{K} = \sum_{i=0}^{\infty} \boldsymbol{A}^i \boldsymbol{b}\boldsymbol{b}^T (\boldsymbol{A}^T)^i.$$

From this expression, it is easily verified that Eq. 6.13.11 is satisfied. Numerically, the convergence of this series is quadratic, and it will converge to machine precision fairly rapidly. This suggests the following algorithm to compute $\boldsymbol{K}$.

Summary

Computation of the matrix $\boldsymbol{K}$ which satisfies

$$\boldsymbol{K} = \boldsymbol{A}\boldsymbol{K}\boldsymbol{A}^T + \boldsymbol{b}\boldsymbol{b}^T.$$

Initialization:

$$\boldsymbol{K}_0 = \boldsymbol{b}\boldsymbol{b}^T$$

$$\boldsymbol{Q}_0 = \boldsymbol{A}.$$

Loop on i:

$$\boldsymbol{K}_{i+1} = \boldsymbol{Q}_i \boldsymbol{K}_i \boldsymbol{Q}_i^T$$

$$\boldsymbol{Q}_{i+1} = \boldsymbol{Q}_i^2$$

Continue until $\boldsymbol{Q}_i \approx \boldsymbol{O}$.

6.14 Scaling and Roundoff Noise

Our study of scaling did not examine the effects of the scaling on the roundoff error performance of the filter. The l^2 scaling paradigm did not take into account the fact that the range of values which can be represented is *quantized*. Rather, we were only concerned with bounding the maximum absolute value of each state within the filter. In actuality, scaling will impact the quantization error behavior of the filter. This can be illustrated by the following simple example. Suppose the filter $H(z)$ is given by

$$H(z) = \frac{1}{1 - az^{-1}}$$

where $|a| < 1$. A state-variable representation for this system is given by

$$\begin{array}{rcl} x(k+1) & = & ax(k) + 1u(k) \\ y(k) & = & ax(k) + 1u(k) \end{array}.$$

The matrix Lyapunov equation for this system is

$$K = aKa + b^2 = a^2K + 1$$

which gives

$$K = \frac{1}{1 - a^2}.$$

Suppose we wish to scale the filter so that for inputs with unity energy, Eq. 6.13.1 is satisfied, *i.e.*,

$$s\sqrt{K} = 1.$$

This means that the transformation T should be chosen according to Eq. 6.13.18 as

$$T = s\sqrt{K} = \frac{s}{\sqrt{1 - a^2}}.$$

The new state variable representation is then given by

$$\begin{array}{rcl} z(k+1) & = & az(k) + s^{-1}\sqrt{1 - a^2}u(k) \\ y(k) & = & \frac{as}{\sqrt{1-a^2}}z(k) + du(k) \end{array}$$

Notice that the new matrix $\bar{b}$ is given by

$$\bar{b} = s^{-1}\sqrt{1 - a^2}.$$

Consider the case where a is close to the unit circle. Then $\bar{b}$ will be close to zero. The impulse response from the input to the state is now given by

$$\bar{f}(k) = \bar{a}^{k-1}\bar{b} = s^{-1}a^{k-1}\sqrt{1 - a^2}.$$

Suppose the quantization step size for the filter is q. For a close to the unit circle, the impulse response of the scaled filter will have a maximum magnitude of $\sqrt{1-a^2}$. For example, suppose $a = 0.99$ and $q = 2^{-8}$ (corresponding to eight bits of wordwidth). Then

$$\bar{f}(k) = s^{-1}0.14(0.99)^{k-1}.$$

The parameter s controls the amount of scaling. For example, $s = 1$ corresponds to bounding the state by unity. In this case, the impulse response will be rounded to the nearest multiple of 2^{-8}. For even moderate k, the impulse response will have decayed to a magnitude which is close to that of q so that large quantization errors will occur. For even larger scaling parameters s, the quantization errors will be even larger since $\bar{f}(k)$ is proportional to s^{-1}.

Obviously, we need to develop a method of analyzing the effect of scaling on the roundoff error performance of a filter. Again, the state variable representation will provide a powerful tool for the analysis of roundoff error.

We begin with some preliminaries. Recall that the quantization operation is modeled as an additive noise source which is white with zero mean, uncorrelated with the signal, and has power $q^2/12$ where q is the quantization step size. The fundamental arithmetic operation in digital filtering is multiplication/accumulation. Consider the direct-II digital filter structure shown in Fig. 6.14.1. During each filter cycle, two sums-of-products of length N must be computed (corresponding to the b_i and the a_i). If the data stored in the shift registers are B bits wide and the coefficients are each B-bits wide, the product of each shift register content with a filter coefficient will be $2B$ bits wide. Eventually, these $2B$-bit words will need to be truncated to B bits. One approach is to truncate the $2B$-bit output of each multiplier to B bits and accumulate the B-bit words two at a time, truncating to B bits after each summation. This is necessary since the sum of two B-bit words will have $B+1$ bits. A better approach is to use an extended-precision accumulator which can accumulate the $2B$-bit outputs of the multipliers and truncate the final accumulated sum.

The overall noise at the output will have contributions from each noise source inside the filter. Consider the noise $\{e_i(k)\}$ which enters at the i-th state variable. Because there are dynamics involved, the manner in which the noise contributes to the filter output is not merely algebraic in nature. Since the filter is recursive, the noise will "recirculate" through the filter. Suppose the impulse response from the i-th state to the output is given by $\boldsymbol{g}_i$. Because the noise is assumed to be white, the output noise power due to $\{e_i(k)\}$ is given by

$$\sigma_i^2 = \frac{q^2}{12}\sum_{k=0}^{\infty} g_i^2(k) = \frac{q^2}{12}\|\boldsymbol{g}_i\|_2^2. \tag{6.14.1}$$

Because all of the noise sources are assumed to be uncorrelated with one another, the overall output noise power due to the internal quantization noises is given by

$$\sum_{i=1}^{N}\sigma_i^2 = \frac{q^2}{12}\sum_{i=1}^{N}\|\boldsymbol{g}_i\|_2^2. \tag{6.14.2}$$

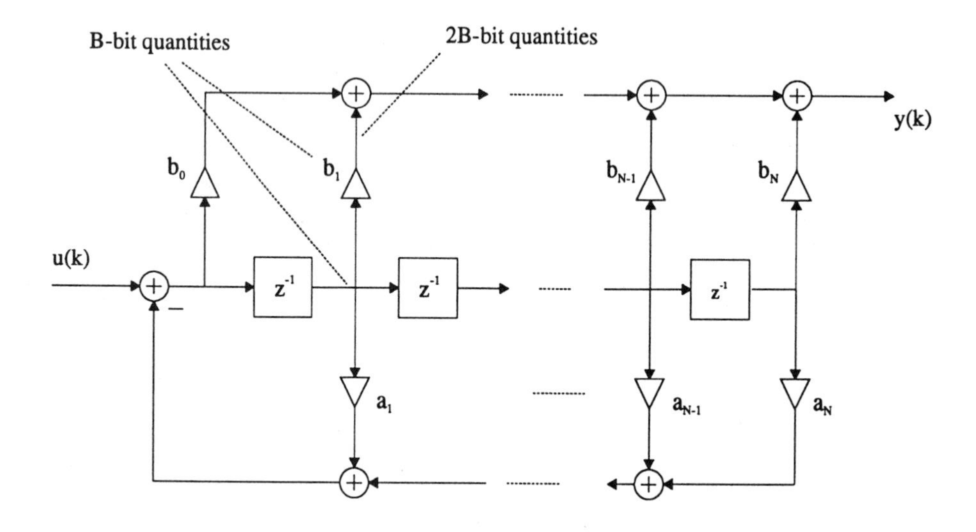

Figure 6.14.1: Direct-II filter structure.

Finally, there will be one additional noise source at the output of the filter which contributes an additional $q^2/12$ to the output noise power. Therefore, the overall output noise power due to quantization is given by

$$\sigma^2 = \frac{q^2}{12}\left[1 + \sum_{i=1}^{N} ||\boldsymbol{g}_i||_2^2\right]. \tag{6.14.3}$$

The l^2 norm $||\boldsymbol{g}_i||_2^2$ can be computed in several ways. The first is to use Parseval's theorem to give

$$||\boldsymbol{g}_i||_2^2 = \frac{1}{2\pi j}\oint_{|z|=1} z^{-1}G_i(z)G_i(z^{-1})\,dz = \frac{1}{2\pi}\int_{-\pi}^{\pi} |G_i(e^{j\theta})|^2\,d\theta.$$

A simpler technique is to use a dual to the matrix Lyapunov equation used for l^2 scaling. We begin with the state variable representation

$$\begin{array}{rclcl} \boldsymbol{x}(k+1) & = & \boldsymbol{A}\boldsymbol{x}(k) & + & \boldsymbol{b}u(k) \\ y(k) & = & \boldsymbol{c}\boldsymbol{x}(k) & + & du(k) \end{array}.$$

Recall that the matrix $\boldsymbol{b}$ describes the coupling between the input and the internal states. In our quantization model, the noise is injected *directly into the states.* Let the noise sources constitute a vector $e(k)$ where

$$e(k) = \begin{bmatrix} e_1(k) \\ e_2(k) \\ \vdots \\ e_N(k) \end{bmatrix}.$$

Ignoring for now the noise which is applied at the output, we can regard the noise $e(k)$ as the input to the system, giving the new system

$$\begin{aligned} x(k+1) &= Ax(k) + Ie(k) \\ y(k) &= cx(k) + 0e(k) \end{aligned} \quad (6.14.4)$$

The transfer function from the noise input vector to the output is given by

$$G(z) = c(zI - A)^{-1}I = c(zI - A)^{-1} \quad (6.14.5)$$

so that

$$Y(z) = G(z)U(z).$$

Because $(zI - A)^{-1}$ is the $\mathcal{Z}$-transform of the matrix sequence

$$A^{k-1}u(k-1),$$

it follows that $G(z)$ is the $\mathcal{Z}$-transform of the sequence

$$g(k) = cA^{k-1}, \quad k = 1, 2, \ldots.$$

Now, consider the product

$$g^T(k)g(k) = (A^T)^{k-1}c^T cA^{k-1}.$$

The i-th diagonal element of $g^T(k)g(k)$ is equal to $g_i^2(k)$. Define the matrix W by

$$W = \sum_{n=0}^{\infty} g^T(n)g(n) = \sum_{n=0}^{\infty} (A^T)^n c^T cA^n. \quad (6.14.6)$$

There is a certain similarity between Eq. 6.14.6 and Eq. 6.13.3. The role of A is now played by A^T and the role of b is now played by c^T. Therefore, W will satisfy the matrix Lyapunov equation

$$W = A^T WA + c^T c. \quad (6.14.7)$$

The squared l^2 norm of the impulse response from the i-th state to the output is then given by the i-th diagonal element of $\boldsymbol{W}$. That is,

$$||\boldsymbol{g}_i||_2^2 = W_{ii}.$$

Therefore, from Eq. 6.14.1, the contribution to the output noise power from the quantization at the i-th state is given by

$$\sigma_i^2 = \frac{q^2}{12} W_{ii}$$

and the overall output noise power from the quantization at all states is

$$\sigma^2 = \frac{q^2}{12} \sum_{i=1}^{N} W_{ii}. \tag{6.14.8}$$

Let's examine the effect of scaling the filter on the output noise power. With the non-singular transformation of the state described by the matrix $\boldsymbol{T}$, the new system matrices involved in the computation of $\boldsymbol{W}$ are

$$\bar{\boldsymbol{A}} = \boldsymbol{T}^{-1}\boldsymbol{A}\boldsymbol{T}, \quad \bar{\boldsymbol{c}} = \boldsymbol{c}\boldsymbol{T}.$$

Therefore, Eq. 6.14.7 becomes

$$\boldsymbol{W} = (\boldsymbol{T}^T)^{-1}\bar{\boldsymbol{A}}^T\boldsymbol{T}^T\boldsymbol{W}\boldsymbol{T}\bar{\boldsymbol{A}}\boldsymbol{T}^{-1} + (\boldsymbol{T}^T)^{-1}\bar{\boldsymbol{c}}^T\bar{\boldsymbol{c}}\boldsymbol{T}^{-1}. \tag{6.14.9}$$

Multiplying both sides of Eq. 6.14.9 on the left by $\boldsymbol{T}^T$ and on the right by $\boldsymbol{T}$, we get

$$\boldsymbol{T}^T\boldsymbol{W}\boldsymbol{T} = \bar{\boldsymbol{A}}^T\boldsymbol{T}^T\boldsymbol{W}\boldsymbol{T}\bar{\boldsymbol{A}} + \bar{\boldsymbol{c}}^T\bar{\boldsymbol{c}}. \tag{6.14.10}$$

This is immediately recognized as the matrix Lyapunov equation for the transformed and we infer that

$$\bar{\boldsymbol{W}} = \boldsymbol{T}^T\boldsymbol{W}\boldsymbol{T}. \tag{6.14.11}$$

The output roundoff noise power of the *scaled* system due to quantization at the states is thus given by

$$\sigma^2 = \frac{q^2}{12} \sum_{i=1}^{N} \bar{W}_{ii}. \tag{6.14.12}$$

Recall that $\boldsymbol{T}$ was chosen as

$$\boldsymbol{T} = \begin{bmatrix} T_{11} & 0 & \cdots & 0 \\ 0 & T_{22} & \cdots & 0 \\ \vdots & \vdots & \ddots & \vdots \\ 0 & 0 & \cdots & T_{NN} \end{bmatrix}$$

where

$$T_{ii} = s\sqrt{K_{ii}}.$$

Therefore,

$$\bar{W}_{ii} = s^2 W_{ii} K_{ii}.$$

This means that the roundoff noise power of the scaled system is given by

$$\sigma^2 = s^2 \frac{q^2}{12} \sum_{i=1}^{N} W_{ii} K_{ii}. \tag{6.14.13}$$

Equation 6.14.13 expresses the roundoff noise power at the output in terms of the *unscaled* parameters K_{ii} and W_{ii}. We can see that the noise power is proportional to s^2. This shows that the scaling parameter s should be chosen large enough to prevent overflow, but not larger. If too large an s is chosen, the filter output will lose all significance because it is dominated by quantization error from the internal states. The quantity

$$G_N = \sum_{i=1}^{N} W_{ii} K_{ii}$$

is known as the *noise gain* of the filter and expresses the amplification of the quantization noise by the filter. Thus, the noise power at the output is given by

$$\sigma^2 = G_N \frac{s^2 q^2}{12}.$$

It is interesting to note that under a nonsingular transformation of the state, the product of $\boldsymbol{K}$ and $\boldsymbol{W}$ undergoes a similarity transformation. To see this, consider the product

$$\bar{\boldsymbol{K}}\bar{\boldsymbol{W}} = \boldsymbol{T}^{-1}\boldsymbol{K}(\boldsymbol{T}^T)^{-1}\boldsymbol{T}^T\boldsymbol{W}\boldsymbol{T} = \boldsymbol{T}^{-1}\boldsymbol{K}\boldsymbol{W}\boldsymbol{T}.$$

Therefore, the product $\bar{\boldsymbol{K}}\bar{\boldsymbol{W}}$ has the same eigenvalues as the product $\boldsymbol{K}\boldsymbol{W}$. These eigenvalues are important in the study of minimum roundoff noise filters.

6.15 Minimum Roundoff Noise Filters

In the previous two sections, we examined both scaling and the roundoff noise due to scaling. For convenience, we repeat the important equations. The noise power at the output due to rounding is equal to

$$\sigma^2 = s^2 \frac{q^2}{12} \sum_{i=1}^{N} K_{ii} W_{ii} \tag{6.15.1}$$

where the matrix $\boldsymbol{K}$ is the solution to the matrix Lyapunov equation

$$\boldsymbol{K} = \boldsymbol{A}\boldsymbol{K}\boldsymbol{A}^T + \boldsymbol{b}\boldsymbol{b}^T$$

and the matrix $\boldsymbol{W}$ is the solution to the matrix Lyapunov equation

$$\boldsymbol{W} = \boldsymbol{A}^T\boldsymbol{W}\boldsymbol{A} + \boldsymbol{c}^T\boldsymbol{c}.$$

Given these equations, an important problem is to start with a transfer function and determine an architecture $(\boldsymbol{A}, \boldsymbol{b}, \boldsymbol{c}, d)$ which *minimizes* the output roundoff noise power σ^2. Such filters are called *minimum roundoff noise* filters.

Classically, there are two cases of interest when designing minimum roundoff noise filters. The first is where we have a fixed number of bits B which can be distributed *unevenly* across the filter states. That is, certain states are allotted more bits than other states. The other case, which will be the one of interest to us, is where each of the filter states is allotted the same number of bits, B.

We have seen that for a wordwidth of B bits, the quantization step size is equal to

$$q = 2^{-B+1}.$$

Thus, Eq. 6.15.1 becomes

$$\sigma^2 = \frac{1}{3}\left(\frac{s}{2^B}\right)^2 \sum_{i=1}^{N} K_{ii}W_{ii}. \tag{6.15.2}$$

Therefore, minimization of the roundoff error power requires that we minimize the sum

$$\sum_{i=1}^{N} K_{ii}W_{ii}.$$

The minimization of this sum is not trivial. Because $\boldsymbol{K}$ and $\boldsymbol{W}$ are positive definite and symmetric, the eigenvalues of $\boldsymbol{K}\boldsymbol{W}$ will all be positive. Thus, let the eigenvalues of $\boldsymbol{K}\boldsymbol{W}$ be denoted by μ_i^2, $i = 1, 2, \ldots, N$. The following theorem [MR76] can be used to find the minimum value of σ^2.

Theorem 6 *If $\boldsymbol{K}$ and $\boldsymbol{W}$ are positive definite and symmetric, then*

$$\sum_{i=1}^{N} K_{ii}W_{ii} \geq \frac{1}{N}\left[\sum_{i=1}^{N} \mu_i\right]^2$$

with equality if and only if

$$\boldsymbol{K} = \boldsymbol{D}\boldsymbol{W}\boldsymbol{D}$$

for some diagonal matrix $\boldsymbol{D}$ *with positive entries and the products of the diagonal elements of* $\boldsymbol{K}$ *and* $\boldsymbol{W}$ *are all equal. That is,*

$$K_{ii}W_{ii} = K_{jj}W_{jj} \quad \textit{for all } i, j.$$

According to the theorem, the minimum roundoff noise power is given by

$$\sigma^2_{min} = \frac{1}{3N}\left(\frac{s}{2^B}\right)^2 \left[\sum_{i=1}^{N} \mu_i\right]^2 . \tag{6.15.3}$$

Notice that the minimum roundoff noise is determined entirely by the eigenvalues of $\boldsymbol{KW}$.

We have still not specified how to actually *find* the architecture which results in the minimum roundoff noise power as given by Eq. 6.15.3. In general, these architectures will be quite computationally complex. Whereas the architectures we have studied so far (parallel, direct-II, cascade) have a small number of multiplications per output cycle, the minimum roundoff noise filter will have many nonzero or nonunity entries in the $\boldsymbol{A}, \boldsymbol{b}$, and $\boldsymbol{c}$ matrices. Consequently, the minimum roundoff noise architecture for an order-N filter may require as many as $(N+1)^2$ multiplications per output. In many applications, it is questionable whether the improvement in performance is worth this increase in computational complexity.

A suboptimal solution to the minimum roundoff noise problem is to separate the filter into a cascade (or parallel) combination of second-order (and first-order real) subfilters. We have already discussed the benefits of this approach earlier in the chapter. Instead of implementing the lower-order subfilters in direct-II form, they can be implemented as minimum roundoff noise architectures. This will result in a filter whose roundoff noise behavior is not quite as good as an order-N minimum roundoff noise filter, but will require only $4N+1$ multiplications per output. As we shall see, the roundoff noise will still be substantially smaller than for the canonical architectures.

The key to determining the minimum roundoff noise architecture is finding the transformation $\boldsymbol{T}$ which transforms the system. For the suboptimal approach, it is important that the transformation $\boldsymbol{T}$ preserve the topology of the architecture. That is, if the filter is architected as a cascade combination of second-order subfilters, the transformation $\boldsymbol{T}$ should leave this configuration intact and affect only the second-order subfilters individually.

Suppose $H(z)$ is decomposed into a cascade or parallel combination of L subfilters

$$H_1(z), H_2(z), \ldots, H_L(z),$$

and each subfilter $H_i(z)$ is described by the state-variable representation

$$H_i(z) \sim (\boldsymbol{A}_i, \boldsymbol{b}_i, \boldsymbol{c}_i, d_i).$$

We have already seen how the overall state-variable representation $(\boldsymbol{A}, \boldsymbol{B}, \boldsymbol{c}, d)$ is computed from the subfilters' state variable matrices. The matrices $\boldsymbol{K}$ and $\boldsymbol{W}$ for the overall system then satisfy

$$\boldsymbol{K} = \boldsymbol{A}\boldsymbol{K}\boldsymbol{A}^T + \boldsymbol{b}\boldsymbol{b}^T$$

and

$$\boldsymbol{W} = \boldsymbol{A}^T\boldsymbol{W}\boldsymbol{A} + \boldsymbol{c}^T\boldsymbol{c}.$$

The l^2 norms of the states are located on the diagonal of the matrix $\boldsymbol{K}$. Thus, the 2×2 matrix $\boldsymbol{K}^{(i)}$ which contains on its diagonal the l^2 norms of the two states within subfilter $H_i(z)$ can be extracted as a 2×2 block from the matrix $\boldsymbol{K}$. It is important to note that the matrix $\boldsymbol{K}^{(i)}$ does *not* satisfy a matrix Lyapunov matrix equation involving $\boldsymbol{A}_i$ and $\boldsymbol{b}_i$. That is,

$$\boldsymbol{K}^{(i)} \neq \boldsymbol{A}_i\boldsymbol{K}^{(i)}\boldsymbol{A}_i^T + \boldsymbol{b}_i\boldsymbol{b}_i^T.$$

The same can be said for the matrix $\boldsymbol{W}^{(i)}$. When the transformation $\boldsymbol{T}$ preserves the topology of the system, however, the eigenvalues of $\boldsymbol{K}\boldsymbol{W}$ are invariant, and therefore so are those of $\boldsymbol{K}^{(i)}\boldsymbol{W}^{(i)}$. Unfortunately, the eigenvalues of $\boldsymbol{K}^{(i)}\boldsymbol{W}^{(i)}$ will not in general be equal to any of the eigenvalues of $\boldsymbol{K}\boldsymbol{W}$. Since the minimum roundoff noise is a function of the eigenvalues of $\boldsymbol{K}\boldsymbol{W}$, the minimum roundoff noise for the cascade filter and the overall minimum roundoff noise filter will be different. This type of structure, where the topology of the filter is left intact, is called a *block-optimal* structure.

A second approach to simplifying the design of minimum roundoff noise filters is to optimize each subfilter in isolation through the use of individual transformations $\boldsymbol{T}^{(i)}$. This type of filter is known as an *section optimal* structure. Again, the roundoff noise performance will not be as good as overall minimum roundoff noise filter (or as good as the block optimal structure), but the behavior may still be quite acceptable and the design is greatly simplified.

An important property of minimum roundoff noise filters is that the roundoff noise behavior is independent of the filter's bandwidth. It is known that the noise gain for direct forms is inversely proportional to bandwidth. Thus, the roundoff noise will be unacceptable for narrow bandpass filters. This can be tempered somewhat by separating closely spaced poles into cascaded subfilters, but if all of the poles are tightly clustered (as is the case for narrow bandpass filters), the roundoff noise will still be unacceptable. The minimum roundoff noise approaches are very useful in this situation.

For the reasons we have discussed, we will concentrate on the roundoff noise minimization for isolated second-order filters (corresponding to the sectional optimal structure). According to the theorem, we need to determine an architecture $(\boldsymbol{A}, \boldsymbol{b}, \boldsymbol{c}, d)$ such that

$$K_{ii}W_{ii} = K_{jj}W_{jj}$$

and

$$\boldsymbol{K} = \boldsymbol{DWD}$$

for some positive diagonal matrix $\boldsymbol{D}$. Jackson has shown [Jac79] that these conditions are equivalent to the following: the filter is l^2 scaled and

$$a_{11} = a_{22} \quad \text{and} \quad b_1 c_1 = b_2 c_2. \tag{6.15.4}$$

Furthermore, since the conditions in Eq. 6.15.4 are not affected by diagonal transformations, the l^2 scaling can be applied after they are met. Starting with the transfer function

$$H(z) = d + \frac{q_1 z^{-1} + q_2 z^{-2}}{1 + p_1 z^{-1} + p_2 z^{-2}}$$

it is possible to derive by brute force a system of equations based on the transfer function coefficients which gives the minimum roundoff noise filter. A more elegant approach can be used which gives a clear geometric picture of the problem and its solution.

Suppose the poles of $H(z)$ are given by

$$\lambda, \lambda^* = \alpha \pm j\beta.$$

This means that

$$1 + p_1 z^{-1} + p_2 z^{-2} = (1 - (\alpha + j\beta) z^{-1})(1 - (\alpha - j\beta) z^{-1}).$$

Thus, the denominator coefficients are related to α and β through

$$p_1 = -2\alpha, \quad p_2 = \alpha^2 + \beta^2.$$

This allows us to write down the direct-II representation for $H(z)$ as

$$\boldsymbol{A} = \begin{bmatrix} 0 & 1 \\ -(\alpha^2 + \beta^2) & 2\alpha \end{bmatrix}, \quad \boldsymbol{b} = \begin{bmatrix} 0 \\ 1 \end{bmatrix}, \quad \boldsymbol{c} = \begin{bmatrix} q_2 & q_1 \end{bmatrix}, \quad d = d.$$

Let us bring the system into normal form by applying the transformation $\boldsymbol{T}_N$ where

$$\boldsymbol{T}_N = \begin{bmatrix} -1/\beta & 0 \\ -\alpha/\beta & 1 \end{bmatrix}.$$

The new state variable representation is then given by $(\boldsymbol{A}_N, \boldsymbol{b}_N, \boldsymbol{c}_N, d_N)$ where

$$\boldsymbol{A}_N = \begin{bmatrix} \alpha & -\beta \\ \beta & \alpha \end{bmatrix}, \quad \boldsymbol{b}_N = \begin{bmatrix} 0 \\ 1 \end{bmatrix}, \quad \boldsymbol{c}_N = \begin{bmatrix} -(q_2 + q_1\alpha)/\beta & q_1 \end{bmatrix}, \quad d_N = d.$$

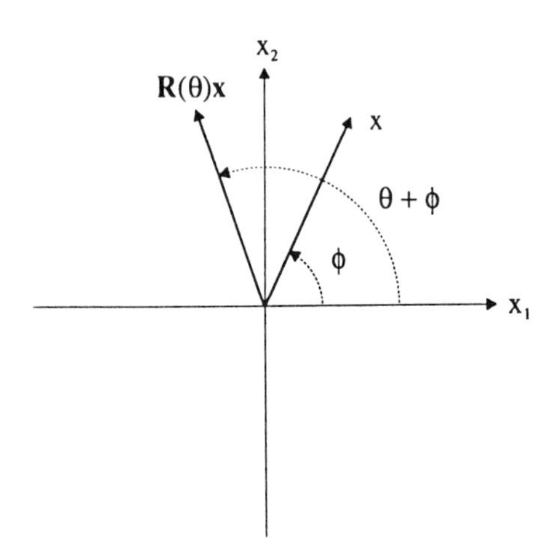

Figure 6.15.1: Rotation via a rotation matrix.

Thus, we have met the first condition $a_{11} = a_{22}$. Next, we need to meet the condition $b_1c_1 = b_2c_2$. This can be accomplished simply if we adopt a polar notation. The vector $\boldsymbol{c}_N$ can be written as

$$\boldsymbol{c}_N = r\begin{bmatrix} \cos\theta & \sin\theta \end{bmatrix}$$

where

$$r = \sqrt{c_{11}^2 + c_{12}^2}, \quad \theta = \tan^{-1}\frac{c_{12}}{c_{11}}.$$

A *rotation matrix* is a matrix of the form

$$\boldsymbol{R}(\theta) = \begin{bmatrix} \cos\theta & -\sin\theta \\ \sin\theta & \cos\theta \end{bmatrix}.$$

Pre-multiplying a vector $\boldsymbol{x}$ by $\boldsymbol{R}(\theta)$ has the effect of "rotating" $\boldsymbol{x}$ through an angle θ. To see this,

$$\boldsymbol{R}(\theta)\begin{bmatrix} x_1 \\ x_2 \end{bmatrix} = \begin{bmatrix} x_1\cos\theta - x_2\sin\theta \\ x_1\sin\theta + x_2\cos\theta \end{bmatrix}.$$

As shown in Fig. 6.15.1, we can see how the vector is rotated by $\boldsymbol{R}(\theta)$. Obviously, the matrix $(\boldsymbol{R}(\theta))^{-1}$ has the effect of rotating through $-\theta$. Thus,

$$(\boldsymbol{R}(\theta))^{-1} = \boldsymbol{R}(-\theta).$$

Similarly, if a row vector is *postmultiplied* by $\boldsymbol{R}(\theta)$, it will be rotated through $-\theta$. Thus, postmultiplying by $\boldsymbol{R}(-\theta)$ will rotate through θ.

Using the rotation matrix $\boldsymbol{R}(\theta/2)$, where

$$\boldsymbol{R}(\theta/2) = \begin{bmatrix} \cos\theta/2 & -\sin\theta/2 \\ \sin\theta/2 & \cos\theta/2 \end{bmatrix},$$

we transform the system defined by $(\boldsymbol{A}_N, \boldsymbol{b}_N, \boldsymbol{c}_N, d_N)$ to the new system given by $(\bar{\boldsymbol{A}}, \bar{\boldsymbol{b}}, \bar{\boldsymbol{c}}, \bar{d})$. Then

$$\bar{\boldsymbol{A}} = \boldsymbol{R}(-\theta/2)\boldsymbol{A}_N\boldsymbol{R}(\theta/2)$$

and because the rotations have the effect of "undoing" one another, we obviously have

$$\bar{\boldsymbol{A}} = \boldsymbol{A}_N = \begin{bmatrix} \alpha & -\beta \\ \beta & \alpha \end{bmatrix}.$$

Next,

$$\bar{\boldsymbol{b}} = \boldsymbol{R}(-\theta/2)\boldsymbol{b}_N = \begin{bmatrix} \sin\theta/2 \\ \cos\theta/2 \end{bmatrix}.$$

Similarly,

$$\bar{\boldsymbol{c}} = \boldsymbol{c}_N\boldsymbol{R}(\theta/2) = r\begin{bmatrix} \cos\theta/2 & \sin\theta/2 \end{bmatrix}$$

since postmultiplication by $\boldsymbol{R}(\theta/2)$ will rotate $\boldsymbol{c}_N$ through $-\theta/2$. We can see that the condition

$$b_1c_1 = b_2c_2$$

is now met. To see why this is so, a geometric picture of the rotations of $\boldsymbol{b}_N$ and $\boldsymbol{c}_N$ induced by $\boldsymbol{R}(\theta/2)$ is shown in Fig. 6.15.2. Finally, $\bar{d} = d$.

Thusfar, we have a state variable representation $(\bar{\boldsymbol{A}}, \bar{\boldsymbol{b}}, \bar{\boldsymbol{c}}, \bar{d})$ which meets the requirements $a_{11} = a_{22}$ and $b_1c_1 = b_2c_2$. We now need only make sure that the filter is l^2 scaled. Thus, the matrix $\boldsymbol{K}$ which satisfies

$$\boldsymbol{K} = \bar{\boldsymbol{A}}\boldsymbol{K}\bar{\boldsymbol{A}}^T + \bar{\boldsymbol{b}}\bar{\boldsymbol{b}}^T$$

is computed. Using the diagonal transformation

$$\boldsymbol{T}_s = s\begin{bmatrix} \sqrt{K_{11}} & 0 \\ 0 & \sqrt{K_{22}} \end{bmatrix},$$

the system described by $(\bar{\boldsymbol{A}}, \bar{\boldsymbol{b}}, \bar{\boldsymbol{c}}, \bar{d})$ is transformed to one which meets the l^2 scaling requirement. The first two optimality criteria are still satisfied since the matrix $\boldsymbol{T}_s$ is diagonal, and we have the second-order minimum roundoff noise filter.

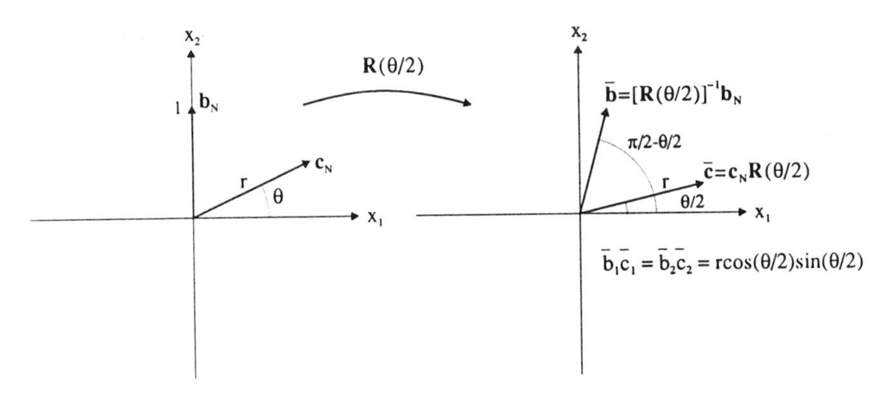

Figure 6.15.2: Rotating to meet the requirement $b_1c_1 = b_2c_2$.

Example 6.14

Suppose

$$H(z) = 1 + \frac{z^{-1} + 2z^{-2}}{1 - \sqrt{2}/2z^{-1} + 0.25z^{-2}}.$$

The direct-II representation for $H(z)$ is given by

$$\boldsymbol{A} = \begin{bmatrix} 0 & 1 \\ -0.25 & \sqrt{2}/2 \end{bmatrix}, \quad \boldsymbol{b} = \begin{bmatrix} 0 \\ 1 \end{bmatrix}, \quad \boldsymbol{c} = \begin{bmatrix} 1 & 2 \end{bmatrix}, \quad d = 1.$$

The matrices $\boldsymbol{K}$ and $\boldsymbol{W}$ are given by

$$\boldsymbol{K} = \begin{bmatrix} 1.569 & 0.887 \\ 0.887 & 1.569 \end{bmatrix}, \quad \boldsymbol{W} = \begin{bmatrix} 1.7120 & -0.011 \\ -0.011 & 11.39 \end{bmatrix}$$

For the direct-II architecture, the noise gain is given by

$$N = K_{11}W_{11} + K_{22}W_{22} = 20.556.$$

Since the poles of the filter are given by

$$0.3536 \pm j0.3536,$$

the transformation $\boldsymbol{T}_N$ is given by

$$\boldsymbol{T}_N = \begin{bmatrix} -2.8284 & 0 \\ -1 & 1 \end{bmatrix}.$$

Applying the transformation $\boldsymbol{T}_N$ yields the normal form

$$A_N = \begin{bmatrix} 0.354 & -0.354 \\ 0.354 & 0.354 \end{bmatrix}, \quad b_N = \begin{bmatrix} 0 \\ 1 \end{bmatrix}, \quad c_N = \begin{bmatrix} -4.828 & 2 \end{bmatrix}, \quad d_N = 1.$$

Notice that $a_{11} = a_{22}$. In polar form, c_N is given by

$$c_N = r \begin{bmatrix} \cos(\theta) & \sin(\theta) \end{bmatrix}$$

where

$$r = 5.2263, \quad \theta = -0.3927$$

so that the transformation $R(\theta/2)$ is given by

$$R(\theta/2) = \begin{bmatrix} 0.981 & 0.195 \\ -0.195 & 0.981 \end{bmatrix}.$$

Applying the transformation $R(\theta/2)$ gives

$$\bar{A} = \begin{bmatrix} 0.354 & -0.354 \\ 0.354 & 0.354 \end{bmatrix}, \quad \bar{b} = \begin{bmatrix} -0.195 \\ 0.981 \end{bmatrix}, \quad \bar{c} = \begin{bmatrix} -5.126 & 1.02 \end{bmatrix}, \quad \bar{d} = 1.$$

At this point, we have $b_1 c_1 = b_2 c_2$. Finally, we must l^2-scale the filter. The matrix K which satisfies

$$K = \bar{A} K \bar{A}^T + \bar{b}\bar{b}^T$$

is found as

$$K = \begin{bmatrix} 0.277 & -0.289 \\ -0.289 & 1.056 \end{bmatrix}.$$

Choosing for this example $s = 1$, the scaling transformation T_s is given by

$$T_s = \begin{bmatrix} \sqrt{K_{11}} & 0 \\ 0 & \sqrt{K_{22}} \end{bmatrix} = \begin{bmatrix} 0.526 & 0 \\ 0 & 1.028 \end{bmatrix}.$$

Therefore, the l^2-scaled minimum roundoff noise filter is given by

$$\hat{A} = \begin{bmatrix} 0.354 & -0.691 \\ 0.181 & 0.354 \end{bmatrix}, \quad \hat{b} = \begin{bmatrix} -0.371 \\ 0.954 \end{bmatrix}, \quad \hat{c} = \begin{bmatrix} -2.697 & 1.048 \end{bmatrix}, \quad \hat{d} = 1.$$

For the minimum roundoff noise filter, we find that

$$K = \begin{bmatrix} 1 & -0.534 \\ -0.534 & 1 \end{bmatrix}, \quad W = \begin{bmatrix} 7.99 & -4.266 \\ -4.266 & 7.99 \end{bmatrix}$$

so that the noise gain is given by

$$N = 15.99.$$

In applying the sectional-optimal approach, the filter $H(z)$ is decomposed into a cascade of second-order subfilters. Each second-order transfer function is implemented as a minimum roundoff noise filter, and the overall filter is obtained by cascading these minimum roundoff noise subfilters. As we have already mentioned, this approach is suboptimal and will not result in the minimum possible roundoff noise. Additionally, when the filters are cascaded, all of the states will not be properly l^2-scaled. The reason for this is simple. In isolation, the subfilters *are* properly l^2-scaled. Recall the connection between the computation of the matrix $\boldsymbol{K}$ and the state covariance for a white noise input. When white noise is applied to the individual subfilters, the l^2 bound will hold. However, when in cascade, the noise is "colored" as it passes through one subfilter to another. In practice, the deviation of the l^2 norms of the states will be tolerable.

6.16 A Comparison of Architectures

Consider the filter $H(z)$ where

$$H(z) = d + \frac{q_1 z^{-1} + q_2 z^{-2} + q_3 z^{-3} + q_4 z^{-4} + q_5 z^{-5} + q_6 z^{-6}}{1 + p_1 z^{-1} + p_2 z^{-2} + p_3 z^{-3} + p_4 z^{-4} + p_5 z^{-5} + p_6 z^{-6}}$$

and the coefficients are given by

$$\begin{aligned} q_1 &= 0.0744 & p_1 &= -2.538 \\ q_2 &= -0.0427 & p_2 &= 3.263 \\ q_3 &= 0.0858 & p_3 &= -2.370 \\ q_4 &= 0.0162 & p_4 &= 1.047 \\ q_5 &= 0.0136 & p_5 &= -0.252 \\ q_6 &= 0.0259 & p_6 &= 0.0276 \end{aligned}$$

and

$$d = 0.0266.$$

This transfer function corresponds to a inverse Chebyshev filter with sampling frequency 20000 Hz and a passband from dc to 2000 Hz, and a transition band out to 3500 Hz. The direct-II realization of $H(z)$ is described by the matrices

$$\boldsymbol{A} = \begin{bmatrix} 0 & 1 & 0 & 0 & 0 & 0 \\ 0 & 0 & 1 & 0 & 0 & 0 \\ 0 & 0 & 0 & 1 & 0 & 0 \\ 0 & 0 & 0 & 0 & 1 & 0 \\ 0 & 0 & 0 & 0 & 0 & 1 \\ -p_6 & -p_5 & -p_4 & -p_3 & -p_2 & -p_1 \end{bmatrix}, \quad \boldsymbol{b} = \begin{bmatrix} 0 \\ 0 \\ 0 \\ 0 \\ 0 \\ 1 \end{bmatrix},$$

and

$$c = \begin{bmatrix} q_1 & q_2 & q_3 & q_4 & q_5 & q_6 \end{bmatrix}, \quad d =$$

Using the algorithm for computing $\boldsymbol{K}$ and $\boldsymbol{W}$, we find that

$$\begin{aligned} K_{11} &= 37.69 & W_{11} &= 8.67 \times 10^{-4} \\ K_{22} &= 37.69 & W_{22} &= 0.0153 \\ K_{33} &= 37.69 & W_{33} &= 0.177 \\ K_{44} &= 37.69 & W_{44} &= 0.718 \\ K_{55} &= 37.69 & W_{55} &= 0.758 \\ K_{66} &= 37.69 & W_{66} &= 0.259 \end{aligned}$$

For the direct-II architecture, the noise gain is therefore given by

$$G_N = \sum_{i=1}^{6} K_{ii} W_{ii} = 72.69$$

Notice that the values of K_{ii} are the same for all states in the direct-II filter. This is not surprising, since the shift register contents are all delayed versions of one another. Recall that $\sqrt{K_{ii}}$ gives a bound for the i-th state for unit energy inputs. Thus, for unit energy inputs, $\log_2 \sqrt{K_{ii}} = 2.61$ so that three integer bits should be allocated.

Assuming the filter is l^2-scaled with $s = 1$, the output roundoff noise is given by

$$\sigma^2 = \frac{q^2}{12} G_N.$$

For unit-energy inputs, the scaling ensures that the magnitude of each state within the filter never exceeds 1 for unit-energy inputs. For unit variance white noise inputs, this is a moderately weak approach to bounding the states by unity. A more conservative approach would be to choose s equal to three or four, but we have chosen $s = 1$ for clarity. It should be noted, however, that the filter must first be protected from overflow for the roundoff noise analysis to have any meaning. Continuing with $s = 1$, all of the bits can be allocated to the fractional part of the data so that

$$q = 2^{-B}.$$

The noise gain G_N should be interpreted as a quantity which magnifies the noise power generated by the quantization within the filter. For the direct-II filter, the noise power is amplified by 72.69.

Next, we use the sectional-optimal approach. The transfer function $H(z)$ is decomposed into three order-2 subfilters $H_1(z), H_2(z)$, and $H_3(z)$. The subfilters are given by

$$H_1(z) = 0.497 + \frac{0.448z^{-1} - 0.161z^{-2}}{1 - 0.529z^{-1} + 0.0989z^{-2}},$$

and

$$H_2(z) = 0.318 + \frac{0.201z^{-1} + 0.171z^{-2}}{1 - 0.822z^{-1} + 0.368z^{-2}},$$

and

$$H_3(z) = 0.168 + \frac{0.041z^{-1} + 0.434z^{-2}}{1 - 1.187z^{-1} + 0.758z^{-2}},$$

where the leading numerator coefficient for each section was chosen so that the subfilter has unity gain in the passband. The direct-II state variable representation for $H_1(z)$ is given by the matrices

$$\boldsymbol{A}_1 = \begin{bmatrix} 0 & 1 \\ -0.0989 & 0.529 \end{bmatrix}, \quad \boldsymbol{b}_1 = \begin{bmatrix} 0 \\ 1 \end{bmatrix}, \quad \boldsymbol{c}_1 = \begin{bmatrix} 0.448 & -0.161 \end{bmatrix}, \quad d_1 = 0.497.$$

The matrices $\boldsymbol{K}_1$ and W_1 are found to be equal to

$$\boldsymbol{K}_1 = \begin{bmatrix} 1.313 & 0.632 \\ 0.632 & 1.313 \end{bmatrix}, \quad \boldsymbol{W}_1 = \begin{bmatrix} 0.202 & -0.075 \\ -0.075 & 0.202 \end{bmatrix}.$$

The minimum roundoff noise subfilter is given by

$$\bar{\boldsymbol{A}}_1 = \begin{bmatrix} 0.264 & -0.930 \\ 0.0313 & 0.264 \end{bmatrix}, \quad \bar{\boldsymbol{b}}_1 = \begin{bmatrix} 0.178 \\ 0.965 \end{bmatrix}, \quad \bar{\boldsymbol{c}}_1 = \begin{bmatrix} -0.452 & -0.0833 \end{bmatrix}, \quad \bar{d}_1 = 0.497.$$

The direct-II state variable representation for $H_2(z)$ is given by the matrices

$$\boldsymbol{A}_2 = \begin{bmatrix} 0 & 1 \\ -0.368 & 0.822 \end{bmatrix}, \quad \boldsymbol{b}_2 = \begin{bmatrix} 0 \\ 1 \end{bmatrix}, \quad \boldsymbol{c}_2 = \begin{bmatrix} 0.201 & 0.171 \end{bmatrix}, \quad d_2 = 0.318.$$

The matrices $\boldsymbol{K}_2$ and W_2 are found to be equal to

$$\boldsymbol{K}_2 = \begin{bmatrix} 1.809 & 1.087 \\ 1.087 & 1.809 \end{bmatrix}, \quad \boldsymbol{W}_2 = \begin{bmatrix} 0.068 & -0.0193 \\ -0.0193 & 0.068 \end{bmatrix}.$$

The minimum roundoff noise subfilter is given by

$$\bar{\boldsymbol{A}}_2 = \begin{bmatrix} 0.411 & -0.745 \\ 0.267 & 0.411 \end{bmatrix}, \quad \bar{\boldsymbol{b}}_2 = \begin{bmatrix} -0.211 \\ 0.918 \end{bmatrix}, \quad \bar{\boldsymbol{c}}_2 = \begin{bmatrix} -0.405 & 0.0932 \end{bmatrix}, \quad \bar{d}_2 = 0.318.$$

The direct-II state variable representation for $H_3(z)$ is given by the matrices

$$\boldsymbol{A}_3 = \begin{bmatrix} 0 & 1 \\ -0.758 & 1.187 \end{bmatrix}, \quad \boldsymbol{b}_3 = \begin{bmatrix} 0 \\ 1 \end{bmatrix}, \quad \boldsymbol{c}_3 = \begin{bmatrix} 0.0406 & 0.434 \end{bmatrix}, \quad d_3 = 0.168.$$

The matrices $\boldsymbol{K}_3$ and W_3 are found to be equal to

$$\boldsymbol{K}_3 = \begin{bmatrix} 4.326 & 2.922 \\ 2.922 & 4.326 \end{bmatrix}, \quad \boldsymbol{W}_3 = \begin{bmatrix} 0.534 & -0.464 \\ -0.464 & 0.534 \end{bmatrix}.$$

The minimum roundoff noise subfilter is given by

$$\bar{\boldsymbol{A}}_3 = \begin{bmatrix} 0.594 & -0.661 \\ 0.614 & 0.594 \end{bmatrix}, \quad \bar{\boldsymbol{b}}_3 = \begin{bmatrix} -0.259 \\ 0.636 \end{bmatrix}, \quad \bar{\boldsymbol{c}}_3 = \begin{bmatrix} -0.839 & 0.342 \end{bmatrix}, \quad \bar{d}_3 = 0.168.$$

The minimum roundoff noise subfilters are all properly l^2 scaled, as can be verified by computing $\bar{\boldsymbol{K}}_i$ and $\bar{\boldsymbol{W}}_i$ for each subfilter. Now, we must determine the state variable representation for the cascade combination of subfilters. As we saw earlier,

$$\bar{\boldsymbol{A}} = \begin{bmatrix} \bar{\boldsymbol{A}}_1 & \boldsymbol{O} & \boldsymbol{O} \\ \bar{\boldsymbol{b}}_2\bar{\boldsymbol{c}}_1 & \bar{\boldsymbol{A}}_2 & \boldsymbol{O} \\ \bar{\boldsymbol{b}}_3\bar{d}_2\bar{\boldsymbol{c}}_1 & \bar{\boldsymbol{b}}_3\bar{\boldsymbol{c}}_2 & \bar{\boldsymbol{A}}_3 \end{bmatrix}, \quad \bar{\boldsymbol{b}} = \begin{bmatrix} \bar{\boldsymbol{b}}_1 \\ \bar{\boldsymbol{b}}_2\bar{d}_1 \\ \bar{\boldsymbol{b}}_3\bar{d}_2\bar{d}_1 \end{bmatrix}$$

and

$$\bar{\boldsymbol{c}} = \begin{bmatrix} \bar{d}_3\bar{d}_2\bar{\boldsymbol{c}}_1 & \bar{d}_3\bar{\boldsymbol{c}}_2 & \bar{\boldsymbol{c}}_3 \end{bmatrix}, \quad \bar{d} = \bar{d}_1\bar{d}_2\bar{d}_3.$$

The diagonal elements of the matrix $\bar{\boldsymbol{K}}$ which satisfies

$$\bar{\boldsymbol{K}} = \bar{\boldsymbol{A}}\bar{\boldsymbol{K}}\bar{\boldsymbol{A}}^T + \bar{\boldsymbol{b}}\bar{\boldsymbol{b}}^T$$

are given by

$$\begin{aligned} \bar{K}_{11} &= 1 \\ \bar{K}_{22} &= 1 \\ \bar{K}_{33} &= 0.431 \\ \bar{K}_{44} &= 0.334 \\ \bar{K}_{55} &= 0.239 \\ \bar{K}_{66} &= 0.0912 \end{aligned}$$

showing that the filter is *approximately* l^2-scaled. The diagonal elements of the matrix $\bar{\boldsymbol{W}}$ which satisfies

$$\bar{\boldsymbol{W}} = \bar{\boldsymbol{A}}^T\bar{\boldsymbol{W}}\bar{\boldsymbol{A}} + \bar{\boldsymbol{c}}^T\bar{\boldsymbol{c}}$$

are given by

$$\begin{aligned} \bar{W}_{11} &= 0.198 \\ \bar{W}_{22} &= 0.215 \\ \bar{W}_{33} &= 0.330 \\ \bar{W}_{44} &= 0.450 \\ \bar{W}_{55} &= 1.744 \\ \bar{W}_{66} &= 1.744 \end{aligned}$$

Architecture	Noise Gain G_N
Direct-II	72.69
Cascade	2.17
Parallel	6.36
Lattice-Ladder	1.29
Sectional Optimal	1.28

Table 6.1: Summary of noise gain performance.

Thus, the noise gain of the sectional-optimal filter is given by

$$G_N = \sum_{i=1}^{6} \bar{K}_{ii}\bar{W}_{ii} = 1.281.$$

Notice the substantial improvement over the noise gain for the direct-II filter. To be complete, we should include the contribution to the roundoff noise power induced by the nodes *between* the cascaded sections. It turns out that this is actually a small contribution to the overall noise power.

For purpose of comparison, the same filter was implemented in cascade, parallel, and lattice ladder architectures. The noise gain is summarized in Table 1.

Let's interpret the results of Table 1. Assuming the filter is adequately scaled with $s = 1$, the noise power for the direct-II filter is given by

$$\sigma^2 = \frac{q^2}{12} \cdot 72.69.$$

Suppose 16-bit arithmetic is used. Since the filter is properly scaled, the states are all bounded by unity and we can allocate most of the bits as fractional bits. Because signed data must be represented, 15 bits can be allocated for fractional precision which means that the quantization step size is given by

$$q = 2^{-15}$$

and the noise power is thus given by

$$\sigma^2 = 5.64 \times 10^{-9}.$$

Therefore, the standard deviation of the roundoff noise is

$$\sigma = 7.51 \times 10^{-5}.$$

The number of quantization steps traversed by one standard deviation of roundoff noise is given by

$$\frac{\sigma}{q} = 2.46,$$

and because

$$2^1 < 2.46 < 2^2,$$

roughly two bits of precision are lost to each standard deviation of roundoff noise.

The other filter architectures can be seen to perform considerable better than the direct-II architecture, with the sectional optimal minimum roundoff noise performing the best. At this point, the user needs to consider the tradeoffs of roundoff noise performance and filter complexity. The direct-II implementation has the worst roundoff noise performance, but requires the least amount of computation per filter cycle. This translates into higher throughput so that higher real-time bandwidths can be achieved. The other architectures require many more computations per filter cycle and as such, can not attain the same throughput rate as the direct-II filter. These attributes must be considered in a balanced manner.

Fixed-point DSP processors remain an inexpensive solution to many filtering and signal processing problems. For applications requiring high precision and high throughput, floating-point DSP processors are an attractive technology. At this point in time, floating-point processors are in general more expensive than fixed-point processors, but are frequently the only logical option. It should be noted, however, that floating-point processors suffer from finite wordlength effects of their own. This is due to the fact that the mantissa is typically limited to 24 bits in width. In general, though, the overflow and roundoff noise problems are drastically reduced.

6.17 Coefficient Quantization Effects

Until now, we have not discussed the effects of coefficient quantization on the behavior of a fixed-point filter. In the simplest sense, the quantization errors in the filter coefficients be viewed as altering the pole and zero locations. Geometrically, we have seen how the pole and zero locations determine the filter's magnitude response. Suppose the denominator polynomial is given by

$$A(z) = 1 + \sum_{k=1}^{N} a_k z^{-k}$$

and the quantized coefficients are given by

$$a_k^q = a_k + \Delta a_k$$

where Δa_k is the coefficient quantization error. Let the transfer function of the system be given by

$$H(z) = \frac{B(z)}{A(z)}$$

where $B(z)$ is the numerator polynomial. The error in a given coefficient impacts *all* of the pole locations. Assume that the poles are given by $p_1, p_2, \ldots p_N$ so that

$$A(z) = \prod_{k=1}^{N} (1 - p_k z^{-1}).$$

The denominator polynomial of the quantized system is given by

$$A^q(z) = 1 + \sum_{k=1}^{N} a_k^q z^{-k}$$

and suppose the roots of $A^q(z)$ are denoted by $p_k^q = p_k + \Delta p_k$. The errors in the roots must be related somehow to the coefficient errors. To this end, the error in each pole location can be expressed as

$$\Delta p_n = \sum_{k=1}^{N} \frac{\partial p_n}{\partial a_k} \Delta a_k, \quad n = 1, 2, \ldots, N. \tag{6.17.1}$$

In order to make use of Eq. 6.17.1, let's rewrite $A(z)$ in terms of z in two different ways:

$$A(z) = z^N + a_1 z^{N-1} + \cdots + a_{N-1} z + a_N \tag{6.17.2}$$

and

$$A(z) = (z - p_1)(z - p_2) \cdots (z - p_N). \tag{6.17.3}$$

Taking the derivative of Eq. 6.17.2 with respect to a_k gives

$$\frac{\partial A(z)}{\partial a_k} = z^{N-k}. \tag{6.17.4}$$

Taking the derivative of Eq. 6.17.3 with respect to p_n gives

$$\frac{\partial A(z)}{\partial p_n} = -\prod_{j \neq n} (z - p_j). \tag{6.17.5}$$

Application of the chain rule yields

$$\frac{\partial A(z)}{\partial a_k} = \frac{\partial A(z)}{\partial p_n}\frac{\partial p_n}{\partial a_k}. \tag{6.17.6}$$

Equations 6.17.4 and 6.17.5 may be substituted into Eq. 6.17.6, from which it follows that

$$\frac{\partial p_n}{\partial a_k} = -\frac{p_n^{N-k}}{\prod_{k \neq n}(p_n - p_k)}. \tag{6.17.7}$$

Equation 6.17.7 can be substituted into Eq. 6.17.1 to determine the overall change in a given pole due to all of the coefficient perturbations. Examining Eq. 6.17.7, it can be seen qualitatively that the pole locations are particularly sensitive to coefficient perturbations when the poles are tightly clustered (as is the case for narrowband filters). This further illustrates why the filter should be decomposed into second-order subfilters: the pole perturbations will be smaller for $N = 2$, especially since the poles can be isolated between subfilters so they are not as proximate *within* subfilters. The same analysis can be performed for the filter zeros.

The analysis we have just presented does not provide a clear picture of the distortion induced on the magnitude response. In practice, this is easily measured experimentally by simply quantizing the coefficients and plotting the frequency response. For FIR filters, the analysis is more straightforward. As a rule of thumb, the zeros of a linear-phase FIR are not tightly clustered in the complex plane and are hence less vulnerable to coefficient perturbations. Analytically, suppose the FIR has $N+1$ coefficients h_k and the coefficients are perturbed by Δh_k. The perturbed coefficients are thus given by

$$\boldsymbol{h}_k^q = h_k + \Delta h_k.$$

Therefore, the perturbed magnitude response is given by

$$H^q(e^{j\theta}) = H(e^{j\theta}) + \Delta H(e^{j\theta})$$

where

$$\Delta H(e^{j\theta}) = \sum_{k=0}^{N} \Delta h_k e^{-jk\theta}.$$

The magnitude of $\Delta H(e^{j\theta})$ is easily bounded:

$$|\Delta H(e^{j\theta})| \leq \sum_{k=0}^{N} |\Delta h_k||e^{-jk\theta}| = \sum_{k=0}^{N} |\Delta h_k|.$$

Therefore, if the perturbations are bounded by ϵ (for a B-bit representation, $|\epsilon| < 2^{-B}$),

$$|\Delta H(e^{j\theta})| < (N+1)\epsilon.$$

The magnitude distortion is thus easily analyzed and can be controlled by sufficiently large wordwidth B.

Chapter 7

MULTIRATE SIGNAL PROCESSING

7.1 Introduction

Multirate signal processing is an area which has received a tremendous amount of attention in recent years, both in the literature and in practice. As the name implies, multirate signal processing is concerned with systems in which there are several sampling rates. We will see that there are a number of advantages to using multirate systems, including signal quality and decreased system cost. These are advantages which have been widely exploited in the area of commercial electronics.

We will study the fundamental operations of multirate signal processing: decimation and interpolation, whereby the sampling rate of a discrete-time signal is decreased or increased, respectively, entirely in the discrete-time domain. We will study a mathematical tool known as the polyphase decomposition which greatly simplifies the analysis of decimation and interpolation and allows us to derive efficient structures to perform these operations. We will also study an important class of multirate filter known as the *quadrature mirror filter* (QMF). The QMF will be seen to be an important building block for many multirate systems.

Another field which is closely related to multirate systems is time-varying spectral analysis, which has also received a flurry of attention recently. We will study both the short-time Fourier transform (STFT) and the wavelet transform, which have shown great promise for the analysis of signals whose spectral content vary with time. In particular, we will examine the connection between multirate filter banks, the STFT, and the discrete-time wavelet transform (DTWT).

7.2 The Polyphase Decomposition

The M-component polyphase decomposition [BBC76] provides a convenient representation of $X(z)$ which will be very useful when discussing decimation, interpolation, and changing the sampling rate by a non-integer ratio.

Suppose $\boldsymbol{x}$ is a signal with $\mathcal{Z}$-transform

$$X(z) = \sum_{k=-\infty}^{\infty} x(k)z^{-k}.$$

Our end goal is to find a convenient expression for the $\mathcal{Z}$-transform of $\boldsymbol{x}$ when the sampling rate is either increased or decreased by a factor of M. As a first step, we can break the signal into a disjoint collection of elements whose indices are separated by M. To this end, rewrite $X(z)$ as

$$\begin{aligned} X(z) = & \cdots + x(0) + x(M)z^{-M} + x(2M)z^{-2M} + \cdots \\ & \cdots + x(1)z^{-1} + x(M+1)z^{-(M+1)} + x(2M+1)z^{-(2M+1)} + \cdots \\ & \cdots + x(2)z^{-2} + x(M+2)z^{-(M+2)} + x(2M+2)z^{-(2M+2)} + \cdots \\ & \cdots \\ & \cdots + x(M-1)z^{-(M-1)} + x(2M-1)z^{-(2M-1)} + x(3M-1)z^{-(3M-1)} + \cdots \end{aligned}$$

We next proceed by factoring z^{-i} from the i-th row of the above set of equations, which gives

$$\begin{aligned} X(z) = & \cdots + x(0) + x(M)z^{-M} + x(2M)z^{-2M} + \cdots \\ & z^{-1}(\cdots + x(1) + x(M+1)z^{-M} + x(2M+1)z^{-2M} + \cdots) \\ & z^{-2}(\cdots + x(2) + x(M+2)z^{-M} + x(2M+2)z^{-2M} + \cdots) \\ & \cdots \\ & z^{-(M-1)}(\cdots + x(M-1) + x(2M-1)z^{-2M} + x(3M-1)z^{-3M} + \cdots). \end{aligned} \tag{7.2.1}$$

The i-th row of this expression can be written as

$$z^{-i} \sum_{k=-\infty}^{\infty} x(kM+i)(z^M)^{-k}. \tag{7.2.2}$$

The summation in Eq. 7.2.2 is simply the $\mathcal{Z}$-transform of the elements of $\boldsymbol{x}$ which are separated by M. If we define the polyphase component $P_i(z)$ by

$$P_i(z) = \sum_{k=-\infty}^{\infty} x(kM+i)z^{-k} \tag{7.2.3}$$

and substitute Eq. 7.2.3 into Eq. 7.2.2, we have

$$z^{-i} \sum_{k=-\infty}^{\infty} x(kM+i)(z^M)^{-k} = z^{-i}P_i(z^M).$$

Finally, from Eq. 7.2.1, we have

$$X(z) = P_0(z^M) + z^{-1}P_1(z^M) + z^{-2}P_2(z^M) + \cdots + z^{-(M-1)}P_{M-1}(z^M),$$

which gives the M-component polyphase decomposition

$$X(z) = \sum_{i=0}^{M-1} z^{-i}P_i(z^M). \tag{7.2.4}$$

Example 7.1

Let $X(z)$ be the simple FIR transfer function

$$X(z) = 1 + 2z^{-1} + 1z^{-2} + 3z^{-3}.$$

If we wish to perform a two-component polyphase decomposition, $X(z)$ can be decomposed as

$$X(z) = (1 + z^{-2}) + (2z^{-1} + 3z^{-3})$$

Factoring z^{-1} from the second term, we have

$$X(z) = (1 + z^{-2}) + z^{-1}(2 + 3z^{-2}).$$

If $P_0(z)$ and $P_1(z)$ are defined by

$$P_0(z) = 1 + z^{-1}$$

and

$$P_1(z) = 2 + 3z^{-1},$$

it follows that

$$X(z) = P_0(z^2) + z^{-1}P_1(z^2).$$

The polyphase decomposition expressed by Eq. 7.2.4 will prove to be very useful for deriving computationally efficient structures for decimation (sampling rate reduction). A slight variation of Eq. 7.2.4 results if we define the transposed polyphase components $Q_i(z)$ by

$$Q_i(z) = P_{M-1-i}(z), \quad i = 0, 1, \ldots, M-1. \tag{7.2.5}$$

In this case, the transposed polyphase decomposition is given by

$$X(z) = \sum_{i=0}^{M-1} z^{-(M-1-i)}Q_i(z^M). \tag{7.2.6}$$

This transposed polyphase representation will be used to derive efficient structures for interpolation (increasing the sampling rate). Block diagrams for both the ordinary and transposed polyphase representations are shown in Fig. 7.2.1.

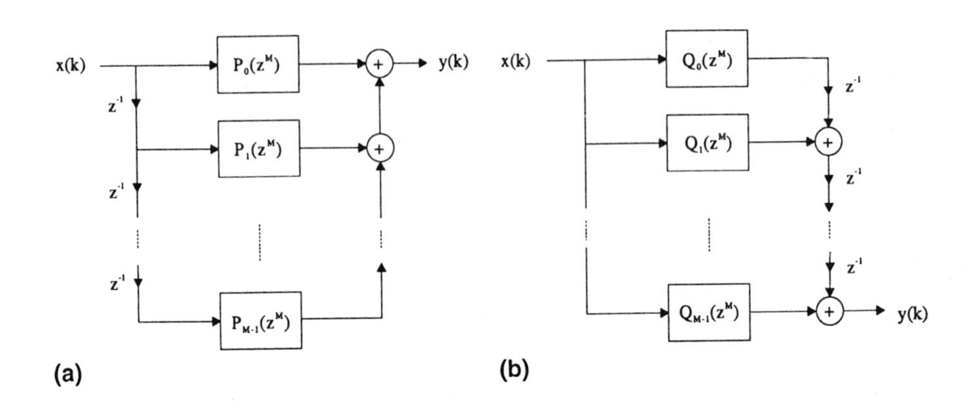

Figure 7.2.1: (a) Ordinary polyphase decomposition; (b) transposed polyphase decomposition.

7.3 Decimation

Suppose we have a sampled version of an analog signal which has a sampling rate which is too high. This can arise for a number of reasons. For instance, the data may have been sampled by a data acquisition system which has a fixed sampling rate, or we may wish to examine the spectral content of the signal over a range of frequencies which is much lower than half the sampling frequency. For reasons of data storage or real-time bandwidth requirements, it may be necessary to lower the sampling rate of the signal. One solution is to convert the signal back to analog and then resample at the new rate. Another solution, which is much more practical, is to perform the sampling rate conversion in the discrete-time domain.

Decimation is the process of reducing the sampling rate by an integer factor, M. In the discrete-time domain, decimation of a signal $\boldsymbol{x}$ by M is performed by discarding all but every M-th sample of $\boldsymbol{h}$. If we denote the decimated signal by $\boldsymbol{x}_d$, it follows that

$$x_d(k) = x(Mk).$$

In other words, only every M-th sample of the original signal is retained. Using the polyphase decomposition, let's obtain an expression for the $\mathcal{Z}$-transform of $\boldsymbol{x}_d$. To begin, we wish to find the value of the summation

$$X_d(z) = \sum_{k=-\infty}^{\infty} x_d(k) z^{-k}.$$

But this is equivalent to

$$X_d(z) = \sum_{k=-\infty}^{\infty} x(Mk)z^{-k}.$$

According to Eq. 7.2.3, however, this is simply the first component of the polyphase decomposition of $X(z)$ so that

$$X_d(z) = P_0(z).$$

Define the *principal M-th root of unity*, W_M by $W_M = e^{-j2\pi/M}$ (this should be familiar from the FFT). Now, consider the expression

$$\sum_{k=0}^{M-1} X(W_M^k z).$$

This expression is the key to evaluating the $\mathcal{Z}$-transform of $x_d(k)$ if we utilize the polyphase decomposition for $X(z)$. Remember from Eq. 7.2.4 that

$$X(z) = \sum_{i=0}^{M-1} z^{-i} P_i(z^M).$$

Thus,

$$\sum_{k=0}^{M-1} X(W_M^k z) = \sum_{k=0}^{M-1} \left(\sum_{i=0}^{M-1} (W_M^k z)^{-i} P_i((W_M^k z)^M) \right). \tag{7.3.1}$$

Because $W_M^{kM} = 1$ for all k, Eq. 7.3.1 can be rewritten as

$$\sum_{k=0}^{M-1} X(W_M^k z) = \sum_{k=0}^{M-1} \left(\sum_{i=0}^{M-1} W_M^{-ik} z^{-i} P_i(z^M) \right). \tag{7.3.2}$$

Reversing the order of summation in Eq. 7.3.2 gives

$$\sum_{k=0}^{M-1} X(W_M^k z) = \sum_{i=0}^{M-1} z^{-i} P_i(z^M) \sum_{k=0}^{M-1} W_M^{-ik}. \tag{7.3.3}$$

Recall from our discussion of the FFT that

$$\sum_{k=0}^{M-1} W_M^{-ik} = M\delta(i)$$

and hence Eq. 7.3.3 becomes

$$\sum_{k=0}^{M-1} X(W_M^k z) = \sum_{i=0}^{M-1} z^{-i} P_i(z^M) M\delta(i),$$

which gives

$$\sum_{k=0}^{M-1} X(W_M^k z) = M P_0(z^M). \tag{7.3.4}$$

Therefore, we conclude that

$$P_0(z^M) = \frac{1}{M} \sum_{k=0}^{M-1} X(W_M^k z). \tag{7.3.5}$$

Since it's $P_0(z)$ we want, Eq. 7.3.5 evaluated at $z^{1/M}$ gives

$$X_d(z) = P_0(z) = \frac{1}{M} \sum_{k=0}^{M-1} X(W_M^k z^{1/M}). \tag{7.3.6}$$

Example 7.2

Let $h(k) = a^k u(k)$, so that

$$X(z) = \frac{1}{1 - az^{-1}}.$$

We will decimate the signal by $M = 2$, giving

$$x(k) = h(2k).$$

We can evaluate $X_d(z)$ directly using

$$X_d(z) = \sum_{k=0}^{\infty} a^{2k} z^{-k} = \sum_{k=-\infty}^{\infty} (a^2)^k z^{-k}.$$

Thus,

$$X_d(z) = \frac{1}{1 - a^2 z^{-1}}.$$

Next, we can obtain the same expression using Eq. 7.3.6. In this case, $W_2 = -1$ so that Eq. 7.3.6 reduces to

$$X_d(z) = \frac{1}{2}(X(z^{1/2}) + X(-z^{1/2}))$$

which gives

$$X_d(z) = \frac{1}{2}\left(\frac{1}{1 - az^{-1/2}} + \frac{1}{1 + az^{-1/2}}\right).$$

Simplifying, we have

$$X_d(z) = \frac{1}{1 - a^2 z^{-1}},$$

which is what we expected.

Now that we have an expression for the $\mathcal{Z}$-transform of a decimated signal in terms of the $\mathcal{Z}$-transform of the original signal, we need a similar expression for the DTFT. Equation 7.3.6 gives

$$X_d(e^{j\theta}) = \frac{1}{M}\sum_{k=0}^{M-1} X(e^{j(\theta/M - 2\pi k/M)}). \tag{7.3.7}$$

Hence, the spectrum of the decimated signal consists of a sum of frequency-scaled and shifted copies of $X(e^{j\theta})$ (because $X(e^{j(\theta/M-2\pi k/M)})$ is simply $X(e^{j\theta})$ scaled in frequency by M and shifted by $2\pi k$). To interpret Eq. 7.3.7, we can make an appeal to common sense. Decimating $x(k)$ consists of discarding all but every M-th sample. This can be interpreted in the context of sampling the analog signal as an *undersampling* of $x_c(t)$. Therefore, decimating $x(k)$ by M will produce the same collection of samples as if $x_c(t)$ had been sampled at a rate M times lower, and we can expect aliasing to occur if the decimation rate M is too large.

Recall that if $x_c(t)$ is bandlimited to ω_N, it must be sampled at a frequency ω_s such that

$$\omega_s > 2\omega_N.$$

Decimating by M is equivalent to sampling the analog signal $h_c(t)$ at the new sampling frequency

$$\omega_s' = \omega_s/M.$$

To avoid aliasing, it is still necessary that

$$\omega_s' = \omega_s/M > 2\omega_N.$$

Thus, the maximum allowable decimation rate satisfies

$$M < \frac{\pi}{\omega_N T}.$$

In terms of θ, we thus have

$$M < \frac{\pi}{\theta_N}.$$

Therefore, the ratio of the digital frequency, θ_N to the Nyquist frequency, $\theta = \pi$, determines the maximum decimation.

We will now show how the same result can be obtained using only discrete-time signals. Equation 7.3.7 states that the DTFT of the decimated signal, $x(k)$, consists of a sum of shifted copies of $X(e^{j\theta})$ which have been frequency-scaled by M. Figure 7.3.1 shows this for the case $M = 2$. Referring to this figure, if the shifted components of the summation do not overlap, there will be no aliasing. The lower edge of the shifted copy is given by

$$\theta_l = 2\pi - \theta_N/M.$$

The upper edge of the baseband copy is given by

$$\theta_u = \theta_N/M.$$

For there to be no aliasing, we require that

$$\omega_u > \omega_l,$$

which gives

$$M < \frac{\pi}{\theta_N}.$$

This is the same result we obtained using the analog signal argument. In other words, if we wish to decimate a discrete-time signal $\boldsymbol{x}$ by a factor M, the bandwidth of $\boldsymbol{x}$ must satisfy

$$\theta_N < \frac{\pi}{M}$$

if no aliasing is to be introduced. If only the low frequency information is significant, the signal $\boldsymbol{x}$ can be lowpass-filtered to limit the signal to a bandwidth of π/M. Then decimation can be performed.

Example 7.3

Suppose $x_c(t)$ is an analog signal with bandwidth $\omega_N = 1000$ rad/s. Assume that the signal has been sampled at $\omega_s = 4000$. Then

$$\theta_N = \omega_N T = 1000\frac{2\pi}{4000} = \frac{\pi}{2}.$$

Therefore, the signal can be decimated by a factor of at most $M = 2$. Suppose, however, that we are only interested in the spectral content of the signal between d.c. and 200 rad/s. Then the discrete-time signal can first be bandlimited to 200 rad/s by lowpass-filtering in discrete time by a lowpass filter with cutoff frequency

$$\theta_c = 200\frac{2\pi}{4000} = \pi/10.$$

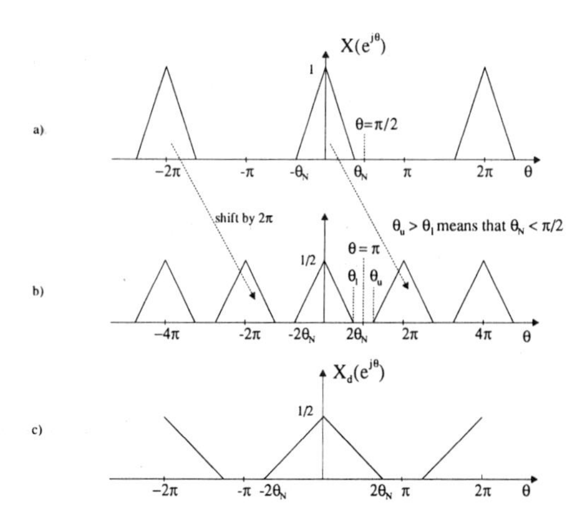

Figure 7.3.1: (a) $X(e^{j\theta})$; (b) frequency-shifted copies of $X(e^{j\theta})$ which are summed to produce $X_d(e^{j\theta})$; (c) $X_d(e^{j\theta})$.

Upon exiting the lowpass filter, the signal will be bandlimited to $\pi/10$ so that decimation by $M = 10$ can be tolerated without introducing any aliasing. Notice that the original sampling rate is T so that $\theta = \pi$ corresponds to the analog frequency $\omega = \pi/T = 2000$ rad/s. After decimation by M, the new sampling rate is MT so that $\theta = \pi$ corresponds to the analog frequency $\omega = \pi/(MT) = 200$ rad/s.

An additional benefit of decimation in this case is that it will increase the resolution of an FFT. If we were interested in the baseband spectral content of the signal, the resolution of an N-point FFT would be

$$\Delta\omega = \frac{4000}{N}.$$

After decimation, however, the resolution of an N-point FFT is increased to

$$\Delta\omega = \frac{400}{N}.$$

Thus, with the same computational complexity, we achieve a ten-fold increase in frequency resolution.

Another significant byproduct of decimation is reduced computational burden on the digital hardware. For instance, consider the previous example. After decimation by $M = 10$, it may be necessary to process the signal further, such as computing FFTs or correlation. If it is necessary that these computations occur in real-time, it will now be simpler since the data rate has been decreased by a factor of 10. Additionally, if a signal can be decimated by a factor of M and the relevant information in the signal preserved, significant data compression can be achieved. This is important in applications where it is difficult to transmit data at high rates (*i.e.*, limited channel capacity).

For certain bandpass signals, it is still possible to perform decimation without introducing any aliasing. In fact, decimation may be used to bring the signal to baseband without the need for any modulation. Consider the spectrum shown in Fig. 7.3.2a. It is assumed that the spectrum is nonzero only in the range

$$\frac{k\pi}{M} \leq |\theta| \leq \frac{(k+1)\pi}{M}$$

where M is the decimation rate and k is a positive integer. If this restriction is not met, the signal must be bandpass filtered to eliminate any signal energy outside this range. It is fairly simple to show that decimation by M results in the spectrum in Fig. 7.3.2b for k even and in Fig. 7.3.2c for k odd. For k odd there is a reflection of the spectrum which can be put back into the correct orientation if the decimated signal is multiplied by the sequence $(-1)^k$. To see how this happens, suppose that $x(k)$ is bandlimited to the range $k\pi/M \leq |\theta| \leq (k+1)\pi/M$ and we decimate by M. Then the spectrum of the decimated signal $x_d(k)$ consists of a sum of frequency-shifted copies of $X(e^{j\theta/M})$. But $X(e^{j\theta/M})$ is a frequency-scaled version of $X(e^{j\theta})$ and hence is non-zero only over the range $k\pi \leq |\theta| \leq (k+1)\pi$, with a width equal to π. Consequently, the frequency-shifted images will not overlap, and only one of the frequency-shifted images will occupy the baseband.

Structures for decimation

The paradigm for decimation which we have just discussed requires that the signal first be bandlimited by lowpass filtering, and then decimated. Consider the FIR decimation system shown in Fig. 7.3.3. This system consists of an FIR of length N followed by a decimator of rate M. The system only needs to compute the output samples $y(kM)$. Because the FIR precedes the decimator, however, we require that N multiplications be performed during the clock cycle when $y(kM)$ is being computed in order to maintain real-time data flow. During the other clock cycles, the system is idle. This is clearly a waste of computational resources. This problem can be rectified in an elegant and simple manner using the polyphase decomposition.

Let $H(z)$ be a rational transfer function. Consider the two systems in Fig. 7.3.4. The first of these systems consists of a decimator of rate M followed by $H(z)$. The second system consists of $H(z^M)$ followed by a decimator of rate M. We claim that these systems are equivalent. To prove this, we derive the transfer function of the first system. According to Eq. 7.3.6, if the input to the decimator has $\mathcal{Z}$-transform $X(z)$ then the output of the

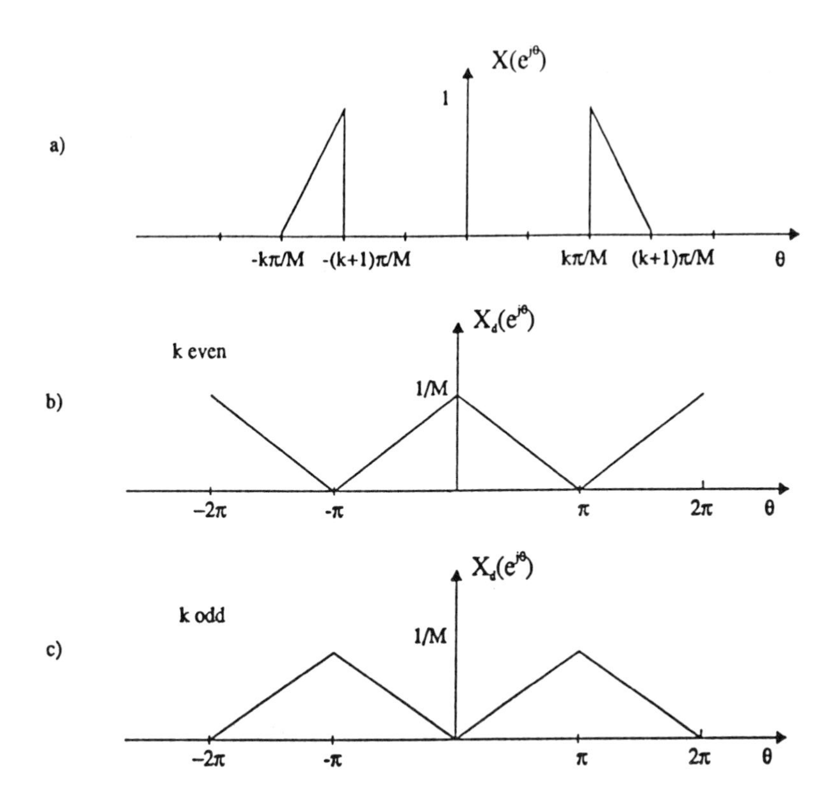

Figure 7.3.2: (a) Bandpass signal; (b) spectrum of decimated signal for k even; (c) spectrum of decimated signal for k odd.

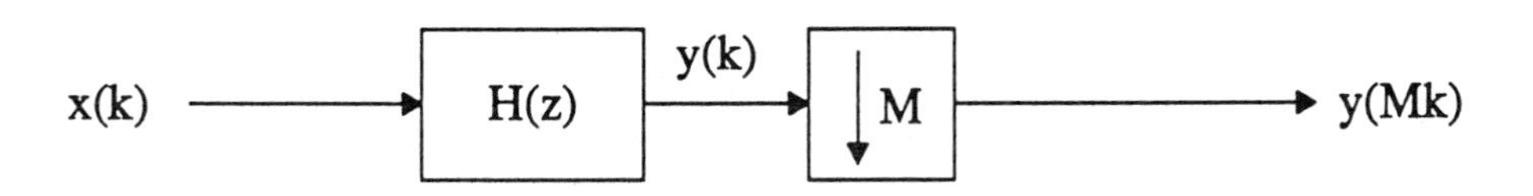

Figure 7.3.3: One possible structure for a FIR decimation filter.

decimator has a $\mathcal{Z}$-transform given by

$$X_d(z) = \sum_{k=0}^{M-1} X(z^{1/M} W_M^k).$$

Therefore, the output of the first system, $y_1(k)$, has $\mathcal{Z}$-transform

$$Y_1(z) = \sum_{k=0}^{M-1} H(z) X(z^{1/M} W_M^k).$$

Now, look at the second system. The output of $H(z^M)$ has $\mathcal{Z}$-transform $H(z^M)X(z)$. Thus, the $\mathcal{Z}$-transform of the output of the decimator is obtained by substituting $H(z^M)X(z)$ into Eq. 7.3.6, which gives

$$Y_2(z) = \frac{1}{M} \sum_{k=0}^{M-1} H((z^{1/M} W_M^k)^M) X(z^{1/M} W_M^k),$$

which, because $W_M^{kM} = 1$, becomes

$$Y_2(z) = \frac{1}{M} \sum_{k=0}^{M-1} H(z) X(z^{1/M} W_M^k).$$

Thus, $Y_1(z) = Y_2(z)$ and the systems are equivalent.

Clearly, the first system in Fig. 7.3.4 is more efficient than the second. The transfer function $H(z^M)$, although of higher degree than $H(z)$, will have the *same number of nonzero coefficients* as $H(z)$. Thus, $H(z^M)$ requires the same number of multiplications per cycle as $H(z)$. Notice, however, that the data rate is much higher for the configuration in which filtering is performed before decimation. If the filter is *preceded* by the decimator, the data arrives at the filter at a data rate which is M times slower.

To see how this result can be used to derive an efficient structure for decimation, assume we wish to filter by $H(z)$ and then decimate by M as in Fig. 7.3.3. According to Eq. 7.2.4, $H(z)$ has the polyphase decomposition given by

$$H(z) = \sum_{i=0}^{M-1} z^{-i} P_i(z^M).$$

Thus, one possible structure for the decimation/filtering system is given in Fig. 7.3.5a. An equivalent structure can be built using the identity we just derived: filtering by $P_i(z^M)$ then decimating by M is equivalent to decimating by M then filtering by $P_i(z)$. Therefore, we can replace the polyphase filters $P_i(z^M)$ with the filters $P_i(z)$ and decimate after the filters, as shown in Fig. 7.3.5b. When $H(z)$ is FIR of length N, the polyphase components will

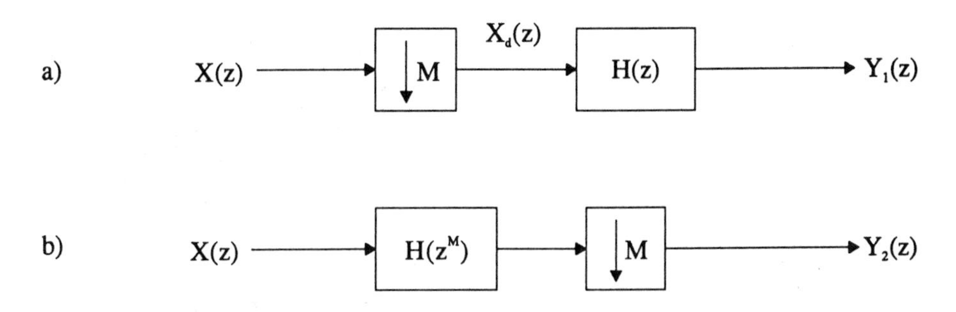

Figure 7.3.4: Equivalent systems for decimation.

each have at most N/M nonzero multiplications so that the new architecture will require a total of $(N/M)M = N$ multiplications per output sample. However, the input to the filters arrives at $1/M$ the clock speed. Thus, the computational complexity has been reduced by a factor of M.

Example 7.4

Suppose $H(z) = 2 + 3z^{-1} + 3z^{-2} + 2z^{-3}$. We wish to filter by $H(z)$ and decimate by $M = 2$. Then

$$H(z) = P_0(z^2) + z^{-1}P_1(z^2)$$

where $P_0(z) = 2 + 3z^{-1}$ and $P_1(z) = 3 + 2z^{-1}$. If filtering is performed prior to decimation, we have the system shown in Fig. 7.3.6a (notice the delay elements are described by z^{-2}). Because P_0 and P_1 are both second-order, this configuration requires that four multiplies be performed per unit time. If, instead, the configuration in Fig. 7.3.6b is used, these four multiplies can be performed in *twice* the time.

Consider again the reduced-complexity decimation structure in Fig. 7.3.5b for the particular case $M = 3$. Let's analyze the data flow at the input to each decimator. The table below illustrates the situation.

Vertical columns correspond to the inputs to the decimators at each instant in time. Every third column of data actually gets to the filters $P_i(z)$ because of the decimators. If every third column is read from the bottom up, we can see that each data sample is sent

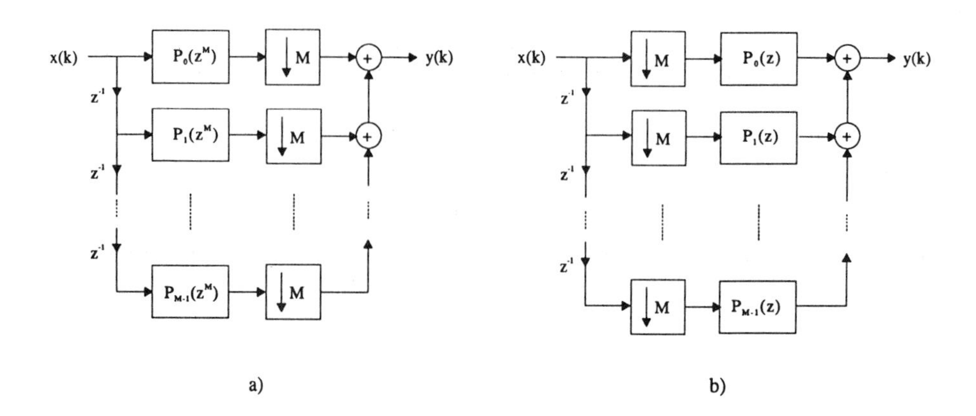

Figure 7.3.5: (a) Decimation followed by filtering; (b) simplified decimation structure.

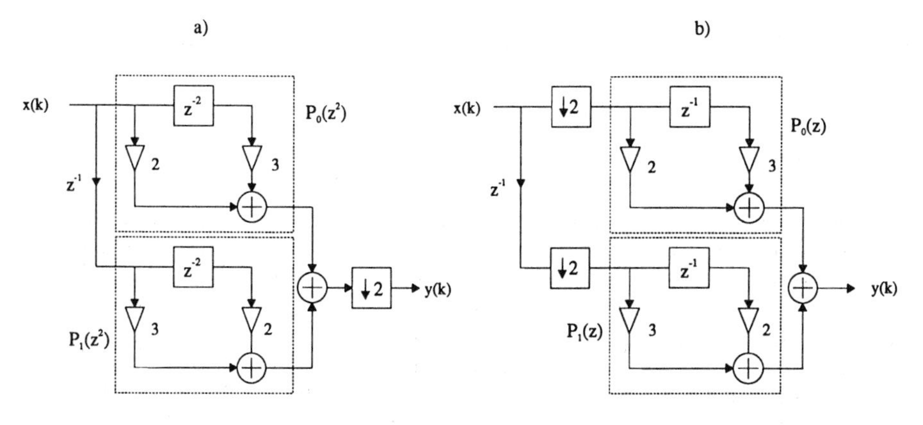

Figure 7.3.6: Decimation structures for Example 7.4.

	$k=0$	$k=1$	$k=2$	$k=3$	$k=4$	$k=5$	$k=6$	$k=7$	$k=8$
Tap 0	$x(0)$	$x(1)$	$x(2)$	$x(3)$	$x(4)$	$x(5)$	$x(6)$	$x(7)$	$x(8)$
Tap 1		$x(0)$	$x(1)$	$x(2)$	$x(3)$	$x(4)$	$x(5)$	$x(6)$	$x(7)$
Tap 2			$x(0)$	$x(1)$	$x(2)$	$x(3)$	$x(4)$	$x(5)$	$x(6)$

to *one and only one* of the filters $P_i(z)$. In general, this process can be realized using the *commutator* structure as shown in Fig. 7.3.7. Beginning with $x(0)$ being fed to the filter $P_0(z)$, subsequent samples are delivered to the remaining filters by a commutator which rotates counterclockwise, moving from one filter to the next for each sample at the original sample rate T. The commutator structure gives a clear conceptual picture of how data should be addressed and filtered in order to actually implement the decimation filter. If $H(z)$ is an FIR of length N, then each $P_i(z)$ will have length N/M. Examining the commutator structure, filtering by each $P_i(z)$ requires N/M multiplications to be performed before a new sample arrives every M cycles. Thus, the computational complexity for each $P_i(z)$ is N/M^2 multiplications per cycle, for a total of N/M multiplications per filter cycle.

7.4 Interpolation

Interpolation is the inverse operation of decimation. By interpolation, we are trying to generate intermediate samples of a discrete-time signal, $x(k)$. This corresponds to increasing the sampling rate. One approach to interpolation would be to reconstruct the analog signal $x_c(t)$ from the samples $x(k)$ and then resample at a higher rate. This does not need to be done, however. Interpolation can be performed entirely in the discrete-time domain, as we will see.

Given an interpolation rate which is an integer, M, define the signal $x_e(k)$ by

$$x_e(k) = \begin{cases} x(k/M), & k = 0, \pm 1, \pm 2, \ldots \\ 0, & \text{otherwise} \end{cases} \tag{7.4.1}$$

The signal $x_e(k)$ is derived from $x(k)$ by *zero-filling* which is also known as *sampling rate expanding*. That is, between every sample of $x(k)$, we insert $M-1$ zeros to form $x_e(k)$. This is shown in Fig. 7.4.1. In order to maintain the same time-scale, the sampling rate at this point is increased by a factor of M.

Another useful expression for $x_e(k)$ is

$$x_e(k) = \sum_{n=-\infty}^{\infty} x(n)\delta(k - nM). \tag{7.4.2}$$

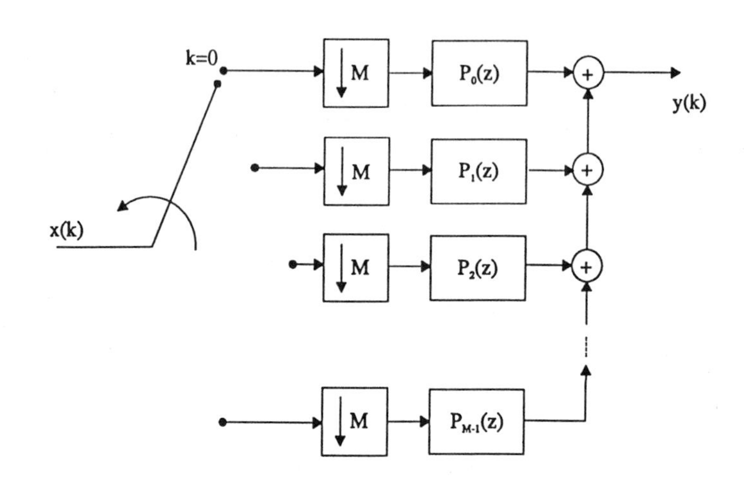

Figure 7.3.7: Commutator structure for decimation.

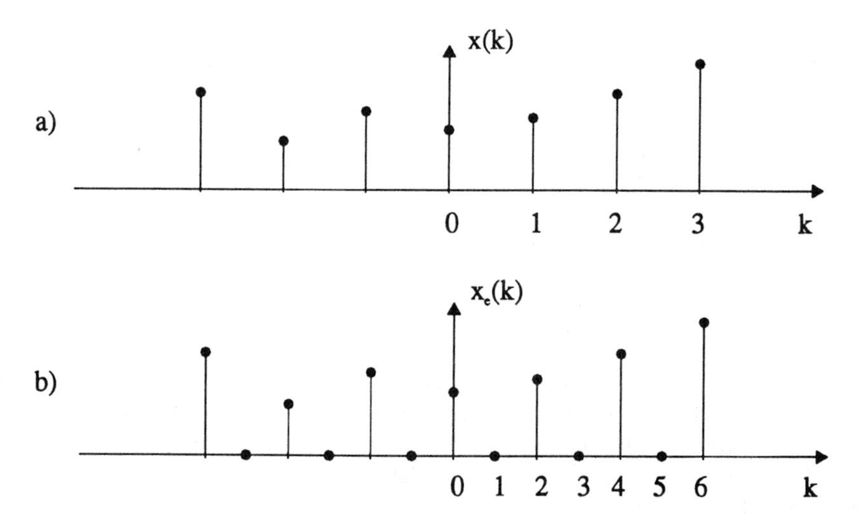

Figure 7.4.1: Sampling rate expansion of a signal $x(k)$.

Taking the $\mathcal{Z}$-transform of Eq. 7.4.2, we find that

$$X_e(z) = \sum_{k=-\infty}^{\infty} z^{-k} \left(\sum_{n=-\infty}^{\infty} x(n)\delta(k-nM) \right). \tag{7.4.3}$$

Reversing the order of summation of Eq. 7.4.3,

$$X_e(z) = \sum_{n=-\infty}^{\infty} x(n) \sum_{k=-\infty}^{\infty} z^{-k}\delta(k-nM) = \sum_{n=-\infty}^{\infty} x(n)z^{-nM}$$

which simply becomes

$$X_e(z) = \sum_{n=-\infty}^{\infty} x(n)(z^M)^{-n}$$

so that

$$X_e(z) = X(z^M). \tag{7.4.4}$$

The corresponding DTFT relationship is

$$X_e(e^{j\theta}) = X(e^{jM\theta}) \tag{7.4.5}$$

which states that the DTFT of the zero-filled signal is equal to the DTFT of the original signal, frequency-scaled by M. This is shown in Fig. 7.4.2b.

Now, suppose $x_e(k)$ is passed through an ideal lowpass filter $h_{LP}(k)$ with cutoff frequency π/M and gain M. Define the *interpolated* signal $x_i(k)$ by

$$x_i(k) = h_{LP}(k) * x_e(k).$$

This has the effect of removing all of the content of $X_e(e^{j\theta})$ between $\theta = \pi/M$ and $\theta = \pi$ and changing the amplitude of the spectrum by a factor of M. Referring to Fig. 7.4.2 it is clear that $X_i(e^{j\theta})$ is the spectrum of a sampled version of $x_c(t)$. Because the frequency ω_N now corresponds to $\theta = \theta_N/M$, the sampling rate for this signal must have been

$$T' = \frac{\theta_N/M}{\omega_N} = \frac{T}{M}.$$

Thus, the elements of $x_i(k)$ are given by

$$x_i(k) = x_c(kT/M).$$

The derivation we just gave is based on frequency-domain arguments. This does not, however, provide any feel for how the intermediate samples of the signal $x_c(t)$ were computed

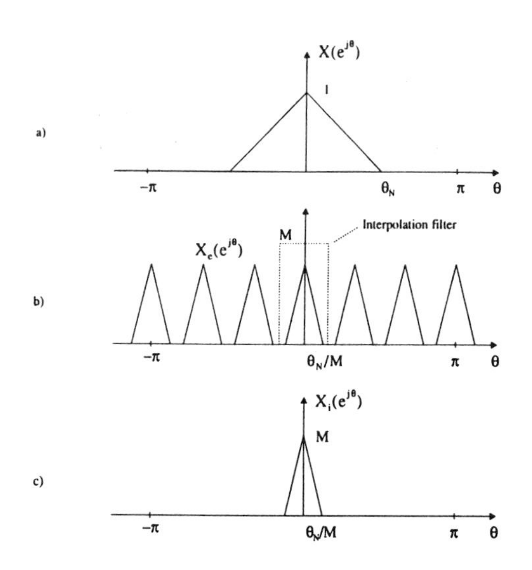

Figure 7.4.2: (a) DTFT of original signal; (b) DTFT of expanded signal; (c) DTFT of interpolated signal.

entirely from the signal $x(k)$ without analog reconstruction and resampling. First, $x_e(k)$ was created from $x(k)$ by decreasing the time between samples from T to T/M and inserting zeros between the samples of $x(k)$. Next, $x_i(k)$ is generated according to

$$x_i(k) = h_{LP}(k) * x_e(k).$$

Because h_{LP} is an ideal lowpass filter with cutoff frequency π/M, we have

$$x_i(k) = \sum_{i=-\infty}^{\infty} \frac{\sin(\pi/M(k-i))}{\pi(k-i)}.$$

That is, the samples of the ideal lowpass filter serve to "interpolate" between the samples of $x(k)$. In reality, however, the ideal lowpass filter is noncausal. Thus, we must resort to an approximation of the ideal lowpass filter for interpolation. From our frequency domain argument, this will still produce acceptable results.

Decimation of a signal served to decrease the computational burden of signal processing systems and achieve data compression. Why then would we want to perform interpolation? The answer is that interpolation can greatly simplify the design of the analog components of a signal processing system. Because analog components tend to be expensive and digital components inexpensive, it is frequently worthwhile to increase the computational burden of the digital hardware with the attendant benefit of simplification of the analog hardware. An example will illustrate.

Example 7.5

This example illustrates the benefits of interpolation in the design of a compact disc (CD) audio playback system. An analog audio signal $x_c(t)$ typically has a bandwidth which is limited by $f_N = 20$ KHz. During the recording process, the analog signal is sampled at $f_s = 44.1$ KHz and "printed" to the CD. The analog spectrum, $X_c(j\omega)$ and the sampled-signal spectrum, $X(e^{j\theta})$ are shown in Fig. 7.4.3. Notice that because the sampling rate is more than twice the highest frequency, there will be no aliasing and there will be a small amount of separation between images in the analog spectrum. To compute the amount of separation, the upper edge of the baseband image is at 20 KHz. The left edge of the first image is located at $f_s - 20$ KHz so that

$$\Delta f = f_s - 2 \cdot (20,000) = 4100 \text{ Hz}.$$

Hence, the analog reconstruction filter must have nearly flat response over the range from d.c. to 20 KHz and then make the transition from flatness to nearly zero over the next 4100 Hz. This requires an analog filter of fairly high order. A side effect of this sharp lowpass characteristic is fairly nonlinear phase toward the transition region, which will result in phase distortion for high frequencies (an effect which is claimed to be quite noticeable by some audiophiles). Thus, the design of the analog reconstruction filter for this system is quite difficult and expensive.

Suppose instead that we create the interpolated signal $x_i(k)$ by expanding $x(k)$ by a factor of four to $x_e(k)$ and digitally lowpass filtering. As we have seen, this effectively increases the sampling rate to $4f_s$ so that the aliases of $X(j\omega)$ are spaced by $4f_s$ in the spectrum $X_e(e^{j\theta})$. The separation between these components is seen to be

$$\Delta f = 4f_s - f_N - f_N = 137.4 \text{ KHz}.$$

For this case, the analog reconstruction filter needs to be flat between d.c. and 20 KHz and can roll off to zero over the 137.4 KHz range between 20 KHz and 157.4 KHz. Clearly, this eliminates the need for a high-order analog filter. Also, the phase distortion around 20 KHz will be virtually eliminated. This analog reconstruction filter will be *significantly* cheaper and simpler than the previous analog reconstruction filter. This is also shown in Fig. 7.4.3

What we just considered is known as *oversampling*. If the data had been available at a higher sampling rate, we would not have needed to perform interpolation digitally. Because the data already arrived from the record store as a 44.1 KHz sampled time series, we had no choice. The only additional expense in the design was in the digital lowpass filter, which is typically realized as a FIR lowpass filter. When realized in VLSI, such a lowpass filter is extremely simple and inexpensive to implement, and there exist a number of monolithic oversamplers and D/A converters which have oversamplers built in.

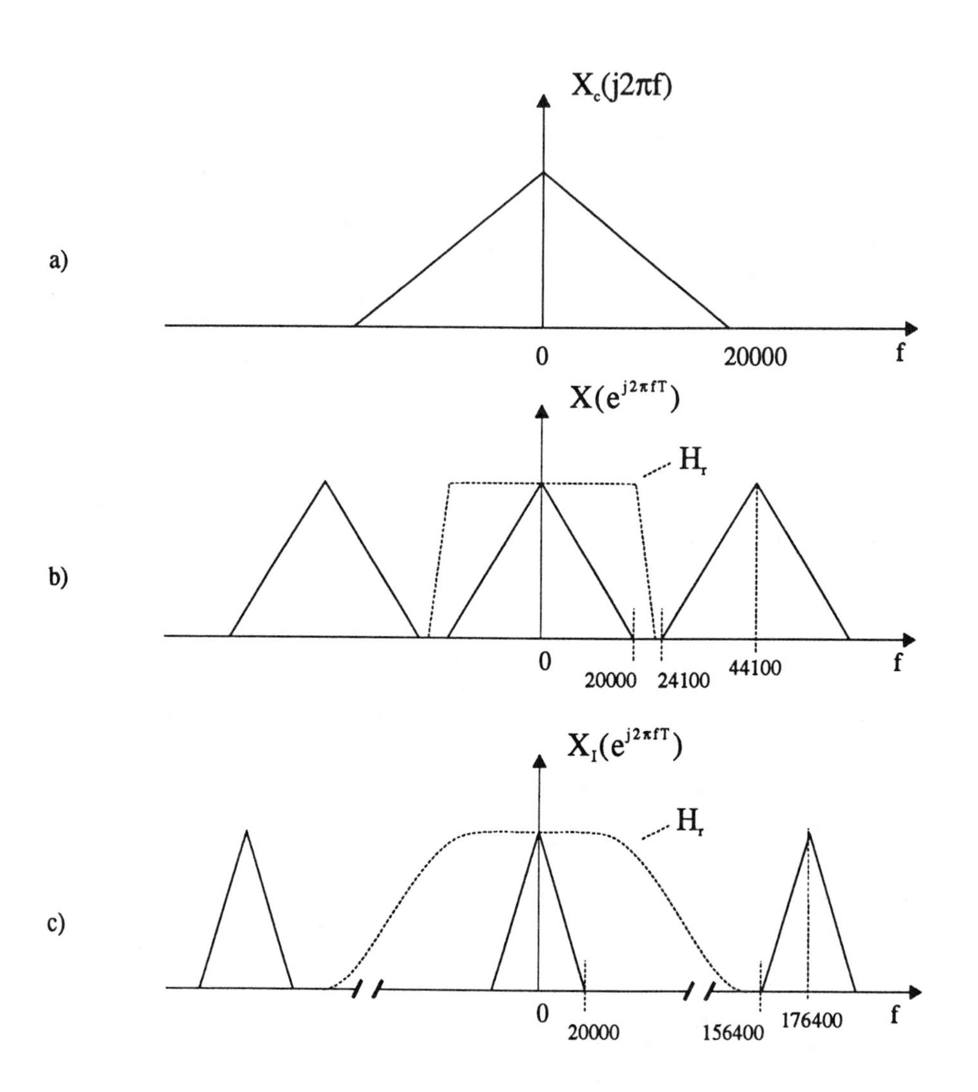

Figure 7.4.3: (a) Spectrum of analog audio signal; (b) spectrum of CD signal and required analog reconstruction filter; (c) spectrum of interpolated (oversampled) CD signal and required analog reconstruction filter.

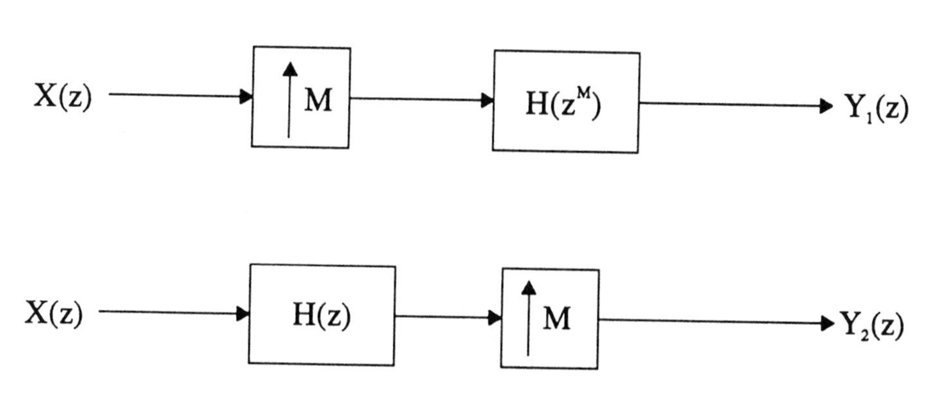

Figure 7.4.4: Equivalent systems for interpolation.

Structures for interpolation

Just as with decimation, the polyphase representation may be used to reduce the computational complexity of interpolation. It is simple to show that the two systems in Fig 7.4.4 have the same input-output behavior. According to Eq. 7.4.4, if the input to the sample-rate expander of the first system is $\{x(k)\}$, the output of the expander has $\mathcal{Z}$-transform $X(z^M)$. Thus, the output of the first system has the $\mathcal{Z}$-transform $H(z^M)X(z^M)$. Examining the second system, the output of the filter is $H(z)X(z)$, and again according to Eq. 7.4.4, the output of the expander is given by $H(z^M)X(z^M)$. Therefore, the two systems are equivalent.

Consider the problem of implementing interpolation in practice. Our theoretical model was to first expand the signal by M by zero-filling and then lowpass filtering at the increased sampling rate T/M. If the lowpass filter is an FIR of length N, each output sample of the filter requires N multiplications per T/M units of time. For even modest interpolation rates and FIR lengths, this may not be possible using affordable (or even existing) hardware. Fortunately, the polyphase representation can be used to lessen the computational complexity of the interpolator.

This time, the transposed polyphase decomposition can be used to realize an efficient structure for interpolation. Figure 7.4.5a shows the sampling rate expander *prior* to the transposed polyphase network. As we have already said, this model requires N multiplications per T/M seconds. Instead, the sampling rate expander can be moved to the right of the polyphase filters using the identity from Fig. 7.4.4. This is shown in Fig. 7.4.5b. In this network, each polyphase filter requires N/M multiplications per T seconds, for a total of N

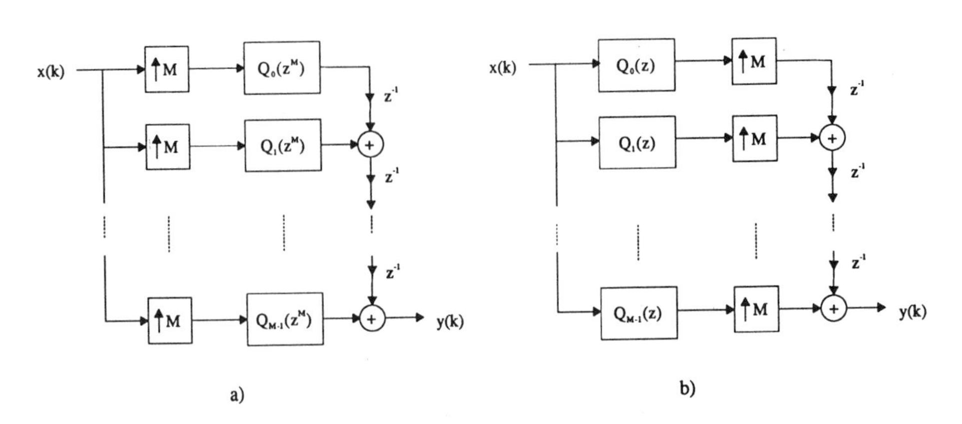

Figure 7.4.5: (a) Sampling rate expansion followed by lowpass filtering; (b) reduced-complexity structure for interpolation.

multiplications per T seconds. This represents a reduction in complexity by a factor of M.

Examining the filter structure in Fig. 7.4.5b, we can see that the outputs of sampling rate expanders are all equal to zero except for every M-th sample. Because each branch is delayed by a unique lag between 0 and $M-1$ before being summed to form the final output, at any given time, the output consists of a *single* output of one of the branches. Specifically, at time zero, the expanders have nonzero outputs, and the final output is given by the undelayed bottom branch. At $k=1$, the outputs of the expanders are all zero and the delayed output of the branch which is second from the bottom appears at the output, and so on. This suggests the commutator structure shown in Fig. 7.4.6. The commutator rotates clockwise and switches from one branch to the next at a rate of M times the input sample rate.

7.5 Non-Integer Sampling Rate Changes

We have already seen how to increase or decrease the sampling rate of a discrete-time signal by an integer factor. There are situations where it is necessary to change the sampling rate by a non-integer factor. For instance, compact disc (CD) and digital audio tape (DAT)

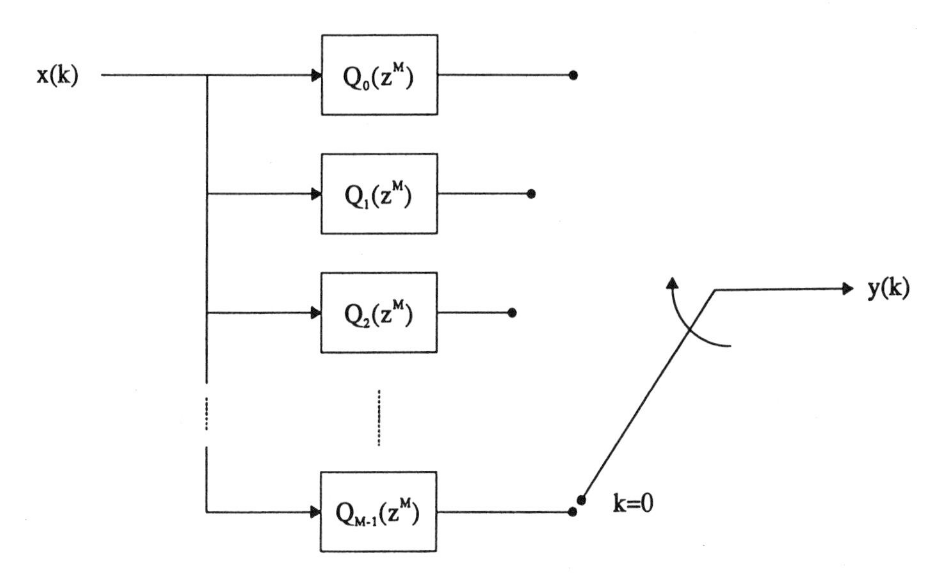

Figure 7.4.6: Commutator model for interpolation.

are based on different sampling rates. If we wish to perform a CD to DAT transfer, the record companies would prefer that it be done by CD-to-analog followed by analog-to-DAT, resulting in a loss of audio fidelity. Instead, we will show the sampling rate conversion can be performed entirely in the discrete-time domain.

Because the ratio of two sampling rates will always be rational, it is not restrictive to consider only the case where the sampling rate must be changed by a rational number. Thus, suppose we wish to change the sampling rate from T to

$$T' = T\frac{M}{L}.$$

This can be accomplished in two steps. First, the sampling rate is converted from T to T/L by interpolating. This consists of expanding the signal by L followed by filtering with a lowpass filter with gain L and cutoff frequency π/L. Next, the signal with sample rate T/L is decimated by M. This is performed by first filtering the signal through a lowpass filter with cutoff frequency π/M and then retaining only every M-th sample. The net result will be a signal whose sampling rate is $T' = TM/L$. This is shown schematically in Fig. 7.5.1a.

If $M > L$, the net effect will be to reduce the sampling rate. If $L > M$, the sampling

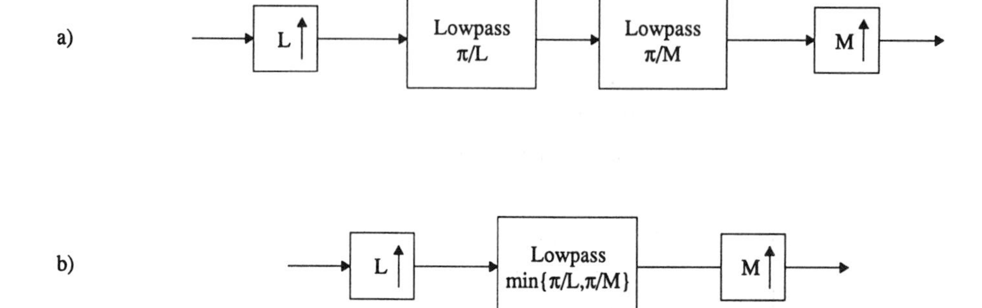

Figure 7.5.1: (a) System for non-integer sampling rate conversion; (b) same system with lowpass filters combined.

rate will be increased. The cascade of lowpass filters in the sampling-rate converter can be combined into one lowpass filter with gain L and cutoff frequency equal to the minimum of π/M and π/L. This is depicted in Fig. 7.5.1b.

7.6 Analysis and Synthesis Filters

As a tool for spectral analysis, it is sometimes useful to break a signal into *subbands*. These subbands are ranges of frequency over which we are interested in the spectral content of a signal. This can be done by passing the signal through a collection of filters,

$$H_0(z), H_1(z), \ldots, H_{M-1}(z),$$

each of which passes only the frequencies of interest. The collection of filters is known as an *analysis filter bank*, shown in Fig. 7.6.1. These filters can be FIR or IIR, and can have characteristics which depend on the type of analysis which needs to be performed. In any case, the analysis has as input $x(k)$ and produces the outputs

$$\hat{x}_0(k), \hat{x}_1(k), \ldots, \hat{x}_{M-1}(k)$$

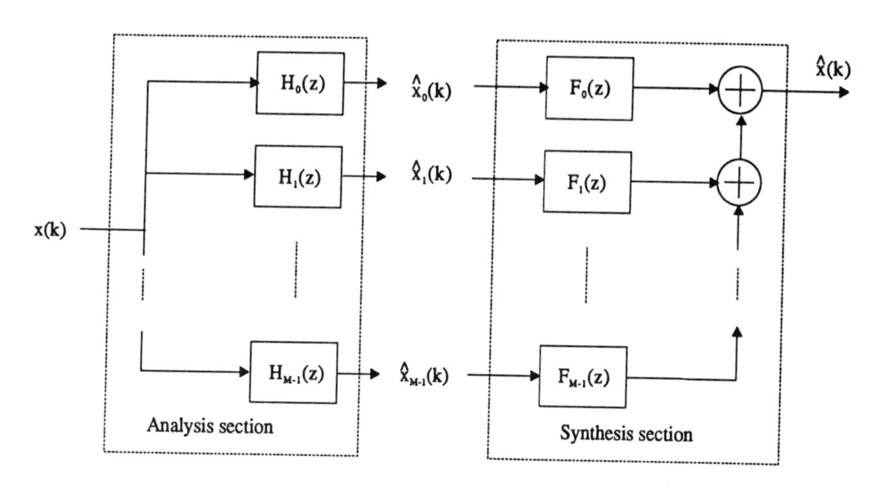

Figure 7.6.1: Analysis and synthesis filters.

where $\hat{x}_i(k) = h_i(k) * x(k)$.

Similarly, we have *synthesis filter banks*. A synthesis bank is used to combine input signals by filtering and summation of the filter outputs. The synthesis filter consists of a collection of filters

$$F_0(z), F_1(z), \ldots F_{M-1}(z)$$

which act on the inputs

$$\hat{x}_0(k), \hat{x}_1(k), \ldots, \hat{x}_{M-1}(k)$$

to produce the outputs $y_i(k)$ according to $y_i(k) = f_i(k) * \hat{x}_i(k)$. The outputs of the filters are then summed to produce $y(k)$. A synthesis bank is shown in Fig. 7.6.1.

One particularly useful analysis bank is known as a *uniform DFT bank*. A collection of filters $H_0(z), H_1(z), \ldots, H_{M-1}(z)$ is called *uniform DFT* if the k-th filter can be obtained from $H_0(z)$ according to

$$H_k(z) = H_0(W_M^k z), \quad k = 1, 2, \ldots, M-1.$$

In terms of frequency response, this means that

$$H_k(e^{j\theta}) = H_0(e^{j(\theta - 2\pi k/M)}).$$

In other words, the frequency response of the k-th filter is the same as that of $H_0(e^{j\theta})$, shifted by π/M. For instance, if $H_0(z)$ is a lowpass filter with cutoff frequency π/M, the

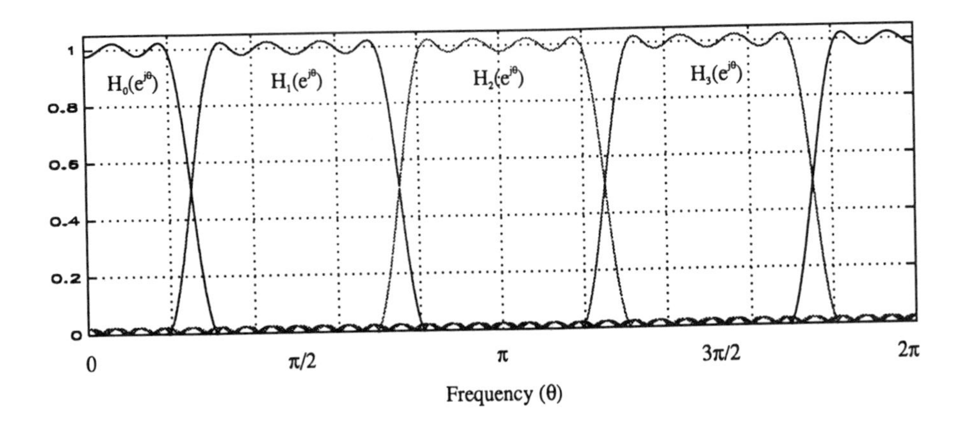

Figure 7.6.2: Uniform DFT filter characteristics for $M = 4$.

subsequent synthesis filters will be bandpass filters of bandwidth $2\pi/M$, centered at $2\pi k/M$. This is shown in Fig. 7.6.2 for the case $M = 4$. Referring to Fig. 7.6.1, it would appear that we need to compute the outputs of M filters per unit time to obtain the complete analysis output. Again, the polyphase representation will provide a drastic reduction in computational complexity for the analysis filter for uniform DFT analysis bank.

Suppose $H_0(z)$ has the polyphase decomposition

$$H_0(z) = \sum_{i=0}^{M-1} z^{-i} P_{0i}(z^M).$$

Because of the uniform DFT relation $H_k(z) = H_0(W_M^k z)$, it follows that

$$H_k(z) = \sum_{i=0}^{M-1} (W_M^k z)^{-i} P_{0i}((W_M^k z)^M).$$

Again, since $W_M^{kM} = 1$, we have

$$H_k(z) = \sum_{i=0}^{M-1} W_M^{-ik} z^{-i} P_{0i}(z^M).$$

Notice that this has the structure of a DFT. To compute the outputs of the analysis filters, we can compute the outputs of the filters described by $z^{-i}P_{0i}(z^M)$ and perform a DFT on them to obtain the analysis outputs. This is illustrated in Fig. 7.6.3. For certain choices of M, the DFT can be computed by the FFT and can even be made multiplierless. If the analysis filters are FIR, the reduction in complexity can be substantial. Supposing the analysis filters are of length N, computing the output of each $H_i(z)$ directly requires N multiplies per unit time, for a total of NM multiplies per unit time for the entire analysis bank. Using the DFT approach, however, reduces the overall complexity. Each polyphase filter $P_{0i}(z)$ is of length approximately N/M and requires N/M multiplies per unit time. Thus, the collection of M polyphase filters requires $NM/M = N$ multiplies per unit time, plus the overhead of the M-point DFT operation.

For example, suppose we are interested in designing a 16-band uniform DFT bank based on a filter $H_0(z)$ which is FIR of length 128. Direct implementation of the uniform DFT bank requires on the order of 2048 multiplications per cycle (in actuality, some of these multiplications are complex since the $H_i(z)$ in general will have some complex coefficients). Next, suppose the polyphase implementation is used. Each of the constituent polyphase filters $P_{0i}(z)$ will require 8 nonzero multiplications for a total of 128 multiplications. If a radix-4 FFT is used for the 16-point DFT, the DFT can be computed with roughly 16 multiplications. Therefore, the overall computational requirement of the uniform DFT bank is $128 + 16 = 134$ multiplications per unit time.

Because the bandwidths of the outputs of the bandpass filters in the uniform DFT bank are bandlimited to $2\pi/M$, this suggests that it may be desirable to decimate the outputs by a factor M. If this is the case, the polyphase representation may be used to further reduce the complexity of the filter bank. This is shown in Fig. 7.6.4. Notice that the number of multiplications per unit time has been reduced further by a factor of M.

M-th band filters

A particularly useful choice for the subfilters in an analysis bank is known as M-th *band filters* [Mue73]. M-th band filters are characterized by

$$h(Mk) = \begin{cases} 1/M, & k = 0 \\ 0, & k \neq 0. \end{cases} \tag{7.6.1}$$

In other words, the zeroth coefficient is a constant and all other coefficients corresponding to indices which are multiples of M are equal to zero. Recall that the zeroth polyphase component of $H(z)$ is defined by

$$P_0(z) = \sum_{k=0}^{\infty} h(Mk)z^{-k}.$$

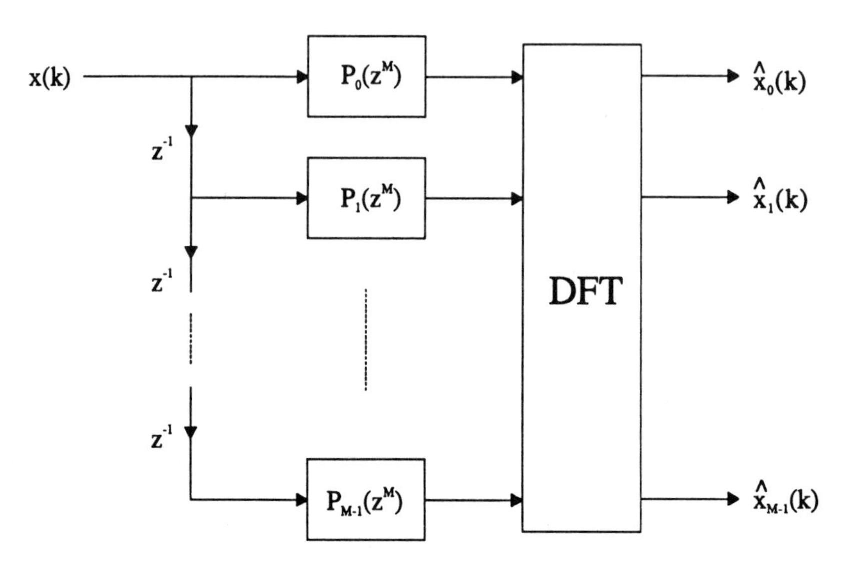

Figure 7.6.3: Analysis filter based on uniform DFT filters.

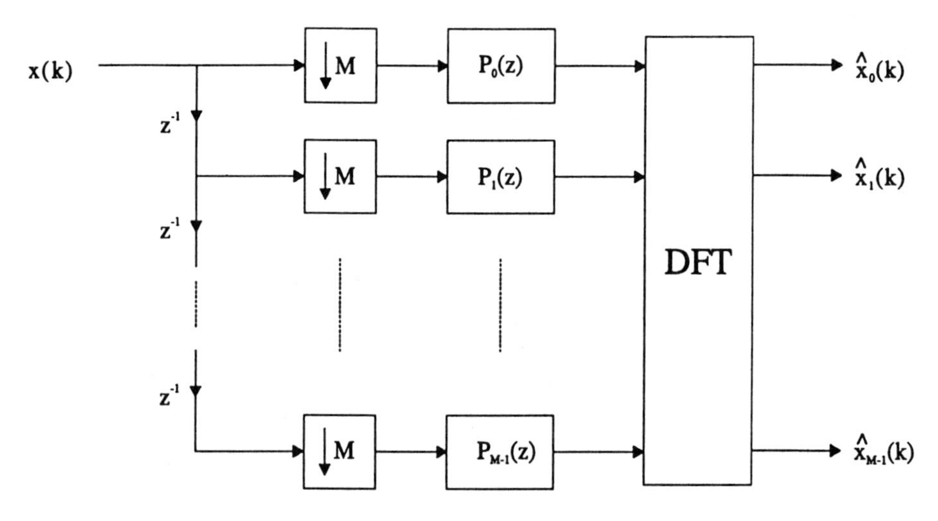

Figure 7.6.4: Decimated uniform DFT filter bank.

For an M-th band filter, it thus follows that $P_0(z) = 1/M$. Recall from Eq. 7.3.4 that

$$\frac{1}{M}\sum_{k=0}^{M-1} H(W_M^k z) = P_0(z^M).$$

Therefore, for an M-th band filter we have

$$\sum_{k=0}^{M-1} H(W_M^k z) = 1. \tag{7.6.2}$$

On the unit circle, this becomes

$$\sum_{k=0}^{M-1} H(e^{j(\theta-2\pi k/M)}) = 1. \tag{7.6.3}$$

What this means is that for any θ, the frequency response at points θ, $\theta + 2\pi/M$, $\ldots \theta + 2\pi(M-1)/M$ all sum to unity. If $H(z)$ is a lowpass M-th band filter, this has an important interpretation. Consider, for example, $M = 2$, which gives a *half-band filter*. Equation 7.6.3 says that

$$H(e^{j\theta}) + H(e^{j(\theta-\pi)}) = 1.$$

In particular, this implies symmetry about the point $\theta = \pi/2$, for

$$H(e^{j(\pi/2-\theta)}) = H(e^{j(\pi/2+\theta)}) = 1.$$

This condition is shown in Fig. 7.6.5

For the more general case of M-th band filters, this same type of lowpass symmetry can be guaranteed if we can generate a lowpass filter with cutoff frequency π/M which also satisfies Eq. 7.6.1. This is simple. Recall that the impulse response of the ideal lowpass filter with cutoff frequency π/M is

$$h(k) = \frac{\sin(\pi k/M)}{\pi k}.$$

This clearly satisfies the requirements, for $h(0) = 1/M$ by L'Hospital's rule, and $h(Mk) = 0$. To make the filter FIR, simply apply a finite-duration window, $w(k)$ so that

$$h(k) = \frac{\sin(\pi k/M)}{\pi k} w(k).$$

The choice of window will determine the sharpness of the cutoff and the amount of ripple in the pass and stopbands.

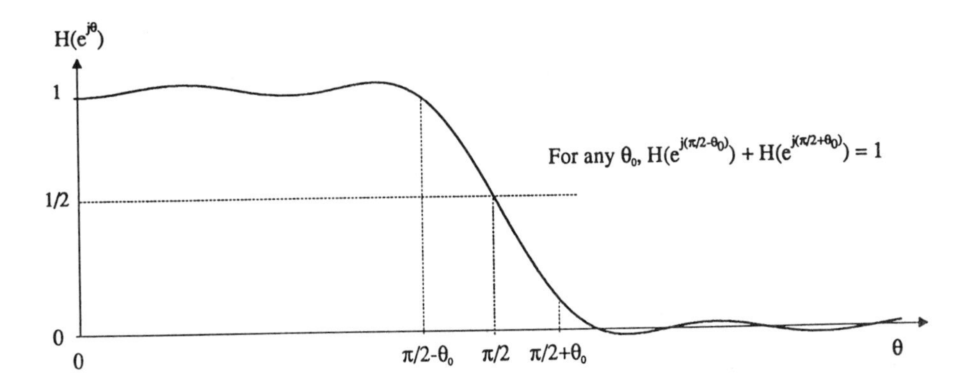

Figure 7.6.5: Half-band filter magnitude response.

The use of half-band filters in analysis banks simplifies the computation since, for a given filter order, half of the coefficients are zero. M-th band filters are also quite useful in analysis filters because they allow a particularly simple reconstruction of the original signal from the analysis outputs for certain filter banks. To see this, suppose $H_0(z)$ is an M-th band filter and let the other analysis filters be given by

$$H_k(z) = H_0(W_M^k z)$$

so that the collection is uniform DFT. This will provide a coverage of the frequency axis by bandpass filters with bandwidth $2\pi/M$. Because of the relationship in Eq. 7.6.2, it follows that

$$\sum_{k=0}^{M-1} H(W_M^k z) = 1.$$

But $H(W_M^k z)$ is simply $H_k(z)$ so that

$$\sum_{k=0}^{M-1} H_k(z) = 1.$$

Let $x(k)$ be the common input to each of the analysis filters. Thus, if the output of the i-th analysis filter is $\hat{x}_i(k)$, it follows that

$$x(k) = \sum_{i=0}^{M-1} \hat{x}_i(k).$$

Therefore, the original signal $x(k)$ can be recovered simply by summing the outputs of the individual analysis filters. This implies that the corresponding synthesis filters are unity.

M-th band filters are extremely useful as interpolation filters. Recall that interpolation consists of first expanding the signal by zero-filling and then lowpass filtering to remove images of the baseband spectrum between π/M and π. Therefore, the interpolation filter should be lowpass with cutoff frequency π/M. The interpolated signal is given by

$$x_i(k) = h_i(k) * x_e(k) \tag{7.6.4}$$

where $h_i(k)$ is the impulse response of the interpolation filter. If the interpolation filter is an M-th band lowpass filter satisfying $h(0) = 1$ and $h(Mk) = 0$, it then follows that $H(z)$ has a zeroth polyphase component $P_0(z) = 1$, which means that the $(M-1)$-th transposed polyphase component is given by $Q_{M-1}(z) = 1$. Referring to the commutator structure shown in Fig. 7.4.6, the output at every M-th sample is given by the output of $Q_{M-1}(z)$, which equals unity, so that

$$x_i(Mk) = x(k).$$

Thus, the interpolated signal exactly matches the original signal at every M-th sample, regardless of whether the interpolation filter is ideal or not.

7.7 Quadrature Mirror Filters

The two-channel quadrature mirror filter (QMF) is an important class of multirate filter which serves as the fundamental building block for a number of multirate systems. Essentially, the QMF is used to split a signal into subbands (typically highpass and lowpass) and then recover the signal from the subband signals. A two-channel quadrature mirror filter (QMF) is shown in Fig. 7.7.1. The type of processing which occurs between the analysis and synthesis sections of the QMF can vary. Typically, there is some coding/decoding, or the subband signals are used purely for analysis purposes. We will discuss some applications of QMFs later.

The QMF consists of an analysis section which is built from a lowpass filter $H_0(z)$, a highpass filter $H_1(z)$, and a pair of decimators, and a synthesis section which is built from a lowpass filter $G_0(z)$, a highpass filter $G_1(z)$, and a pair of upsamplers. The highpass/lowpass pair H_0, H_1 serves to split the input into subbands which are then decimated. Because of the decimation, a certain amount of aliasing will be introduced in the decimated signals since the filters are non-ideal. The beauty of the QMF approach is that the synthesis filters can be chosen so that this aliasing is canceled in the reconstruction process.

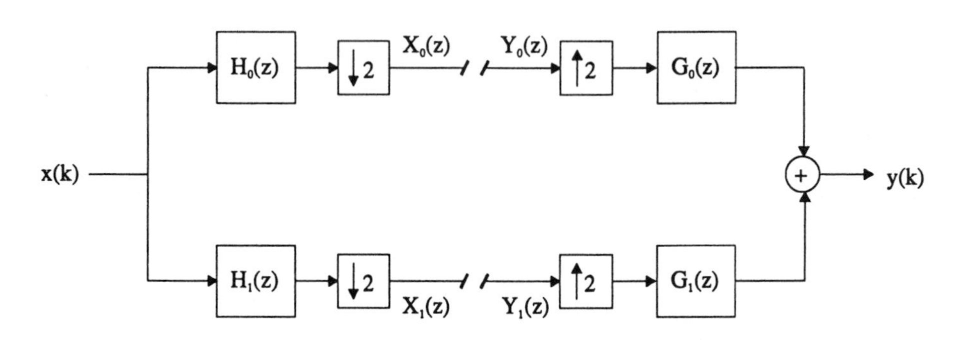

Figure 7.7.1: Two-channel QMF.

Let the outputs of the decimators be denoted by $X_0(z)$ and $X_1(z)$, respectively. It then follows that

$$X_0(z) = \frac{1}{2}\left[X(z^{1/2})H_0(z^{1/2}) + X(-z^{1/2})H_0(-z^{1/2})\right] \tag{7.7.1}$$

and

$$X_1(z) = \frac{1}{2}\left[X(z^{1/2})H_1(z^{1/2}) + X(-z^{1/2})H_1(-z^{1/2})\right]. \tag{7.7.2}$$

Next, let $Y_0(z)$ and $Y_1(z)$ denote the inputs to the upsamplers. The outputs of the upsamplers are then given by $Y_0(z^2)$ and $Y_1(z^2)$ respectively, and hence the output of the QMF is given by

$$Y(z) = G_0(z)Y_0(z^2) + G_1(z)Y_1(z^2). \tag{7.7.3}$$

Suppose that the outputs of the analysis section are fed to the inputs of the synthesis section. Then substituting Eqs. 7.7.1 and 7.7.2 into Eq. 7.7.3 gives

$$\begin{aligned} Y(z) \;=\; & \tfrac{1}{2}\left[H_0(z)G_0(z) + H_1(z)G_1(z)\right]X(z) \\ & + \tfrac{1}{2}\left[H_0(-z)G_0(z) + H_1(-z)G_1(z)\right]X(-z). \end{aligned} \tag{7.7.4}$$

The first term in Eq. 7.7.4 is the desired output of the QMF. The second term is an aliasing term which we would like to remove. This is accomplished by requiring that

$$H_0(-z)G_0(z) + H_1(-z)G_1(z) = 0. \tag{7.7.5}$$

This is satisfied by choosing

$$G_0(z) = H_1(-z) \tag{7.7.6}$$

and

$$G_1(z) = -H_0(-z). \tag{7.7.7}$$

With the aliasing term eliminated, the output of the QMF is thus given by

$$Y(z) = \frac{1}{2}\left[H_0(z)H_1(-z) - H_1(z)H_0(-z)\right]X(z) \tag{7.7.8}$$

and the transfer function of the QMF is given by

$$T(z) = \frac{1}{2}\left[H_0(z)H_1(-z) - H_1(z)H_0(-z)\right] \tag{7.7.9}$$

The filters $H_0(z), H_1(z)$ determine the type of subband splitting performed by the QMF. One popular method is to choose $H_0(z)$ as a lowpass filter and $H_1(z)$ as a "mirror image" highpass filter. That is,

$$H_1(z) = H_0(-z),$$

which means that

$$H_1(e^{j\theta}) = H_0(e^{j(\theta-\pi)}).$$

This ensures that if $H_0(z)$ is a good lowpass filter, then $H_1(z)$ will be a good highpass filter. In fact, these filters will be the mirror image of one another about the frequency $\theta = \pi/2$, as shown in Fig. 7.7.2. To eliminate aliasing and compensate for the magnitude scaling by 1/2 due to the decimation, the synthesis filters are chosen according to Eqs. 7.7.6 and 7.7.7 as

$$G_0(z) = 2H_0(z) \tag{7.7.10}$$

and

$$G_1(z) = -2H_0(-z) \tag{7.7.11}$$

(most of the time, we will not be explicitly concerned with the scaling at the output). With $G_0(z)$ and $G_1(z)$ thus chosen, aliasing due to decimation is completely eliminated. Substituting Eqs. 7.7.10 and 7.7.11 into Eq. 7.7.4, the output of the QMF is given by

$$Y(z) = \left[H_0^2(z) - H_0^2(-z)\right]X(z) \tag{7.7.12}$$

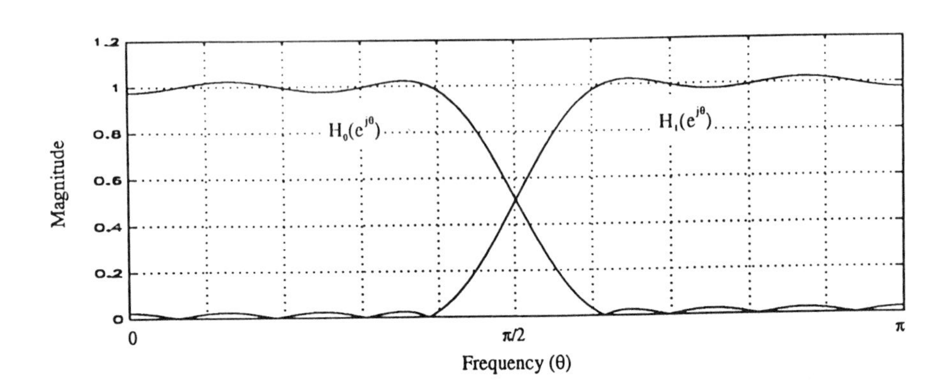

Figure 7.7.2: Mirror-image filters.

or in terms of Fourier transforms,

$$Y(e^{j\theta}) = \left[H_0^2(e^{j\theta}) - H_0^2(e^{j(\theta-\pi)})\right] X(e^{j\theta}). \tag{7.7.13}$$

Let's take a closer look at the manner in which aliasing is eliminated at the output of the QMF. According to Eq. 7.7.4, the aliasing inside the QMF is due to the term

$$[H_0(-z)G_0(z) + H_1(-z)G_1(z)]\, X(-z). \tag{7.7.14}$$

Consider the case where $X(z)$ is as shown in Fig. 7.7.3a and the filters $H_0(z)$ and $H_1(z)$ form a mirror-image lowpass/highpass pair as also shown in Fig. 7.7.3a. The spectra $H_0(z)X(z)$ and $H_1(z)X(z)$ are shown in Fig. 7.7.3b. Because of the relationship

$$X(-z)|_{z=e^{j\theta}} = X(e^{j(\theta-\pi)}),$$

$H_0(-z)X(-z)$ and $H_1(-z)X(-z)$ are as shown in Fig. 7.7.3c. Figures 7.7.3d and 7.7.3e show the magnitudes of $H_0(-z)X(-z)G_0(z)$ and $H_1(-z)X(-z)G_1(z)$. It should now be easy to see how the filters $G_0(z)$ and $G_1(z)$ can be made to cancel these aliasing terms.

Returning to the mirror-image lowpass/highpass-pair QMF, from Eq. 7.7.12 it immediately follows that the transfer function is given by

$$T(z) = H_0^2(z) - H_0^2(-z). \tag{7.7.15}$$

Ideally, we would like $T(z)$ to be equal to unity, *i.e.*, to have perfect reconstruction, or to at least have a flat magnitude repsonse. There are a number of constraints which must be met for this to be possible. For instance, suppose we wish to use a mirror-image pair *and* require that the analysis filters be linear phase. We will now show that perfect reconstruction is for all intents and purposes impossible, and that requiring flat magnitude response renders the filters $H_0(z)$ and $H_1(z)$ useless for splitting the input into subbands.

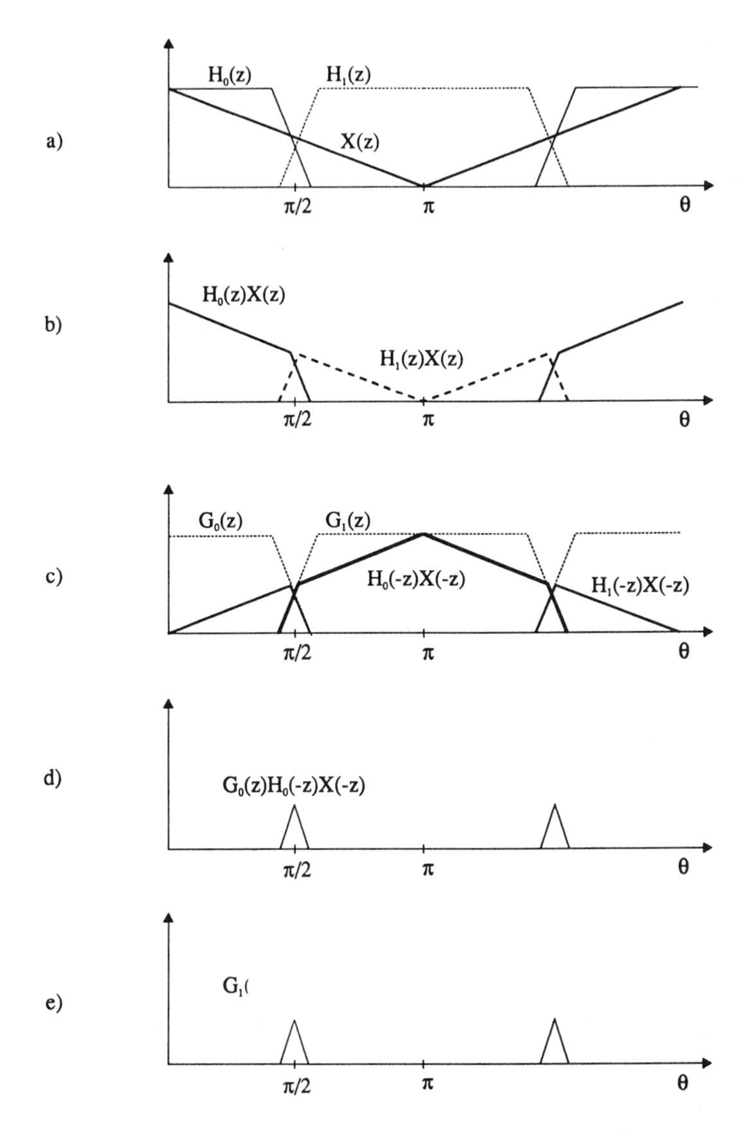

Figure 7.7.3: Illustration of aliasing cancellation in the QMF

Linear-phase QMFs

Let $H_0(z)$ be a linear-phase FIR of length N, which hence can be expressed as

$$H_0(e^{j\theta}) = H(\theta)e^{-j(N-1)\theta/2}.$$

Then Eq. 7.7.15 shows that $T(e^{j\theta})$ is given by

$$T(e^{j\theta}) = \left[|H(\theta)|^2 - (-1)^{N-1}|H(\theta - \pi)|^2\right] e^{-j(N-1)\theta}.$$

Thus, the QMF is linear-phase and has a magnitude response given by

$$|T(e^{j\theta})| = |H(\theta)|^2 - (-1)^{N-1}|H(\theta - \pi)|^2.$$

When N is odd, it follows that

$$|T(e^{j\theta})| = |H(\theta)|^2 - |H(\theta - \pi)|^2$$

and since $|H(\pi/2)| = |H(3\pi/2)|$, it follows that the magnitude response has a null at $\theta = \pi/2$. This is an undesirable property for an analysis/synthesis bank since certain frequencies will be completely eliminated and accurate reconstruction will be impossible. Therefore, odd-length linear-phase FIRs cannot be used if it is desired that $|T(e^{j\theta})|$ be flat.

When N is even, however, we have

$$|T(e^{j\theta})| = |H(\theta)|^2 + |H(\theta - \pi)|^2. \tag{7.7.16}$$

Let's see if it is possible to obtain $|T(e^{j\theta})| = 1$ for all frequencies. Assume $H_0(z)$ is FIR and we are using the mirror-image pair $H_1(z) = H_0(-z)$. If $H_0(z)$ has the polyphase decomposition

$$H_0(z) = P_0(z^2) + z^{-1}P_1(z^2).$$

Then the transfer function $T(z)$ from Eq. 7.7.15 becomes

$$T(z) = 2z^{-1}P_0(z^2)P_1(z^2).$$

The condition $|T(e^{j\theta})| = 1$ means that the FIR $T(z)$ is a perfect delay, so that $T(z) = cz^{-n}$, which, from the above expression, means that the polyphase components $P_0(z)$ and $P_1(z)$ must be pure delays, as well, *i.e.*,

$$P_0(z) = c_0z^{-n_0}, \quad P_1(z) = c_1z^{-n_1}.$$

Therefore, the filters $H_0(z)$ and $H_1(z)$ will be two-coefficient FIR filters given by

$$H_0(z) = c_0z^{-2n_0} + c_1z^{-2(n_1+1)}, \quad H_1(z) = c_0z^{-2n_0} - c_1z^{-2(n_1+1)}.$$

Hence, the filters $H_0(z), H_1(z)$ will not be useful in splitting the input signal into subbands. This shows that, even with even-length FIRs, it is still not possible to obtain a flat magnitude response if the analysis FIRs are anything other than a trivial sum of two delays. Therefore, any linear-phase FIR will induce some amplitude distortion on the overall QMF if the perfect mirror image condition is $H_1(z) = H_0(-z)$ is retained. The amount of distortion can be minimized, at best, through an appropriate optimization method. If we are willing to drop the perfect mirror constraint $H_1(z) = H_0(-z)$ or the linear phase constraint on the analysis/synthesis filters, as we shall see, it is possible to eliminate magnitude *and* phase distortions entirely for the overall transfer function $T(z)$. Such a QMF is known as a *perfect reconstruction* QMF.

Perfect reconstruction QMFs

As the name implies, the output of a perfect reconstruction QMF is equal to the input with some time delay. The following method for designing perfect reconstruction QMFs is due to Smith and Barnwell [SB84]. Suppose the analysis filters $H_0(z)$ and $H_1(z)$ must be of order $N-1$. We begin by designing a zero-phase half-band filter $F(z)$ of order $2(N-1)$. Let the magnitude response of $F(z)$ be as shown in Fig. 7.7.4a, with a peak stopband ripple of δ. From $F(z)$, form the half-band filter

$$F_+(z) = F(z) + \delta. \tag{7.7.17}$$

$F_+(z)$ is obtained from $F(z)$ simply by adding δ to the FIR coefficient $f(0)$ so $F_+(z)$ has a peak stopband ripple of 2δ, as shown in Fig. 7.7.4b. Then $F_+(e^{j\theta})$ is real and nonnegative so that $F_+(z)$ has the spectral factorization

$$F_+(z) = H(z)H(z^{-1}) \tag{7.7.18}$$

for some FIR $H(z)$ with real coefficients (that this is so may be shown heuristically by factoring such an $F_+(z)$. Because $F_+(z)$ is linear-phase, its roots fall not only in complex-conjugate pairs, but in conjugate-reciprocal pairs, as well. $H(z)$ may be taken as the polynomial formed from the complex conjugate root pairs within the unit circle, and $H(z^{-1})$ from those outside the unit circle).

Because $F_+(z)$ is half-band, the coefficients are of the form

$$\ldots, f_+(-5), 0, f_+(-3), 0, f_+(-1), f_+(0), f_+(1), 0, f_+(3), 0, f_+(5), 0, \ldots.$$

It can be seen that

$$F_+(z) + F_+(-z) = \alpha \tag{7.7.19}$$

where $\alpha = 2f_+(0)$ is a constant. Substituting Eq. 7.7.18 into Eq. 7.7.19, we have

$$H(z)H(z^{-1}) + H(-z)H(-z^{-1}) = \alpha. \tag{7.7.20}$$

If both sides of Eq. 7.7.20 are multiplied by $z^{-(N-1)}$, it follows that

$$z^{-(N-1)}H(z)H(z^{-1}) + z^{-(N-1)}H(-z)H(-z^{-1}) = \alpha z^{-(N-1)}. \tag{7.7.21}$$

The objective of perfect reconstruction filtering is to choose $H_0(z)$ and $H_1(z)$ so that $T(z)$ as given by Eq. 7.7.15 will be equal to a perfect delay. Recall from Eq. 7.7.9 that

$$T(z) = \frac{1}{2}\left[H_0(z)H_1(-z) - H_1(z)H_0(-z)\right] \tag{7.7.22}$$

Comparing Eq. 7.7.22 and Eq. 7.7.21, we make the choices

$$H_0(z) = H(z), \quad H_1(-z) = z^{-(N-1)}H(z^{-1}) \tag{7.7.23}$$

which further implies

$$H_1(z) = (-1)^{N-1}z^{-(N-1)}H(-z^{-1}). \tag{7.7.24}$$

If these expressions for $H_0(z)$ and $H_1(z)$ are substituted into Eq. 7.7.22, we have

$$T(z) = \frac{1}{2}\left[z^{-(N-1)}H(z^{-1})H(z) + (-1)^N z^{-(N-1)}H(-z)H(-z^{-1})\right]$$

which, for even N, becomes

$$T(z) = \frac{1}{2}\left[z^{-(N-1)}H(z^{-1})H(z) + z^{-(N-1)}H(-z)H(-z^{-1})\right]. \tag{7.7.25}$$

According to Eq. 7.7.21, however, this simply means that

$$T(z) = \beta z^{-(N-1)} \tag{7.7.26}$$

for some constant β. This means that if the aliasing component in the QMF is eliminated according to the choices dictated by Eqs. 7.7.6 and 7.7.7, then the output of the QMF is simply a delayed and scaled version of the input!

To guarantee that aliasing is eliminated, we first use Eq. 7.7.6 for $G_0(z)$, giving

$$G_0(z) = H_1(-z)$$

which, according to Eq. 7.7.23 becomes

$$G_0(z) = z^{-(N-1)}H(z^{-1}). \tag{7.7.27}$$

Next, Eq. 7.7.7 says that $G_1(z)$ is chosen as

$$G_1(z) = -H(-z) \tag{7.7.28}$$

which, according to Eq. 7.7.23 becomes

$$G_1(z) = -z^{-(N-1)}H_1(z^{-1}). \tag{7.7.29}$$

This completes the design of the perfect reconstruction QMF. To summarize, we first find the causal spectral factor $H(z)$ of a zero-phase FIR $F_+(z)$. The constituent filters of the QMF are then chosen according to Eqs. 7.7.23, 7.7.27 and 7.7.29. Furthermore, observe that since $F_+(z)$ was a lowpass filter and $H_0(z)$ is a spectral factor of $F_+(z)$, it follows that $H_0(z)$ is a lowpass filter, as well. Examining the expression for $H_1(-z)$ in Eq. 7.7.23, we can see that

$$|H_1(e^{j\theta})| = |H(e^{j(\theta-\pi)})|$$

so that $H_1(z)$ is a highpass filter with mirror image magnitude response.

In practice, there are several algorithms for extracting the spectral factor $H(z)$. Finding $H(z)$ from a factorization of the polynomial $F_+(z)$ is impractical for large filter lengths N. More efficient algorithms have been developed which are based on the use of the complex cepstrum [MN82].

Example 7.6

A 14-th order (length-15) half-band equiripple lowpass FIR is given by

$$F(z) = f_7(z^7 + z^{-7}) + f_5(z^5 + z^{-5}) + f_3(z^3 + z^{-3}) + f_1(z + z^{-1}) + f_0$$

(corresponding to $(N-1) = 7$) where

$$\begin{aligned} f_7 &= -0.02648 \\ f_5 &= 0.04411 \\ f_3 &= -0.09340 \\ f_1 &= 0.3139 \\ f_0 &= 0.5000 \end{aligned}$$

The frequency response is as shown in Fig. 7.7.4a. It can be seen that the peak stopband ripple is equal to $\delta = 0.0238$. Therefore, we form the new half-band filter

$$F_+(z) = F(z) + 1.01\delta$$

which has the frequency response shown in Fig. 7.7.4b (we have added slightly more than the ripple δ so that the response is strictly greater than zero. This avoids having to deal with zeros of $F_+(z)$ on the unit circle). Using a simple root-finding technique, the zeros of $F_+(z)$ are found and those inside the unit circle are ascribed to the spectral factor $H(z)$. Indeed, it is readily verified that $H(z)$ as given by

$$\begin{aligned} H(z) &= 1.0000 + 1.3403z^{-1} + 0.6851z^{-2} - 0.2444z^{-3} \\ &\quad - 0.3410z^{-4} + 0.0991z^{-5} + 0.2399z^{-6} - 0.1790z^{-7} \end{aligned}$$

satisfies $F_+(z) = H(z)H(z^{-1})$. Next, we choose the filters in the $H_0(z)$ and $H_1(z)$ according to Eqs. 7.7.23 and 7.7.24 as

$$H_0(z) = H(z), \quad H_1(z) = -z^{-(N-1)}H(-z^{-1})$$

and the filters $G_0(z)$ and $G_1(z)$ are given by Eqs. 7.7.27 and 7.7.28 as

$$G_0(z) = z^{-(N-1)}H(z^{-1}) \quad G_1(z) = -H(-z).$$

This results in the following filters:

$$\begin{aligned} H_0(z) &= 1.0000 + 1.3403z^{-1} + 0.6851z^{-2} - 0.2444z^{-3} \\ &\quad - 0.3410z^{-4} + 0.0991z^{-5} + 0.2399z^{-6} - 0.1790z^{-7} \\ H_1(z) &= -0.1790 - 0.2399z^{-1} + 0.0991z^{-2} + 0.3140z^{-3} \\ &\quad - 0.2444z^{-4} - 0.6851z^{-5} + 1.3403z^{-6} - z^{-7} \\ G_0(z) &= -0.1790 + 0.2399z^{-1} + 0.0991z^{-2} - 0.3140z^{-3} \\ &\quad - 0.2444z^{-4} + 0.6851z^{-5} + 1.3403z^{-6} + z^{-7} \\ G_1(z) &= -1.0000 + 1.3403z^{-1} - 0.6851z^{-2} - 0.2444z^{-3} \\ &\quad + 0.3410z^{-4} + 0.0991z^{-5} - 0.2399z^{-6} - 0.1790z^{-7} \end{aligned}$$

Observe that the analysis/synthesis filters are not linear-phase. The frequency responses of these filters are shown in Figs. 7.7.4c. It can be verified after some algebraic manipulation that the QMF described by these filters has no aliasing and has an overall transfer function given equal to αz^{-7} for some constant α.

7.8 Interpolated FIR Filters

There are a number of efficient techniques for implementing narrowband FIR filters. Narrowband lowpass filters are necessary to bandlimit a signal to π/M if the signal must be decimated by a factor of M. Since FIRs have desirable features such as linear phase and good fixed-point behavior, it would be advantageous to use an FIR as a decimation filter. The problem with FIR filters, however, is the high order which must be used to meet a desired magnitude profile. The *interpolated FIR* (IFIR) [NDM84] approach provides simple solution to this problem.

Suppose we wish to design a FIR with the magnitude response $|H(e^{j\theta})|$ shown in Fig. 7.8.1a, resulting in an FIR of order N. Consider the magnitude response $|G(e^{j\theta})|$ shown in Fig. 7.8.1b. This frequency response is simply a "stretched" version of $H(e^{j\theta})$ with a

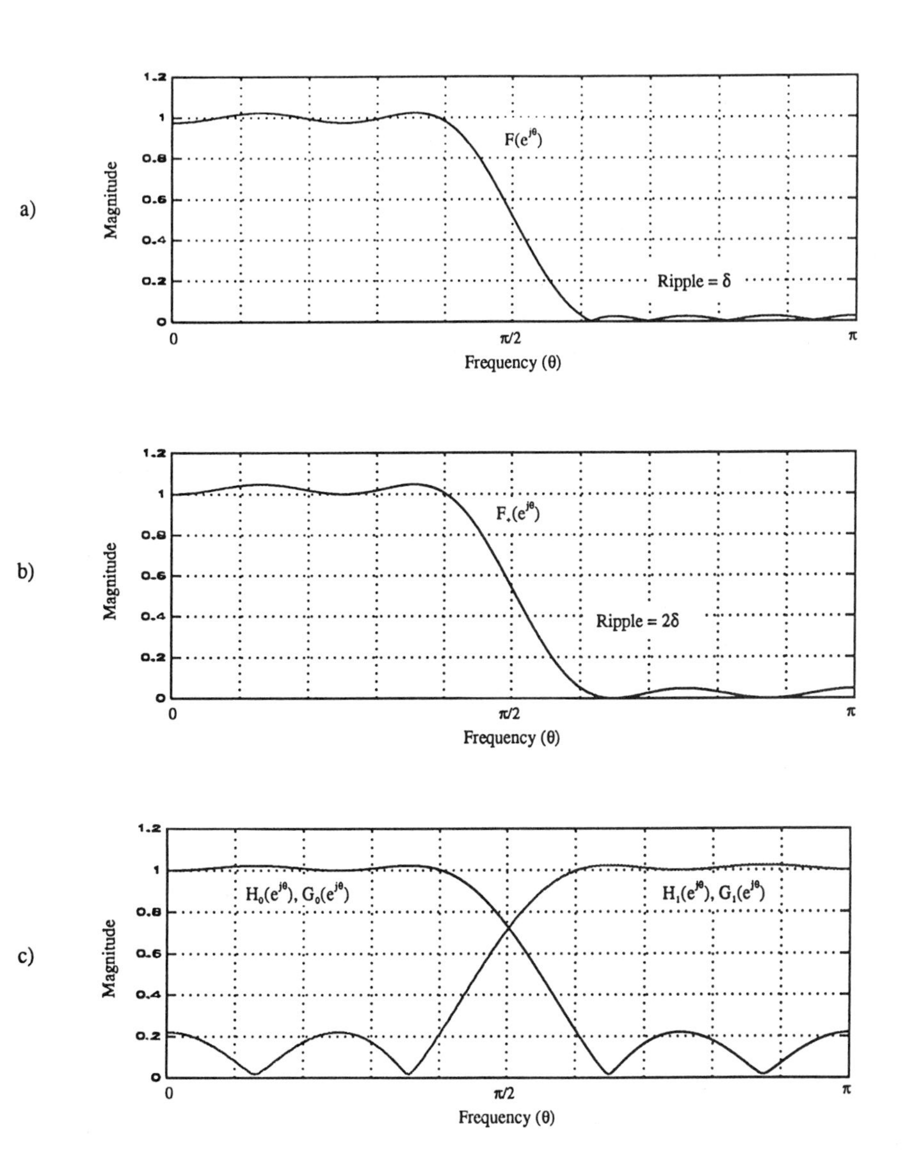

Figure 7.7.4: (a) Zero-phase FIR $F(z)$; (b) $F_+(z)$; (c) $H_0(z)$, $H_1(z)$, $G_0(z)$ and $G_1(z)$.

normalized transition band which is twice that of $H(e^{j\theta})$. Therefore, the FIR order required to meet $|G(e^{j\theta})|$ will be $N/2$.

If we expand the impulse response of $G(z)$ by a factor of two, we have a filter $G(z^2)$ of length N where only $N/2$ of the coefficients are nonzero. This is done by replacing each delay with two delays. The frequency response of this FIR will be $G(e^{j2\theta})$, as shown in Fig. 7.8.1c. In order to make the filter $G(z^2)$ meet the magnitude response $|H(e^{j\theta})|$, we only need eliminate the passband near $\theta = \pi$. It is seen that this can be accomplished with a lowpass filter $L(z)$ which has a very wide transition band (see Fig. 7.8.1c) and hence is of very low order. The lowpass filter $L(z)$ acts to interpolate the impulse response of $G(z^2)$. Thus, we can implement the interpolated FIR with $N/2$ multiplies per output point plus the overhead incurred by $L(z)$. For the situation where $H(z)$ is extremely narrowband, the response can be stretched by more than a factor of two, resulting in further reduction of the multiply count.

If the FIR filter $H(z)$ is to be used as a decimation filter, the IFIR approach provides an even larger decrease in complexity. Suppose the order-N FIR $H(z)$ is used to bandlimit an input signal to π/R and the output of $H(z)$ is then decimated by M where $R > M$ (we assume this so that the cutoff frequency of $H(z)$ is well below π/M). Let $G(z)$ be an M-fold stretched version of $H(z)$ so that $G(z)$ has order N/M. The expanded FIR $G(z^M)$ is of length N but has only N/M nonzero coefficients. Finally, a lowpass filter $L(z)$ must be used to eliminate $M-1$ of the passbands of $G(z^M)$. Now, we can reverse the order in which filtering is performed and first filter with $L(z)$ and then by $G(z^M)$. If the output of the filter is to be decimated by M, we follow $G(z^M)$ with a decimator. Recall, however, that the operation of filtering by $G(z^M)$ then decimating by M is equivalent to the operation of first decimating by M *then* filtering by $G(z)$ at the lower sample rate. This IFIR scheme is depicted in Fig. 7.8.2.

Let's analyze the complexity of this IFIR approach. Direct application of $H(z)$ requires N multiplications per output point. Using $L(z)$ then $G(z^M)$ followed by decimation requires N/M multiplications per output point (plus the overhead of $L(z)$). If we decimate after $L(z)$, the order-N/M FIR $G(z)$ now operates at $1/M$ of the input sample rate so that we need only perform $1/M^2$ as many multiplications as $H(z)$ in the same unit of time.

7.9 The Short-Time Fourier Transform

Up to this point, the principal tool we have used for analyzing the frequency content of discrete-time signals has been the discrete-time Fourier transform (DTFT). The DTFT is described by the analysis equation

$$X(e^{j\theta}) = \sum_{k=-\infty}^{\infty} x(k)e^{-jk\theta}$$

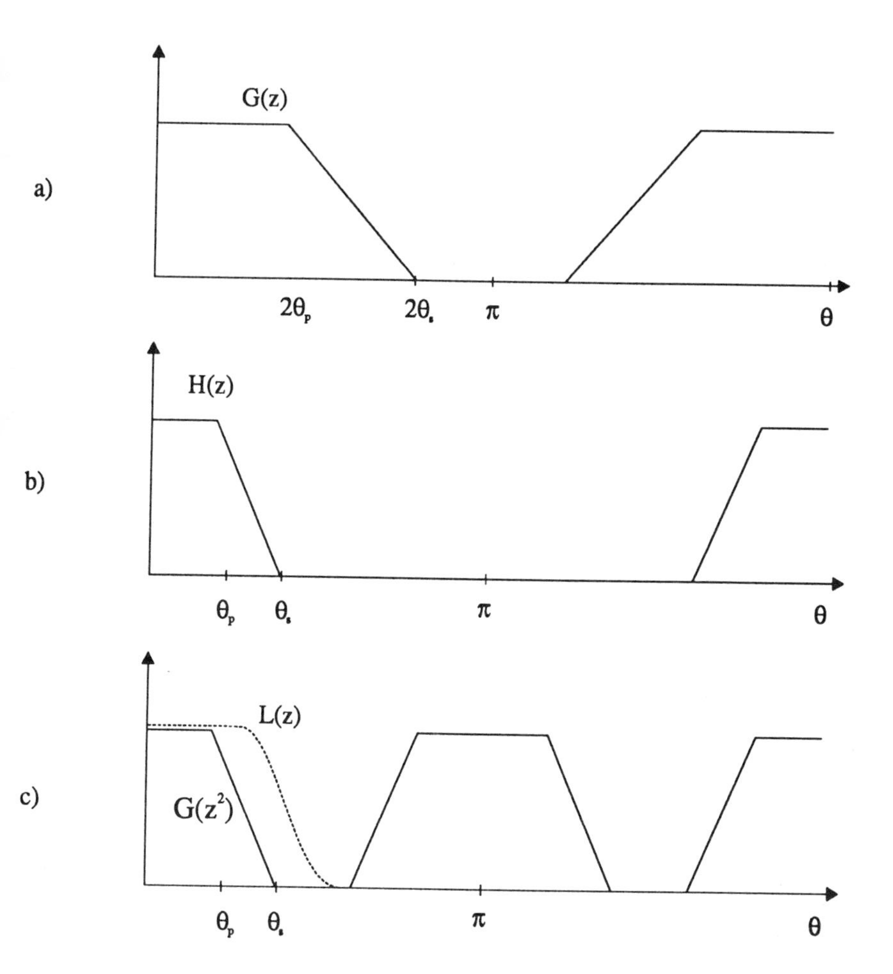

Figure 7.8.1: (a) Desired FIR lowpass response; (b) stretched lowpass response; (c) expanded lowpass response and lowpass filter to remove unwanted passband.

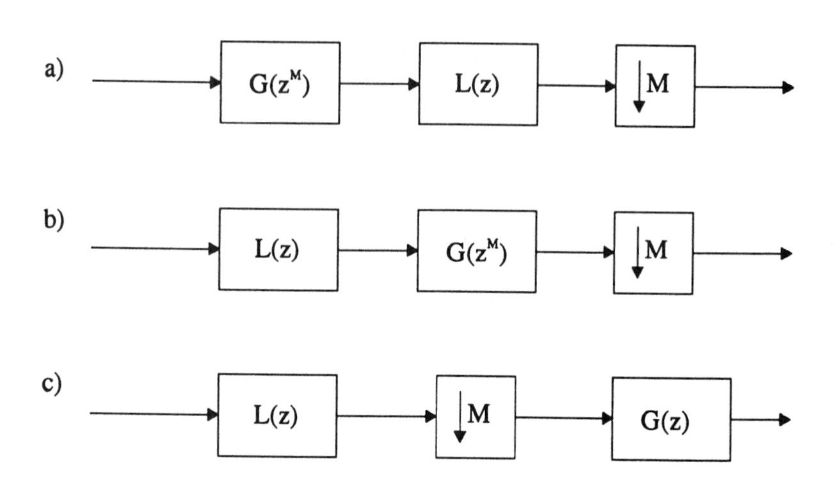

Figure 7.8.2: Replacing a decimation filter with an interpolated FIR: (a) FIR, IIR, then decimator; (b) reversing order of FIR and IIR; (c) moving decimator before FIR.

and the synthesis equation

$$x(k) = \frac{1}{2\pi} \int_{-\pi}^{\pi} X(e^{j\theta}) e^{jk\theta} \, d\theta.$$

The analysis equation yields a function $X(e^{j\theta})$ which is supposed to give a measure of the frequency content of $x(k)$ at the frequency θ. This is a satisfactory paradigm for signals whose frequency content does not vary with time – for instance, simple sinusoids. Consider, however, a signal which changes its frequency content with time. For instance, a musical passage which changes pitch has frequency content which varies as time progresses. DTFT analysis of such a signal would yield a transform which has content at an infinite number of frequencies, whereas we intuitively understand that there are only discrete frequencies present at any given time, and these frequencies evolve with time.

The problem with the DTFT for the analysis of such signals is due to the fact that a single-frequency DTFT concentrated at θ_0 is implicitly associated with an *infinite duration* time-domain signal $x(k) = e^{j\theta_0 k}$. In other words, the transform is *localized* at θ_0 only if $x(k)$ is infinite in time extent. This can also be seen in the case of a rectangular pulse which, as we know, has a DTFT which for small pulse widths is wide in the frequency-domain and narrows only as the pulse width increases in the time-domain. This is a manifestation of the *uncertainty principle* which says quantitatively that if $x(k)$ is of short duration then $X(e^{j\theta})$ has wide support.

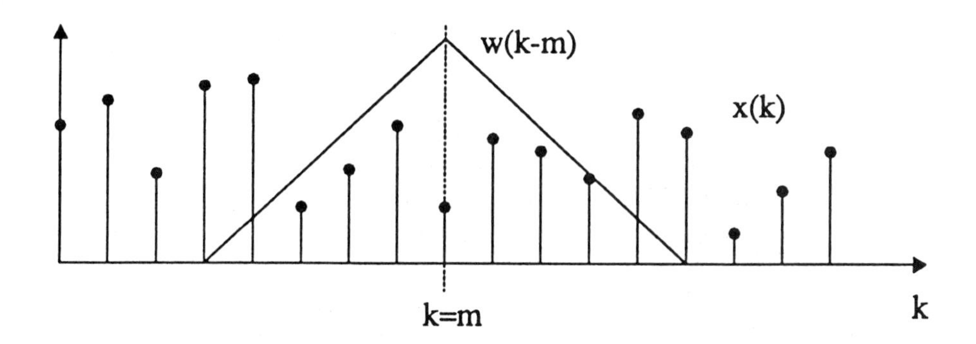

Figure 7.9.1: Forming the products for analysis with the STFT.

In order to better analyze signals with time-varying frequency content, a transform representation which jointly considers the time-domain and frequency-domain properties of signals is needed. This is the motivation behind both the short-time Fourier transform (STFT).

Heuristically, the STFT is a windowed version of the DTFT which "looks" at the signal $x(k)$ through a sliding window, giving a transform which is indexed by both time and frequency. Given some window $w(k)$ centered at $k = 0$, we form the product $x(k)w(k-m)$ and compute its DTFT. This gives a collection of DTFTs, one for each time lag m, as shown in Fig. 7.9.1. In this manner, we can examine the frequency content at $x(k)$ in a "local" fashion around the time instant m by capturing the time-domain properties of $x(k)$ only in a region around time m. Obviously, the choice of the window function $w(k)$ will play an important role in the quality of the localization. We will discuss this issue later.

Formally, the STFT is given by

$$X_{STFT}(e^{j\theta}, m) = \sum_{k=-\infty}^{\infty} x(k)w(k-m)e^{-jk\theta}. \tag{7.9.1}$$

We can see from Eq. 7.9.1 that the STFT at time m is indeed computed by sliding the window $w(k)$ to the new center-point m, forming the product with $x(k)$, and computing the traditional DTFT. Clearly, when the window function is taken to be a rectangular window of infinite duration (*i.e.*, $w(k) = 1$ for all k), $X_{STFT}(e^{j\theta}, m)$ is equal to the DTFT $X(e^{j\theta})$ for all m. The STFT is a complex-valued function of two variables, θ and m, and its magnitude can be visualized as a surface in the time-frequency plane with axes (θ, m). For instance,

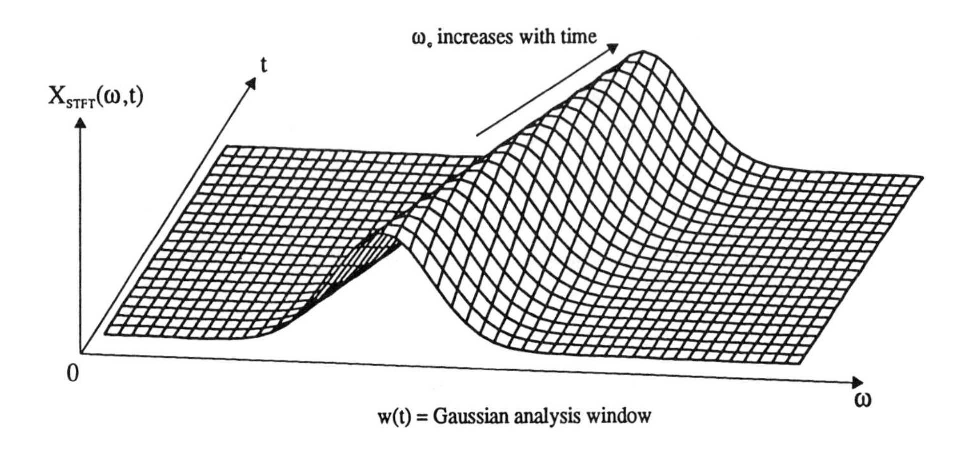

Figure 7.9.2: STFT of a chirp signal.

consider a sampled version $x(k)$ of the signal

$$x_c(t) = \sin(\theta(t))$$

where

$$\theta(t) = \int_0^t \gamma\tau \, d\tau.$$

The signal $x_c(t)$ is known as a "chirp" signal and can be seen to have an instantaneous frequency which grows linearly with t at a rate determined by γ. When viewed in the time-frequency plane, we would see $X_{STFT}(e^{j\theta}, m)$ as a concentrated region centered at the instantaneous frequency which migrates to increasing frequency as we move in the direction of increasing m. The rate at which the migration occurs is determined by the rate parameter γ. This is illustrated in Fig. 7.9.2.

Referring to Eq. 7.9.1, the function $X_{STFT}(e^{j\theta}, m)$ is seen to be equal to the DTFT of the sequence $x(k)w(k-m)$. Consequently, this sequence can be recovered from $X_{STFT}(e^{j\theta}, m)$ by using the DTFT inversion formula

$$x(k)w(k-m) = \frac{1}{2\pi}\int_{-\pi}^{\pi} X_{STFT}(e^{j\theta}, m)e^{jk\theta} \, d\theta. \tag{7.9.2}$$

Provided that $w(0) \neq 0$, we can let $k = m$ in Eq. 7.9.2 to obtain

$$x(m) = \frac{1}{2\pi w(0)}\int_{-\pi}^{\pi} X_{STFT}(e^{j\theta}, m)e^{jm\theta} \, d\theta. \tag{7.9.3}$$

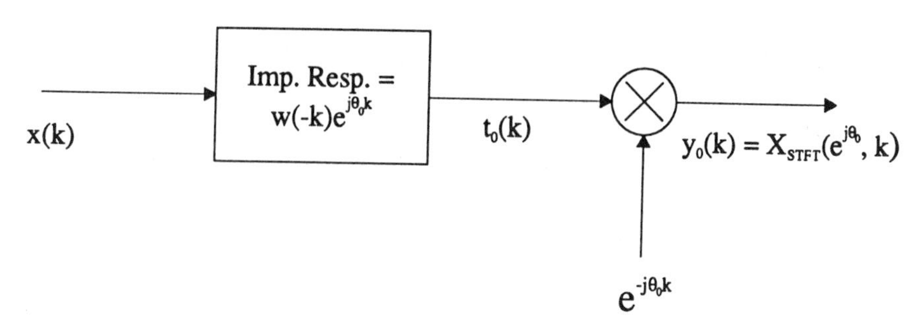

Figure 7.9.3: Obtaining the STFT as the modulated output of a linear system.

If $w(0) = 0$, another value of k can be used.

Returning to Eq. 7.9.1, for most cases of interest to us the window $w(k)$ will be of finite duration. Consequently, the mathematical delicacies concerning the DTFT (such as absolute summability) will be of no concern since the products $x(k)w(k-m)$ will also be of finite duration and hence absolute-summable. Typically, the lag m will be taken to be a multiple of some integer M. The choice of M heuristically determines the temporal resolution of the STFT and corresponds to a decimation of the STFT coefficients $X_{STFT}(e^{j\theta}, m)$. We will see later how this affects the invertibility of the STFT.

An illuminating view of the STFT is provided by relating it to the concept of filter banks. Beginning with Eq. 7.9.1, we can multiply inside the summation by $e^{jm\theta}$ and outside the summation by $e^{-jm\theta}$ giving

$$X_{STFT}(e^{j\theta}, m) = e^{-jm\theta} \sum_{k=-\infty}^{\infty} x(k)w(k-m)e^{j(m-k)\theta}. \tag{7.9.4}$$

Equation 7.9.4 can be viewed as the convolution of $x(k)$ with the sequence $w(-k)e^{jk\theta}$, followed by modulation with the sequence $e^{-jk\theta}$. Accordingly, for a particular frequency θ_0 and time m, $X_{STFT}(e^{j\theta_0}, m)$ can be obtained as the modulated output at time m of a filter with impulse response $w(-k)e^{jk\theta_0}$ when driven by the input $x(k)$. This is shown schematically in Fig. 7.9.3.

Consider the case where the window function $w(k)$ is a lowpass filter with DTFT $W(e^{j\theta})$. The DTFT of $w(-k)$ is then given by $W(e^{-j\theta})$ and hence the DTFT of $w(-k)e^{jk\theta_0}$ is given by $W(e^{-j(\theta-\theta_0)})$. Therefore, the analysis filter is a frequency-shifted version of the lowpass filter $W(e^{j\theta})$ and is hence bandpass centered at θ_0. The bandpass filter extracts the frequency content of $x(k)$ around the frequency θ_0 and the modulator recenters the bandpass output back to zero frequency. This is shown in Fig. 7.9.4. Referring to Fig. 7.9.3, the output of the bandpass filter is denoted by $t_0(k)$ and has a bandpass DTFT $T_0(e^{j\theta})$ as shown in Fig.

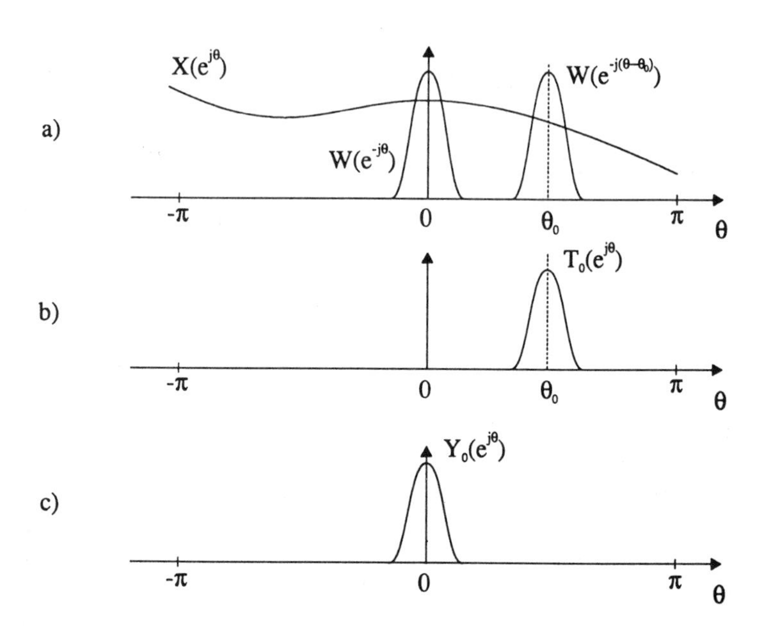

Figure 7.9.4: (a) $X(e^{j\theta})$, lowpass analysis window $W(e^{j\theta})$, and frequency-shifted analysis window $W(e^{-j(\theta-\theta_0)})$; (b) DTFT of the output of frequency-shifted analysis window; (c) DTFT of output of modulator.

7.9.4b. The output of the modulator is the sequence $y_0(k) = X_{STFT}(e^{j\theta_0}, k)$ which, because of the modulator, has the DTFT $Y_0(e^{j\theta})$ shown in Fig. 7.9.4c.

The filtering/modulation scheme depicted in Fig. 7.9.3 can be used to produce the STFT for all frequencies so that the STFT can be viewed as an uncountably infinite bank of filter to compute the STFT at each θ_0. In practice, we are often satisfied with computing the STFT at a finite set of M frequencies, in which case the STFT can be viewed as an analysis filter bank with M filters followed by M modulators. Let the frequencies of interest be

$$0 \leq \theta_0 < \theta_1 < \cdots < \theta_{M-1} < 2\pi.$$

The window centered at zero frequency is $W(e^{-j\theta})$ and the remaining frequency-shifted analysis windows are described by $W(e^{-j(\theta-\theta_0)})$. Consequently, we have an analysis bank where the base lowpass analysis filter is given by

$$H(e^{j\theta}) = W(e^{-j\theta})$$

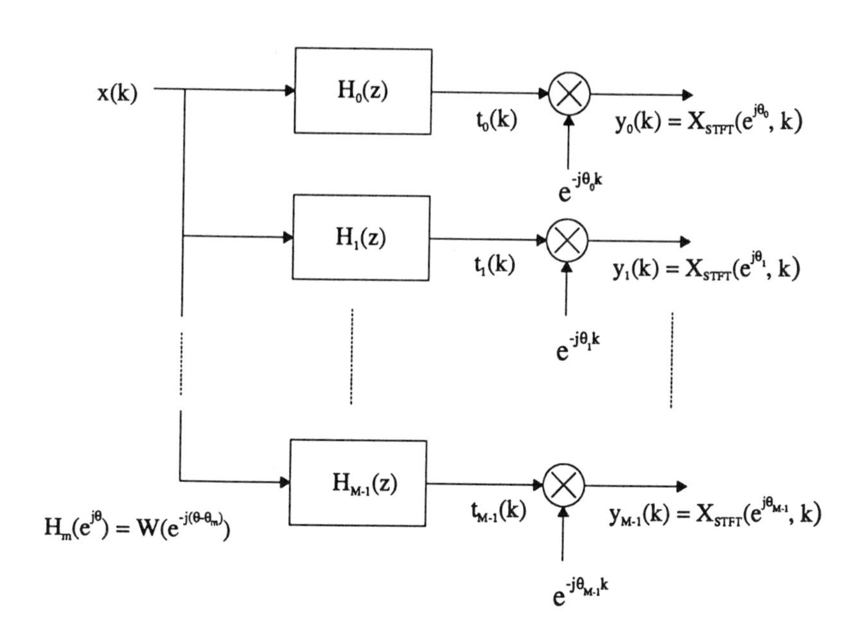

Figure 7.9.5: Computing the STFT at a set of discrete frequencies using a filter bank.

and the analysis filters centered at each θ_m given by

$$H_m(e^{j\theta}) = H(e^{j(\theta-\theta_m)}), \quad m = 0, 2, \ldots, M-1$$

followed by modulators $e^{-jk\theta_m}$. This is shown in Fig. 7.9.5.

A familiar case arises if we choose the frequencies θ_m to be uniformly spaced along the frequency axis, *i.e.*, $\theta_m = m\theta_0$. In this case, the analysis filters are related to the base filter $H_0(e^{j\theta})$ by

$$H_m(e^{j\theta}) = H_0(e^{j(\theta-2\pi m/M)}), \quad m = 0, 1, \ldots M-1.$$

We have seen that this is simply a uniform DFT collection of filters so that

$$H_m(z) = H_0(W^m z)$$

where $W = e^{-j2\pi/M}$. Consider the case where the base analysis filter $H_0(z)$ is taken to be a rectangular window of length M (which has a lowpass response). We have seen that the outputs of the analysis bank can be computed by taking the DFT of the outputs of the polyphase filters for $H_0(z)$. Since $H_0(z)$ is a rectangular window, it is simple to see that the polyphase components $P_{0,m}(z) = 1$ for all m and hence, referring to Fig. 7.9.5, the output of the m-th analysis filter is the m-th harmonic of the DFT of a block of M consecutive samples of the input $x(k)$. Again, the modulators simply serve to recenter the analysis outputs about zero frequency.

We have already alluded to the fact that the choice of the window $w(k)$ plays an important role in the quality of the time-frequency analysis given by the STFT. The window $w(k)$ serves to localize the frequency content in time. In Fig. 7.9.5, the sequence $y_m(k)$ gives a measure of the frequency content near θ_m of the input signal around time k. Here is where the interplay between temporal resolution and frequency resolution becomes important. The signal $t_m(k)$ is the output of a frequency-shifted version of the analysis filter $W(e^{-j\theta})$. As the support of $W(e^{-j\theta})$ gets narrower, the frequency-domain information about $x(k)$ gets more accurately localized in time. However, in order for the window width in the frequency-domain to get narrower, the window must be wider in time; this results in a decrease in time localization. Unfortunately, the objectives of time and frequency localization are conflicting in the STFT paradigm of time-frequency analysis. This is the principal motivation for the wavelet transform, which we will soon discuss.

Returning to the STFT, we have seen that the sequences $y_m(k)$ have lowpass Fourier transforms, which means that they are slowly varying in time. Suppose the sequences $y_m(k)$ are decimated by M, giving the analysis bank shown in Fig. 7.9.6a (where the decimators have been moved to the left of the modulators). This is equivalent to evaluating the STFT at times kM, *i.e.*, the analysis window $w(k)$ is slid M samples at a time. The resulting STFT will produce M STFT samples per M time instants, which gives the same data rate as the signal $x(k)$. The decimated STFT provides samples of the STFT which are spaced in time and frequency as shown in Fig. 7.9.6b. Whether $x(k)$ is recoverable from this decimated STFT representation is another question. Heuristically, we can see from Fig. 7.9.1 that if the window is slid by an amount larger than the window's width in time, some information will be lost in the STFT representation and will not be recoverable. We will not study the inversion problem in depth. Rather, we are primarily concerned with the STFT as an analysis tool.

For a cursory explanation of how the STFT can be inverted, suppose no decimation is performed, and the analysis filters are a uniform DFT collection generated from an M-th band analysis window $w(k)$. We have already seen that the input to a uniform DFT analysis bank based on an M-th band filter can be recovered by simple summation of the outputs. Since the STFT bank follows the analysis filters with modulators, we can simply demodulate and sum to recover the input. That is,

$$x(k) = \sum_{m=0}^{M-1} e^{jk\theta_m} y_m(k).$$

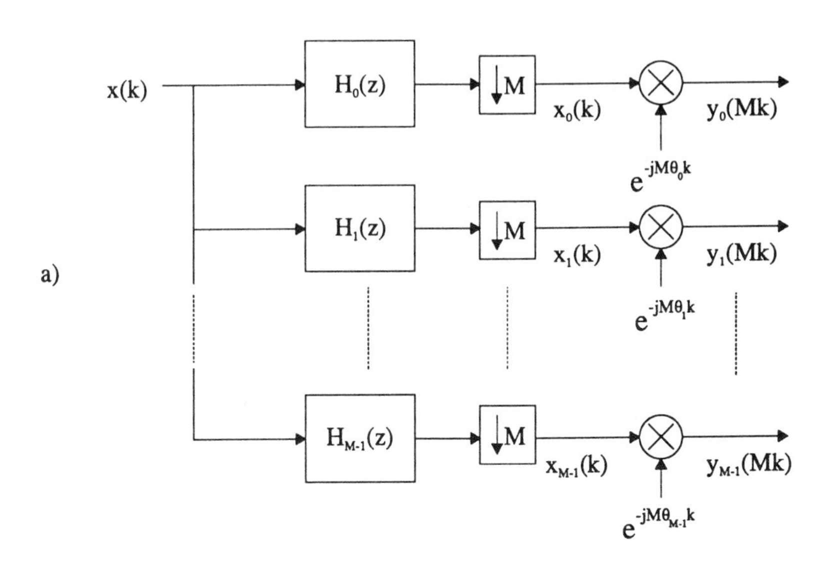

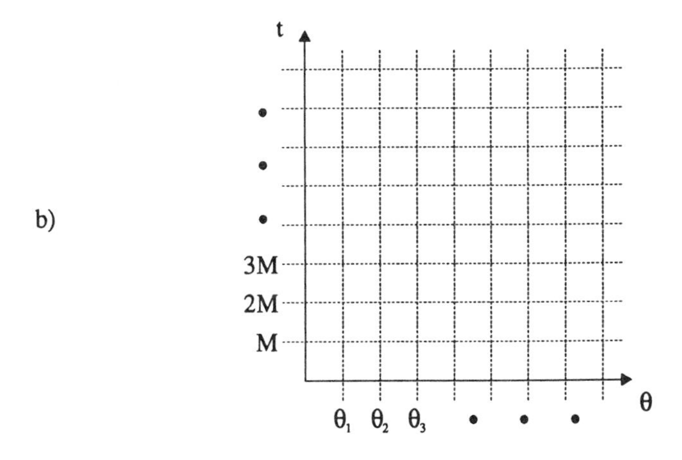

Figure 7.9.6: (a) Filter bank representation of the decimated STFT; (b) time-frequency grid for the decimated STFT.

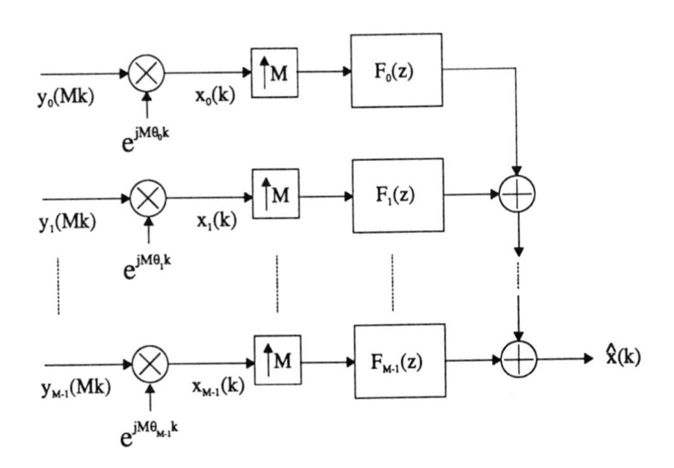

Figure 7.9.7: Synthesis bank to recover $x(k)$ from the decimated STFT coefficients.

Consider now the more general synthesis bank shown in Fig. 7.9.7. The modulators "undo" the effect of the modulation at the output of the analysis bank, and the reconstructed output is given by

$$\hat{X}(z) = \sum_{m=0}^{M-1} F_m(z) X_m(z^M), \tag{7.9.5}$$

which, in the time-domain, is given by

$$\hat{x}(k) = \sum_{m=0}^{M-1} \sum_{r=-\infty}^{\infty} x_m(r) f_m(k - Mr). \tag{7.9.6}$$

It can be seen from Fig. 7.9.7 that the sequence $x_m(k)$ is equal to $e^{jMk\theta_m} y_m(k)$ so that Eq. 7.9.6 becomes

$$\hat{x}(k) = \sum_{m=0}^{M-1} \sum_{r=-\infty}^{\infty} y_m(Mr) e^{jMr\theta_m} f_m(k - Mr). \tag{7.9.7}$$

Ideally, we would like to find *stable* analysis filters $F_m(z)$ such that $\hat{x}(k) = x(k)$, in which case Eq. 7.9.7 gives a stable (perfect) reconstruction of $x(k)$ from the decimated STFT coefficients $y_m(Mk)$.

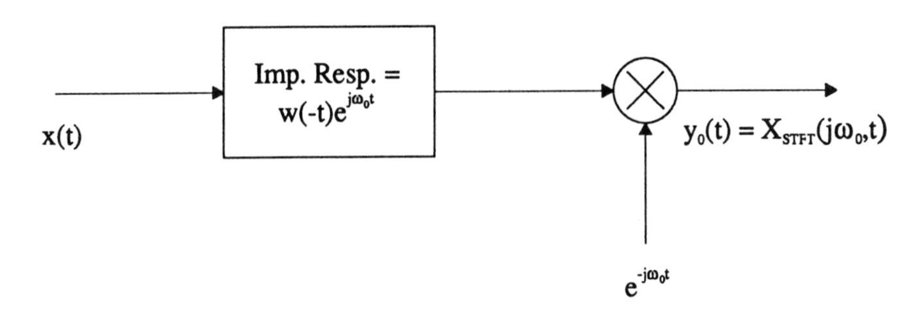

Figure 7.10.1: Computing the CTSTFT as the modulated output of a linear system.

7.10 The Continuous-Time STFT

We will now study the continuous-time STFT (CTSTFT) as a bridge to the study of wavelets. The CTSTFT is similar in form to the discrete-time STFT. Given a signal $x(t)$ and a lowpass window $w(t)$, we have

$$X_{STFT}(j\omega, \tau) = \int_{-\infty}^{\infty} x(t)w(t-\tau)e^{-j\omega t}\,dt \tag{7.10.1}$$

and the inversion formula

$$x(\tau) = \frac{1}{2\pi w(0)} \int_{-\infty}^{\infty} X_{STFT}(j\omega, \tau)e^{j\omega\tau}\,d\omega \tag{7.10.2}$$

again, provided $w(0) \neq 0$. As with the discrete-time STFT, we can provide a filter bank interpretation of the CTSTFT. For a given frequency ω_0, we can rewrite Eq. 7.10.1 as

$$X_{STFT}(j\omega_0, \tau) = e^{-j\omega_0\tau} \int_{-\infty}^{\infty} x(t)w(t-\tau)e^{j\omega_0(\tau-t)}\,dt. \tag{7.10.3}$$

As before, this can be viewed as the modulated output of a filter with impulse response $w(-t)e^{j\omega_0 t}$ at time τ when driven by the input $x(t)$. Specifically,

$$X_{STFT}(j\omega_0, \tau) = [e^{-j\omega_0 t}(h(t) * x(t))]\Big|_{t=\tau}$$

where $h(t) = w(-t)e^{j\omega_0 t}$. This is shown schematically in Fig. 7.10.1. As with the discrete-time STFT, the filter described by $h(t)$ will be a bandpass filter centered at ω_0 which is obtained by frequency-shifting $W(-j\omega)$, and the modulation at the output of the filter brings the output of the filter back to zero frequency.

Again, the output $y_0(t)$ in Fig. 7.10.1 can be regarded as a measure of the frequency content of $x(t)$ around the frequency ω_0 near time $t = \tau$. As with the STFT, we are left with the problem of choosing a window $w(t)$ to meet the conflicting objectives of time and frequency localization. In the discrete-time case, it can be shown (in a somewhat complicated fashion) that the optimal window is a prolate spheroidal window. For the continuous-time case, we will defer discussion until later.

Returning to the filtering interpretation of the CTSTFT, we can compute the STFT at a set of uniformly-spaced frequencies $\omega_m = m\omega_0$ using a bank comprised of filters like the one in Fig. 7.10.1. After modulation at the outputs of the filters, the signals will be narrowband lowpass and can be sampled with some period T to give the two-dimensional sequence

$$X(m,k) = X_{STFT}(jm\omega_0, kT)$$

which is a sampled version of $X_{STFT}(j\omega, \tau)$. Using Eq. 7.10.3, we have

$$X(m,k) = e^{-jmk\omega_0 T} \int_{-\infty}^{\infty} x(t)w(t-kT)e^{jm\omega_0(kT-t)}\,dt. \tag{7.10.4}$$

This is shown in Fig. 7.10.2.

The reconstruction of $x(t)$ from the sampled CTSTFT can be performed using an analysis filter bank. In order to stably reconstruct the signal $x(t)$ from the sampled CTSTFT, it can been shown that the condition $\omega_0 T < 2\pi$ is necessary [Dau90]. Notice that we have not explicitly imposed any bandlimiting on $x(t)$ in order to allow reconstruction; this is implicit in the condition $\omega_0 T < 2\pi$. Consider the case where ω_0 approaches infinity. In this case, there will only be one analysis filter and T will need to approach zero in order to meet the constraint $\omega_0 T < 2\pi$. Therefore, the samples at the output of the filter become arbitrarily close together, and we essentially have $x(t)$.

7.11 The Wavelet Transform

In the previous sections, we examined the STFT and how it can be used to analyze signals whose spectral content vary with time. Although the STFT provides a useful extension of the conventional Fourier transform, it still has some shortcomings which we will soon make clear. A number of alternative techniques have arisen in an attempt to overcome these problems, and the one which has received the most attention of late has been *wavelet analysis*. For a detailed treatment of wavelets, the reader is referred to the books by Daubechies [Dau92] and Chui [Chu92], and for a tutorial review, Rioul and Vetterli's article [RV91] can be consulted. As with Fourier analysis, there are a number of variants on the basic wavelet analysis theory. The one with which we will be most concerned is the discrete-time wavelet transform (DTWT). We will briefly study the discrete wavelet transform (DWT) and the

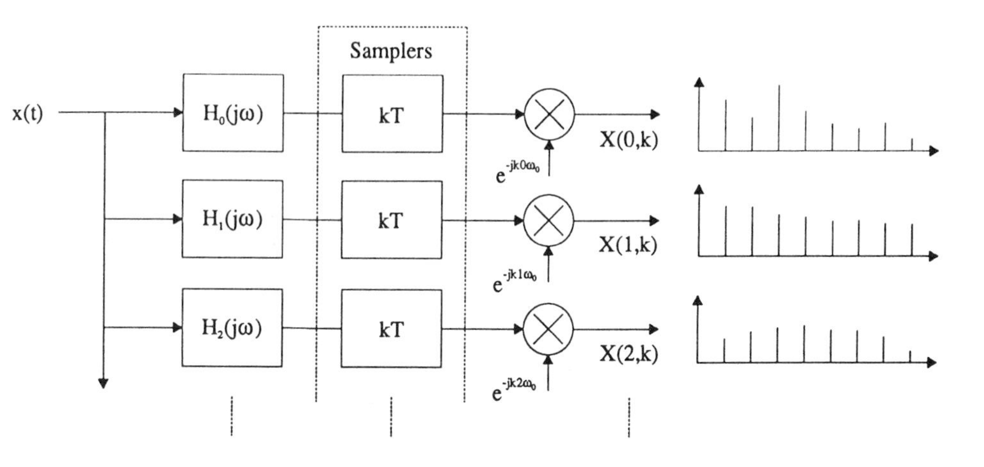

Figure 7.10.2: Sampling the CTSTFT.

continuous wavelet transform (CWT), but mainly for the purpose of developing the DTWT. The existing literature on wavelets typically requires more mathematical sophistication than that possessed by most signal processing professionals. We will give a presentation which is easily understood in the context of multirate systems.

Many of the STFT's shortcomings are a result of the fact that the time-frequency grid is uniform for all time and frequency. To appreciate why this is a problem, consider the problem of estimating the frequency content at both high and low frequencies. Because the analysis window $w(t)$ has a fixed width in the STFT analysis equation, the window will be able to capture many more periods of a sinusoid at a high frequency than at a low frequency. Consequently, the spectral estimate given by the STFT will be good for high frequencies and increasingly poorer for lower frequencies.

For example, suppose we are interested in analyzing a signal of the form

$$x(t) = \begin{cases} \sin(2\pi \times 60t), & t < t_0 \\ \sin(2\pi \times 5000t), & t_0 \leq t \leq t_1 \\ \sin(2\pi \times 60t), & t > t_1 \end{cases}$$

In order to capture the sudden change in frequency in $x(t)$, it is desirable to have the analysis window $v(t)$ very narrow in time in order to capture the transient nature of the signal. For the low-frequency portion of the signal, the narrow window will provide a poor estimate of the signal's spectral content. The wavelet transform [Dau90] provides a solution to this problem by using an analysis window which depends on both time *and* frequency: the window gets wider in time for lower frequencies. Thus, the window captures in time the same number of periods of any frequency sine wave. In addition, because the bandwidth of the filters gets smaller for lower frequencies (due to the fact the the window is wider in time), the outputs in the corresponding filter bank can be decimated by higher rates for lower frequencies. These characteristics constitute the essence of the wavelet transform: analysis windows which depend on both time and frequency, and nonuniform decimation rates.

The filter bank which was used to compute the STFT was seen to consist of analysis filters which were frequency-shifted versions of a base window; consequently, they all have equal bandwidth. The wavelet transform instead uses what are known as *constant-Q* filters. Constant-Q filters are filters which have a constant bandwidth to center-frequency ratio. To see how constant-Q filters can be generated, consider the bandpass filter $H(j\omega)$ shown in Fig. 7.11.1. The center frequency of such a filter is defined as the center of the bandpass region when the frequency response is plotted with a logarithmic frequency axis. Namely,

$$\log(\omega_c) = \frac{\log(\omega_1) + \log(\omega_2)}{2}.$$

This means that

$$\omega_c = \sqrt{\omega_1 \omega_2} \tag{7.11.1}$$

so that the center frequency is the geometric mean of the cutoff frequencies. With the bandwidth given by $\omega_2 - \omega_1$, the *quality factor* Q is given by

$$Q = \frac{\text{bandwidth}}{\text{centerfrequency}} = \frac{\omega_2 - \omega_1}{\sqrt{\omega_1 \omega_2}} \tag{7.11.2}$$

(technically speaking, the quality factor is actually the inverse of the quantity Q we just defined). Now, consider the filter $H_m(j\omega)$ in Fig. 7.11.1 which is obtained from $H(j\omega)$ according to

$$H_m(j\omega) = H(ja^m\omega)$$

where $a > 1$. The new cutoff frequencies are $a^{-m}\omega_1$ and $a^{-m}\omega_2$, respectively so that the center frequency is given by $a^{-m}\sqrt{\omega_1\omega_2}$. The bandwidth is simply $a^{-m}(\omega_2 - \omega_1)$ so that the quality factor for this filter is given by

$$Q_m = \frac{a^{-m}(\omega_2 - \omega_1)}{a^{-m}\sqrt{\omega_1\omega_2}} = \frac{\omega_2 - \omega_1}{\sqrt{\omega_1\omega_2}},$$

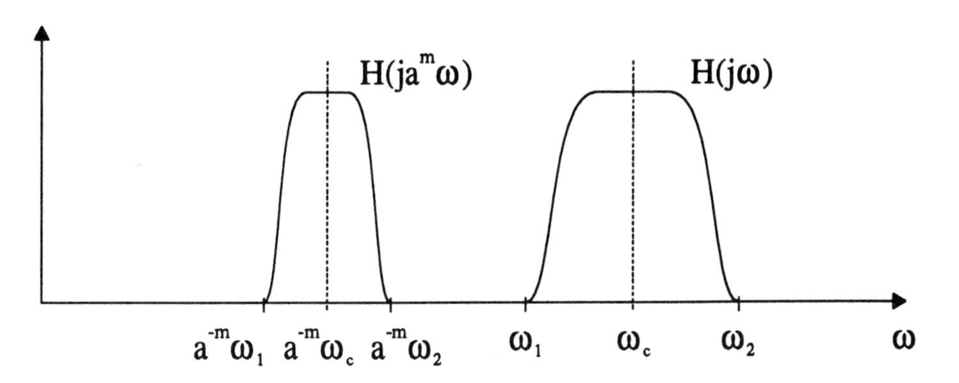

Figure 7.11.1: Prototype bandpass filter and frequency-scaled bandpass filter.

which is the same as the quality factor of $H(j\omega)$. This shows how constant-Q filters can be generated by frequency-scaling a prototype bandpass filter.

If the filter $H(j\omega)$ has impulse response $h(t)$, it follows from the frequency-scaling property of the Fourier transform that

$$h_m(t) = a^{-m} h(a^{-m} t). \tag{7.11.3}$$

Since the constant-Q filters will be used as analysis filters, it is desirable that they all have the same energy, namely

$$\int_{-\infty}^{\infty} h_m^2(t)\, dt = \int_{\infty}^{\infty} h^2(t)\, dt, \qquad \text{for all } m.$$

This normalization can be accomplished by taking

$$h_m(t) = a^{-m/2} h(a^{-m} t) \tag{7.11.4}$$

in which case

$$H_m(j\omega) = a^{m/2} H(j a^m \omega). \tag{7.11.5}$$

This can be visualized in the frequency domain as a "heightening" of the filters as m increases in order to maintain the same energy in the filter as the bandwidth decreases with increasing m, as shown in Fig. 7.11.2. Qualitatively, we can see from Eq. 7.11.4 that as m increases,

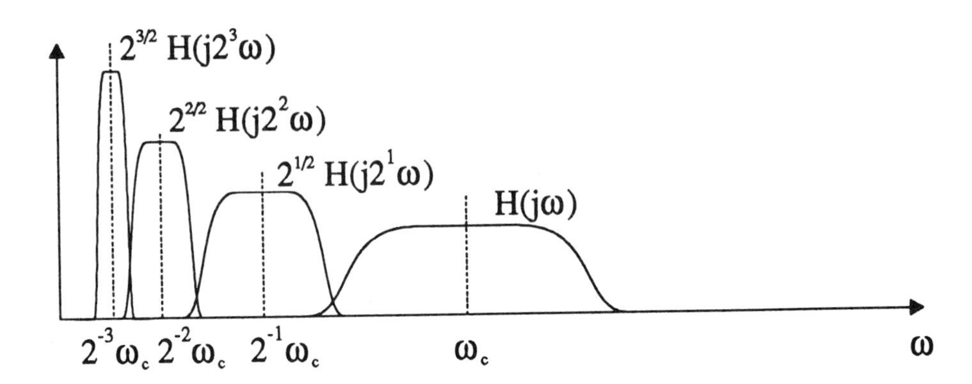

Figure 7.11.2: Frequency responses of successive constant-Q filters obtained by frequency-scaling and height-normalizing (shown for $a = 2$).

the impulse response $h_m(t)$ becomes more spread out in time and hence more concentrated in frequency, as illustrated by Eq. 7.11.5.

The first step in obtaining the wavelet transform is replacing the STFT analysis filter $w(t)$ in Eq. 7.10.3 with the filter $h_m(t)$ and dropping the modulation by $e^{-j\omega_m t}$ (since it is absorbed by the demodulator in the synthesis bank), giving a convolution integral of the form

$$\int_{-\infty}^{\infty} x(t)h_m(\tau - t)\, dt \tag{7.11.6}$$

which, according to Eq. 7.11.4, is equal to

$$a^{-m/2}\int_{-\infty}^{\infty} x(t)h(a^{-m}(\tau - t))\, dt. \tag{7.11.7}$$

Equation 7.11.7 gives the output of the filter $h_m(t)$ when driven by the input $x(t)$. Now, recall that the window $h_m(t)$ becomes more spread out in time as m increases and hence the bandwidth of $H_m(j\omega)$ decreases. Therefore, it seems plausible that the outputs of the analysis filters can be sampled with increasingly larger periods (which corresponds to larger window movement for larger m). Assuming that the output of $H(j\omega)$ is sampled with period T, let's sample the output of $H_m(j\omega)$ with period $a^m T$, which means that we are computing Eq. 7.11.7 at times $\tau = a^m kT$, giving the *discrete wavelet transform* (DWT),

$$X_{DWT}(m, k) = \int_{-\infty}^{\infty} x(t)h_m(a^m kT - t)\, dt. \tag{7.11.8}$$

Using the expression in Eq. 7.11.4 for $h_m(t)$ gives the formula

$$X_{DWT}(m,k) = a^{-m/2} \int_{-\infty}^{\infty} x(t)h(kT - a^{-m}t)\,dt. \tag{7.11.9}$$

The DWT is seen to be a mapping from a one-dimensional signal $x(t)$ to a two-dimensional sequence $X_{DWT}(m,k)$, as shown in Fig. 7.11.3a. The index m in essence corresponds to the center frequency of the bandpass analysis filters, and corresponds to a non-uniform partitioning of the frequency axis. For example, when the frequency scaling parameter a is taken equal to 2, the center frequency is halved each time m is increased by 1. Furthermore, since the filters are sampled increasingly slower with larger m, the index k corresponds to the multiple of the sampling period a^mT at which the output of filter m is sampled. This gives rise to the time-frequency grid for the DWT shown in Fig. 7.11.3b. Notice the difference from the time-frequency grid for the STFT. In the DWT, the frequency samples get closer for lower frequencies while the time samples get farther apart.

For completeness, it should be noted that the DWT is a special case of the *continuous wavelet transform* (CWT), given by

$$X_{CWT}(p,q) = |p|^{-1/2} \int_{-\infty}^{\infty} x(t)w(p^{-1}(t-q))\,dt \tag{7.11.10}$$

where p and q are now taken as real variables rather than integers, as in the case of the DWT. The DWT can be regarded as a sampled version of the CWT if we take $h(t) = w(-t)$, $p = a^m$, and $q = a^mkT$.

Figure 7.11.3a gave a schematic depiction of how the DWT can be computed using an analysis filter bank. A natural question which arises is whether the original signal $x(t)$ can be recovered from the DWT. This problem can be put in terms of designing a synthesis filter bank with inputs equal to the DWT coefficients and making the overall analysis/synthesis bank perfect reconstruction. A synthesis filter bank is shown in Fig. 7.11.4 where the synthesis filters are given by $F_m(j\omega)$. As with the discrete-to-continuous conversion problem, the DWT sequence first needs to be converted to an impulse train. Recall that the sequence $X_{DWT}(m,k)$ corresponds to samples of the m-th analysis filter taken at time instants a^mkT. Therefore, the proper impulse train is of the form

$$\sum_{k=-\infty}^{\infty} X_{DWT}(m,k)\delta(t - a^mkT). \tag{7.11.11}$$

This means that the output of the analysis filter $F_m(j\omega)$ when driven by the impulse train is equal to

$$\sum_{k=-\infty}^{\infty} X_{DWT}(m,k)f_m(t - a^mkT) \tag{7.11.12}$$

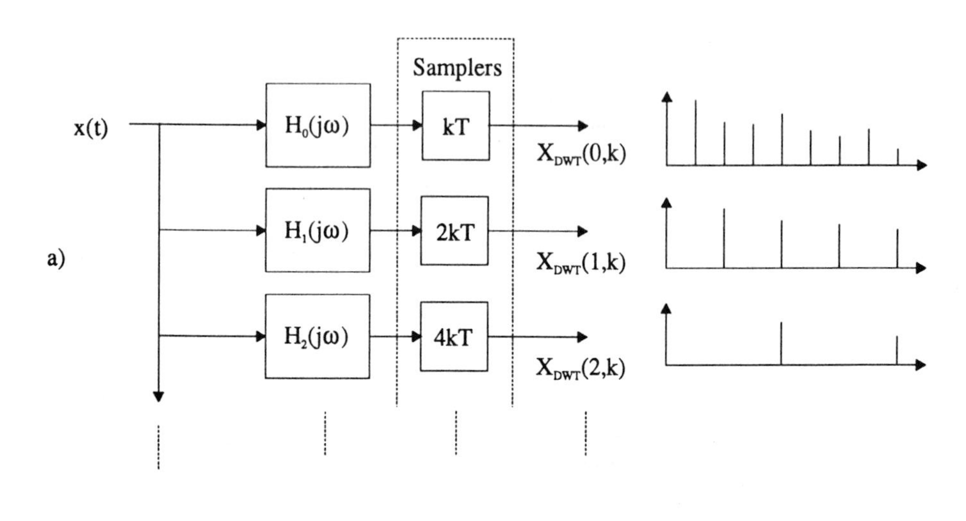

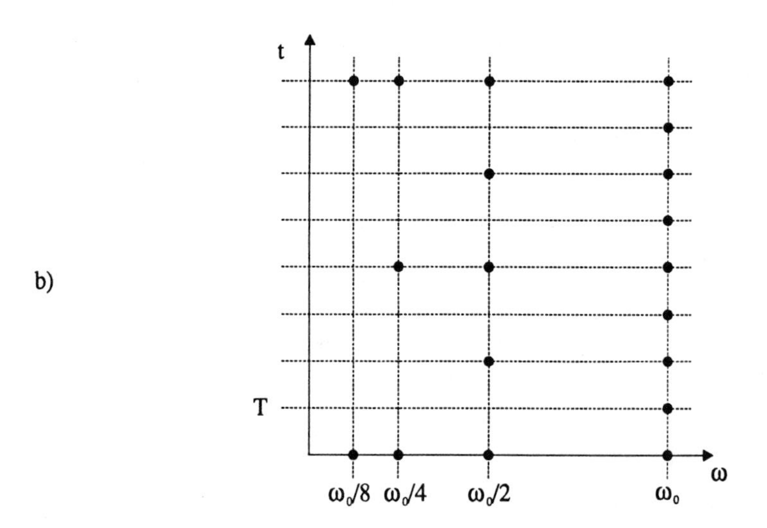

Figure 7.11.3: (a) Schematic illustration of the DWT with $a = 2$; (b) time-frequency grid for the DWT with $a = 2$.

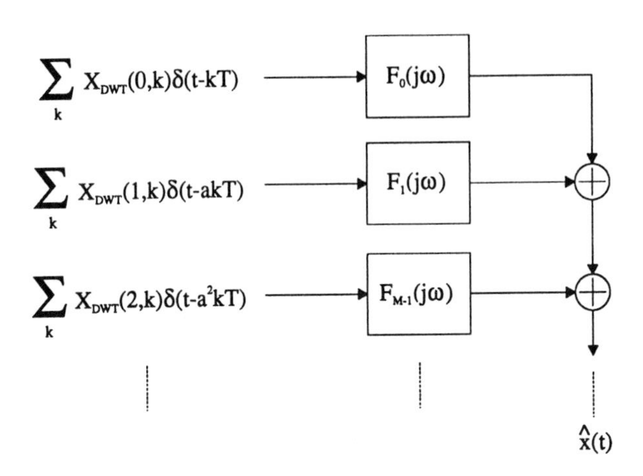

Figure 7.11.4: Synthesis bank to reconstruct $x(t)$ from $X_{DWT}(m,k)$.

and hence the output of the analysis bank is given by

$$\hat{x}(t) = \sum_m \sum_{k=-\infty}^{\infty} X_{DWT}(m,k) f_m(t - a^m kT). \tag{7.11.13}$$

Remember that the DWT analysis filters were related to one another by Eqs. 7.11.4 and 7.11.5. Since the inputs to the synthesis filters are bandlimited to the region passed by the analysis filters, let's assume a similar relationship between the synthesis filters. That is, assume

$$f_m(t) = a^{-m/2} f(a^{-m} t) \tag{7.11.14}$$

for some filter $f(t)$. Assuming we have perfect reconstruction, Eq. 7.11.13 then becomes

$$x(t) = \sum_m \sum_{k=-\infty}^{\infty} X_{DWT}(m,k) a^{-m/2} f(a^{-m}(t - a^m kT)) \tag{7.11.15}$$

which simplifies to

$$x(t) = \sum_m \sum_{k=-\infty}^{\infty} X_{DWT}(m,k) f(a^{-m} t - kT). \tag{7.11.16}$$

Now, let's define a collection of functions $\{\varphi_{mk}(t)\}$ by

$$\varphi_{mk}(t) = a^{-m/2} \varphi(a^{-m}(t - a^m kT)) \tag{7.11.17}$$

where $\varphi(t) = f(t)$. Then Eq. 7.11.15 becomes

$$x(t) = \sum_{m} \sum_{k=-\infty}^{\infty} X_{DWT}(m,k)\varphi_{mk}(t). \tag{7.11.18}$$

Because the $f_m(t)$ are related as in Eq. 7.11.14, it is simple to see from Eq. 7.11.17 that $\varphi_{mk}(t)$ is related to $f_m(t)$ by

$$\varphi_{mk}(t) = f_m(t - a^m kT). \tag{7.11.19}$$

Equation 7.11.18 expresses $x(t)$ as a linear combination of basis functions φ_{mk}. What is significant about this decomposition is that the basis functions are all related in a simple way. The function $\varphi(t)$ is known as a *mother wavelet* and the φ_{mk} are obtained from $\varphi(k)$ through *dilation* and *translation*. The dilation step scales t by $a^{-m}t$ and the translation replaces replaces t with $t - a^m kT$.

So far, we have only addressed the computation of the DWT and how the inverse DWT would be computed, if inversion were at all possible. As with the STFT, this depends on both the basis functions $\{\varphi_{mk}(t)\}$ and the time and frequency sampling parameters a and T [Dau90]. This is a fairly sophisticated matter which we will not pursue further. Rather, we have only discussed the basics as a model for and in preparation for the discrete-time wavelet transform, which we will soon discuss in detail.

A simplification of the DWT results if the basis functions $\{\varphi_{mk}(t)\}$ are *orthonormal, i.e.*,

$$\int_{-\infty}^{\infty} \varphi_{mk}(t)\varphi_{nl}(t)\,dt = \delta(m-n)\delta(k-l). \tag{7.11.20}$$

Assuming this to be the case, multiply Eq. 7.11.18 on both sides by $\varphi_{nl}(t)$, which gives

$$x(t)\varphi_{nl}(t) = \sum_{m} \sum_{k=-\infty}^{\infty} X_{DWT}(m,k)\varphi_{mk}(t)\varphi_{nl}(t). \tag{7.11.21}$$

Now, integrating both sides of Eq. 7.11.21 yields

$$\int_{-\infty}^{\infty} x(t)\varphi_{nl}(t)\,dt = \sum_{m} \sum_{k=-\infty}^{\infty} X_{DWT}(m,k) \int_{-\infty}^{\infty} \varphi_{mk}(t)\varphi_{nl}(t)\,dt \tag{7.11.22}$$

which, according to the orthonormality condition (Eq. 7.11.20) gives

$$\int_{-\infty}^{\infty} x(t)\varphi_{nl}(t)\,dt = \sum_{m} \sum_{k=-\infty}^{\infty} X_{DWT}(m,k)\delta(m-n)\delta(k-l). \tag{7.11.23}$$

Simplifying Eq. 7.11.23, we thus have the relationship

$$\int_{-\infty}^{\infty} x(t)\varphi_{nl}(t)\,dt = X_{DWT}(n,l). \tag{7.11.24}$$

This shows that the DWT coefficients can be computed as simple inner products between $x(t)$ and the wavelet basis functions $\varphi_{mk}(t)$.

The orthonormality condition also gives a simple relationship between the analysis and synthesis filters $h_m(t)$ and $f_m(t)$. Comparing Eqs. 7.11.24 and 7.11.8, we see that

$$\varphi_{mk}(t) = h_m(a^m kT - t). \tag{7.11.25}$$

Because of the relationship between the $\varphi_{mk}(t)$ expressed by Eq. 7.11.17, it follows that $\varphi_{00}(t) = \varphi(t)$, which, by construction, is equal to $f(t)$. Equation 7.11.25 shows further that $\varphi_{00}(t) = h(-t)$. Therefore, for the case of orthonormal wavelets, it follows that

$$f(t) = h(-t)$$

and hence, $f_m(t) = h_m(-t)$, giving a very simple relationship between the analysis and synthesis filters. Again, we will not discuss how to generate an orthonormal basis for the DWT, but will for the discrete-time wavelet transform.

7.12 The Discrete-Time Wavelet Transform

We are now in a position to discuss the discrete-time wavelet transform (DTWT). Unlike the DWT, we will actually see how to actually design the filter banks for the transform and for the inversion, as well as how to generate orthonormal wavelet bases.

We will attempt to mirror the frequency-domain properties of the DWT as a starting point for the DTWT. The reason why we do not instead begin from the time-domain properties is that the time dilation step $t \to a^{-m}t$ will not in general give integer samples $a^{-m}k$. Instead, let's try to generate a collection of filters which have frequency responses analogous to those shown in Fig. 7.11.2. Suppose $H(z)$ is a highpass filter with cutoff frequency $\pi/2$ and $G(z)$ is a lowpass filter with cutoff frequency $\pi/2$. Figure 7.12.1 shows the frequency responses of $H(z)$, $G(z)$, $H(z^2)$, $G(z^2)$, $H(z^4)$, and $G(z^4)$.

Now, we can see that the desired responses are obtained by using the filters

$$\begin{aligned} H_3(z) &= G(z)G(z^2)G(z^4) \\ H_2(z) &= G(z)G(z^2)H(z^4) \\ H_1(z) &= G(z)H(z^2) \\ H_0(z) &= H(z) \end{aligned} \tag{7.12.1}$$

These filters will have the frequency responses shown in Fig. 7.12.1 and 7.12.2c. Given $G(z)$ and $H(z)$, it is simple to show that the tree-structured filter bank in Fig. 7.11.4a will produce these transfer functions. For example, consider the output $y_3(k)$. Starting from the left-hand side of the filter bank, we can move the decimator to the right of the middle $G(z)$, replace this

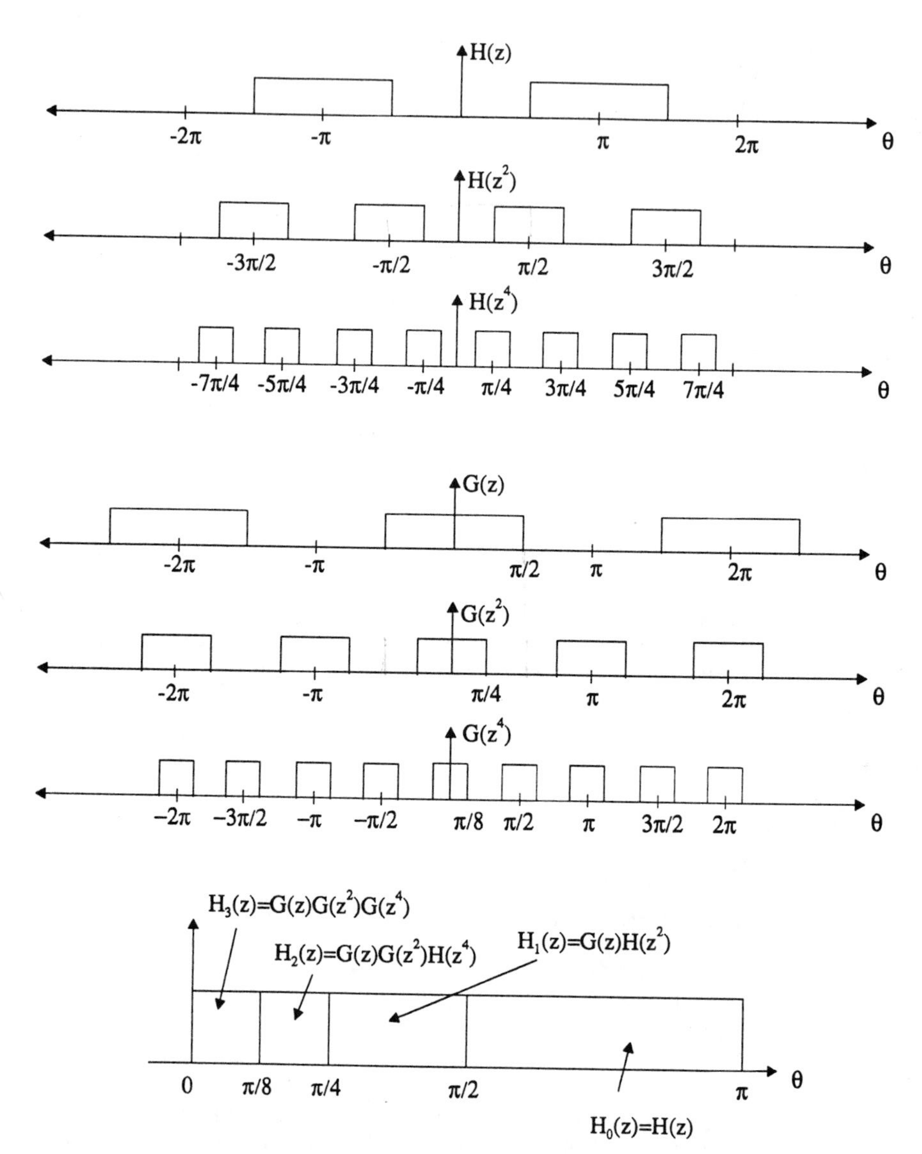

Figure 7.12.1: Frequency-scaled replicas of $H(z)$ and $G(z)$.

$G(z)$ with $G(z^2)$, and combine the two decimators to form one decimator with a rate equal to 4. Next, the decimator of rate 4 is moved to the right of the right-most $G(z)$, this $G(z)$ is replaced with $G(z^4)$, and the two decimators are combined to form one decimator with rate equal to eight. In a similar manner, this is performed for each branch of the tree-structured filter bank, giving the ordinary filter bank with nonuniform decimation ratios shown in Fig. 7.12.2b. The frequency responses of the $H_m(z)$ are as shown in Fig. 7.12.2c.

Notice that the signals $x_m(k)$ in Fig. 7.12.2b are bandlimited by the filters $H_m(z)$ and that the amount of decimation at the filter outputs is proportional to the bandwidth of the filters. Furthermore, it is simple to see that the filters $H_m(z)$ are constant-Q (measured over the range $(0, \pi)$, of course). Now, the output $x_m(k)$ is given by

$$x_m(k) = \sum_{l=-\infty}^{\infty} x(l) h_m(k-l). \tag{7.12.2}$$

The discrete-time wavelet coefficients are given by the decimated signals $y_m(k)$. Notice from Fig. 7.12.2b that the decimation rate for the m-th filter is 2^{m+1} for $m = 0, 1, \ldots, M-2$ and 2^{M-1} for the $(M-1)$-st filter. Therefore, we have

$$y_m(k) = \sum_{l=-\infty}^{\infty} x(l) h_m(2^{m+1}k - l), \quad m = 0, 1, \ldots, M-2 \tag{7.12.3}$$

and

$$y_{M-1}(k) = \sum_{l=-\infty}^{\infty} x(l) h_{M-1}(2^{M-1}k - l). \tag{7.12.4}$$

Equations 7.12.3 and 7.12.4 constitute the DTWT.

The issue of inversion of the DTWT is simpler than DWT. We have already seen how to generate two-channel perfect reconstruction filter banks. Consider the synthesis filter bank in Fig. 7.12.3a. If the filters

$$\{G(z), H(z), G_s(z), H_s(z)\}$$

form a two-channel perfect reconstruction bank, it is easy to argue inductively that the overall tree-structured bank will also have the perfect reconstruction property. This is simply due to the fact that path from the input to the output of each two-channel bank is perfect reconstruction and the tree is comprised of a set of nested two-channel perfect reconstruction banks.

As with the tree-structured analysis bank, the tree-structured synthesis bank can be put in the form shown in Fig. 7.12.3b. Like we did earlier, it is easily shown that the synthesis

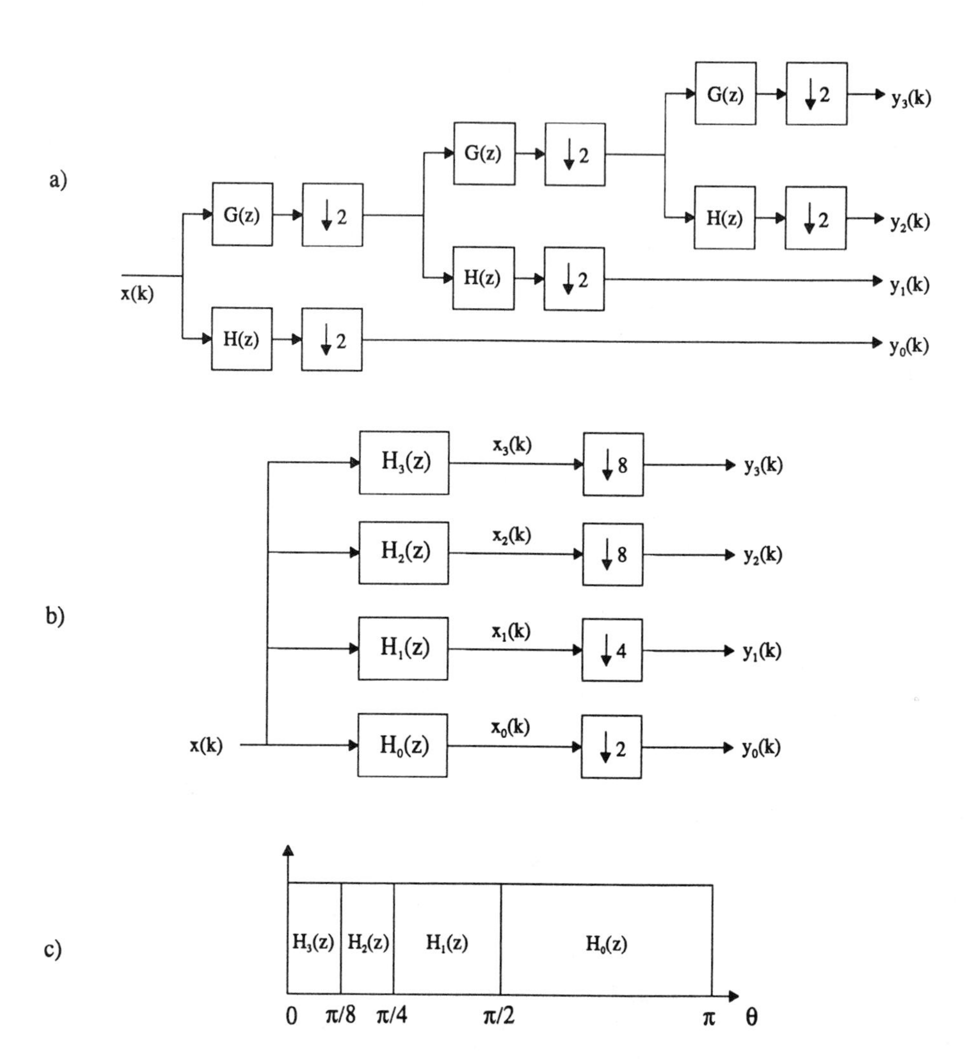

Figure 7.12.2: (a) Tree-structured analysis filter bank; (b) equivalent analysis bank; (c) frequency responses of analysis filters.

filters $F_m(z)$ are given by

$$\begin{aligned} F_3(z) &= G_s(z^4)G_s(z^2)G_s(z) \\ F_2(z) &= H_s(z^4)G_s(z^2)G_s(z) \\ F_1(z) &= H_s(z^2)G_s(z) \\ F_0(z) &= H_s(z) \end{aligned} \tag{7.12.5}$$

The analysis filters will have frequency responses as shown in Fig. 7.12.3c.

With the synthesis filter bank as shown in Fig. 7.12.3b, the reconstruction process is described by

$$\begin{aligned} X(z) &= F_0(z)Y_0(z^2) + F_1(z)Y_1(z^4) + \cdots + F_{M-2}(z)Y_{M-2}(z^{2^{M-1}}) \\ &\quad + F_{M-1}(z)Y_{M-2}(z^{2^{M-1}}) \end{aligned} \tag{7.12.6}$$

In the time domain, the output $v_m(k)$ of the m-th synthesis filter is given by

$$v_m(k) = \sum_{l=-\infty}^{\infty} y_m(l) f_m(k - 2^{m+1}l), \quad m = 0, 1, \ldots, M-2 \tag{7.12.7}$$

and the output of the $(M-1)$-st filter is given by

$$v_{M-1}(k) = \sum_{l=-\infty}^{\infty} y_{M-1}(l) f_{M-1}(k - 2^{M-1}l). \tag{7.12.8}$$

The output $x(k)$ is equal to the sum of the $v_m(k)$, so we have from Eqs. 7.12.7 and 7.12.8 that

$$x(k) = \sum_{m=0}^{M-2} \sum_{l=-\infty}^{\infty} y_m(l) f_m(k - 2^{m+1}l) + \sum_{l=-\infty}^{\infty} y_{M-1}(l) f_{M-1}(k - 2^{M-1}l). \tag{7.12.9}$$

Let's define the basis functions $\{\varphi_{ml}\}$ by

$$\begin{aligned} \varphi_{ml}(k) &= f_m(k - 2^{m+1}l), \quad m = 0, 1, \ldots, M-2 \\ \varphi_{M-1,l}(k) &= f_{M-1}(k - 2^{M-1}l). \end{aligned} \tag{7.12.10}$$

Comparing Eqs. 7.12.9 and 7.12.10, we see immediately that

$$x(k) = \sum_{m=0}^{M-1} \sum_{l=-\infty}^{\infty} y_m(l) \varphi_{ml}(k). \tag{7.12.11}$$

Equation 7.12.11 is the inverse DTWT equation and expresses $x(k)$ as a decomposition of $x(k)$ into DTWT coefficients $\{y_m(l)\}$ which are weights for the basis functions $\{\varphi_{ml}(k)\}$.

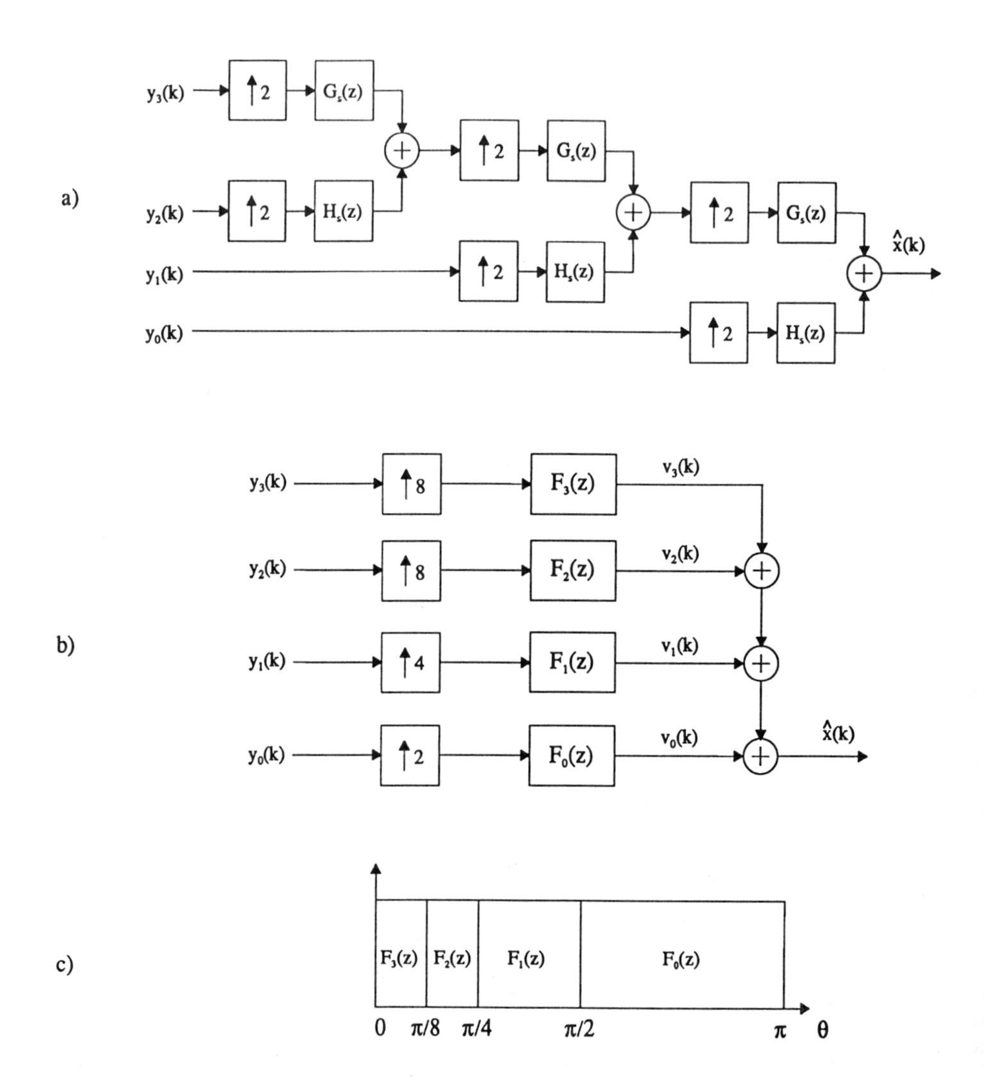

Figure 7.12.3: (a) Tree-structured synthesis filter bank; (b) equivalent synthesis bank; (c) frequency responses of synthesis filters.

As a brief side note, we can discuss one popular application of the DTWT: multiresolution analysis. Referring to Figs. 7.12.2 and 7.12.3, we can see how the input signal and the DTWT coefficients are filtered by the analysis and synthesis filters. The signal $v_3(k)$ can be regarded as a lowpass filtered (smoothed) version of $x(k)$ and is a first approximation to $x(k)$. The signal $v_2(k)$ is a bandpass filtered version of $x(k)$ and adds slightly more detail to the output. The same is true for $v_1(k)$. Finally, $v_0(k)$ adds the highest-frequency detail to the output. The signals $v_m(k)$ are referred to as the *multiresolution components* [Mal89] of $x(k)$ and contribute increasingly finer detail to the output of the synthesis bank as m decreases. In practice, this can be exploited to obtain data compression: the multiresolution components which contribute as much detail as desired are stored or transmitted (*i.e.* the higher resolution components can be omitted or coded with fewer bits). This techniques has been used successfully in the video field.

Orthonormal DTWT basis

As with the DWT, if the basis functions $\{\varphi_{ml}(k)\}$ can be made orthonormal, the situation is simplified. Orthonormality means that

$$\sum_{k=-\infty}^{\infty} \varphi_{ml}(k)\varphi_{nr}(k) = \delta(m-n)\delta(l-r). \tag{7.12.12}$$

Just as we showed with DWT, in a similar fashion it is simple to show that orthonormality of the DTWT basis functions implies that the DTWT coefficients can be computed according to

$$y_m(l) = \sum_{k=-\infty}^{\infty} x(k)\varphi_{ml}(k). \tag{7.12.13}$$

Comparing Eqs. 7.12.13 and 7.12.3, it is clear that

$$\varphi_{ml}(k) = h_m(2^{m+1}l - k). \tag{7.12.14}$$

Furthermore, from Eq. 7.12.10, we have

$$\varphi_{ml}(k) = f_m(k - 2^{m+1}l). \tag{7.12.15}$$

Therefore, if the orthonormality condition is satisfied, it follows immediately from Eqs. 7.12.14 and 7.12.15 that the analysis and synthesis filters are related by

$$f_m(k) = h_m(-k). \tag{7.12.16}$$

We have seen so far how to compute the DTWT and the inverse DTWT and how the orthonormality condition simplifies the relationship between the analysis and synthesis filters.

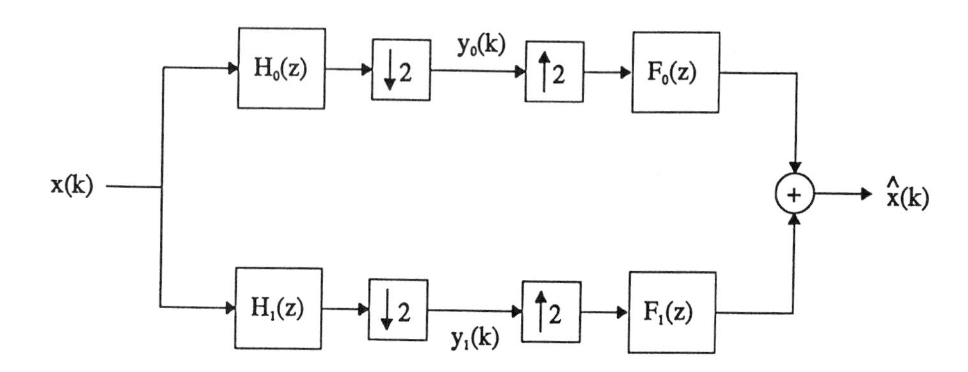

Figure 7.12.4: Two-channel QMF bank.

The next problem is how to actually generate an orthonormal DTWT basis. We will show that this can be accomplished from a tree-structured filter bank using our earlier results from perfect reconstruction two-channel QMF banks.

Figure 7.12.4 shows, repeated for convenience, the two-channel QMF, with analysis filters $H_0(z)$ and $H_1(z)$ and synthesis filters $F_0(z)$ and $F_1(z)$. This is a simple system for computing a DTWT, and the DWT coefficients are given by

$$y_0(k) = \sum_{l=-\infty}^{\infty} x(l)h_0(2k-l) \qquad (7.12.17)$$

and

$$y_1(k) = \sum_{l=-\infty}^{\infty} x(l)h_1(2k-l) \qquad (7.12.18)$$

If the filter bank is perfect reconstruction, then the output is given by

$$x(k) = \sum_{l=-\infty}^{\infty} y_0(l)f_0(k-2l) + \sum_{l=-\infty}^{\infty} y_1(l)f_1(k-2l). \qquad (7.12.19)$$

Comparing Eq. 7.12.19 with Eq. 7.12.9, we can see that the basis functions are given by

$$\varphi_{0l}(k) = f_0(k-2l), \quad \varphi_{1l}(k) = f_1(k-2l).$$

The orthonormality condition expressed by Eq. 7.12.12 means that we require

$$\sum_{k=-\infty}^{\infty} f_m(k-2l)f_n(k-2r) = \delta(m-n)\delta(l-r).$$

If we make the change of summation $q = k - 2l$, the above equation becomes

$$\sum_{q=-\infty}^{\infty} f_m(q) f_n(q + 2(l - r)) = \delta(m - n)\delta(l - r). \tag{7.12.20}$$

Finally, let $l - r = s$, in which case Eq. 7.12.20 reduces to

$$\sum_{q=-\infty}^{\infty} f_m(q) f_n(q + 2s) = \delta(m - n)\delta(s). \tag{7.12.21}$$

Equation 7.12.21 tells us that $f_m(k)$ and $f_n(k)$ are orthogonal for even time shifts s. Now, we recognize the left- hand side of Eq. 7.12.21 as the cross-correlation between $f_m(k)$ and $f_n(k)$ evaluated at even time-lag $2s$. The $\mathcal{Z}$-transform of the cross-correlation is given by $F_m(z)F_n(z^{-1})$ and extracting the even lags is equivalent to decimating the cross-correlation sequence by two. Therefore, the $\mathcal{Z}$-transform of Eq. 7.12.21 is given by

$$\frac{1}{2}[F_m(z^{1/2})F_n(z^{-1/2}) + F_m(-z^{1/2})F_n(-z^{-1/2})] = \delta(m - n)$$

which simplifies to

$$F_m(z)F_n(z^{-1}) + F_m(-z)F_n(-z^{-1}) = 2\delta(m - n) \tag{7.12.22}$$

This gives us a $\mathcal{Z}$-transform-domain description of the conditions which must be satisfied by the two-channel QMF for a orthonormal DTWT basis.

Substituting $m, n = 0, 1$ into Eq. 7.12.22 gives us four equations which must be satisfied:

$$\begin{aligned} F_0(z)F_0(z^{-1}) + F_0(-z)F_0(-z^{-1}) &= 2 \\ F_1(z)F_1(z^{-1}) + F_1(-z)F_1(-z^{-1}) &= 2 \\ F_0(z)F_1(z^{-1}) + F_0(-z)F_1(-z^{-1}) &= 0 \\ F_1(z)F_0(z^{-1}) + F_1(-z)F_0(-z^{-1}) &= 0 \end{aligned} \tag{7.12.23}$$

Recall the perfect reconstruction QMF which was described by the four filters

$$\begin{array}{ll} H_0(z) = H(z) & H_1(z) = -z^{-(N-1)}H(-z^{-1}) \\ F_0(z) = z^{-(N-1)}H(z^{-1}) & F_1(z) = z^{-(N-1)}H_1(z^{-1}) \end{array} \tag{7.12.24}$$

where $H(z)$ satisfies

$$H(z)H(z^{-1}) + H(-z)H(-z^{-1}) = \alpha \tag{7.12.25}$$

and we showed how $H(z)$ could be obtained as the spectral factor of a positive-definite FIR. Let's make two simple modifications to this scheme. First, take $\alpha = 2$ in Eq. 7.12.25. Second, let's allow the the synthesis filters in Eq. 7.12.24 to be noncausal (this will not affect the perfect reconstruction property; it will simply make it a delay-free perfect reconstruction). Therefore, we have the analysis/synthesis bank described by

$$H(z)H(z^{-1}) + H(-z)H(-z^{-1}) = 2 \tag{7.12.26}$$

and

$$\begin{array}{ll} H_0(z) = H(z) & H_1(z) = -z^{-(N-1)}H(-z^{-1}) \\ F_0(z) = H(z^{-1}) & F_1(z) = H_1(z^{-1}). \end{array} \tag{7.12.27}$$

We can see that the condition $f_m(k) = h_m(-k)$ from Eq. 7.12.16 is clearly met. Furthermore, it is a trivial exercise to show that this collection of filters satisfies Eq. 7.12.23. Therefore, the QMF bank is perfect reconstruction *and* has an orthonormal DTWT basis!

All that remains to be shown is how to generate a M-channel bank with an orthonormal DTWT basis. We will proceed by an inductive argument. Namely, we will show that given a tree-structured filter bank with L levels which has an orthonormal DTWT basis, it is simple to force a tree with $L+1$ levels to have an orthonormal DTWT basis. We have shown how to generate a two-channel ($L = 1$) tree-structured bank with an orthonormal DTWT basis (see Eqs. 7.12.24 and 7.12.25). Suppose now that we have a L-level tree with orthonormal basis. Two of the branches of the synthesis bank are shown in Fig. 7.12.5a, where we will assume without loss of generality that $n_m \geq n_n$. The orthonormality condition for the L-level tree means that the condition

$$\sum_{k=-\infty}^{\infty} f_m(k - 2^{n_m}l)f_n(k - 2^{n_n}r) = \delta(m-n)\delta(l-r) \tag{7.12.28}$$

is satisfied. It can be shown [Vai93] that this is equivalent to

$$\sum_{k=-\infty}^{\infty} f_m(k)f_n(k + 2^{n_n}s) = \delta(m-n)\delta(s). \tag{7.12.29}$$

The left-hand side of Eq. 7.12.29 is seen to be equal to the cross-correlation between $f_m(k)$ and $f_n(k)$ for lags $2^{n_n}s$. Consequently, we can view the summation in Eq. 7.12.29 as the cross-correlation between $f_m(k)$ and $f_n(k)$, decimated by 2^{n_n}. The $\mathcal{Z}$-transform of the cross-correlation is given by $F_m(z)F_n(z^{-1})$ and thus taking the $\mathcal{Z}$-transform of both sides of Eq. 7.12.29 gives

$$F_m(z)F_n(z^{-1})\Big|_{\downarrow 2^{n_n}} = \delta(m-n) \tag{7.12.30}$$

where we have used the notation "$\downarrow 2^{2^{n_n}}$" to indicate that we are interested in the $\mathcal{Z}$-transform of the decimated-by-2^{n_n} sequence.

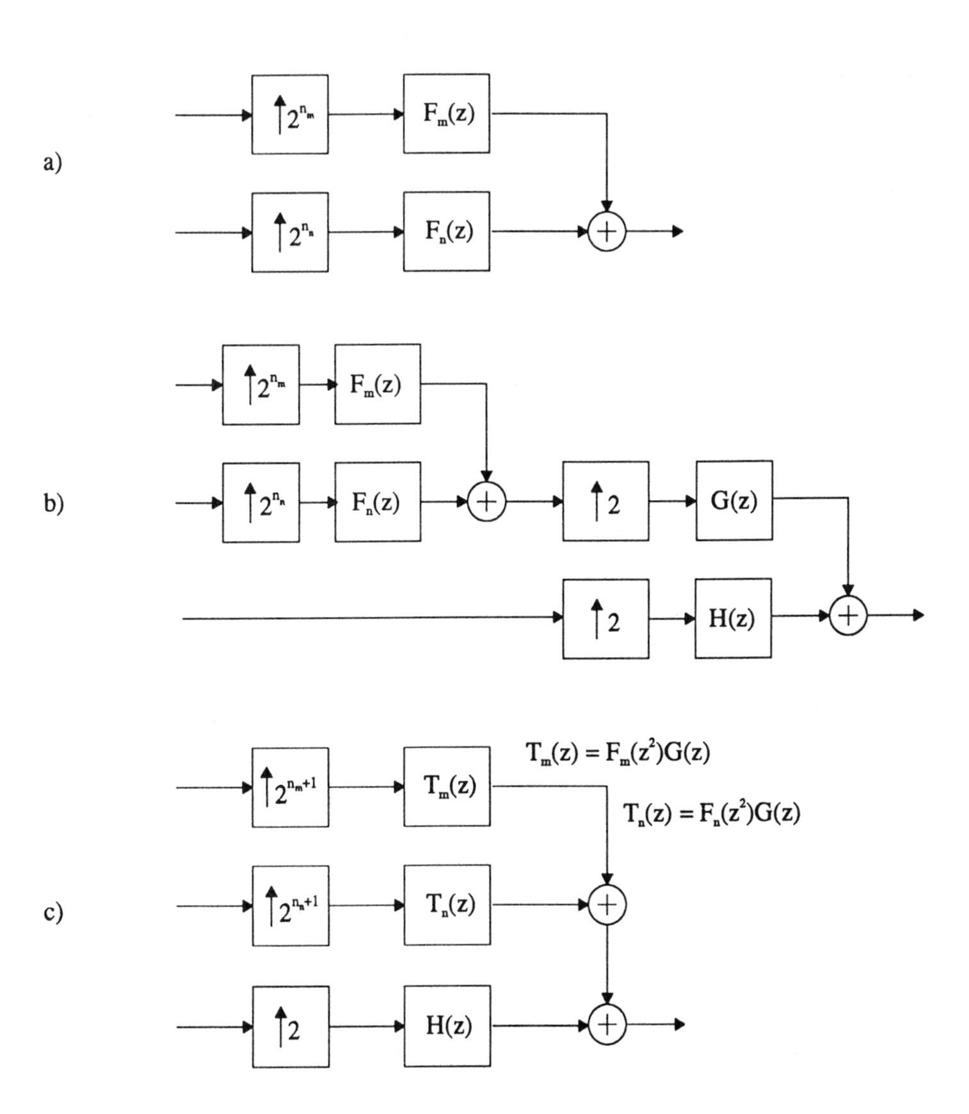

Figure 7.12.5: (a) Two branches in the L-level synthesis bank; (b) adding another level to the tree; (c) Filter bank which is equivalent to (b).

Now, Fig. 7.12.5b shows how a new level is added to the tree structure. At this point, suppose the filters $H_s(z)$ and $G_s(z)$ satisfy Eqs. 7.12.23. This can be put in the more compact notation

$$G_s(z)G_s(z^{-1})\Big|_{\downarrow 2} = 1, \quad H_s(z)H_s(z^{-1})\Big|_{\downarrow 2} = 1, \quad G_s(z)H_s(z^{-1})\Big|_{\downarrow 2} = 0. \tag{7.12.31}$$

Moving the upsamplers in Fig. 7.12.5b, we obtain the rearrangement shown in Fig. 7.12.5c. Clearly, the filters $T_m(z)$ and $T_n(z)$ are given by

$$T_m(z) = F_m(z^2)G_s(z), \quad T_n(z) = F_n(z^2)G_s(z). \tag{7.12.32}$$

To prove orthonormality, Eq. 7.12.30 states that it is sufficient to show that

$$T_m(z)T_n(z^{-1})\Big|_{\downarrow 2^{n_n+1}} = \delta(m-n) \tag{7.12.33}$$

and

$$T_m(z)H_s(z^{-1})\Big|_{\downarrow 2} = 0, \quad T_n(z)H_s(z^{-1})\Big|_{\downarrow 2} = 0. \tag{7.12.34}$$

First, we cite the simple identity [Vai93]

$$\left(A(z^2)B(z)\right)\Big|_{2^{N+1}} = \left(A(z)(B(z)|_{\downarrow 2})\right)\Big|_{\downarrow 2^N} \tag{7.12.35}$$

and use this identity to show Eq. 7.12.33 is true. First, using Eq. 7.12.32, we have

$$T_m(z)T_n(z^{-1}) = F_m(z^2)F_m(z^{-2})G_s(z)G_s(z^{-1}). \tag{7.12.36}$$

Using the identity in Eq. 7.12.35 gives

$$F_m(z^2)F_n(z^{-2})G_s(z)G_s(z^{-1})\Big|_{\downarrow 2^{n_n+1}} = \left(T_m(z)T_n(z^{-1})(G_s(z)G_s(z^{-1})\Big|_{\downarrow 2})\right)\Big|_{\downarrow 2^{n_n}} \tag{7.12.37}$$

and from Eq. 7.12.31, the above becomes

$$\left(F_m(z^2)F_n(z^{-2})G_s(z)G_s(z^{-1})\right)\Big|_{2^{n_n+1}} = F_m(z)F_n(z^{-1})\Big|_{\downarrow 2^{n_n}}. \tag{7.12.38}$$

Now, the orthogonality assumption for the L-level tree yielded Eq. 7.12.30, which, when substituted into the above gives

$$\left(F_m(z^2)F_n(z^{-2})G_s(z)G_s(z^{-1})\right)\Big|_{2^{n_n+1}} = \delta(m-n). \tag{7.12.39}$$

Comparing Eqs. 7.12.36 and 7.12.39 thus gives

$$T_m(z)T_n(z^{-1})\Big|_{2^{n_n+1}} = \delta(m-n). \tag{7.12.40}$$

Therefore, we have proved that Eq. 7.12.33 is true. The conditions in Eq. 7.12.34 are shown to be true in a similar fashion. This means that the $L+1$ level tree has an orthonormal wavelet basis.

We now know how to generate an orthonormal wavelet basis. We simply build a tree-structured filter bank where the analysis/synthesis pairs at each stage are perfect reconstruction and satisfy the constraints in Eq. 7.12.31. We know that the filters described by Eqs. 7.12.26 and 7.12.27 meet these needs. In this case, the overall filter bank will have perfect reconstruction and an orthonormal DTWT basis.

7.13 Time-Frequency Localization

Until now, we have not provided quantitative measures of the time-frequency localization of the STFT and wavelet transform. Given a window $w(t)$, we define the *center* by

$$t_* = \frac{1}{||w||_2^2} \int_{\infty}^{\infty} t|w(t)|^2 \, dt \tag{7.13.1}$$

and the *radius* by

$$\Delta_t = \frac{1}{||w||_2} \left\{ \int_{-\infty}^{\infty} (t-t_*)^2 |w(t)|^2 \, dt \right\}^{1/2} \tag{7.13.2}$$

where

$$||w||_2^2 = \int_{-\infty}^{\infty} |w(t)|^2 \, dt. \tag{7.13.3}$$

The norm $||w||_2$ is the L^2 norm of $w(t)$, which gives the energy of $w(t)$. The quantity t_* is the temporal center of the window, and for even functions of time, it is clear that the center is $t_* = 0$. The radius Δ_t is also known as the *RMS duration* of the window. Similarly, for the Fourier transform $W(j\omega)$ of $w(t)$, we define the center by

$$\omega_* = \frac{1}{||W||_2^2} \int_{\infty}^{\infty} \omega |W(j\omega)|^2 \, d\omega \tag{7.13.4}$$

and the radius by

$$\Delta_\omega = \frac{1}{||W||_2} \left\{ \int_{-\infty}^{\infty} (\omega-\omega_*)^2 |W(j\omega)|^2 \, d\omega \right\}^{1/2} \tag{7.13.5}$$

where

$$||W||_2^2 = \int_{-\infty}^{\infty} |W(j\omega)|^2 \, d\omega. \tag{7.13.6}$$

From Parseval's theorem, it immediately follows that

$$\int_{\infty}^{\infty} |w(t)|^2\, dt = \frac{1}{2\pi}\int_{-\infty}^{\infty} |W(j\omega)|^2\, d\omega$$

so that Eqs. 7.13.3 and 7.13.6 imply that

$$||W||_2^2 = 2\pi ||w||_2^2.$$

The quantity Δ_ω is also known as the *RMS bandwidth* of $W(j\omega)$. The RMS duration and RMS bandwidth give a measure of time and frequency localization provided by the window $w(t)$, and taken together, they measure time-frequency localization. We will make this notion precise shortly.

Recall that we defined the CSTFT by

$$X_{STFT}(j\omega, \tau) = \int_{\infty}^{\infty} x(t)w(t-\tau)e^{-j\omega t}\, dt.$$

At a particular time-frequency point (ω_0, t_0), the CTSTFT is given by

$$X_{STFT}(j\omega_0, t_0) = \int_{\infty}^{\infty} x(t)w(t-t_0)e^{-j\omega_0 t}\, dt.$$

The conventional Fourier transform $X(j\omega_0)$ at a frequency ω_0 of $x(t)$ is given by

$$X(j\omega_0) = \int_{-\infty}^{\infty} x(t)e^{-j\omega_0 t}\, dt.$$

This may be regarded as the inner product of $x(t)$ and the function $\varphi(t) = e^{j\omega_0 t}$,

$$X(j\omega) = \langle x(t), \varphi(t)\rangle = \int_{-\infty}^{\infty} x(t)\bar{\varphi}(t)\, dt.$$

The time-frequency of the Fourier transform is poor because the RMS duration of $e^{j\omega_0 t}$ is infinite. In a similar manner, the CTSTFT can viewed as the inner product of $x(t)$ with $w(t-t_0)e^{j\omega_0 t}$. The time localization will be improved because the window $w(t-t_0)$ decreases the RMS duration. Suppose the window $w(t)$ has center t_* and RMS duration Δ_t. What can be said of the center and RMS duration of $w(t-t_0)e^{j\omega_0 t}$? Let's define the function $w_{t_0,\omega_0}(t)$ by

$$w_{t_0,\omega_0}(t) = w(t-t_0)e^{j\omega_0 t}. \tag{7.13.7}$$

Then it is trivial to show that the energy of w_{t_0,ω_0} is given by

$$||w_{t_0,\omega_0}||_2^2 = ||w||_2^2. \tag{7.13.8}$$

The center of w_{t_0,ω_0} is given by

$$t_*^{t_0,\omega_0} = \frac{1}{||w_{t_0,\omega_0}||} \int_{-\infty}^{\infty} t|w_{t_0,\omega_0}(t)|^2 \, dt.$$

Using Eq. 7.13.7 for w_{t_0,ω_0}, we find that

$$t_*^{t_0,\omega_0} = t_* + t_0, \tag{7.13.9}$$

which should come as no surprise since the term $w(t-t_0)$ moves the window by t_0. Similarly, the RMS duration is given by

$$\Delta_t^{t_0,\omega_0} = \frac{1}{||w_{t_0,\omega_0}||} \left\{ \int_{\infty}^{\infty} (t - t_*^{t_0,\omega_0})^2 |w_{t_0,\omega_0}(t)|^2 \, dt \right\}^{1/2},$$

which is simple to show gives

$$\Delta_t^{t_0,\omega_0} = \Delta_t. \tag{7.13.10}$$

We say that the the STFT at (t_0, ω_0) localizes $x(t)$ in the time interval centered at $t_*^{t_0,\omega_0}$ with a radius of $\Delta_t^{t_0,\omega_0}$, so the time localization interval is given by

$$[t_*^{t_0,\omega_0} - \Delta_t^{t_0,\omega_0}, t_*^{t_0,\omega_0} + \Delta_t^{t_0,\omega_0}] = [t_* + t_0 - \Delta_t, t_* + t_0 + \Delta_t].$$

The time-localization width for the STFT is thus a constant $2\Delta_t$.

Next, we consider the frequency localization. Assume that $w(t)$ has center ω_* and RMS bandwidth Δ_ω. We denote the Fourier transform of $w_{t_0,\omega_0}(t)$ by $W_{t_0,\omega_0}(j\omega)$, which is related to $W(j\omega)$ by

$$W_{t_0,\omega_0}(j\omega) = e^{-j(\omega-\omega_0)t} G(j(\omega - \omega)).$$

In a manner analogous to the time-domain quantities, it is simple to prove that the center of G_{t_0,ω_0} is given by

$$\omega_*^{t_0,\omega_0} = \omega_* + \omega_0$$

and that the RMS bandwidth is given by

$$\Delta_\omega^{t_0,\omega_0} = \Delta_\omega.$$

Therefore, the frequency localization interval is given by

$$[\omega_* + \omega_0 - \Delta_\omega, \omega_* + \omega_0 + \Delta_\omega].$$

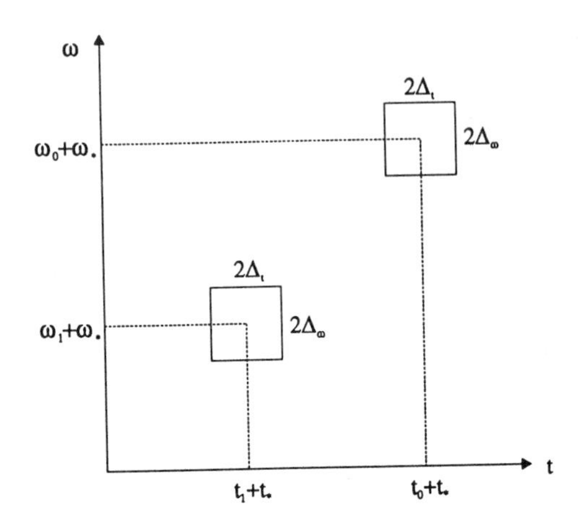

Figure 7.13.1: Time-frequency localization provided by the STFT.

The frequency localization width for the STFT is thus a constant $2\Delta_\omega$.

For any time-frequency point (t_0, ω_0), the time-frequency localization provided by the STFT is over the rectangle

$$[t_* + t_0 - \Delta_t, t_* + t_0 + \Delta_t] \times [\omega_* + \omega_0 - \Delta_\omega, \omega_* + \omega_0 + \Delta_\omega]. \tag{7.13.11}$$

The time-localization interval has a constant width $2\Delta_t$ and the frequency localization has a constant width $2\Delta_\omega$. Therefore, the time-frequency localization occurs over rectangles with constant area $4\Delta_t\Delta_\omega$. This is shown in Fig. 7.13.1. This indicates what is wrong with the STFT: the time-frequency localization is too "rigid." For any point in the time-frequency plane, the region of time-frequency localization has constant area $4\Delta_t\Delta_\omega$, but also has constant rectangular shape. It would be more desirable if the time localization interval could be made to widen for low frequencies and narrow for high frequencies, yet maintain a constant-area time-frequency localization interval. We will see that the wavelet transform meets this goal.

We have not yet discussed how to choose the STFT analysis window $g(t)$ so as to provide optimum time-frequency localization. Unfortunately, the product $\Delta_t\Delta_\omega$ (which is proportional to the area of the time-frequency localization rectangle) can not be made arbitrarily small. The quantities Δ_t and Δ_ω are related in a manner we might expect; signals which have short duration in the time-domain tend to have wide support in the frequency-domain, and vice-versa. In fact, it can be shown that [Chu92]

$$\Delta_t\Delta_\omega \geq \frac{1}{2}$$

with equality only if $w(t)$ is a Gaussian window of the form

$$w(t) = \alpha e^{-\beta t^2}.$$

Therefore, optimal time-frequency localization for the STFT is obtained when $w(t)$ is a Gaussian window, in which case the time-frequency localization rectangle has an area equal to 2. The STFT computed with a Gaussian window is historically known as the *Gabor transform* [Gab46].

We now consider the time-frequency localization of the wavelet transform. The DWT is computed as the inner product of $x(t)$ and the time-shifted, dilated function

$$h_{m,k}(t) = a^{-m/2} h(a^{-m}(t - a^m kT)).$$

Suppose the function $h(t)$ has center t_* and RMS duration Δ_t. By construction, we forced the condition

$$||h_{m,k}||_2 = ||h||_2$$

so that the center of $h_{m,k}(t)$ is given by

$$t_*^{m,k} = \frac{1}{||h||_2} \int_{\infty}^{\infty} t|a^{-m/2} h(a^{-m}(t - a^m kT))|^2 \, dt. \tag{7.13.12}$$

Making the change of variables $\lambda = a^{-m}(t - a^m kT)$, it is simple to show that Eq. 7.13.12 becomes

$$t_*^{m,k} = a^m t_* + a^m kT||h||_2^2$$

and if the wavelet is normalized so that $||h||_2 = 1$, we get

$$t_*^{m,k} = a^m t_* + a^m kT. \tag{7.13.13}$$

Likewise, the RMS duration is given by

$$\Delta_t^{m,k} = \frac{1}{||h||_2} \left\{ \int_{-\infty}^{\infty} (t - t_*^{m,k})^2 |h_{m,k}(t)|^2 \, dt \right\}^{1/2}.$$

Again using the substitution $\lambda = a^{-m}(t - a^m kT)$, we get

$$\Delta_t^{m,k} = a^m \Delta_t. \tag{7.13.14}$$

Therefore, the time-localization occurs on the interval

$$[t_*^{m,k} - \Delta_t^{m,k}, t_*^{m,k} + \Delta_t^{m,k}] = [a^m(t_* + kT - \Delta_t), a^m(t_* + kT + \Delta_t)]$$

which has width $2a^m\Delta_t$. Since larger m correspond to lower window center frequencies, we can see that the width of the time localization interval increases for lower frequencies (because $a > 1$).

Next, we consider the frequency localization of the DWT. Suppose $H(j\omega)$ has center ω_* and RMS bandwidth Δ_ω. It is simple to show that the Fourier transform of $h_{m,k}(t)$ is given by

$$H_{m,k}(j\omega) = a^{m/2}e^{-j\omega a^m kT}H(ja^m\omega).$$

From this, we can easily derive that

$$\omega_*^{m,k} = a^{-m}\omega_*$$

and

$$\Delta_\omega^{m,k} = a^{-m}\Delta_\omega.$$

Thus, the frequency localization occurs over the interval

$$[a^{-m}(\omega_* - \Delta_\omega), a^{-m}(\omega_* + \Delta_\omega)].$$

The frequency localization width is equal to $2a^{-m}\Delta_\omega$ and can be seen to narrow for lower frequencies. The time-frequency localization of the DWT occurs over the rectangle

$$[a^m(t_* + kT - \Delta_t), a^m(t_* + kT + \Delta_t)] \times [a^{-m}(\omega_* - \Delta_\omega), a^{-m}(\omega_* + \Delta_\omega)]$$

which has constant area $4\Delta_t\Delta_\omega$, just like the STFT. However, the width of the rectangle is seen to narrow for low frequencies, while the height increases in order to keep the area constant. This is shown in Fig. 7.13.2.

The constant-Q property of the DWT is simply illustrated by this discussion. For any (m, k), we have seen that the center of the frequency localization interval is given by $a^m\omega_*$. The width of the interval is equal to $2a^m\Delta_t$. Therefore, the ratio of the width to the center is given by

$$\frac{2a^m\Delta_t}{a^m\omega_*} = \frac{2\Delta_t}{\omega_*}.$$

This shows that the ratio of the interval width to the interval center is *independent* of frequency, hence the constant-Q property.

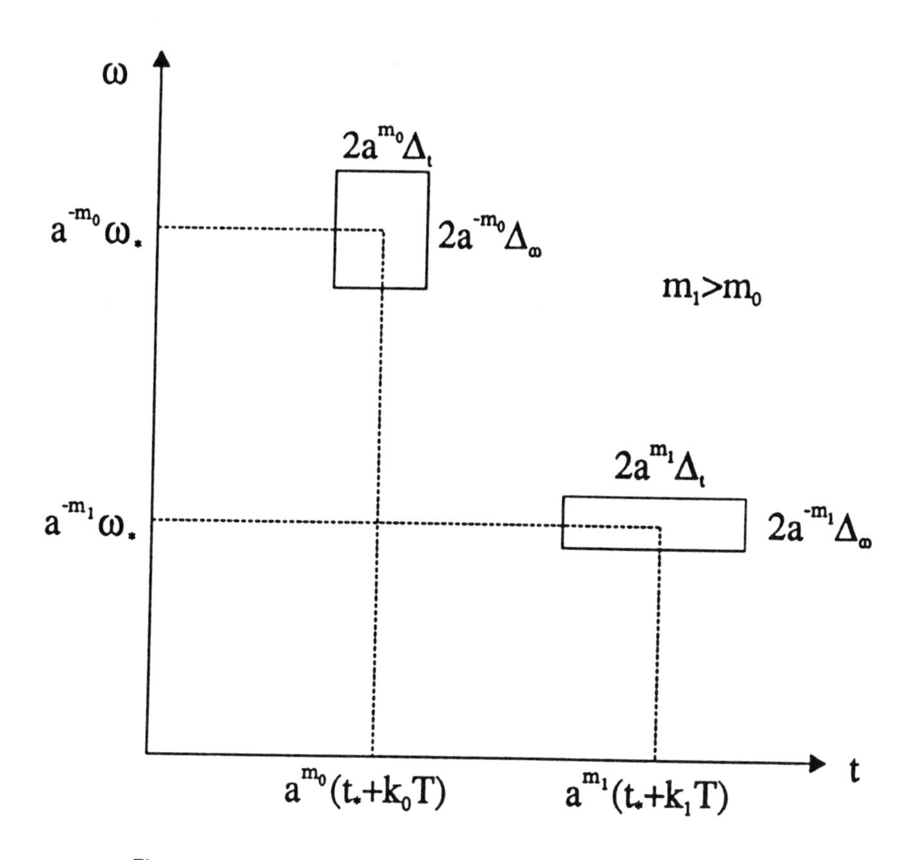

Figure 7.13.2: Time-frequency localization provided by the DWT.

Chapter 8

WIENER FILTERING

8.1 Introduction

The Wiener filter, which is diagrammed in Fig. 8.1.1, is an important class of optimum linear filter. In its most general form, the Wiener filter consists of an input signal, $x(k)$, a desired response, $d(k)$, and a linear filter with impulse response $h(k)$ which is fed by $x(k)$ to produce the output $y(k)$. The difference between the output of the Wiener filter, $y(k)$, and the desired response, $d(k)$, is denoted by the estimation error, $e(k)$.

The objective of Wiener filtering is to determine the impulse response $h(k)$ which makes the estimation error $e(k)$ "small" in some statistical sense. There are several possible choices as to what constitutes "small." The one which is most mathematically tractable, however, is that we wish to minimize the mean-squared value of $e(k)$. This is what we will use as the index of performance for the Wiener filter.

There are several structures which the Wiener filter is allowed to assume. We will begin with the case where the Wiener filter is allowed to be non-causal and of infinite duration. We will then impose the constraint of causality, which leads to a different solution. Finally, we will consider the case where the Wiener filter is constrained to be an FIR of length M. In each case, there will be an optimum solution among filters of each particular class. The FIR solution, however, has proved to be the most popular for several reasons, the most significant of which is the ability to implement *adaptive* solutions to the Wiener filtering problem with an FIR structure.

An example of Wiener filtering is provided by the following. Consider the communication system shown in Fig. 8.1.2a. A signal $d(k)$ is transmitted over the communication channel which is described by the (possibly unknown) transfer function $C(z)$. The model $C(z)$ can incorporate the effects of channel distortion. Furthermore, we assume that there is channel noise, $v(k)$, which further corrupts the received signal, $x(k)$. We wish to design an equalizer, $H(z)$, which attempts to "undo" the effects of $C(z)$ and $v(k)$. As shown in Fig. 8.1.2b, the

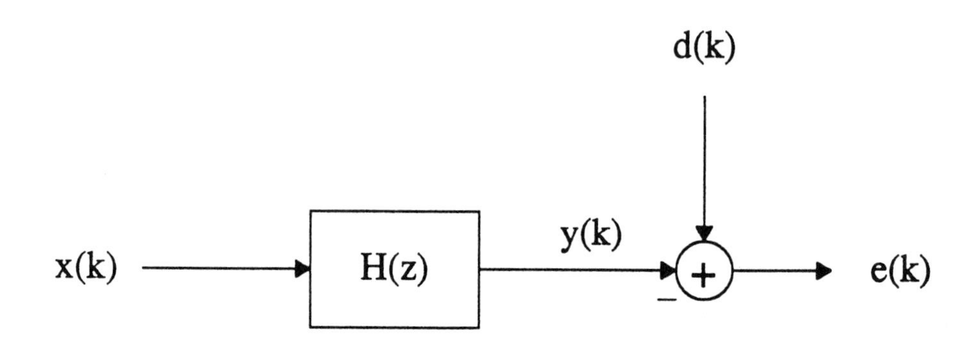

Figure 8.1.1: Basic model for Wiener filtering.

equalizer has as its input the received signal $x(k)$ and produces the output $y(k)$. The desired signal is the transmitted signal $d(k)$. We will a Wiener filter $H(z)$ for the equalizer, which minimizes the mean-squared error between $y(k)$ and $d(k)$.

Solution of this problem requires a statistical description of the transmitted signal, the channel noise, and the received signal. Depending on whether the equalizer is allowed to be causal or non-causal, we will obtain different solutions. For physical implementation, however, we must impose causality. Among the class of causal linear filters, we can allow the equalizer to be FIR or IIR. It may turn out that the optimal causal linear filter is IIR. In many cases, though, an FIR with enough taps may provide an adequate solution.

8.2 The Principle of Orthogonality

We assume that the input $x(k)$ and the desired response $d(k)$ are jointly WSS. For the present discussion, no assumptions are made about the nature of the filter (*i.e.*, causal or non-causal, FIR or IIR) other than linearity. The output of the filter is given by

$$y(k) = \sum_{n=-\infty}^{\infty} h_n x(k-n) \tag{8.2.1}$$

and the error between the desired response and the output is

$$e(k) = d(k) - y(k)..$$

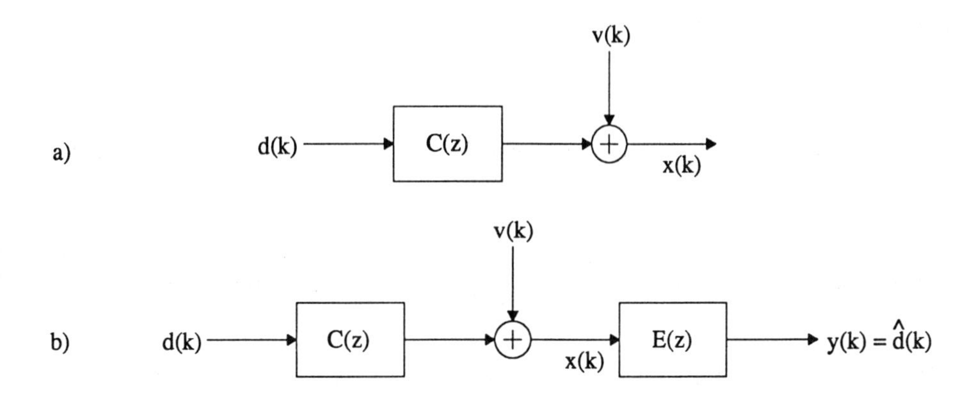

Figure 8.1.2: Using a Wiener filter for channel equalization: (a) Model of communication system; (b) Communication system with equalizer.

The objective of Wiener filtering is to determine the values of the filter coefficients $\{h_n\}$ which minimize the performance index J where

$$J = \mathcal{E}[e^2(k)]. \tag{8.2.2}$$

In other words, the Wiener filter will minimize the mean-squared error between the desired response and the output of the filter. The performance index J is a function of the impulse response, $\boldsymbol{h}$ and its minimization can be achieved by setting the gradient of J with respect to $\boldsymbol{h}$ equal to zero. The the n-th component of ∇J is given by

$$[\nabla J]_n = \frac{\partial J}{\partial h_n}.$$

Using the chain rule for differentiation,

$$\frac{\partial J}{\partial h_n} = \mathcal{E}\left[2\frac{\partial e(k)}{\partial h_n} e(k)\right]. \tag{8.2.3}$$

But using Eq. 8.2.1, we find that

$$\frac{\partial e(k)}{\partial h_n} = -\frac{\partial y(k)}{\partial h_n} = -x(k-n)$$

so that

$$\frac{\partial J}{\partial h_n} = -2\mathcal{E}[x(k-n)e(k)]. \tag{8.2.4}$$

Because each component of the gradient must be equal to zero for optimality, we find that

$$\mathcal{E}[x(k-n)e_o(k)] = 0 \quad \text{for all } n \tag{8.2.5}$$

where $e_o(n)$ refers to the error when the filter is operating in the *optimal* condition. Equation 8.2.5 is known as the *principle of orthogonality.* What it indicates is that when the filter coefficients assume their optimal values, the error between the output and the desired response is uncorrelated with every input sample which is used to compute the output. The principle of orthogonality actually provides necessary and sufficient conditions for optimality.

It is easily shown as a consequence of the principle of orthogonality that if the filter is operating in the optimal condition, then the error is also orthogonal to the output of the filter,

$$\mathcal{E}[y_o(k)e_o(k)] = 0. \tag{8.2.6}$$

The value of J when the filter is optimal is given by

$$J_{min} = \mathcal{E}[e_o^2(k)].$$

By definition, $e_o(k) = d(k) - y_o(k)$ so that

$$d(k) = y_o(k) + e_o(k). \tag{8.2.7}$$

Using Eq. 8.2.7,

$$\mathcal{E}[d^2(k)] = \sigma_d^2 = \mathcal{E}[y_o^2(k) + e_o^2(k) + 2e_o(k)y_o(k)].$$

Because of Eq. 8.2.7, $e_o(k)$ and $y_o(k)$ are orthogonal so that the above becomes

$$\sigma_d^2 = \sigma_{y0}^2 + J_{min}$$

so that

$$J_{min} = \sigma_d^2 - \sigma_{y0}^2. \tag{8.2.8}$$

We now need to determine how to solve for the optimal filter parameters. The principle of orthogonality states that

$$\mathcal{E}[x(k-n)e_o(k)] = 0. \tag{8.2.9}$$

The optimal error can be expressed as

$$e_o(k) = d(k) - \sum_{i=-\infty}^{\infty} h_{oi} x(k-i)$$

where the h_{oi} indicate the optimal filter parameters. Substituting this into Eq. 8.2.9, we have

$$\mathcal{E}\left[x(k-n)(d(k) - \sum_{i=-\infty}^{\infty} h_{oi} x(k-i))\right] = 0. \tag{8.2.10}$$

This means that

$$\sum_{i=-\infty}^{\infty} h_{oi} \mathcal{E}[x(k-n)x(k-i)] = \mathcal{E}[x(k-n)d(k)]. \tag{8.2.11}$$

But

$$\mathcal{E}[x(k-n)x(k-i)] = r_{xx}(n-i),$$

and

$$\mathcal{E}[x(k-n)d(k)] = r_{xd}(n).$$

Therefore, Eq. 8.2.11 becomes

$$\sum_{i=-\infty}^{\infty} h_{oi} r_{xx}(n-i) = r_{xd}(n), \qquad \text{for all} n. \tag{8.2.12}$$

Equation 8.2.12 is known as the discrete-time *Wiener-Hopf* equation and implicitly gives the optimal $\{h_i\}$.

8.3 IIR Wiener Filters

We first consider the simple case where the Wiener filter is allowed to be IIR and non-causal. Namely, the filter coefficients h_i are allowed to be nonzero for *all* i in the Wiener-Hopf equation. The solution to the Wiener-Hopf equation for this case is simple to compute in the frequency domain. The $\mathcal{Z}$-transform relationship corresponding to Eq. 8.2.12 is

$$H(z)P_{xx}(z) = P_{xd}(z).$$

Thus, the Wiener filter $H(z)$ is given by

$$H(z) = \frac{P_{xd}(z)}{P_{xx}(z)}. \tag{8.3.1}$$

If the spectral densities $P_{xd}(z)$ and $P_{xx}(z)$ are not known, they can be estimated from measured data. Because we have placed no temporal constraints on the filter coefficients, the solution can be non-causal.

When $H(z)$ is equal to the Wiener solution, the mean-squared error is a minimum. To find its value, we have

$$J_{min} = \mathcal{E}[(d(k) - y(k))^2] = \mathcal{E}[d^2(k)] - 2\mathcal{E}[d(k)y(k)] + \mathcal{E}[y^2(k)],$$

which we can write as

$$J_{min} = \sigma_d^2 + r_{yy}(0) - 2r_{dy}(0). \tag{8.3.2}$$

This expression is best evaluated in the frequency domain. Using contour integration to invert $\mathcal{Z}$-transforms, Eq. 8.3.2 becomes

$$J_{min} = \sigma_d^2 + \frac{1}{2\pi j} \oint [P_{yy}(z) - 2P_{dy}(z)] z^{-1}\, dz. \tag{8.3.3}$$

Because $y(k)$ is generated by filtering $x(k)$ through $H(z)$, it follows that

$$P_{dy}(z) = H(z) P_{dx}(z)$$

and

$$P_{yy}(z) = H(z) H(z^{-1}) P_{xx}(z).$$

Therefore, Eq. 8.3.3 becomes

$$J_{min} = \sigma_d^2 + \frac{1}{2\pi j} \oint [H(z^{-1}) P_{xx}(z) - 2P_{dx}(z)] H(z) z^{-1}\, dz. \tag{8.3.4}$$

Equivalently, because $P_{dx}(z) = P_{xd}(z^{-1})$ and $P_{xx}(z^{-1}) = P_{xx}(z)$, we can also express J_{min} as

$$J_{min} = \sigma_d^2 + \frac{1}{2\pi j} \oint [H(z) P_{xx}(z) - 2P_{xd}(z)] H(z^{-1}) z^{-1}\, dz. \tag{8.3.5}$$

Either of Eqs. 8.3.4 or 8.3.5 may be used to evaluate the mean-squared error produced by the Wiener filter.

Let's obtain some physical insight into what the Wiener filter actually does. Consider again the communication system from the first section in this chapter. The received signal is given by

$$x(k) = \sum_{i=-\infty}^{\infty} c(i)d(k-i) + v(k)$$

where we assume that $v(k)$ is a zero-mean white noise process with power σ_v^2 and is uncorrelated with the transmitted signal $d(k)$. After some manipulation, we find that

$$P_{xd}(z) = C(z^{-1})P_{dd}(z) + P_{dv}(z)$$

and because $d(k)$ and $v(k)$ are assumed to be uncorrelated, we have

$$P_{xd}(z) = C(z^{-1})P_{dd}(z).$$

Also, it is easily shown that

$$P_{xx}(z) = C(z)C(z^{-1})P_{dd}(z) + \sigma_v^2.$$

Therefore, the Wiener filter is given by

$$H(z) = \frac{P_{xd}(z)}{P_{xx}(z)} = \frac{C(z^{-1})P_{dd}(z)}{C(z)C(z^{-1})P_{dd}(z) + \sigma_v^2}.$$

In the limiting case where σ_v^2 equals zero, we have

$$H(z) = \frac{1}{C(z)}$$

so that the Wiener filter acts as the inverse filter for the communication channel $C(z)$.

Another useful interpretation of the Wiener filter is that it acts as a *correlation canceler.* According to the principle of orthogonality, the output $y(k)$ of the Wiener filter is produced from the signal $x(k)$ resulting in an error $e(k)$ which is uncorrelated with $x(k)$. Because $e(k) = d(k) - y(k)$ and $e(k)$ is uncorrelated with $x(k)$, we can say that the correlation between $e(k)$ and $x(k)$ has been *canceled* by subtracting $y(k)$. In this sense, we can think of $y(k)$ as the optimal estimate of the part of $d(k)$ which is correlated with $x(k)$. Consequently, if $x(k) = x_1(k) + x_2(k)$ where $x_2(k)$ and $d(k)$ are uncorrelated, the Wiener filter will be the same as when $x(k) = x_1(k)$ alone. This property will be useful in applications such as noise and echo cancellation.

We now consider the solution of the *causal* Wiener filtering problem, which is slightly more complicated than the non-causal counterpart we just solved. We can use the spectral

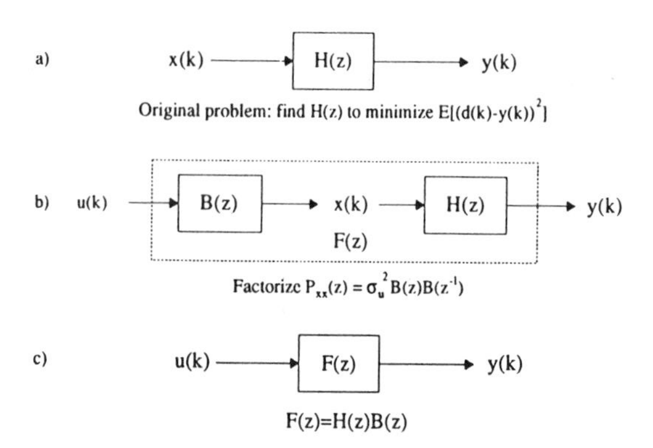

Figure 8.3.1: Wiener filtering by prewhitening.

factorization theorem to simplify the causal Wiener filtering problem. This procedure is known as *pre-whitening*. Specifically, we can factorize $P_{xx}(z)$ as

$$P_{xx}(z) = \sigma_u^2 B(z)B(z^{-1})$$

where $B(z)$ is causal and minimum phase. In this sense, we model the stochastic process $x(k)$ as the output of the filter $B(z)$ when driven by the white noise process $u(k)$. The problem then becomes one of estimating $d(k)$ in terms of the white noise sequence $u(k)$, as shown in Fig. 8.3.1. The overall transfer function from $u(k)$ to $y(k)$ is

$$F(z) = B(z)H(z).$$

If we can find a causal $F(z)$, then we can solve for the Wiener filter $H(z)$ as

$$H(z) = \frac{F(z)}{B(z)} \tag{8.3.6}$$

which is also causal because $B(z)$ is causal.

To determine $F(z)$, we can write the Wiener-Hopf equations for the impulse response $f(k)$ as

$$\sum_{i=0}^{\infty} f_i r_{uu}(n-i) = r_{ud}(n), \quad n \geq 0.$$

Notice that the summation runs from *zero* to infinity because of the assumed causality of $F(z)$. Because $u(k)$ is white,

$$r_{uu}(n-i) = \delta(n-i)$$

and the Wiener-Hopf equations reduce to

$$r_{ud}(n) = f_n,$$

which gives the impulse response of $F(z)$ as

$$f_n = r_{ud}(n), \quad n \geq 0.$$

We compute the transfer function $F(z)$ as

$$F(z) = \sum_{n=0}^{\infty} f_n z^{-n} = \sum_{n=0}^{\infty} r_{ud}(n) z^{-n}.$$

The summation is recognized as the *causal* part of $P_{ud}(z)$, which we denote this by $[P_{ud}(z)]_+$. Therefore,

$$F(z) = [P_{ud}(z)]_+. \tag{8.3.7}$$

We next need to determine the relationship between $P_{xd}(z)$ and $P_{ud}(z)$. The first step is to determine the relationship between $r_{xd}(k)$ and $r_{ud}(k)$. Recall that

$$r_{ud}(k) = \mathcal{E}[u(n)d(n+k)]$$

and

$$r_{xd}(k) = \mathcal{E}[x(n)d(n+k)].$$

Since $x(k)$ is generated by filtering $u(k)$ through $B(z)$, it follows that

$$x(n) = \sum_{i=0}^{\infty} b_i u(n-i).$$

Therefore,

$$r_{xd}(k) = \mathcal{E}\left[\sum_{i=0}^{\infty} b_i u(n-i) d(n+k)\right] = \sum_{i=0}^{\infty} b_i r_{ud}(k+i).$$

Taking $\mathcal{Z}$-transforms, we get

$$P_{xd}(z) = \sum_{k=-\infty}^{\infty} \sum_{i=0}^{\infty} b_i r_{ud}(k+i) z^{-k}.$$

Reversing the summation and simplifying, we find that

$$P_{xd}(z) = \sum_{i=0}^{\infty} b_i z^i \left(\sum_{k=-\infty}^{\infty} r_{ud}(k+i) z^{-(k+i)} \right) = P_{ud}(z) \sum_{i=0}^{\infty} b_i z^i.$$

The last summation on the right is recognized as $B(z^{-1})$ so that

$$P_{xd}(z) = P_{ud}(z)B(z^{-1}).$$

Therefore, the relationship we seek is given by

$$P_{ud}(z) = \frac{P_{xd}(z)}{B(z^{-1})}. \tag{8.3.8}$$

Because of Eq. 8.3.7, the filter $F(z)$ is given by

$$F(z) = [P_{ud}(z)]_+ = \left[\frac{P_{xd}(z)}{B(z^{-1})}\right]_+.$$

Finally, the solution to the causal Wiener filtering problem is given by Eq. 8.3.6 as

$$H(z) = \frac{1}{B(z)}\left[\frac{P_{xd}(z)}{B(z^{-1})}\right]_+. \tag{8.3.9}$$

Because $B(z)$ is minimum-phase, the solution $H(z)$ will also be stable if the causal part of $P_{xd}(z)$ is stable (as is the case in any problem of interest). Thus, we have solved the causal Wiener filtering problem. The only real difficulty lies in determining the causal part of a transfer function. Frequently, we can use the residue theorem for contour integration.

Example 8.1

Suppose we have the input signal

$$x(k) = d(k) + v(k)$$

where $v(k)$ is white noise with $\sigma_v^2 = 1$ which is uncorrelated with the signal $d(k)$. The signal $d(k)$ is given by the model

$$d(k+1) = 0.5d(k) + w(k)$$

where $w(k)$ is white noise with power $\sigma_w^2 = 0.75$. We first note that $d(k)$ is generated by the transfer function

$$Q(z) = \frac{1}{z - 0.5}$$

so that

$$P_{dd}(z) = \sigma_w^2 Q(z)Q(z^{-1}) = \frac{0.75}{(1-0.5z^{-1})(1-0.5z)}.$$

The function $P_{xd}(z)$ is given by

$$P_{xd}(z) = P_{dd}(z) + P_{dv}(z),$$

and because $v(k)$ is assumed to be uncorrelated with $d(k)$,

$$P_{xd}(z) = P_{dd}(z).$$

Also,

$$P_{xx}(z) = P_{dd}(z) + P_{vv}(z) + P_{dv}(z) + P_{vd}(z)$$

which gives

$$P_{xx}(z) = P_{dd}(z) + P_{vv}(z) = 1 + P_{dd}(z).$$

We find that $P_{xx}(z)$ can be factorized as

$$P_{xx}(z) = (8/7)\frac{(1 - 0.4375z^{-1})(1 - 0.4375z)}{(1 - 0.5z^{-1})(1 - 0.5z)}$$

so that we can take as $B(z)$ the function

$$B(z) = \sqrt{8/7}\frac{(1 - 0.4375z^{-1})}{(1 - 0.5z^{-1})}.$$

Thus, we must compute the causal part of

$$G(z) = \frac{P_{xd}(z)}{B(z^{-1})} = \frac{0.75\sqrt{8/7}}{(1 - 0.5z^{-1})(1 - 0.4375z)}.$$

That is,

$$F(z) = [G(z)]_{+}.$$

This is accomplished by using the contour integral to find $f(k)$. The causal part is determined by integrating along the unit circle, which isolates the causal, stable poles. We have

$$f(k) = \oint_{|z|=1} G(z)z^{k-1}\, dz = \oint_{|z|=1} \frac{0.75\sqrt{8/7}z^{k}}{(z - 0.5)(1 - 0.4375z)}\, dz.$$

Using the residue theorem, we find that the pole inside the unit circle is at $z = 0.5$ and hence,

$$f(k) = 12\sqrt{8/7}(0.5)^{k}, \quad k \geq 0.$$

Thus,

$$F(z) = \frac{12\sqrt{8/7}}{1 - 0.5z^{-1}}.$$

Finally, the Wiener filter $H(z)$ is given by

$$H(z) = \frac{F(z)}{\sigma_u^2 B(z)} = \frac{10.5}{1 - 0.4375z^{-1}}.$$

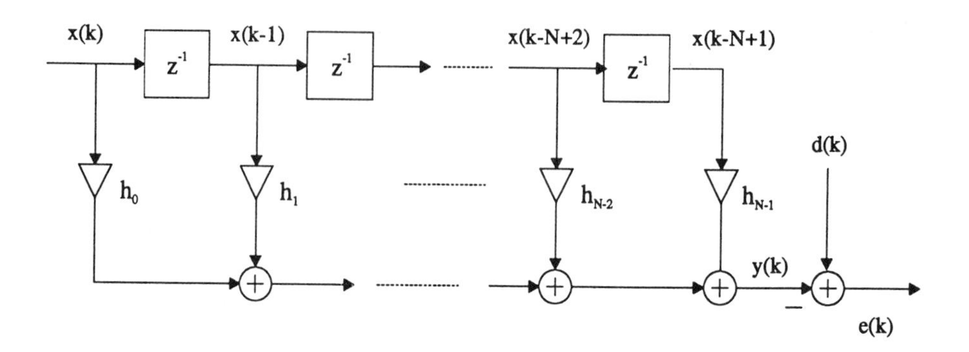

Figure 8.4.1: FIR Wiener filter.

8.4 FIR Wiener Filters

Up to this point, we have considered the general case where the Wiener filter is allowed to assume the form of an IIR filter. We have solved both the non-causal and the causal Wiener filtering problems. We now consider the case where the Wiener filter is constrained to be a causal finite impulse response filter of length N, as shown in Fig. 8.4.1. This is the most popular structure for adaptive filtering and will be the only structure we will consider from here on.

Let $H(z)$ be a transversal filter with N taps, denoted by the vector $\boldsymbol{h}$, where

$$\boldsymbol{h} = [h_0, h_1, \ldots, h_{N-1}]^T.$$

The Wiener-Hopf equation then states that

$$\sum_{i=0}^{N-1} h_{oi} r_{xx}(n-i) = r_{xd}(n), \quad n = 0, 1, \ldots, N-1 \tag{8.4.1}$$

because there are only N taps and only the N most recent input samples are used in the optimization. Equation 8.4.1 can be put in matrix form. Let $\boldsymbol{x}(k)$ be the vector of the N most recent samples,

$$\boldsymbol{x}(k) = [x(k), x(k-1), \ldots, x(k-N+1)]^T$$

so that $x(k-i)$ represents the contents of the i-th shift register in the transversal filter at time k. Recall that the autocorrelation matrix of the vector $\boldsymbol{x}(k)$ was defined by

$$\boldsymbol{R} = \begin{bmatrix} r(0) & r(1) & \cdots & r(N-1) \\ r(1) & r(0) & \cdots & r(N-2) \\ \vdots & \vdots & \ddots & \vdots \\ r(N-1) & r(N-2) & \cdots & r(0) \end{bmatrix}. \tag{8.4.2}$$

Define the cross-correlation vector $\boldsymbol{p}$ by

$$\boldsymbol{p} = \mathcal{E}[\boldsymbol{x}(k)d(k)] = \begin{bmatrix} r_{xd}(0) \\ r_{xd}(1) \\ \vdots \\ r_{xd}(M-1) \end{bmatrix}. \tag{8.4.3}$$

Then the Wiener-Hopf equation can be written in matrix form as

$$\boldsymbol{Rh} = \boldsymbol{p} \tag{8.4.4}$$

which has the optimal solution given by

$$\boldsymbol{h}_o = \boldsymbol{R}^{-1}\boldsymbol{p}. \tag{8.4.5}$$

The output of the transversal filter can be described in vector form by

$$y(k) = \boldsymbol{h}^T\boldsymbol{x}(k). \tag{8.4.6}$$

Consequently, the error may be described as

$$e(k) = d(k) - \boldsymbol{h}^T\boldsymbol{x}(k).$$

Recall that the performance index for the Wiener filter is

$$J(\boldsymbol{h}) = \mathcal{E}[e^2(k)]$$

which, using Eq. 8.4.6 can be expressed by

$$J(\boldsymbol{h}) = \sigma_d^2 - \boldsymbol{h}^T\mathcal{E}[\boldsymbol{x}(k)d(k)] - \mathcal{E}[\boldsymbol{x}^T(k)d(k)]\boldsymbol{h} + \boldsymbol{h}^T\mathcal{E}[\boldsymbol{x}(k)\boldsymbol{x}^T(k)]\boldsymbol{h}. \tag{8.4.7}$$

Using Eqs. 8.2.3 and 8.2.4, we have

$$J = \sigma_d^2 - 2\boldsymbol{h}^T\boldsymbol{p} + \boldsymbol{h}^T\boldsymbol{Rh}. \tag{8.4.8}$$

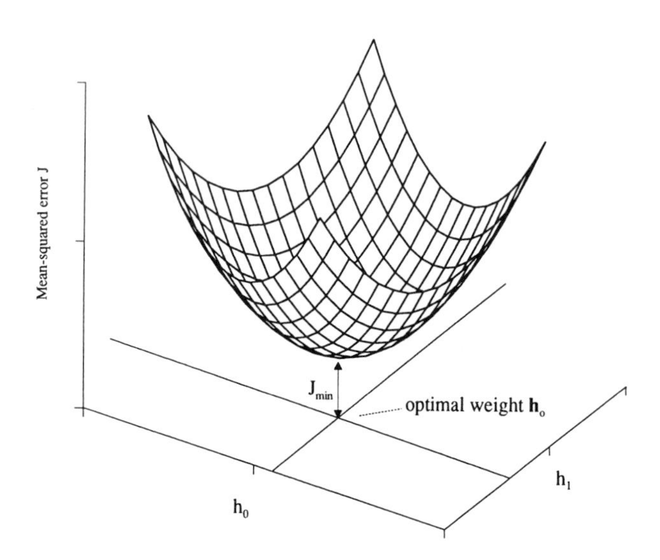

Figure 8.4.2: Quadratic error performance surface for FIR Wiener filter.

The minimum value of J occurs when $\boldsymbol{h} = \boldsymbol{h}_o$ where $\boldsymbol{h}_o = \boldsymbol{R}^{-1}\boldsymbol{p}$. Substituting this into Eq. 8.4.8, we find that

$$J_{min} = \sigma_d^2 - \boldsymbol{h}_o^T \boldsymbol{p}. \tag{8.4.9}$$

Equation 8.4.8 describes a paraboloid, as shown in Fig. 8.4.2 for the easily visualized case of a two-dimensional weight vector. It is significant that this error performance has a *global* minimum at $\boldsymbol{h} = \boldsymbol{h}_o$ and no other local minima. This admits a *unique* solution to the FIR Wiener filtering problem, a property which is not always shared by the IIR Wiener filter.

To gain better geometric insight into the error performance surface, Eq. 8.4.8 is a quadratic form in $\boldsymbol{h}$ which can be put in the standard form (see Appendix A)

$$J(\boldsymbol{h}) = J_{min} + (\boldsymbol{h} - \boldsymbol{h}_o)^T \boldsymbol{R} (\boldsymbol{h} - \boldsymbol{h}_o). \tag{8.4.10}$$

Because $\boldsymbol{R}$ is a correlation matrix, we have the decomposition

$$\boldsymbol{R} = \boldsymbol{Q} \boldsymbol{\Lambda} \boldsymbol{Q}^H$$

where $\boldsymbol{Q}$ is orthogonal with columns equal to the eigenvectors of $\boldsymbol{R}$ and

$$\boldsymbol{\Lambda} = \mathrm{diag}(\lambda_1, \lambda_2, \ldots, \lambda_N)$$

where the λ_i are the eigenvalues corresponding to the eigenvectors. Then Eq. 8.4.10 becomes

$$J = J_{min} + (\boldsymbol{h} - \boldsymbol{h}_o)^T \boldsymbol{Q} \boldsymbol{\Lambda} \boldsymbol{Q}^H (\boldsymbol{h} - \boldsymbol{h}_o). \quad (8.4.11)$$

This equation lends a simple geometric interpretation of the error surface described by the quadratic form. Let's perform a transformation of the weight-space by first shifting the origin to the optimal weight $\boldsymbol{h}_0$ and then performing a change of basis where the new basis is taken as the eigenvectors of the correlation matrix $\boldsymbol{R}$. In other words, let $\boldsymbol{z}$ be given by the affine transformation

$$\boldsymbol{h} = \boldsymbol{Q}\boldsymbol{z} + \boldsymbol{h}_o.$$

Because $\boldsymbol{Q}$ is orthogonal, this means that

$$\boldsymbol{z} = \boldsymbol{Q}^H (\boldsymbol{h} - \boldsymbol{h}_o). \quad (8.4.12)$$

Substituting Eq. 8.4.12 into Eq. 8.4.11, we find that

$$J = J_{min} + \boldsymbol{z}^T \boldsymbol{\Lambda} \boldsymbol{z} = J_{min} + \sum_{i=1}^{N} \lambda_i |z_i|^2. \quad (8.4.13)$$

This expression provides a clear picture of the error surface. Recall that the error surface is a quadratic form in $\boldsymbol{h}$ with a global minimum equal to J_{min} occurring at $\boldsymbol{h} = \boldsymbol{h}_0$. In the transformed weight-space, we have a quadratic form in the transformed weight-vector $\boldsymbol{z}$ which assumes the global minimum J_{min} at the origin, $\boldsymbol{z} = \mathbf{0}$.

A useful picture is obtained if we look at cross-sections of the performance surface. In this case, we will have contours of constant error which have the shape of ellipsoids. The major axes of the ellipse are the eigenvectors of the correlation matrix $\boldsymbol{R}$ and the eccentricity is determined by the eigenvalues of the correlation matrix, $\boldsymbol{R}$. This is illustrated in Fig. 8.4.3. If the ratio of the largest to smallest eigenvalue is large, the contours of constant error will be highly eccentric. When all of the eigenvalues are equal, the contours of constant error will be perfectly circular.

8.5 Linear Prediction

One of the fundamental applications of Wiener filtering is linear prediction. As the name implies, the role of linear prediction is to determine the future value of a time series based on a linear function of past values. The particular structure we will use is the N-th order transversal filter. In this case, we are trying to predict the next value of a time series using a linear combination of the N most recent samples.

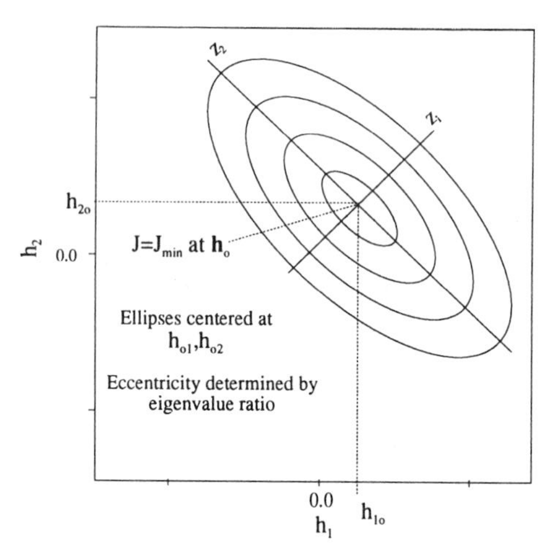

Figure 8.4.3: Contours of constant error for two-dimensional weight space and transformed weight space.

8.5.1 Forward Prediction

Given $x(k-1), x(k-2), \ldots, x(k-N)$, we form an estimate of $x(k)$, denoted $\hat{x}(k)$, according to

$$\hat{x}(k) = h_{f1}x(k-1) + h_{f2}x(k-2) + \cdots + h_{fN}x(k-N). \tag{8.5.1}$$

If we define the input vector $\boldsymbol{x}(k-1)$ by

$$\boldsymbol{x}(k-1) = [x(k-1), x(k-2), \ldots, x(k-N)]^T$$

and the forward predictor tap weight vector $\boldsymbol{h}_f$ by

$$\boldsymbol{h}_f = [h_{f1}, h_{f2}, \ldots, h_{fN}]^T,$$

we then have

$$\hat{x}(k) = \boldsymbol{h}_f^T \boldsymbol{x}(k-1). \tag{8.5.2}$$

In the Wiener filtering framework, the desired response is

$$d(k) = x(k).$$

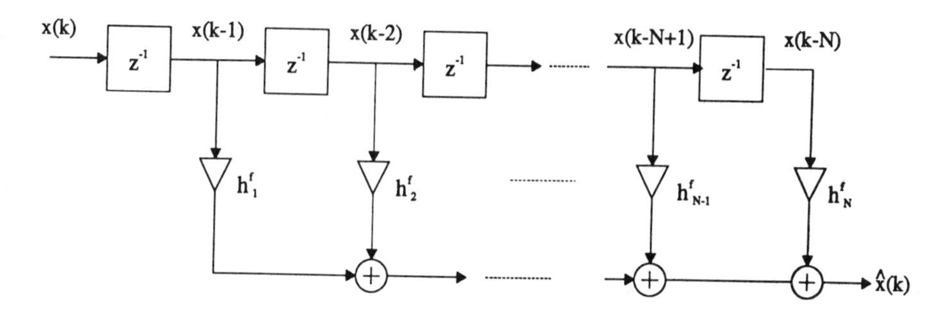

Figure 8.5.1: Transversal forward prediction filter.

We call the difference between the desired response and the predictor output the *forward prediction error*, $e^f_N(k)$, where

$$e^f_N(k) = x(k) - \hat{x}(k) = x(k) - \boldsymbol{h}_f^T \boldsymbol{x}(k-1). \tag{8.5.3}$$

A transversal forward prediction filter is shown in Fig. 8.5.1.

In keeping with the Wiener filtering theory, our criterion of optimization for the forward predictor is to minimize the mean-squared value of the forward prediction error, so that

$$J = \mathcal{E}[(e^f_N(k))^2]. \tag{8.5.4}$$

This problem is easily solved using the results from the previous section. The input correlation matrix is given by

$$\mathcal{E}[\boldsymbol{x}(k-1)\boldsymbol{x}^T(k-1)] = \mathcal{E}[\boldsymbol{x}(k)\boldsymbol{x}^T(k)] = \boldsymbol{R}$$

because of the stationarity of $x(k)$. The crosscorrelation between the input and the desired response is given by

$$\boldsymbol{p} = \mathcal{E}[\boldsymbol{x}(k-1)x(k)] = \begin{bmatrix} r(1) \\ r(2) \\ \vdots \\ r(N) \end{bmatrix}, \tag{8.5.5}$$

which we have seen is nothing more than the vector $\boldsymbol{r}$ in Eq. 5.5.3. Therefore, the Wiener-Hopf equation for the forward predictor is

$$\boldsymbol{R}\boldsymbol{h}_f = \boldsymbol{r} \tag{8.5.6}$$

which has the solution

$$\boldsymbol{h}_f = \boldsymbol{R}^{-1}\boldsymbol{r}. \tag{8.5.7}$$

According to Eq. 8.4.9, when we have optimized the filter, the performance index satisfies

$$J_{min} = \sigma_d^2 - \boldsymbol{p}^T\boldsymbol{h}. \tag{8.5.8}$$

Because the desired response is $x(k)$, we have

$$\sigma_d^2 = \mathcal{E}[x^2(k)] = r(0).$$

For the forward prediction filter, we choose to denote J_{min} by the symbol P_a. Thus, Eq. 8.5.8 becomes

$$P_a = r(0) - \boldsymbol{h}_f^T\boldsymbol{r}. \tag{8.5.9}$$

Given an N-th order forward predictor $\boldsymbol{h}_f$, we define the *forward prediction error filter* $\boldsymbol{a}$ by

$$\boldsymbol{a} = \begin{bmatrix} a_0 \\ a_1 \\ \vdots \\ a_N \end{bmatrix} = \begin{bmatrix} 1 \\ -\boldsymbol{h}_f \end{bmatrix}. \tag{8.5.10}$$

It is seen that for the forward prediction error filter, we have

$$\begin{cases} a_0 &= 1 \\ a_i &= -h_{f,i}, \quad i = 1, 2 \ldots, N. \end{cases}$$

It follows that the forward prediction error $e_N^f(k)$ can be computed according to

$$e_N^f(k) = \boldsymbol{a}^T \begin{bmatrix} x(k) \\ \boldsymbol{x}(k-1) \end{bmatrix}. \tag{8.5.11}$$

A forward prediction error filter is shown in Fig. 8.5.2.

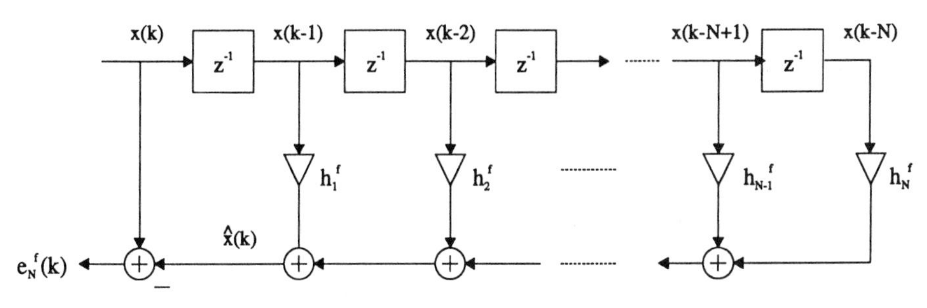

Figure 8.5.2: Transversal forward prediction error filter.

Recall from Eq. 5.5.4 that the input correlation matrix of dimension $N+1$ can be artitioned as

$$\boldsymbol{R}_{N+1} = \begin{bmatrix} r(0) & \boldsymbol{r}^T \\ \boldsymbol{r} & \boldsymbol{R}_N \end{bmatrix}.$$

quations 8.5.9 and 8.5.6 can be combined into the single *augmented normal equation* given y

$$\begin{bmatrix} r(0) & \boldsymbol{r}^T \\ \boldsymbol{r} & \boldsymbol{R} \end{bmatrix} \begin{bmatrix} 1 \\ -\boldsymbol{h}_f \end{bmatrix} = \begin{bmatrix} P_a \\ \boldsymbol{0} \end{bmatrix}, \tag{8.5.12}$$

hich can be succinctly expressed by

$$\boldsymbol{R}_{N+1}\boldsymbol{a} = \begin{bmatrix} P_a \\ \boldsymbol{0} \end{bmatrix}. \tag{8.5.13}$$

xample 8.2

Suppose $\{x(k)\}$ is an AR(N) process given by

$$x(k) = \sum_{i=1}^{N} a_i x(k-i) + v(k)$$

where $v(k)$ white noise with power σ_v^2. The N-th order forward predictor $\boldsymbol{h}_f$ is computed according to

$$\begin{bmatrix} r(0) & r(1) & \cdots & r(N-1) \\ r(1) & r(0) & \cdots & r(N-2) \\ \vdots & \vdots & \ddots & \vdots \\ r(N-1) & r(N-2) & \cdots & r(0) \end{bmatrix} \begin{bmatrix} h_{f1} \\ h_{f2} \\ \vdots \\ h_{fN} \end{bmatrix} = \begin{bmatrix} r(1) \\ r(2) \\ \vdots \\ r(N) \end{bmatrix}.$$

It can be seen from Eq. 5.4.17 that this system of equations is structurally identical to the Yule-Walker equations for the AR process. The tap weights satisfy

$$h_{fi} = -a_i$$

Where the a_i are the AR parameters. Therefore, the forward prediction error is given by

$$e_N^f(k) = x(k) - \boldsymbol{h}_f \boldsymbol{x}(k-1) = x(k) + \sum_{i=1}^{N} a_i x(k-i),$$

which is seen to be equal to the white noise $v(k)$ used to generate the AR process. For this reason, the forward prediction error filter for an AR process is sometimes referred to as a *whitening filter*. Furthermore, according to Eq. 8.5.9, the forward prediction error power is given by

$$P_a = r(0) - \boldsymbol{h}_f^T \boldsymbol{r} = \sum_{i=0}^{N} a_i r(i).$$

But Eq. 5.4.19 says that

$$\sum_{i=0}^{N} a_i r(i) = \sigma_v^2$$

which gives

$$P_a = \sigma_v^2.$$

This is not surprising, since the prediction error is simply the white noise $v(k)$ which generates the process.

The previous example illustrated the fact that the prediction error filter coefficients are identical to the AR process parameters if the predictor is equal to the order of the AR process. It then follows that the *zeros of the prediction error filter are identical to the poles of the AR process generation filter.*

Example 8.3

This example will examine the error performance surface for a linear prediction Wiener filter. Suppose $x(k)$ is an AR(2) process which is described by the equation

$$x(k) = v(k) + \frac{3}{4}x(k-1) + \frac{1}{8}x(k-2)$$

where $v(k)$ is a zero-mean white noise process with

$$\sigma_v^2 = 1.$$

Suppose we wish to design a two-coefficient predictor for the AR process $x(k)$. We already know that the optimum tap-weight for the forward predictor is equal to the negative of the AR parameter vector. This AR(2) process has the AR parameters

$$a_0 = 1, \quad a_1 = -\frac{3}{4}, \quad a_2 = -\frac{1}{8}$$

so that the optimum prediction coefficients are

$$h_{f1} = \frac{3}{4}, \quad h_{f2} = \frac{1}{8}.$$

Since we wish to examine the error performance surface, we need the matrices $\boldsymbol{R}$ and $\boldsymbol{p}$. This means that we need the first three values of the autocorrelation sequence. The Yule-Walker equations are given by

$$\begin{bmatrix} r(0) & r(1) \\ r(1) & r(0) \end{bmatrix} \begin{bmatrix} -a_1 \\ -a_2 \end{bmatrix} = \begin{bmatrix} r(1) \\ r(2) \end{bmatrix}.$$

This gives two equations in the three unknown autocorrelation values. The third equation can be obtained from Eq. 5.4.19, which states that

$$r(0) + a_1 r(1) + a_2 r(2) = \sigma_v^2.$$

We thus obtain the following system of equations

$$\begin{array}{rcrcrcl} \frac{3}{4}r(0) & - & \frac{7}{8}r(1) & & & = & 0 \\ \frac{1}{8}r(0) & + & \frac{3}{4}r(1) & - & r(2) & = & 0 \\ r(0) & - & \frac{3}{4}r(1) & - & \frac{1}{8}r(2) & = & 1 \end{array}$$

which has the solution

$$r(0) = 3.8291, \quad r(1) = 3.2821, \quad r(2) = 2.9402.$$

Therefore,

$$\boldsymbol{R} = \begin{bmatrix} 3.8291 & 3.2821 \\ 3.2821 & 3.8291 \end{bmatrix}$$

and

$$p = \begin{bmatrix} 3.2821 \\ 2.9402 \end{bmatrix}.$$

Defining the forward predictor h_f by

$$h_f = \begin{bmatrix} h_{f1} \\ h_{f2} \end{bmatrix},$$

we have the expression for the mean-squared forward prediction error given by Eq. 8.4.8, which states that

$$J = \sigma_d^2 - 2p^T h_f + h_f^T R h_f.$$

For the case of forward prediction, $d(k) = x(k)$ and hence

$$\sigma_d^2 = r(0).$$

Substituting the values of R and p into the equation for J, we find that

$$J = r(0) - 2r(1)h_{f1} - 2r(2)h_{f2} + r(0)h_{f1}^2 + r(0)h_{f2}^2 + 2r(1)h_{f1}h_{f2}.$$

This describes a three-dimensional paraboloid which is centered at the optimal weight, $(3/4, 1/8)$. The minimum value of J is given by

$$J_{min} = \sigma_d^2 - p^T h_{fo} = 1.$$

This value makes sense since the prediction error when the optimal prediction weight is achieved is given by

$$e^f(k) = x(k) - \frac{3}{4}x(k-1) - \frac{1}{8}x(k-2),$$

which, by assumption, is equal to $v(k)$. Therefore,

$$J_{min} = \mathcal{E}[v^2(k)] = \sigma_v^2 = 1.$$

Figure 8.5.3a shows contours of constant mean-squared error for the forward predictor. Notice that the contours are centered at the optimum weight and that they are highly ellipsoidal. This can be explained by examining the eigenstructure of R.

We find that R can be decomposed as

$$R = Q\Lambda Q^H$$

where

$$\Lambda = \begin{bmatrix} 0.5470 & 0 \\ 0 & 7.1111 \end{bmatrix}$$

and

$$Q = \frac{1}{2}\begin{bmatrix} \sqrt{2} & \sqrt{2} \\ -\sqrt{2} & \sqrt{2} \end{bmatrix}.$$

Using the change of coordinates described by Eq. 8.4.12, the mean-squared error can be described by Eq. 8.4.13 as

$$J = J_{min} + z^T \Lambda z = 1 + .5470z_1^2 + 7.111z_2^2$$

and the new minimum occurs at $z_1 = z_2 = 0$. The contours of constant error in this new coordinate system are shown in Fig. 8.5.3b.

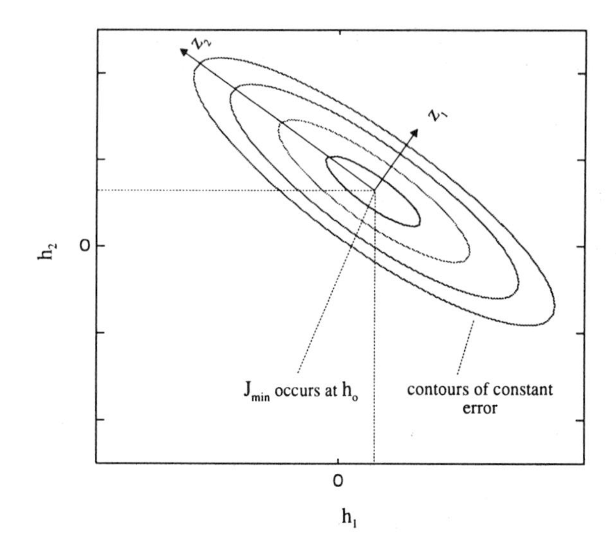

Figure 8.5.3: Contours of constant mean-squared error for Example 8.3 in terms of weight-space coordinates and transformed coordinates.

Minimum-phase property of the forward prediction error filter

It is fairly simple to show that the transfer function of the Wiener forward prediction error filter is *minimum-phase* [Kay88]. To show this, recall that the optimum predictor minimizes the forward prediction error power,

$$P = \mathcal{E}[(e_N^f(k))^2].$$

According to the Wiener-Khinchine theorem, the minimum prediction error power can be expressed as

$$P_{min} = \frac{1}{2\pi}\int_{-\pi}^{\pi} |A(e^{j\theta})|^2 P_{xx}(\theta)\, d\theta \tag{8.5.14}$$

where $A(z)$ is the transfer function of the FIR forward prediction error filter and $P_{xx}(\theta)$ is the PSD of the stochastic process, $\{x(k)\}$. The transfer function $A(z)$ can be expressed as

$$A(z) = \prod_{k=1}^{N}(1 - z_k z^{-1}) \tag{8.5.15}$$

where the z_k are the zeros of the prediction error filter. Now, assume by contradiction that $A(z)$ has a zero, z_i, which is outside the unit circle. Then $A(z)$ can be factorized as

$$A(z) = (1 - z_i z^{-1}) \prod_{k \neq i} (1 - z_k z^{-1}) \tag{8.5.16}$$

where $|z_i| > 1$. Denoting by $A'(z)$ the transfer function

$$A'(z) = \prod_{k \neq i} (1 - z_k z^{-1}),$$

Eq. 8.5.16 can be rewritten as

$$A(z) = (1 - z_i z^{-1}) A'(z). \tag{8.5.17}$$

Therefore, the prediction power can be computed by substituting Eq. 8.5.17 into Eq. 8.5.14 to yield

$$P_{min} = \frac{1}{2\pi} \int_{-\pi}^{\pi} |1 - z_i e^{-j\theta}|^2 |A'(e^{j\theta})|^2 P_{xx}(\theta)\, d\theta. \tag{8.5.18}$$

It is trivial to show that

$$|1 - z_i e^{-j\theta}|^2 = |z_i|^2 \left| 1 - \frac{1}{z_i^*} \right|^2 \geq 0. \tag{8.5.19}$$

Because it was assumed that $|z_i| > 1$, Eq. 8.5.19 is seen to imply that

$$|1 - z_i e^{-j\theta}|^2 > \left| 1 - \frac{1}{z_i^*} \right|^2 \geq 0. \tag{8.5.20}$$

Referring to Eq. 8.5.18, the inequality in Eq. 8.5.20 implies that

$$P_{min} > \frac{1}{2\pi} \int_{-\pi}^{\pi} \left| 1 - \frac{1}{z_i^*} e^{-j\theta} \right|^2 |A'(e^{j\theta})|^2 P_{xx}(\theta)\, d\theta. \tag{8.5.21}$$

Equation 8.5.21 implies that the prediction error power generated by the forward prediction error filter

$$\bar{A}(z) = (1 - z/z_i^*) A'(z)$$

is smaller than P_{min}, which is a contradiction, since $\bar{A}(z)$ and $A(z)$ have the same order. Therefore, it is not possible that the Wiener forward predictor has any zeros outside the unit circle.

8.5.2 Backward Prediction

Given $x(k), x(k-1), \ldots, x(k-N+1)$, we wish to estimate $x(k-N)$ using a transversal filter of order N. The estimate is a linear combination given by

$$\hat{x}(k-N) = h_{b1}x(k) + h_{b2}x(k-1) + \cdots h_{bN}x(k-N+1). \tag{8.5.22}$$

We denote the vector of N most recent samples by $\boldsymbol{x}(k)$ where

$$\boldsymbol{x}(k) = [x(k), x(k-1), \ldots, x(k-N)]^T$$

and the backward predictor tap weight vector by $\boldsymbol{h}_b$ where

$$\boldsymbol{h}_b = [h_{b1}, h_{b2}, \ldots, h_{bN}]^2.$$

We then have

$$\hat{x}(k-N) = \boldsymbol{h}_b^T \boldsymbol{x}(k). \tag{8.5.23}$$

The desired response is $d(k) = x(k-N)$ and we denote the backward prediction error by $e_N^b(k)$, where

$$e_N^b(k) = x(k-N) - \hat{x}(k-N) = x(k-N) - \boldsymbol{h}_b^T \boldsymbol{x}(k). \tag{8.5.24}$$

This time, the Wiener filtering problem is to minimize the mean-squared value of the backward prediction error, giving

$$J = \mathcal{E}[(e_N^b(k))^2]. \tag{8.5.25}$$

A transversal backward predictor is shown in Fig. 8.5.4.

The input correlation matrix for the backward predictor is

$$\mathcal{E}[\boldsymbol{x}(k)\boldsymbol{x}^T(k)] = \boldsymbol{R}$$

and the crosscorrelation between the input and the desired response is

$$\boldsymbol{p} = \mathcal{E}[x(k-N)\boldsymbol{x}(k)] = \begin{bmatrix} r(N) \\ r(N-1) \\ \vdots \\ r(1) \end{bmatrix}, \tag{8.5.26}$$

which we have seen is equal to the vector $\boldsymbol{r}^B$ in Eq. 8.5.26. Thus, the Wiener-Hopf equation for the backward predictor is

$$\boldsymbol{R}\boldsymbol{h}_b = \boldsymbol{r}^B \tag{8.5.27}$$

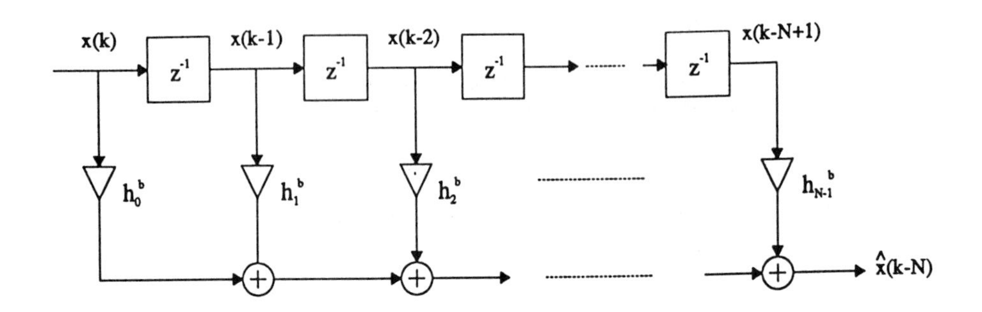

Figure 8.5.4: Transversal backward predictor.

which has the solution

$$h_b = R^{-1} r^B. \tag{8.5.28}$$

For the backward predictor, we choose to refer to the minimum value of J as P_b. Because $x(k)$ is assumed stationary, we have

$$\mathcal{E}[x^2(k-N)] = \mathcal{E}[x^2(k)] = r(0)$$

so that

$$\sigma_d^2 = r(0).$$

In direct analogy with Eq. 8.5.9, it follows that

$$P_b = r(0) - r^{BT} h_b. \tag{8.5.29}$$

Given an N-th order backward prediction filter h_b, we define the *backward prediction error filter* b by

$$b = \begin{bmatrix} b_0 \\ b_1 \\ \vdots \\ b_N \end{bmatrix} = \begin{bmatrix} -h_b \\ 1 \end{bmatrix}. \tag{8.5.30}$$

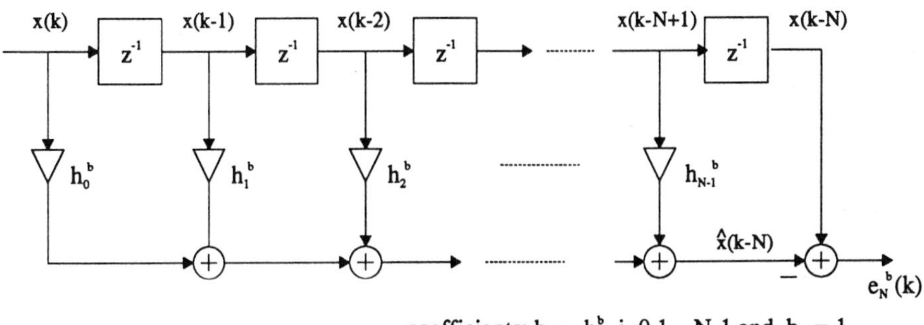

Figure 8.5.5: Transversal backward prediction error filter.

It is seen that for the backward prediction error filter, we have

$$\begin{cases} b_i &= -h_{b,i+1}, \quad i = 0, 1, \ldots, N-1. \\ b_N &= 1 \end{cases}$$

The backward prediction error can then be computed according to

$$\boldsymbol{e}_N^b(k) = \boldsymbol{b}^T \begin{bmatrix} \boldsymbol{x}(k) \\ x(k-N) \end{bmatrix}. \tag{8.5.31}$$

A backward prediction error filter is shown in Fig. 8.5.5.

We can also derive the augmented normal equations for backward prediction. Using Eq. 5.5.5, the matrix R_{N+1} can be partitioned as

$$\boldsymbol{R}_{N+1} = \begin{bmatrix} R & \boldsymbol{r}^B \\ \boldsymbol{r}^{BT} & r(0) \end{bmatrix}.$$

Equations 8.5.30 and 8.5.27 can be put into the augmented normal equation given by

$$\begin{bmatrix} R & \boldsymbol{r}^B \\ \boldsymbol{r}^{BT} & r(0) \end{bmatrix} \begin{bmatrix} -\boldsymbol{h}_b \\ 1 \end{bmatrix} = \begin{bmatrix} \boldsymbol{0} \\ P_b \end{bmatrix}, \tag{8.5.32}$$

which can be succinctly expressed by

$$\boldsymbol{R}_{N+1}\boldsymbol{b} = \begin{bmatrix} \boldsymbol{0} \\ P_b \end{bmatrix}. \tag{8.5.33}$$

There is an important connection between the forward and backward linear predictors when they are optimized in the Wiener sense. To explore this relationship, we first define the *exchange matrix* J by

$$\boldsymbol{J} = \begin{bmatrix} 0 & 0 & \cdots & 0 & 1 \\ 0 & 0 & \cdots & 1 & 0 \\ \vdots & \vdots & \ddots & \vdots & \vdots \\ 0 & 1 & \cdots & 0 & 0 \\ 1 & 0 & \cdots & 0 & 0 \end{bmatrix}.$$

Clearly,

$$\boldsymbol{J}^T = \boldsymbol{J}$$

and

$$\boldsymbol{J}\boldsymbol{J} = \boldsymbol{I}.$$

It is simple to see that for any vector $\boldsymbol{x}$,

$$\boldsymbol{J}\boldsymbol{x} = \boldsymbol{x}^B$$

so that premultiplication by $\boldsymbol{J}$ corresponds to reversing the elements in a column. Postmultiplication by $\boldsymbol{J}$ reverses the elements in a row.

Because of the Toeplitz structure of the matrix $\boldsymbol{R}$, we have

$$\boldsymbol{R}\boldsymbol{J} = \boldsymbol{J}\boldsymbol{R}. \tag{8.5.34}$$

The Wiener-Hopf equation for the forward predictor is

$$\boldsymbol{R}\boldsymbol{h}_f = \boldsymbol{r}.$$

Premultiplying both sides of the above by $\boldsymbol{J}$, we have

$$\boldsymbol{J}\boldsymbol{R}\boldsymbol{h}_f = \boldsymbol{J}\boldsymbol{r}.$$

But $\boldsymbol{J}\boldsymbol{r} = \boldsymbol{r}^B$ and by Eq. 8.5.34, $\boldsymbol{J}\boldsymbol{R} = \boldsymbol{R}\boldsymbol{J}$ so that

$$\boldsymbol{R}\boldsymbol{J}\boldsymbol{h}_f = \boldsymbol{r}^B.$$

The Wiener-Hopf equation for the backward predictor is

$$\boldsymbol{R}\boldsymbol{h}_b = \boldsymbol{r}^B.$$

We thus conclude that

$$\boldsymbol{h}_b = \boldsymbol{J}\boldsymbol{h}_f = \boldsymbol{h}_f^B.$$

Furthermore, it is obvious that the forward and backward prediction error filters satisfy

$$\boldsymbol{b} = \boldsymbol{J}\boldsymbol{a}.$$

Therefore, when the forward and backward predictors are optimized in the Wiener sense, they can be obtained from one another by reversing the tap weights.

Recall that the transfer function of the forward prediction error filter is *minimum-phase.* Because the backward prediction error filter is obtained by reversing the coefficients of the forward prediction error filter, the zeros of the backward prediction error filter are at reciprocal locations from the forward prediction error filter. Therefore, the backward prediction error filter is *maximum phase.* That is, when the backward prediction error filter is optimized in the Wiener sense, all of its zeros lie outside the unit circle.

What about the forward and backward prediction error energies P_a and P_b? Recall that we can compute the backward prediction error energy by

$$P_b = r(0) - \boldsymbol{r}^{BT}\boldsymbol{h}_b.$$

Using the relationships $\boldsymbol{h}_f = \boldsymbol{J}\boldsymbol{h}_b$ and $\boldsymbol{r}^B = \boldsymbol{J}\boldsymbol{r}$, the above becomes

$$P_b = r(0) - \boldsymbol{r}^T\boldsymbol{J}^T\boldsymbol{J}\boldsymbol{h}_f.$$

But $\boldsymbol{J}^T\boldsymbol{J} = \boldsymbol{I}$ so that

$$P_b = r(0) - \boldsymbol{r}^T\boldsymbol{h}_f.$$

From Eq. 8.5.9, this is simply the forward prediction error energy, P_a, so that

$$P_b = P_a. \tag{8.5.35}$$

Therefore, when the forward and backward predictors are optimized, the forward and backward prediction error energies are the same. We will thus be justified in using the single symbol P_N where

$$P_N = P_a = P_b$$

and N signifies N-th order.

8.6 The Levinson-Durbin Algorithm

Direct solution of the Wiener-Hopf equations by techniques such as Gaussian elimination requires on the order of N^3 operations where N is the predictor order. By exploiting the Toeplitz structure of the autocorrelation matrix R, the complexity can be reduced to N^2 operations. The technique we will discuss is called the *Levinson-Durbin* algorithm [Dur60]. The Levinson-Durbin algorithm uses order recursions; that is, the augmented normal equations for an m-th order predictor are used to produce the $m+1$-st order predictor. The recursion continues until the final prediction order, N, is reached. We will see that the computations bear a strong resemblance to the computations for lattice FIR filters, and in fact suggest a useful lattice structure for linear prediction. The real strength of the Levinson-Durbin algorithm is that not only is the computation simpler, but we also obtain predictors of all order between zero and the final prediction order, N.

Recall that the m-th order prediction filter was given by

$$\boldsymbol{h}_a^{(m)} = \boldsymbol{R}_m^{-1}\boldsymbol{r}_m \tag{8.6.1}$$

where the m explicitly indicates the prediction order. We defined the forward prediction error $e_m^f(k)$ by

$$e_m^f(k) = x(k) - \boldsymbol{h}_f^{(m)T}\boldsymbol{x}_m(k-1)$$

and the forward prediction error filter $\boldsymbol{a}^{(m)}$ by

$$\boldsymbol{a}^{(m)} = \begin{bmatrix} 1 \\ -\boldsymbol{h}_a^{(m)} \end{bmatrix}.$$

The notation for backward prediction follows immediately from the above. At each order m, we have the augmented normal equations

$$\boldsymbol{R}_{m+1}\boldsymbol{a}^{(m)} = \begin{bmatrix} P_m \\ \boldsymbol{0} \end{bmatrix} \tag{8.6.2}$$

and

$$\boldsymbol{R}_{m+1}\boldsymbol{b}^{(m)} = \begin{bmatrix} \boldsymbol{0} \\ P_m \end{bmatrix} \tag{8.6.3}$$

where $\boldsymbol{R}_{m+1}$ can be partitioned either as

$$\boldsymbol{R}_{m+1} = \begin{bmatrix} \boldsymbol{r}(0) & \boldsymbol{r}_m^T \\ \boldsymbol{r}_m & \boldsymbol{R}_m \end{bmatrix} \tag{8.6.4}$$

or

$$\boldsymbol{R}_{m+1} = \begin{bmatrix} \boldsymbol{R}_m & \boldsymbol{r}_m^B \\ \boldsymbol{r}_m^{BT} & \boldsymbol{r}(0) \end{bmatrix} \tag{8.6.5}$$

It is important to remember that when the forward and backward predictors are optimized, the predictors and prediction error filters are the reverse of one another. Furthermore, the forward and backward prediction energy are the same.

The Levinson-Durbin algorithm states that we can obtain the forward prediction error filter of order m from the forward and backward prediction error filters of order $m-1$ according to

$$\boldsymbol{a}^{(m)} = \begin{bmatrix} \boldsymbol{a}^{(m-1)} \\ 0 \end{bmatrix} + \kappa_m \begin{bmatrix} 0 \\ \boldsymbol{b}^{(m-1)} \end{bmatrix}. \tag{8.6.6}$$

This corresponds to the $\mathcal{Z}$-transform relationship

$$A_m(z) = A_{m-1}(z) + \kappa_m z^{-1} B_{m-1}(z) \tag{8.6.7}$$

where $A_m(z)$ is the transfer function of the m-th order forward prediction error filter and $B_m(z)$ is the transfer function of the m-th order backwards prediction error filter. Notice the similarity to the lattice FIR. What we must do is establish a relationship between the autocorrelation sequence and the parameters κ_i.

We begin by multiplying both sides of Eq. 8.6.6 by $\boldsymbol{R}_{m+1}$, giving

$$\boldsymbol{R}_{m+1}\boldsymbol{a}^{(m)} = \boldsymbol{R}_{m+1} \begin{bmatrix} \boldsymbol{a}^{(m-1)} \\ 0 \end{bmatrix} + \kappa_m \boldsymbol{R}_{m+1} \begin{bmatrix} 0 \\ \boldsymbol{b}^{(m-1)} \end{bmatrix}. \tag{8.6.8}$$

Using the partition of $\boldsymbol{R}_{m+1}$ from Eq. 8.6.5, the first term on the right becomes

$$\begin{bmatrix} \boldsymbol{R}_m & \boldsymbol{r}_m^B \\ \boldsymbol{r}_m^{BT} & r(0) \end{bmatrix} \begin{bmatrix} \boldsymbol{a}^{(m-1)} \\ 0 \end{bmatrix} = \begin{bmatrix} \boldsymbol{R}_m \boldsymbol{a}^{(m-1)} \\ \boldsymbol{r}_m^{BT} \boldsymbol{a}^{(m-1)} \end{bmatrix}. \tag{8.6.9}$$

But the augmented normal equations for the forward prediction error filter of order $m-1$ state that

$$\boldsymbol{R}_m \boldsymbol{a}^{(m-1)} = \begin{bmatrix} P_{m-1} \\ \boldsymbol{0} \end{bmatrix}. \tag{8.6.10}$$

Define the quantity Δ_{m-1} by

$$\Delta_{m-1} = \boldsymbol{r}_m^{BT} \boldsymbol{a}^{(m-1)}. \tag{8.6.11}$$

Then Eq. 8.6.9 becomes

$$\boldsymbol{R}_{m+1}\begin{bmatrix} \boldsymbol{a}^{(m-1)} \\ 0 \end{bmatrix} = \begin{bmatrix} P_{m-1} \\ \boldsymbol{0} \\ \Delta_{m-1} \end{bmatrix}. \tag{8.6.12}$$

For the second term on the right of Eq. 8.6.8, we use the partition of $\boldsymbol{R}_{m+1}$ from eq. 8.6.4, giving

$$\begin{bmatrix} r(0) & \boldsymbol{r}_m^T \\ \boldsymbol{r}_m & \boldsymbol{R}_m \end{bmatrix}\begin{bmatrix} 0 \\ \boldsymbol{b}^{(m-1)} \end{bmatrix} = \begin{bmatrix} \boldsymbol{r}_m^T\boldsymbol{b}^{(m-1)} \\ \boldsymbol{R}_m\boldsymbol{b}^{(m-1)} \end{bmatrix}. \tag{8.6.13}$$

The augmented normal equations for the backward prediction error filter of order $m-1$ state that

$$\boldsymbol{R}_m\boldsymbol{b}^{(m-1)} = \begin{bmatrix} \boldsymbol{0} \\ P_{m-1} \end{bmatrix}. \tag{8.6.14}$$

As for the quantity $\boldsymbol{r}_m^T\boldsymbol{b}^{(m-1)}$, it can be rewritten as

$$\boldsymbol{r}_m^T\boldsymbol{b}^{(m-1)} = (\boldsymbol{J}\boldsymbol{r}_m^B)^T\boldsymbol{J}\boldsymbol{a}^{(m-1)} = \boldsymbol{r}_m^{BT}\boldsymbol{a}^{(m-1)} = \Delta_{m-1}. \tag{8.6.15}$$

Therefore,

$$\boldsymbol{R}_{m+1}\begin{bmatrix} 0 \\ \boldsymbol{b}^{(m-1)} \end{bmatrix} = \begin{bmatrix} \Delta_{m-1} \\ \boldsymbol{0} \\ P_{m-1} \end{bmatrix}. \tag{8.6.16}$$

Finally, the left-hand side of Eq. 8.6.8 is simplified as

$$\boldsymbol{R}_{m+1}\boldsymbol{a}^{(m)} = \begin{bmatrix} P_m \\ \boldsymbol{0} \end{bmatrix},. \tag{8.6.17}$$

Substituting Eqs. 8.6.12, 8.6.16, and 8.6.17 into Eq. 8.6.8, we thus have

$$\begin{bmatrix} P_m \\ \boldsymbol{0} \end{bmatrix} = \begin{bmatrix} P_{m-1} \\ \boldsymbol{0} \\ \Delta_{m-1} \end{bmatrix} + \kappa_m \begin{bmatrix} \Delta_{m-1} \\ \boldsymbol{0} \\ P_{m-1} \end{bmatrix}. \tag{8.6.18}$$

From the last row of Eq. 8.6.18, it is clear that in order for Eq. 8.6.6 to hold we must have

$$\kappa_m = -\frac{\Delta_{m-1}}{P_{m-1}}. \tag{8.6.19}$$

The last row of Eq. 8.6.18 says that

$$P_m = P_{m-1} + \kappa_m \Delta_{m-1}. \tag{8.6.20}$$

Substituting Eq. 8.6.19 into Eq. 8.6.20, it follows that

$$P_m = P_{m-1} - \kappa_m^2 P_{m-1} = (1 - \kappa_m)^2 P_{m-1}. \tag{8.6.21}$$

Equation 8.6.21 expresses the evolution of the prediction error energy as the predictor order is increased. The prediction error energy P_0 for the zeroth order predictor is simply the signal power, $r(0)$. At the first order, we have

$$P_1 = (1 - \kappa_1^2) r(0).$$

At the second order,

$$P_2 = (1 - \kappa_2^2) P_1 = (1 - \kappa_2^2)(1 - \kappa_1^2) r(0).$$

In general, we continue to the final predictor order N, giving

$$P_N = r(0) \prod_{m=1}^{N} (1 - \kappa_m^2). \tag{8.6.22}$$

Let's attempt to attribute some physical significance to the quantity Δ_{m-1}. According to Eq. 8.6.15,

$$\Delta_{m-1} = \boldsymbol{r}_m^T \boldsymbol{b}^{(m-1)}$$

where

$$\boldsymbol{r}_m = \mathcal{E}[x(k)\boldsymbol{x}_m(k-1)].$$

Therefore,

$$\Delta_{m-1} = \mathcal{E}[x(k)\boldsymbol{x}_m^T(k-1)\boldsymbol{b}^{(m-1)}].$$

By definition,

$$\boldsymbol{x}_m^T(k-1)\boldsymbol{b}^{(m-1)} = e_{m-1}^b(k-1)$$

and thus

$$\Delta_{m-1} = \mathcal{E}[x(k)e_{m-1}^b(k-1)]. \tag{8.6.23}$$

The forward prediction error for order $m-1$ satisfies

$$e^f_{m-1}(k) = \boldsymbol{a}^{(m-1)T}\boldsymbol{x}_m(k-1)$$

so that $x(k)$ can be expressed by

$$x(k) = e^f_{m-1}(k) - a_1^{(m-1)}x(k-1) - a_2^{(m-1)}x(k-2) - \cdots - a_{m-1}^{(m-1)}x(k-m+1). \quad (8.6.24)$$

The principle of orthogonality guarantees that the backward prediction error at time $k-1$ is orthogonal to the values of $\boldsymbol{x}$ which were used for its computation, namely, $x(k-1), x(k-2), \ldots, x(k-m+1)$. Using this fact and substituting Eq. 8.6.24 into Eq. 8.6.23, we obtain

$$\Delta_{m-1} = \mathcal{E}[e^f_{m-1}(k)e^b_{m-1}(k-1)]. \quad (8.6.25)$$

Equation 8.6.25 can be used to determine the initial value of Δ for the Levinson-Durbin algorithm. Because

$$e^f_0(k) = e^b_0(k) = x(k),$$

the initial value, Δ_0 is given by Eq. 8.6.25 as

$$\Delta_0 = \mathcal{E}[x(k)x(k-1)] = r(1). \quad (8.6.26)$$

According to Eq. 8.6.19, the m-th lattice parameter κ_m is given by

$$\kappa_m = -\frac{\Delta_{m-1}}{P_{m-1}}.$$

The $\{\kappa_m\}$ are typically known as *reflection coefficients* because of the similarity between Eq. 8.6.21 and a fundamental equation from transmission line theory. Because the prediction error power can never be negative, Eq. 8.6.21 implies that

$$|\kappa_m| \leq 1 \quad \text{for all } m.$$

This condition in turn implies that the forward prediction error filter $\boldsymbol{a}^{(m)}$ will be minimum-phase for each order, m.

When the prediction error filters are optimized in the Wiener sense, we showed that

$$\mathcal{E}[(e^f_{m-1}(k))^2] = \mathcal{E}[(e^b_{m-1}(k))^2] = P_{m-1}.$$

Using Eq. 8.6.25, κ_m can then be expressed by

$$\kappa_m = -\frac{\mathcal{E}[e^f_{m-1}(k)e^b_{m-1}(k-1)]}{\mathcal{E}[(e^f_{m-1}(k))^2]}. \quad (8.6.27)$$

Eq. 8.6.27 expresses κ_m as what is known in the statistical literature as a *partial correlation* (PARCOR) coefficient.

Summary

The Levinson-Durbin algorithm is summarized as follows.

$$P_0 = r(0)$$

$$\Delta_0 = r(1)$$

$$\Delta_{m-1} = \boldsymbol{r}_m^T \boldsymbol{b}^{(m-1)}$$

$$\kappa_m = -\frac{\Delta_{m-1}}{P_{m-1}}$$

$$P_m = (1-\kappa_m^2)P_{m-1}$$

$$\boldsymbol{a}^{(m)} = \begin{bmatrix} \boldsymbol{a}^{(m-1)} \\ 0 \end{bmatrix} + \kappa_m \begin{bmatrix} 0 \\ \boldsymbol{b}^{(m-1)} \end{bmatrix}$$

$$\boldsymbol{b}^{(m)} = \boldsymbol{a}^{(m)B}.$$

Example 8.4

Suppose we again have the AR(2) process

$$x(k) = v(k) + \frac{3}{4}x(k-1) + \frac{1}{8}x(k-2)$$

where $v(k)$ is a zero-mean white noise process with variance

$$\sigma_v^2 = 1.$$

Let's use the Levinson-Durbin algorithm to design a second order linear prediction error filter.

We have already showed that

$$r(0) = 3.8291, \quad r(1) = 3.2821, \quad r(2) = 2.9402.$$

We begin with a predictor of order zero. The zeroth order prediction error power is given by

$$P_0 = r(0).$$

The zeroth order forward and backward prediction error filters are given by

$$\boldsymbol{a}^{(0)} = \boldsymbol{b}^{(0)} = 1.$$

The first order crosscorrelation vector $\boldsymbol{r}_1$ is given by

$$\boldsymbol{r}_1 = r(1).$$

According to Eq. 8.6.26,

$$\Delta_0 = r(1) = 3.2821.$$

Next, κ_1 is computed according to Eq. 8.6.19 as

$$\kappa_1 = -\frac{\Delta_0}{P_0} = -0.8572.$$

We then update the prediction error power by Eq. 8.6.21:

$$P_1 = (1 - \kappa_1^2)P_0 = 1.0159.$$

Now, the forward prediction error filter is updated to order one by Eq. 8.6.6:

$$\boldsymbol{a}^{(1)} = \begin{bmatrix} \boldsymbol{a}^{(0)} \\ 0 \end{bmatrix} + \kappa_1 \begin{bmatrix} 0 \\ \boldsymbol{b}^{(0)} \end{bmatrix},$$

which gives

$$\boldsymbol{a}^{(1)} = \begin{bmatrix} 1 \\ 0 \end{bmatrix} + \kappa_1 \begin{bmatrix} 0 \\ 1 \end{bmatrix} = \begin{bmatrix} 1 \\ -0.8572 \end{bmatrix}.$$

The backward prediction error filter is the reverse of $\boldsymbol{a}^{(1)}$, giving

$$\boldsymbol{b}^{(1)} = \begin{bmatrix} -0.8572 \\ 1 \end{bmatrix}.$$

We have thus obtained the forward and backward prediction error filter of first order.

Now the second order prediction error filters are computed. The second order cross-correlation vector is given by

$$\boldsymbol{r}_2 = \begin{bmatrix} r(1) \\ r(2) \end{bmatrix} = \begin{bmatrix} 3.2821 \\ 2.9402 \end{bmatrix}.$$

The quantity Δ_1 is then computed by Eq. 8.6.15:

$$\Delta_1 = \boldsymbol{r}_2^T \boldsymbol{b}^{(1)} = 0.1270.$$

The parameter κ_2 is given by

$$\kappa_2 = -\frac{\Delta_1}{P_1} = -0.125.$$

We can then compute the forward prediction error filter by

$$\boldsymbol{a}^{(2)} = \begin{bmatrix} \boldsymbol{a}^{(1)} \\ 0 \end{bmatrix} + \kappa_2 \begin{bmatrix} 0 \\ \boldsymbol{b}^{(1)} \end{bmatrix},$$

which gives

$$a^{(2)} = \begin{bmatrix} 1 \\ -0.8715 \\ 0 \end{bmatrix} + \kappa_2 \begin{bmatrix} 0 \\ -0.8715 \\ 1 \end{bmatrix} = \begin{bmatrix} 1 \\ -0.75 \\ -0.125 \end{bmatrix}.$$

Finally, the second order prediction error power is computed by

$$P_2 = (1 - \kappa_2^2)P_1 = 1.$$

Notice that $a^{(2)}$ is the correct forward prediction error filter, having tap weights equal to the AR process parameters. Also, the second order prediction error power is seen to equal the white noise power, which is what we expected.

The Levinson-Durbin algorithm is more computationally efficient than direct solution of the Wiener-Hopf equation for the FIR Wiener filter. As such, it is the preferred method of solution. As we have seen, the Levinson-Durbin algorithm assumes explicit knowledge of the autocorrelation values $r(0)$ through $r(M)$. If these values are not available, they can be estimated from the data assuming the stochastic process $\{x(k)\}$ is ergodic. If this is the case, we may estimate $r(k)$ by either the *biased* estimator

$$\hat{r}(k) = \frac{1}{N} \sum_{n=0}^{N-k-1} x(n+k)x(n), \quad k = 0, 1, \ldots, M \tag{8.6.28}$$

or by the *biased* estimator

$$\bar{r}(k) = \frac{1}{N-k} \sum_{n=0}^{N-k-1} x(n+k)x(n), \quad k = 0, 1, \ldots, M. \tag{8.6.29}$$

As we will see later, the biased estimator $\bar{r}(k)$ has smaller variance and is often the preferred estimator.

8.7 Lattice Wiener Filtering

The Levinson-Durbin recursions suggest an alternative architecture for prediction filters. We have shown that the Wiener-Hopf equations for an N-th order predictor can be solved by starting with a zeroth order predictor and performing order recursions until the final order N is reached; this is the essence of the Levinson-Durbin algorithm. This is a very powerful technique, for it allows us to increase the order of the predictor to $N+1$ without rendering the lower-order predictors useless.

Recall that the Levinson-Durbin algorithm allows the prediction error filter of order m to be obtained from the prediction error filter of order $m-1$ by

$$\boldsymbol{a}^{(m)} = \begin{bmatrix} \boldsymbol{a}^{(m-1)} \\ 0 \end{bmatrix} + \kappa_m \begin{bmatrix} 0 \\ \boldsymbol{b}^{(m-1)} \end{bmatrix}. \tag{8.7.1}$$

This corresponds to the $\mathcal{Z}$-transform relationship

$$A_m(z) = A_{m-1}(z) + \kappa_m z^{-1} B_{m-1}(z) \tag{8.7.2}$$

Since the backward prediction error filter is obtained by reversing the coefficients of the forward prediction error filter, it is simple to see from Eq. 8.7.2 that the backward prediction error filter can be updated by

$$\boldsymbol{b}^{(m)} = \begin{bmatrix} 0 \\ \boldsymbol{b}^{(m-1)} \end{bmatrix} + \kappa_m \begin{bmatrix} \boldsymbol{a}^{(m-1)} \\ 0 \end{bmatrix}, \tag{8.7.3}$$

giving the $\mathcal{Z}$-transform relationship

$$B_m(z) = z^{-1} B_{m-1}(z) + \kappa_m A_{m-1}(z). \tag{8.7.4}$$

Equations 8.7.2 and 8.7.4 relate the $\mathcal{Z}$-transforms of the forward and backward prediction errors of the m-th order predictors to the forward and backward prediction errors of the $(m-1)$-st order predictors. Notice the similarity of these equations to those describing an FIR lattice filter. In fact, we can readily deduce a lattice architecture which implements these equations.

$A_m(z)$ is the transfer function from the input to the m-th order forward prediction error, $e_m^f(k)$. $B_m(z)$ is the transfer function from the input to the m-th order backward prediction error, $e_m^b(k)$. Therefore, Eqs. 8.7.2 and 8.7.4 correspond to the pair of equations

$$\begin{aligned} e_m^f(k) &= e_{m-1}^f(k) + \kappa_m e_{m-1}^b(k-1) \\ e_m^b(k) &= e_{m-1}^b(k-1) + \kappa_m e_{m-1}^f(k). \end{aligned} \tag{8.7.5}$$

The initial conditions for these recursions are

$$e_0^f(k) = e_0^b(k) = x(k).$$

One can easily see that the lattice of Fig. 8.7.1 implements these equations.

The reflection coefficients can be related to the predictor coefficients through the Levinson-Durbin algorithm. There are two problems to consider. The first is to determine the final prediction filter and the final prediction error power given the signal power P_0 and the reflection coefficients. The second problem is to determine the reflection coefficients given the

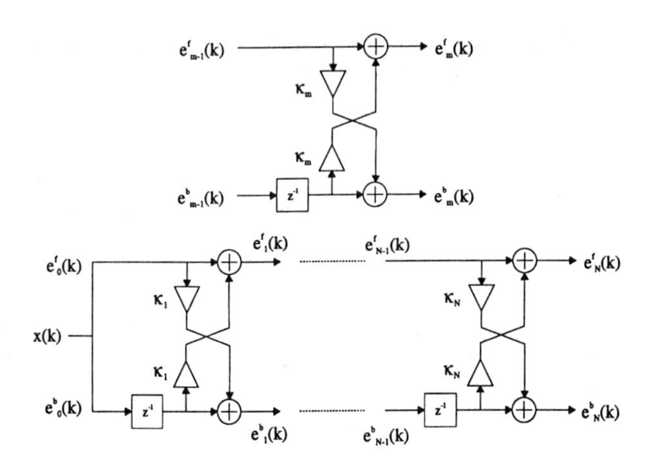

Figure 8.7.1: Lattice prediction error filter.

final predictor. Recall from the Levinson-Durbin algorithm that the forward prediction error filter is order-updated according to

$$\boldsymbol{a}^{(m)} = \begin{bmatrix} \boldsymbol{a}^{(m-1))} \\ 0 \end{bmatrix} + \kappa_m \begin{bmatrix} 0 \\ \boldsymbol{b}^{(m-1))} \end{bmatrix}.$$

Because the last element of $\boldsymbol{b}^{(m-1)}$ is unity, it follows that the last element of $\boldsymbol{a}^{(m)}$ is equal to κ_m. That is,

$$a_m^{(m)} = \kappa_m.$$

Furthermore, from Eqs. 8.7.2 and 8.7.4, we have

$$\begin{aligned} A_m(z) &= A_{m-1}(z) + \kappa_m z^{-1} B_{m-1}(z) \\ B_m(z) &= \kappa_m A_m(z) + z^{-1} B_{m-1}(z). \end{aligned} \tag{8.7.6}$$

Remembering that the forward and backward predictors are the reverse of one another, it also follows that

$$B_m(z) = z^{-m} A_m(z^{-1}).$$

Therefore, we have

$$A_m(z) = A_{m-1}(z) + \kappa_m z^{-1} z^{-(m-1)} A_{m-1}(z^{-1}) \tag{8.7.7}$$

and the backward prediction error filter is obtained by reversing the coefficients of $A_m(z)$. Recall also that the prediction error power is updated according to

$$P_m = (1 - \kappa_m^2)P_{m-1}. \tag{8.7.8}$$

We can use Eqs. 8.7.7 and 8.7.8 iteratively to find the final prediction error filter and final prediction error power from the reflection coefficients and the input power.

Example 8.5

Suppose we are given the reflection coefficients $\kappa_1 = -0.8572$ and $\kappa_2 = -0.125$ along with the input power $P_0 = 3.829$ and we wish to compute the final prediction error filter $A_2(z)$ along with the final prediction error power P_2. We begin with $A_(z) = B_0(z) = 1$. Eq. 8.7.7 then gives

$$A_1(z) = A_0(z) + \kappa_1 z^{-1} = 1 - 0.8572z^{-1}.$$

Also, Eq. 8.7.8 gives

$$P_1 = (1 - \kappa_1^2)P_0 = 1.0156.$$

Next, we have

$$A_2(z) = A_1(z) + \kappa_1 z^{-2} A_1(z^{-1})$$

which gives

$$A_2(z) = 1 - 0.75z^{-1} - 0.125z^{-2}.$$

The final prediction error power is given by

$$P_2 = (1 - \kappa_2^2)P_1 = 1.$$

To solve the inverse problem (finding the reflection coefficients from the final prediction error filter) Eq. 8.7.6 can be solved for $A_{m-1}(z)$, which gives

$$A_{m-1}(z) = \frac{A_m(z) - \kappa_m z^{-m} A_m(z^{-1})}{1 - \kappa_m^2}. \tag{8.7.9}$$

Equation 8.7.9 can be iterated backwards from $A_N(z)$ until $A_1(z)$ and at each step, we have $\kappa_m = a_m^{(m)}$.

Example 8.6

Suppose we have the second-order prediction error filter

$$\boldsymbol{a}^{(2)} = \begin{bmatrix} 1 \\ -0.75 \\ -0.125 \end{bmatrix}.$$

Thus,

$$A_2(z) = 1 - 0.75z^{-1} - 0.125z^{-2}$$

and we have

$$\kappa_2 = -0.125.$$

Next, we have from Eq. 8.7.9

$$A_1(z) = \frac{A_2(z) - \kappa_2 z^{-2} A_2(z^{-1})}{1 - \kappa_2^2}$$

which gives

$$A_1(z) = 1 - 0.8572z^{-1}$$

and hence

$$\kappa_1 = -0.8572.$$

One might wonder why the lattice structure is useful in light of the fact that its complexity is clearly greater than that of a transversal filter. There are several reasons. First of all, the successive stages of the lattice correspond to successive orders in the Levinson-Durbin recursions. As such, the outputs of the m-th stage are the m-th order forward and backward prediction errors, respectively. As we have already mentioned, the Levinson-Durbin algorithm provides prediction filters of all intermediate orders. Consequently, the lattice consists of predictors of *all* intermediate orders. This is significant if we do not know the required order *a priori*. If a lattice is used, we have access to several orders simultaneously and can make the proper choice of which order is correct based on the prediction errors. Another reason for the appeal of the lattice architecture is the regularity and modularity of the architecture. Computations occur locally within each stage and a new stage can be added without modifying the earlier stages.

Beginning with the lattice predictor, it is possible to derive optimal values of the lattice parameters $\{\kappa_m\}$ which minimize some appropriate index of performance. One such performance index is to minimize a weighted sum of the forward and backward prediction error powers at each stage. We can define the performance index J_m for the m-th lattice stage as

$$J_m = \mathcal{E}[(1-a)(e_m^f(k))^2 + a(e_m^b(k))^2], \quad 0 \le a \le 1. \tag{8.7.10}$$

The case $a = 0$ corresponds to a minimization of the forward prediction error power only, and is known as the PARCOR method. When $a = 1$, this corresponds to a minimization of the backward prediction error power only. The choice $a = 1/2$ corresponds to a method of optimization known as the *Burg method*. In this case,

$$J_m = \frac{1}{2}\mathcal{E}[(e_m^f(k))^2 + (e_m^b(k))^2]. \tag{8.7.11}$$

Using Eqs. 8.7.5 to express $(e_m^f(k))^2$ and $(e_m^b(k))^2$, Eq. 8.7.11 becomes

$$\begin{aligned} J_m &= \tfrac{1}{2}\kappa_m^2 \mathcal{E}[(e_{m-1}^f(k))^2 + (e_{m-1}^b(k-1))^2] + 2\kappa_m \mathcal{E}[e_{m-1}^f(k) e_{m-1}^b(k-1)] \\ &\quad + \tfrac{1}{2}\mathcal{E}[(e_{m-1}^b(k-1))^2 + (e_{m-1}^f(k))^2]. \end{aligned} \tag{8.7.12}$$

The optimal choice of κ_m is found by setting the gradient of J_m to zero:

$$\frac{\partial J_m}{\partial \kappa_m} = 0 = \kappa_m \mathcal{E}[(e_{m-1}^f(k))^2 + (e_{m-1}^b(k-1))^2] + 2\mathcal{E}[e_{m-1}^f(k) e_{m-1}^b(k-1)] \tag{8.7.13}$$

which gives

$$\kappa_m = \frac{-2\mathcal{E}[e_{m-1}^f(k) e_{m-1}^b(k-1)]}{\mathcal{E}[(e_{m-1}^f(k))^2 + (e_{m-1}^b(k-1))^2]}. \tag{8.7.14}$$

The choice of κ_m as given by Eq. 8.7.14 minimizes the sum of the forward and backward prediction error powers for the m-th lattice stage.

If, instead, we use $a = 0$ (PARCOR method), the optimal reflection coefficient is found to be

$$\kappa_m = \frac{-2\mathcal{E}[e_{m-1}^f(k) e_{m-1}^b(k-1)]}{\mathcal{E}[(e_{m-1}^f(k))^2]}. \tag{8.7.15}$$

This results in the same value of κ_m found in Eq. 8.6.27. Thus, when the lattice is optimized in the sense that the forward prediction error power is minimized at each stage, the Wiener solution results.

When the autocorrelation sequence of the ergodic process $\{x(k)\}$ is not known explicitly, we can use ergodicity to estimate the reflection coefficients. For the Burg method, we can use

$$\hat{\kappa}_m = -\frac{\sum_{n=m+1}^{L} e_{m-1}^b(k-1) e_{m-1}^f(k)}{\sum_{n=m+1}^{L} [(e_{m-1}^f(k))^2 + (e_{m-1}^b(k-1))^2]}, \quad m = 1, 2, \ldots$$

with a block of data of length L. We begin with $e_0^b(k) = e_0^f(k) = x(k)$ and compute $\hat{\kappa}_1$. Once $\hat{\kappa}_1$ is available, the prediction errors at the second lattice stage, and hence $\hat{\kappa}_2$, can be computed. The procedure continues until the final stage is reached. The reason for the choice of $n = m + 1$ as the lower limit on the summations is because this is the first time at which all input samples contribute to the prediction error outputs at the m-th stage. The choice of how large an L to use is dependent on two important and conflicting factors. L should be large enough so that the time average represents a reasonable approximation to the ensemble average, but not larger than the period over which the input can be assumed to be stationary.

8.8 Lattice Predictor Properties

An important property of the lattice predictor is that the backward prediction errors are *uncorrelated.* That is,

$$\mathcal{E}[e_i^b(k)e_j^b(k)] = P_i\delta(i-j)$$

where P_i is the i-th order prediction error power (recall that for WSS signals the forward and backward prediction error powers are the same). This result is easily proved using the principle of orthogonality.

We can put the backward prediction errors of each order in a vector which can be expressed as follows:

$$\begin{bmatrix} e_0^b(k) \\ e_1^b(k) \\ \vdots \\ e_N^b(k) \end{bmatrix} = \begin{bmatrix} b_0^{(0)} & 0 & 0 & \cdots & 0 \\ b_0^{(1)} & b_1^{(1)} & 0 & \cdots & 0 \\ b_0^{(2)} & b_1^{(2)} & b_2^{(2)} & \cdots & 0 \\ \vdots & \vdots & \vdots & \ddots & \vdots \\ b_0^{(N)} & b_1^{(N)} & b_2^{(N)} & \cdots & b_N^{(N)} \end{bmatrix} \begin{bmatrix} x(k) \\ x(k-1) \\ \vdots \\ x(k-N) \end{bmatrix}, \tag{8.8.1}$$

which we express compactly by

$$\boldsymbol{B}(k) = \boldsymbol{L}\boldsymbol{x}(k). \tag{8.8.2}$$

We have used the notation $b_j^{(m)}$ to denote the j-th coefficient of the m-th order backward prediction error filter, which we have seen is equal to the negative of the $j+1$-st coefficient of the m-th order backward *prediction* filter. Also, the diagonal elements of $\boldsymbol{L}$ are equal to one. Equation 8.8.1 is another statement of the Gram-Schmidt algorithm whereby a linearly independent collection of vectors is transformed to an orthogonal collection of vectors.

Because of the orthogonality of the backward prediction errors, we have

$$\mathcal{E}[\boldsymbol{B}(k)\boldsymbol{B}^T(k)] = \begin{bmatrix} P_0 & 0 & \cdots & 0 \\ 0 & P_1 & \cdots & 0 \\ \vdots & \vdots & \ddots & \vdots \\ 0 & 0 & \cdots & P_N \end{bmatrix}. \tag{8.8.3}$$

We have also just showed that $\boldsymbol{B}(k) = \boldsymbol{L}\boldsymbol{x}(k)$ so that

$$\mathcal{E}[\boldsymbol{B}(k)\boldsymbol{B}^T(k)] = \mathcal{E}[\boldsymbol{L}\boldsymbol{x}(k)\boldsymbol{x}^T(k)\boldsymbol{L}^T] = \boldsymbol{L}\boldsymbol{R}\boldsymbol{L}^T. \tag{8.8.4}$$

Comparing Eqs. 8.8.3 and 8.8.4, we see that

$$\boldsymbol{L}\boldsymbol{R}\boldsymbol{L}^T = \boldsymbol{E} \tag{8.8.5}$$

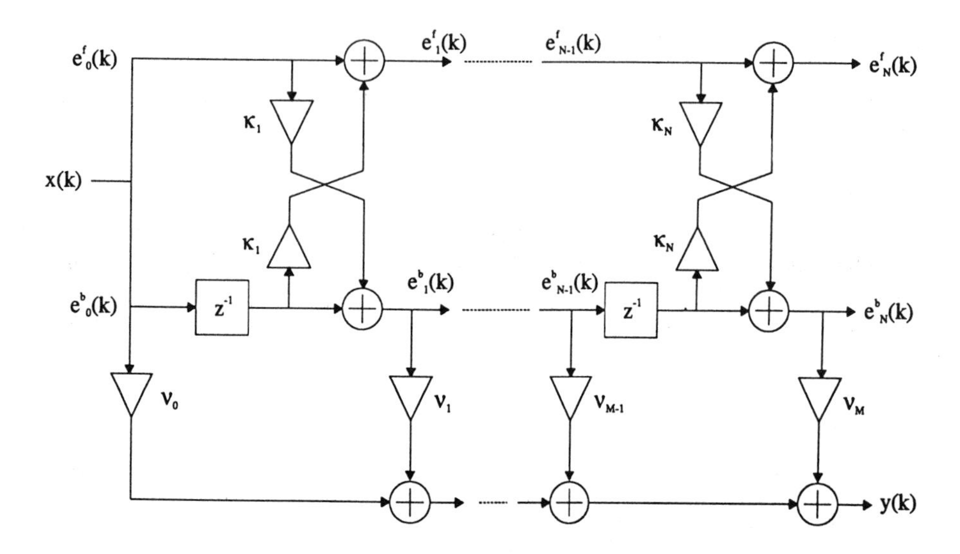

Figure 8.8.1: Using a lattice filter for Wiener filtering.

where $\boldsymbol{E}$ is the diagonal matrix consisting of the prediction error powers.

The fact that the backward prediction errors are uncorrelated is significant because it allows us to use the lattice as a *conditioning filter* for Wiener filtering. To be precise, suppose we have the input signal $x(k)$ and the desired response $d(k)$. Assume that we have obtained the lattice parameters κ_i which generate the forward and backward prediction errors. We wish to approximate the desired response as a linear combination of the backward prediction errors, $e_m^b(k)$. In other words, we form the output $y(k)$ by

$$y(k) = \nu_0 e_0^b(k) + \nu_1 e_1^b(k) + \cdots + \nu_N e_N^b(k),$$

which we can write as

$$y(k) = \boldsymbol{\nu}^T \boldsymbol{B}(k).$$

This is accomplished using the architecture in Fig. 8.8.1. Using the Wiener filter theory we have developed thusfar, it is clear that the optimal value of $\boldsymbol{\nu}$ is given by

$$\boldsymbol{\nu} = (\mathcal{E}[\boldsymbol{B}(k)\boldsymbol{B}^T(k)])^{-1}\mathcal{E}[d(k)\boldsymbol{B}(k)]. \tag{8.8.6}$$

We have seen from Eq. 8.8.5 that

$$\mathcal{E}[\boldsymbol{B}(k)\boldsymbol{B}^T(k) = \boldsymbol{L}\boldsymbol{R}\boldsymbol{L}^T$$

where $\boldsymbol{L}$ is the matrix whose rows are given by the backward prediction error filters. Also, we have

$$\boldsymbol{L}\boldsymbol{R}\boldsymbol{L}^T = \boldsymbol{E} \tag{8.8.7}$$

where $\boldsymbol{E}$ is the diagonal matrix of prediction error powers. Furthermore, using Eq. 8.8.2, it follows that

$$\mathcal{E}[d(k)\boldsymbol{B}(k)] = \boldsymbol{L}\mathcal{E}[d(k)\boldsymbol{x}(k)] = \boldsymbol{L}\boldsymbol{p}.$$

Thus, Eq. 8.8.6 becomes

$$\boldsymbol{\nu} = \boldsymbol{E}^{-1}\boldsymbol{L}\boldsymbol{p}.$$

This solution is extremely simple to compute since $\boldsymbol{E}$ is diagonal, a fact which will be very useful when we study adaptive algorithms to compute the optimal solution. To relate the value of $\boldsymbol{\nu}$ to the Wiener solution for the optimal *transversal* filter, we substitute Eq. 8.8.7 into Eq. 8.8.6, giving

$$\boldsymbol{\nu} = (\boldsymbol{L}\boldsymbol{R}\boldsymbol{L}^T)^{-1}\boldsymbol{L}\boldsymbol{p} = (\boldsymbol{L}^T)^{-1}\boldsymbol{h}_o.$$

Chapter 9

ADAPTIVE FILTERING: GRADIENT DESCENT ALGORITHMS

9.1 Introduction

The explicit solution of the Wiener filtering problem requires knowledge of the input autocorrelation matrix and the crosscorrelation between the input and the desired response. Furthermore, the Wiener-Hopf equations must be solved. In practice, the autocorrelation and crosscorrelation may not be known and solution of the Wiener-Hopf equations in real-time may not be possible. This is especially true if the signals have statistics which vary with time. The purpose of adaptive filtering is to develop a filter which is capable of *adapting* to changing signal statistics.

We will mostly restrict the study of adaptive filters to the transversal structure. There are several reasons for this. First, the mean-squared error for the transversal filter will be a quadratic function of the tap-weight vector. As such, the error surface will be a paraboloid with only one minimum. This makes searching the error surface for the minimum mean-squared error relatively simple. For other filter structures, the error surface may have many local minima. Another reason for using the transversal filter is *stability*. The adaptive transversal filter is guaranteed to be stable, which may not be the case for an adaptive IIR filter.

For our purposes, an adaptive filter can be regarded as a dynamical system which we would like to converge to the Wiener solution. There are essentially three important quantities which measure the effectiveness of an adaptive algorithm. The first of these is computational complexity. Computational complexity measures the amount of computation which must be expended at each time step in order to implement an adaptive algorithm and is often the governing factor in whether real-time implementation is feasible. Next, we have speed of adaptation. The rate at which an adaptive filter converges to the Wiener solution is important, particularly in situations where the signal statistics are varying in time. Unfortunately, speed of adaptation is typically inversely proportional to computational complexity. Finally, we have *misadjustment*, which measures the offset between the actual Wiener solution and the solution produced by the adaptive algorithm. As we shall see, misadjustment is usually inversely proportional to both speed of adaptation and computational complexity.

It can be seen that adaptive filtering involves many trade-offs and is often a choice of complexity vs. speed of adaptation vs. misadjustment. This chapter will attempt to provide a survey of the popular adaptive algorithms and structures and indicate their strengths and weaknesses. The result should be that the reader is capable of making an intelligent choice of which to use based on the particular needs and constraints of the application.

We will proceed by first developing the method of steepest descent, which is a gradient-search type of algorithm. The method of steepest descent will provide the basic model from which other adaptive algorithms can be derived. We will then discuss *stochastic gradient* algorithms, which use available input data to develop an approximation of the signal statistics. The stochastic gradient-based filters have low computational complexity but produce a misadjustment which may be too large for certain applications. This misadjustment can be made small by slowing the speed of adaptation, but this may be unacceptable in situations where the signal statistics vary rapidly with time. Finally, we will discuss *recursive least squares* algorithms, which have higher computational complexity than stochastic gradient algorithms but provide a better tradeoff of speed of adaptation vs. misadjustment

9.2 Examples of Adaptive Filters

Before beginning an in-depth of study of adaptive filtering algorithms and structure, we will give a brief survey of common applications of adaptive filtering.

Channel Equalization

Earlier, we presented a simple model for a communications channel with additive noise. An adaptive equalizer is shown in Fig. 9.2.1. The purpose of the equalizer $E(z)$ is to "undo" the effects of the channel distortion represented by both the channel transfer function $H(z)$ and the additive noise $n(k)$. In many practical situations, the exact model of the channel is unknown or may even be time-varying. The purpose of the equalizer is to process the received signal $y(k)$ and produce as good an estimate of the transmitted signal $x(k)$ as possible. The adaptive equalizer is typically fed with a known signal $x(k)$ as a reference signal and the output of the channel $y(k)$. The filter $E(z)$ produces an output $\hat{x}(k)$ which is an estimate of the signal $x(k)$ and the error signal $e(k)$ is used to update the coefficients of $E(z)$.

We saw that when the noise is white with variance σ_n^2, the Wiener solution of the

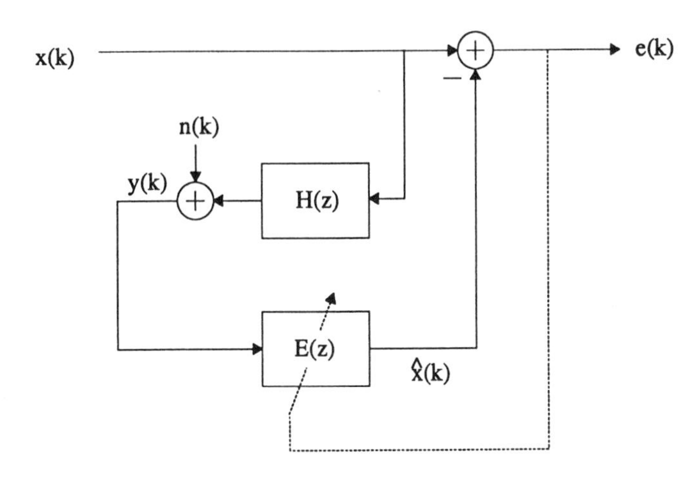

Figure 9.2.1: An adaptive equalizer.

equalization problem is given by

$$E(z) = \frac{\sigma_x^2 H(z^{-1})}{H(z)H(z^{-1})\sigma_x^2 + \sigma_n^2}.$$

This solution assumes knowledge of the signal and noise statistics and allows the equalizer to be IIR and possibly noncausal. In practice, we let the equalizer be an FIR with enough taps to approximate the inverse of the channel. These taps are adjusted adaptively until they converge to the optimal values.

Adaptive Line Enhancement

As we already discussed, the key to Wiener filtering is *correlation canceling.* Suppose we have a broadband signal which is contaminated by a narrowband noise source which has spectral content overlapping the signal's spectral content. In such a case, linear filtering to remove the noise will destroy the signal's spectral content which overlaps that of the noise. Evidently, a conventional filtering approach is not satisfactory. What, then, can we do to remove the noise? Narrowband signals tend to have long-range correlation. That is, there are sinusoidal components which induce autocorrelation sequences that do not decay rapidly. Broadband signals ten to have short-range correlation.

If $x(k)$ is the contaminated signal, we can express $x(k)$ as

$$x(k) = x_N(k) + x_B(k)$$

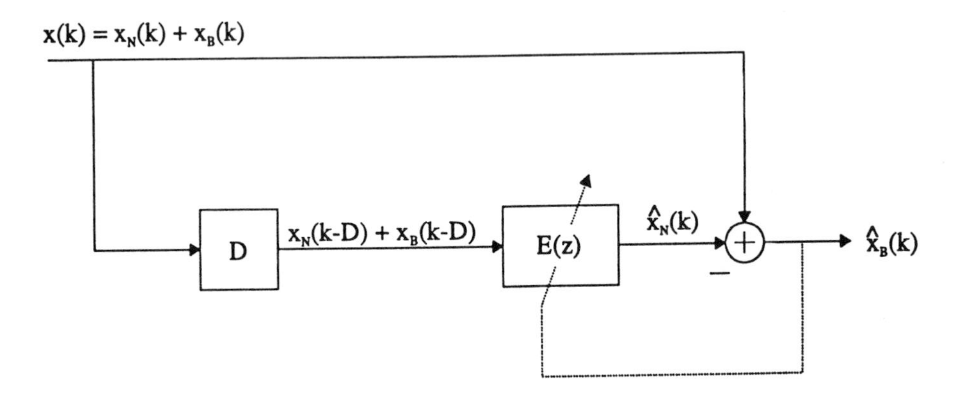

Figure 9.2.2: An adaptive line enhancer.

where $x_N(k)$ is the narrowband component and $x_B(k)$ is the broadband component. Suppose $r_N(k)$ and $r_B(k)$ represent the autocorrelation sequences of $x_N(k)$ and $x_B(k)$, respectively. Let k_N and k_B denote the autocorrelation lags above which $r_N(k)$ and $r_B(k)$ become negligible, respectively. By assumption,

$$k_B < k_N.$$

Consider the arrangement in Fig. 9.2.2. We choose a delay D such that

$$k_B < D < k_N$$

and the output of the delay is

$$x(k-D) = x_N(k-D) + x_B(k-D).$$

Because $D > k_B$, the delayed signal $x_B(k-D)$ is uncorrelated with $x_B(k)$. Also, because $D < k_N$, the delayed signal $x_N(k-D)$ is still correlated with $x_N(k)$. The adaptive filter will adjust its weights so as to cancel the part of the input signal $(x_N(k))$ which is correlated with $x_N(k-D)$. The output of the adaptive filter will be an approximation of $x_N(k)$ which is subtracted from $x(k)$ to give an approximation of $x_B(k)$, which is what we desired.

Adaptive Noise Cancellation

The adaptive noise canceler is a generalization of the adaptive line enhancer. As shown in Fig. 9.2.3, two signals are available: a signal which is contaminated with interference and a

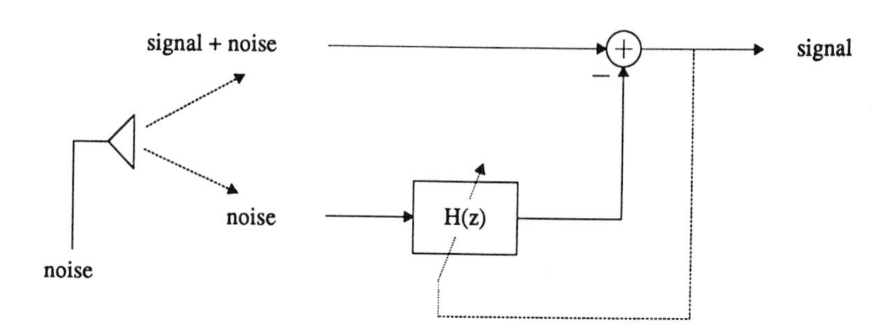

Figure 9.2.3: Adaptive noise cancellation.

noise source which is "similar" to the interference. By similar, we mean either identical or in some way correlated. The adaptive filter acts so as to produce the best possible estimate of the interference which contaminates the signal.

Adaptive Echo Cancellation

Echo cancellation is an important problem in many applications involving two-way communications (particularly in telephone systems). The annoyance of the echo is largely a function of the time delay; the longer the delay between the speech and the echo, the more annoying the echo. Echoes in telephone systems are due in large part to impedance mismatches. To understand how echoes may occur, consider the simple model of a telephone circuit connection shown in Fig. 9.2.4a. Locally, telephones in a given area are connected by two-wire lines which can support two-way communication. For long-distance communication, however, a separate signal path is needed for each direction. This requires a four-wire line. At some point, the two-wire lines need to be connected to the four-wire lines. The connection is made via a *hybrid*. Due to impedance-matching problems, there will be some leakage through the hybrid which can cause echoes.

Consider a speech signal generated at speaker X. After passing through the long-distance channel, the speech is received at the hybrid at speaker Y's side. If there is any leakage through the hybrid, part of the speech from speaker X will be returned to speaker X as though it were part of the speech signal generated by speaker Y. This causes the echo. If the propagation delay of the communication channel is sufficiently long, the echo can become quite a nuisance. For instance, if the communication channel involves transmission to and from a geosynchronous orbit, the total delay will be approximately 540 milliseconds.

The echo can be attenuated by an adaptive echo canceler as shown in Fig. 9.2.4b. The echo canceler produces an approximation of the echo and cancels it from the return path

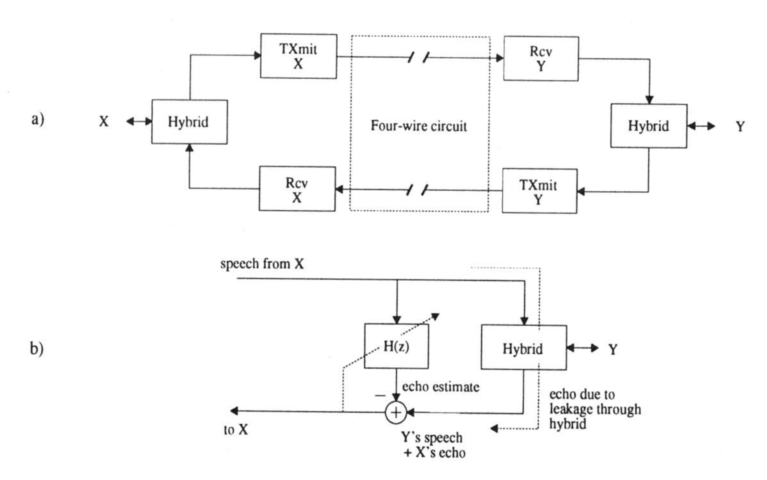

Figure 9.2.4: (a) Simple telephone connection; (b) adaptive echo canceler.

from Y to X. Again, this is a classic example of correlation cancellation. The input to the adaptive filter is the signal appearing at the hybrid for speaker Y and the reference is the the signal produced at Y plus the echo. The adaptive filter attempts to produce a facsimile of the echo, which is correlated with the echo part of overall signal which emerges from speaker Y. This estimate of the echo is subtracted from the output of Y's hybrid and sent back out over the communication path. The order of the adaptive filter needs to be large enough to accommodate the echo path, and in an actual system an echo canceler is present at both X and Y.

Adaptive Prediction

Adaptive prediction is an important application of adaptive filtering which has uses in speech analysis and synthesis, spectral estimation, data transmission, and image compression, to name just a few areas. The problem of linear prediction is simply stated as follows. We are given the N most recent values of a time series $x(k)$ and wish to estimate the next sample. Again, this procedure makes use of the correlation between samples in a stochastic process. The adaptive predictor is shown in Fig. 9.2.5.

Frequently, the purpose of prediction is not so much one of actually *predicting* the next sample, but of data compression. For instance, it is well known that short segments of human speech can be modeled as autoregressive processes. The vocal tract can be approximated as a concatenation of concentric uniform lossless tubes of varying width. There is a direct analogy between this model of the vocal tract and the reflection coefficients of a lattice filter.

The reflection coefficients are estimated from the speech segment, along with the pitch of the signal if the sound is voiced. Linear prediction forms the basis of the method which is used to determine the reflection coefficients. The speech segment can then be reconstructed approximately by exciting an all-pole lattice filter with white noise or a periodic impulse train, depending on whether the speech is voiced or unvoiced. Therefore, the speech can be stored or transmitted by transmitting a small collection of parameters: the reflection coefficients, the pitch period, and the gain. This technique is known as *linear predictive coding* (LPC) [RG78].

Using LPC, the speech segment is transmitted or stored via the reflection coefficients rather than its actual samples. This technique achieves considerable data compression over transmitting the actual speech signal. The order of the lattice is usually no greater than twelve, and the reflection coefficients can usually be coded with a small number of bits. Successful LPC systems which can code and transmit speech at 800 bits per second have been demonstrated, although it is fairly difficult to recognize the speaker at this bit rate. Fairly good speech quality is possible with 2400 bits per second. This should be contrasted with direct transmission or storage of eight-bit speech at an 8 kHz data rate.

Adaptive prediction is also useful in real-time spectral estimation. Many spectral estimation methods rely on fitting an autoregressive model to the input time series. The AR parameters are frequently estimated by determining the optimal predictor coefficients. These predictor coefficients can be estimated, in turn, by an adaptive predictor. The power of this approach lies in the ability of the adaptive predictor to track time-varying statistics of non-stationary signals and allow a time-varying estimate of the signal's power distribution to be computed.

Pulse code modulation (PCM) is a widely used technique for transmitting speech signals. When transmitting speech over telephone channels, the bandwidth of the signals is typically limited to 4 kHz so that the signals can be sampled at 8 kHz. If each speech sample is coded with b bits, the PCM technique requires that b bits be transmitted each second, for a total data rate of $8000b$ bits per second. For high-quality speech at least twelve bits per sample are required, which means that 96,000 bits per second must be transmitted. Obviously, the rate at which bits can be transmitted over a telephone channel depends on the bandwidth of the channel. Hence, the channel bandwidth places a limitation on the quality of transmitted speech.

Direct PCM is memoryless. That is, each sample is encoded independently of every other sample. Speech signals which are sampled at 8 kHz, however, exhibit strong correlation between samples. A technique which is capable of exploiting this correlation can correspondingly reduce the bit rate for speech transmission. This is the premise behind *differential pulse code modulation* (DPCM). Consider the DPCM system shown in Fig. 9.2.6. The encoder consists of a quantizer and a predictor which is in a feedback loop around the quantizer. The prediction $\hat{x}(k)$ is generated as a linear combination of the N previous

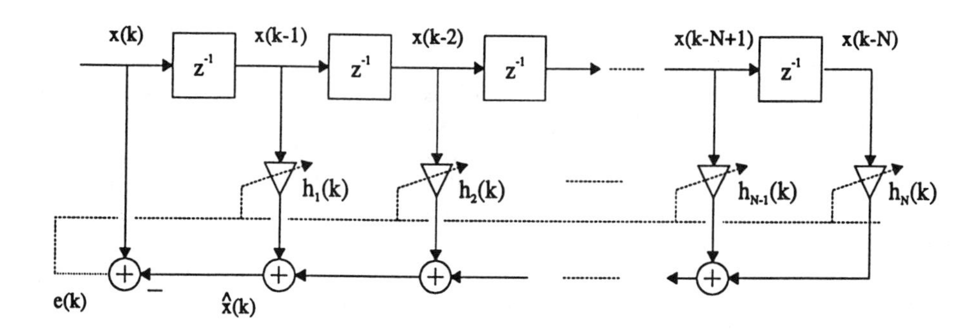

Figure 9.2.5: Adaptive prediction.

samples of the signal $\tilde{x}(k)$. The prediction error is then given by

$$e(k) = x(k) - \hat{x}(k) = x(k) - \sum_{i=1}^{N} a_i \tilde{x}(k-i).$$

The signal $\tilde{x}(k)$ is given by

$$\tilde{x}(k) = \hat{x}(k) + e_q(k)$$

where $e_q(k)$ is the *quantized* prediction error, which differs from the true prediction error by the quantization error. That is,

$$e_q(k) = Q[e(k)] = e(k) + n_q(k)$$

where $n_q(k)$ is the quantization error. The quantized prediction error, $e_q(k)$, is then transmitted. The reason the predictor is in a loop around the quantizer is to avoid accumulation of quantization errors in the decoder. To see this, we have

$$n_q(k) = e_q(k) - e(k)$$

where

$$e(k) = x(k) - \hat{x}(k).$$

Thus,

$$n_q(k) = e_q(k) + \hat{x}(k) - x(k).$$

From the schematic, it is clear that

$$e_q(k) + \hat{x}(k) = \tilde{x}(k).$$

Thus, it follows that

$$\tilde{x}(k) - x(k) = n_q(k).$$

Therefore, the difference between the predictor input and the input sample is due only to the instantaneous quantization error and does not accumulate.

At the receiving end, the signal $\tilde{x}(k)$ is reconstructed by the decoder as shown in Fig. 9.2.6. The decoder consists of a predictor which is identical to the predictor in the encoder. If the encoder and decoder predictors are started from the same initial conditions, the only error in the reconstructed signal will be the quantization error.

The data compression which results from the DPCM system is due to the fact that if the speech signal is highly correlated, the prediction error will have a smaller dynamic range than the signal itself. Consequently, the prediction error can be coded with fewer bits per sample than the actual signal, resulting in fewer bits per second to be transmitted. The amount of compression actually achieved is a function of the quality of the predictor. If the predictor is better able to predict the signal, the prediction error will have a smaller dynamic range. *Adaptive differential pulse code modulation* (ADPCM) simply replaces the fixed predictor in the DPCM system with an adaptive predictor which is capable of adapting to time-varying input signal statistics.

9.3 Method of Steepest Descent

We will first study an algorithm for the iterative solution of the Wiener-Hopf equations which is known as the *steepest descent algorithm.* As the name implies, the steepest descent algorithm is a search algorithm for the Wiener solution which proceeds by moving along the performance surface in the negative direction of the gradient. The steepest descent algorithm assumes complete knowledge of the $\boldsymbol{R}$ and $\boldsymbol{p}$ matrices and hence can not be used when the signal statistics are unknown. The algorithm does, however, provide a basic model on which several important adaptive algorithms are based. These adaptive algorithms essentially rely on an *approximation* of the signal statistics which can be computed from the available data. Depending on the computational effort we are willing to expend on this approximation, the quality of the results will vary.

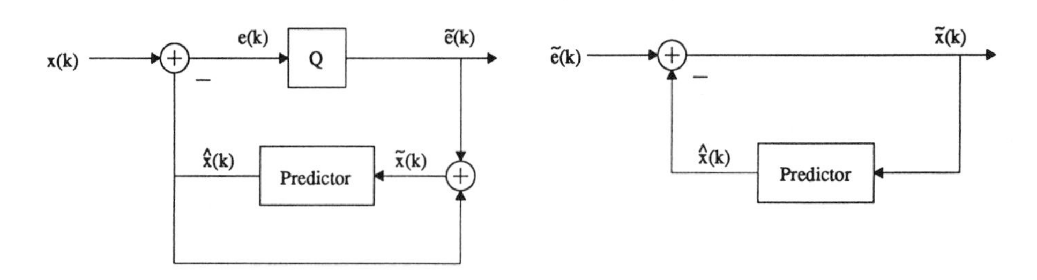

Figure 9.2.6: DPCM encoder and decoder.

The framework is the standard one for Wiener filtering: we have an N-tap transversal filter with input vector $\boldsymbol{x}(k)$ given by

$$\boldsymbol{x}(k) = [x(k), x(k-1), \ldots, x(k-N+1)]^T$$

and a *time-varying* tap-weight vector $\boldsymbol{h}(k)$, where

$$\boldsymbol{h}(k) = [h_0(k), h_1(k), \ldots, h_{N-1}(k)]^T.$$

The output of the adaptive filter is given by

$$y(k) = \boldsymbol{h}^T(k)\boldsymbol{x}(k)$$

and the error between the output and the desired response, $d(k)$ is denoted by $e(k)$ where

$$e(k) = d(k) - y(k) = d(k) - \boldsymbol{h}^T(k)\boldsymbol{x}(k).$$

The goal is to determine an algorithm which updates the time-varying weight $\boldsymbol{h}(k)$ so that it approaches the Wiener solution, $\boldsymbol{h}_0$. Recall that the optimum weight $\boldsymbol{h}_0$ satisfies the Wiener-Hopf equation,

$$\boldsymbol{Rh} = \boldsymbol{p}$$

where $\boldsymbol{R} = \mathcal{E}[\boldsymbol{x}(k)\boldsymbol{x}^T(k)]$ and $\boldsymbol{p} = \mathcal{E}[d(k)\boldsymbol{x}(k)]$. The optimum weight minimizes the mean-squared error,

$$J(\boldsymbol{h}) = \mathcal{E}[e^2(k)] = \sigma_d^2 - 2\boldsymbol{hp} + \boldsymbol{h}^T\boldsymbol{Rh}$$

and we had

$$J_{min} = J(\boldsymbol{h}_0) = \sigma_d^2 - \boldsymbol{p}^T \boldsymbol{h}_0.$$

Accordingly, the mean-squared error is now a function of k:

$$J(k) = \sigma_d^2 - 2\boldsymbol{h}^T(k)\boldsymbol{p} + \boldsymbol{h}^T(k)\boldsymbol{R}\boldsymbol{h}(k) \tag{9.3.1}$$

and we desire

$$\lim_{k\to\infty} \boldsymbol{h}(k) = \boldsymbol{h}_0$$

and

$$\lim_{k\to\infty} J(k) = J_{min}.$$

The principle behind the method of steepest descent is to start from some initial weight, $\boldsymbol{h}(0)$, which has with it some associated mean-squared error, $J(\boldsymbol{h}(0))$. The tap weight is then updated in a manner which causes the mean-squared error to move in the direction of steepest decrease on the performance surface. This direction is determined by the negative of the gradient of the performance surface, $J(\boldsymbol{h})$. The weight is updated according to

$$\boldsymbol{h}(k+1) = \boldsymbol{h}(k) - \frac{1}{2}\mu\nabla_k \tag{9.3.2}$$

where

$$\nabla_k = \frac{\partial J(k)}{\partial \boldsymbol{h}(k)} \tag{9.3.3}$$

(the factor 1/2 is included for mathematical convenience). From Eq. 9.3.1, the gradient is found to be

$$\nabla_k = -2\boldsymbol{p} + 2\boldsymbol{R}\boldsymbol{h}(k)$$

so that Eq. 9.3.2 becomes

$$\boldsymbol{h}(k+1) = (\boldsymbol{I} - \mu\boldsymbol{R})\boldsymbol{h}(k) + \mu\boldsymbol{p}. \tag{9.3.4}$$

Equation 9.3.4 is a simple first-order matrix difference equation whose behavior is controlled by the parameter μ, which we refer to as the *step-size parameter*. Let's examine the behavior of Eq. 9.3.4. If we use the relationship $\boldsymbol{R}\boldsymbol{h}_0 = \boldsymbol{p}$, Eq. 9.3.4 becomes

$$\boldsymbol{h}(k+1) = (\boldsymbol{I} - \mu\boldsymbol{R})\boldsymbol{h}(k) + \mu\boldsymbol{R}\boldsymbol{h}_0. \tag{9.3.5}$$

Now, we subtract $\boldsymbol{h}_0$ from both sides of Eq. 9.3.5, which gives

$$\boldsymbol{h}(k+1) - \boldsymbol{h}_0 = (\boldsymbol{I} - \mu \boldsymbol{R})(\boldsymbol{h}(k) - \boldsymbol{h}_0). \tag{9.3.6}$$

Recall that the autocorrelation matrix has the decomposition

$$\boldsymbol{R} = \boldsymbol{Q}\boldsymbol{\Lambda}\boldsymbol{Q}^H$$

where $\boldsymbol{\Lambda}$ is a real, diagonal matrix and $\boldsymbol{Q}$ satisfies

$$\boldsymbol{Q}^H\boldsymbol{Q} = \boldsymbol{Q}\boldsymbol{Q}^H = \boldsymbol{I}.$$

Using this decomposition of $\boldsymbol{R}$, Eq. 9.3.6 becomes

$$\boldsymbol{h}(k+1) - \boldsymbol{h}_0 = [\boldsymbol{I} - \mu \boldsymbol{Q}\boldsymbol{\Lambda}\boldsymbol{Q}^H](\boldsymbol{h}(k) - \boldsymbol{h}_0). \tag{9.3.7}$$

If we premultiply both sides of the above by $\boldsymbol{Q}^H$, we get

$$\boldsymbol{Q}^H[\boldsymbol{h}(k+1) - \boldsymbol{h}_0] = [\boldsymbol{I} - \mu \boldsymbol{\Lambda}]\boldsymbol{Q}^H(\boldsymbol{h}(k) - \boldsymbol{h}_0). \tag{9.3.8}$$

Notice that this resembles the transformation of the weight-space given by Eq. 8.4.12, where we defined the vector $\boldsymbol{z}$ by

$$\boldsymbol{z} = \boldsymbol{Q}^H(\boldsymbol{h} - \boldsymbol{h}_0).$$

This time, the transformed weight depends on the index k and we have

$$\boldsymbol{z}(k) = \boldsymbol{Q}^H(\boldsymbol{h}(k) - \boldsymbol{h}_0).$$

In this new weight-space, Eq. 9.3.8 becomes

$$\boldsymbol{z}(k+1) = [\boldsymbol{I} - \mu \boldsymbol{\Lambda}]\boldsymbol{z}(k) \tag{9.3.9}$$

and the point $\boldsymbol{z} = \boldsymbol{0}$ coincides with the optimal weight $\boldsymbol{h}_0$. Therefore, convergence of the steepest descent algorithm is assured if we can guarantee that Eq. 9.3.9 converges to zero. Equation 9.3.9 can be transformed to the original weight-space, giving

$$\boldsymbol{h}(k) = [\boldsymbol{I} - \mu \boldsymbol{R}]^k(\boldsymbol{h}(0) - \boldsymbol{h}_o) + \boldsymbol{h}_o.$$

The behavior of the steepest descent is best studied in the transformed weight-space. Notice the simplicity of Eq. 9.3.9. We have a first-order matrix difference equation in which all of the components are decoupled. This implies that the dynamical behavior along each of the coordinate directions is independent. In particular, the n-th component of $\boldsymbol{z}(k)$ evolves according to

$$z_n(k+1) = (1-\mu\lambda_n)z_n(k), \quad n = 1, 2, \ldots, N. \tag{9.3.10}$$

The solution to this equation is

$$z_n(k) = (1-\mu\lambda_n)^k z_n(0), \quad n = 1, 2, \ldots, N \tag{9.3.11}$$

where the $z_n(0)$ are the coordinates of $\boldsymbol{z}(0)$, the initial weight. Examining Eq. 9.3.10, the n-th component of the weight will converge to zero if

$$|1-\mu\lambda_n| < 1 \tag{9.3.12}$$

which means that we must choose μ such that

$$0 < \mu < \frac{2}{\lambda_n}.$$

In order for Eq. 9.3.9 to converge to zero, *every* component z_n must converge to zero. This means that the step size parameter μ must satisfy

$$0 < \mu < \frac{2}{\lambda_n} \quad \text{for all } n = 1, 2, \ldots, N.$$

Therefore, μ is bounded by

$$0 < \mu < \frac{2}{\lambda_{max}}. \tag{9.3.13}$$

If μ satisfies the bound expressed by Eq. 9.3.13, $\boldsymbol{z}(k)$ will reach the origin *regardless of the initial weight* $\boldsymbol{z}(0)$.

The *rate* at which $\boldsymbol{z}(k)$ approaches the origin is a more delicate issue. If we assume that all of the eigenvalues of $\boldsymbol{R}$ are approximately equal, then it is possible to choose a value of μ which forces the quantity

$$(1-\mu\lambda_n)$$

to be small for all n. Therefore, the algorithm can be made to converge almost as quickly as desired since the quantity

$$(1-\mu\lambda_n)^k$$

approaches zero very quickly. If, however, the eigenvalues of $\boldsymbol{R}$ are widely spread, the situation is more difficult. Consider, for example the case where we have a two-weight filter with λ_1 small and λ_2 large. For λ_1, we need a large μ to make $1-\mu\lambda_1$ small. However, this value of μ can not be so large as to make $1-\mu\lambda_2$ larger than one in magnitude. Conversely, we need a small μ to make $1-\mu\lambda_2$ small. This value of μ will render $1-\mu\lambda_1$ close to one so that the weight component in the first coordinate direction will converge slowly. In general, when the eigenvalues of $\boldsymbol{R}$ are widely spread, the rate of convergence is limited by the smallest eigenvalues.

Now that we know how the weights converge, what about the mean-squared error? Equation 9.3.1 can be used to express the mean-squared error in terms of $\boldsymbol{h}(k)$, or, according to Eq. 8.4.13, the mean-squared error can be expressed in terms of the transformed weight-space as

$$J(k) = J_{min} + \boldsymbol{z}^T(k)\boldsymbol{\Lambda}\boldsymbol{z}(k) = J_{min} + \sum_{i=1}^{N} \lambda_i |z_i(k)|^2. \tag{9.3.14}$$

Using Eq. 9.3.11, this simplifies to

$$J(k) = J_{min} + \sum_{i=1}^{N} \lambda_i (1-\mu\lambda_i)^{2k} |z_i(0)|^2. \tag{9.3.15}$$

If μ satisfies the bounds described by Eq. 9.3.13, then $J(k)$ will satisfy

$$\lim_{k\to\infty} J(k) = J_{min}. \tag{9.3.16}$$

Again, the choice of μ will affect the rate at which $J(k)$ approaches J_{min}. For iterative-type algorithms, the evolution of the mean-squared error is often called the *learning curve.* The *time constant* of the i-th mode is defined as the time required for the mean-squared error corresponding to the i-th mode to decay to $1/e$ of its original value. From Eq. 9.3.15, it can be seen that the time constant for the i-th mode is given by

$$\tau_i = \frac{-1}{2\ln(1-\mu\lambda_i)}.$$

For small μ, this is well approximated by

$$\tau_i \approx \frac{1}{2\mu\lambda_i}.$$

When the eigenvalues are widely spread, we have seen that the rate of convergence of the coefficients is determined largely by the mode corresponding to the smallest eigenvalue. The same is true for the convergence of the mean-squared error. Thus, for small μ and large eigenvalue spread, the time constant for the mean-squared error is given approximately by

$$\tau_{MSE} \approx \frac{1}{1-\mu\lambda_{min}}.$$

Example 9.1

Let's use the steepest descent algorithm to find the optimal weight vector for a two-tap predictor. The input signal is zero-mean, unit-variance white noise. This means that the autocorrelation matrix is given by

$$\boldsymbol{R} = \begin{bmatrix} 1 & 0 \\ 0 & 1 \end{bmatrix}$$

and the crosscorrelation vector is

$$\boldsymbol{p} = \begin{bmatrix} 0 \\ 0 \end{bmatrix}.$$

Therefore, the optimal weight is given by $\boldsymbol{h} = \boldsymbol{0}$, which makes sense since this yields a prediction of zero for all time, which is the best guess at a zero-mean white noise sequence. Furthermore, the minimum mean-squared error is equal to the power of the signal itself, which is assumed to be equal to one. This is easily seen by using

$$J = \sigma_d^2 - 2\boldsymbol{h}^T\boldsymbol{p} + \boldsymbol{h}^T\boldsymbol{R}\boldsymbol{h}$$

and recognizing that $\sigma_d^2 = r(0)$ for the case of prediction.

Now, let's look at using the steepest-descent algorithm. The weight updating is performed according to

$$\boldsymbol{h}(k+1) = [\boldsymbol{I} - \mu\boldsymbol{I}]\boldsymbol{h}(k) = (1-\mu)\boldsymbol{h}(k)$$

where we start from some initial weight

$$\boldsymbol{h}(0) = \begin{bmatrix} h_1(0) \\ h_2(0) \end{bmatrix}.$$

Clearly, for stability we must require that

$$0 < \mu < \frac{2}{\lambda_{max}} = 2.$$

The weights will satisfy

$$\begin{aligned} h_1(k) &= (1-\mu)^k h_1(0) \\ h_2(k) &= (1-\mu)^k h_2(0). \end{aligned} \qquad (9.3.17)$$

Therefore, the weights are seen to approach the optimal weight, zero, independent of the initial weight, $\boldsymbol{h}(0)$, at a rate determined by μ. This is shown in Fig. 9.3.1a for $\mu = 0.01$ and a initial weight vector with $h_1(0) = 1, h_2(0) = 1/2$ and in Fig. 9.3.1b for the same initial weight vector and $\mu = 0.05$. Notice that the choice $\mu = 0.05$ leads to damped weight trajectories which approach the optimal weights quicker than when $\mu = 0.01$. Clearly, as $(1-\mu)$ approaches zero, the convergence is more rapid. If μ was such that the term $(1-\mu)$ is negative, the weights would follow oscillatory trajectories.

The mean-squared error is found by substituting Eq. 9.3.17 into Eq. 9.3.1, which gives

$$J(k) = 1 + (1-\mu)^{2k} h_1^2(0) + (1-\mu)^{2k} h_2^2(0).$$

This could also have been obtained from Eq. 9.3.15 if we recognize that the $\boldsymbol{z}$ vectors are the same as the $\boldsymbol{h}$ vectors for this particular example. It is simple to see that when μ is chosen correctly, the mean-squared error will converge to its minimum value, unity, independent of the initial weight $\boldsymbol{h}(0)$. Again, the rate of this convergence is determined by μ. The convergence of the MSE for $\mu = 0.05$ is shown in Fig. 9.3.1.

A useful depiction of the tap-weight evolution is obtained if we plot h_1 versus h_2. Each point in the space described by h_1 and h_2 has associated with it a mean-squared error given by

$$J = \sigma_d^2 - 2\boldsymbol{p}^T\boldsymbol{h} + \boldsymbol{h}^T\boldsymbol{R}\boldsymbol{h} = 1 + h_1^2 + h_2^2.$$

The minimum value of J, as we already have said, is equal to one and occurs at the origin. It is useful to superimpose on the plot of h_1 versus h_2 *contours of constant error.* For this example, these contours are clearly circles in the h_1- h_2 plane. This is illustrated in Fig. 9.3.1 for $\mu = 0.05$. Notice that the weight trajectory always runs perpendicularly to the error contours. This is always true for the steepest descent algorithm – the trajectory runs along the gradient to the error surface, and the gradient is perpendicular to th contours of constant error. As k approaches infinity, the weight trajectory approaches the origin.

Example 9.2

Consider again the problem of designing a two-tap forward predictor for the AR(2) process

$$x(k) = v(k) + \frac{3}{4}x(k-1) + \frac{1}{8}x(k-2)$$

where $v(k)$ is zero mean white-noise with power

$$\sigma_v^2 = 1.$$

We have already seen that

$$\boldsymbol{h}_0 = \begin{bmatrix} 3/4 \\ 1/8 \end{bmatrix}.$$

Also, we know that

$$\boldsymbol{R} = \begin{bmatrix} 3.8291 & 3.2821 \\ 3.2821 & 3.8291 \end{bmatrix}$$

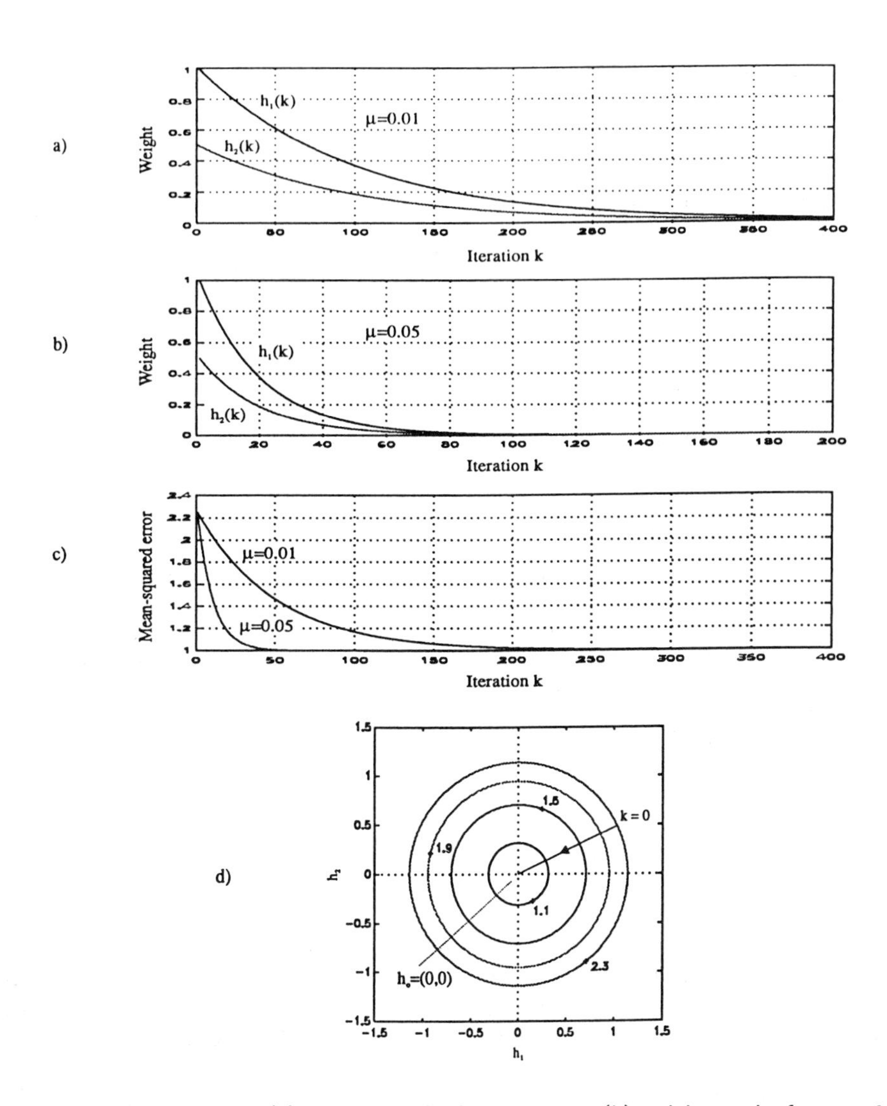

Figure 9.3.1: Example 9.1: (a) Weight tracks for $\mu = 0.01$; (b) weight tracks for $\mu = 0.05$; (c) convergence of mean-squared error; (d) weight evolution in weight-space and contours of constant error.

which has eigenvalues 0.5470 and 7.111, and

$$\boldsymbol{p} = \begin{bmatrix} 3.2821 \\ 2.9402 \end{bmatrix}.$$

Accordingly, the steepest descent algorithm as described by Eq. 9.3.4 becomes

$$\begin{bmatrix} h_1(k+1) \\ h_2(k+1) \end{bmatrix} = \begin{bmatrix} 1-3.8291\mu & -3.2821\mu \\ -3.2821\mu & 1-3.8291\mu \end{bmatrix} \begin{bmatrix} h_1(k) \\ h_2(k) \end{bmatrix} + \begin{bmatrix} 3.2821\mu \\ 2.9402\mu \end{bmatrix}. \tag{9.3.18}$$

The allowable range for μ is given by

$$0 < \mu < \frac{2}{7.1111}.$$

We will examine the behavior with $\mu = 0.05$. Suppose we start with the initial weight

$$\boldsymbol{h}(0) = \begin{bmatrix} -4.5 \\ -4 \end{bmatrix}.$$

Then the behavior of $h_1(k)$ and $h_2(k)$ as given by Eq. 9.3.18 is shown in Fig. 9.3.2a. Notice that both weights approach their optimal values. Another useful picture is obtained if we superimpose the weight evolution over the contours of constant error. This is shown in Fig. 9.3.2b. Observe that the trajectory begins at a point of large mean-squared error and evolves toward the point of minimum mean-squared error, $\boldsymbol{h}_o$. Also, observe that the minimum mean-squared error is equal to 1.0, the power of the noise which drives the AR model.

9.4 The LMS Algorithm

The LMS algorithm [WH60],[WS85] is one of the simplest stochastic gradient algorithms. There are many variants of the LMS algorithm, and we will describe some of the more important ones in detail. The filter structure for the basic LMS algorithm is the transversal filter with time-varying tap-weight vector $\boldsymbol{h}(k)$. Again, we have the input stochastic process $\{x(k)\}$ and the desired response $\{d(k)\}$. The output of the transversal filter is given by

$$y(k) = \boldsymbol{h}^T(k)\boldsymbol{x}(k)$$

where $\boldsymbol{x}(k)$ is the vector of the N most recent samples of $\{x(k)\}$. The error between the output and the desired response is denoted by $e(k)$ where

$$e(k) = d(k) - y(k) = e(k) - \boldsymbol{h}^T(k)\boldsymbol{x}(k).$$

a)

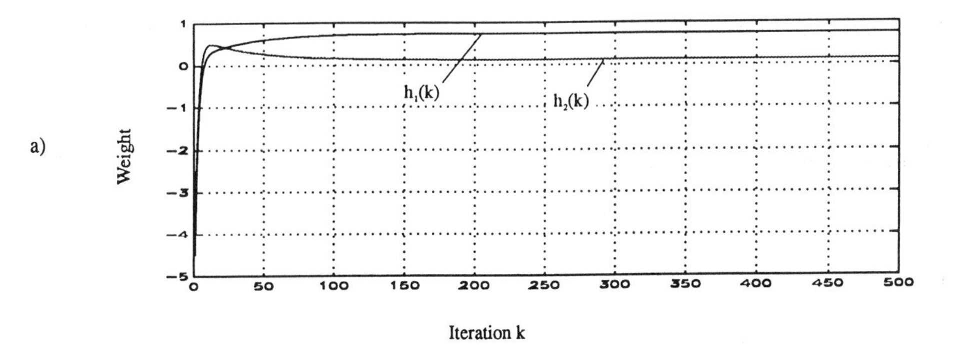

b)

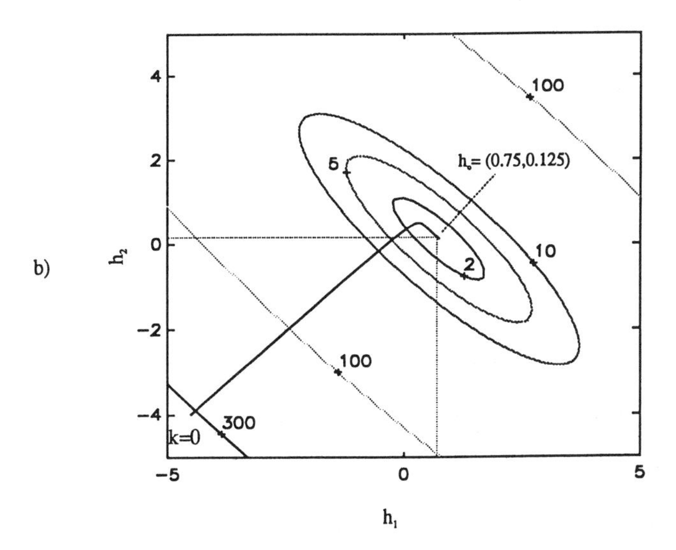

Figure 9.3.2: Behavior of the steepest descent algorithm for Example 9.2: (a) Tap weights for $\mu = 0.05$; (b) mean-squared error evolution for $\mu = 0.05$.

The purpose of the LMS algorithm is to iteratively update the tap-weight vector $\boldsymbol{h}(k)$ so as to minimize the performance criterion

$$J = \mathcal{E}[e^2(k)].$$

Recall that the steepest descent algorithm used the recursion

$$\boldsymbol{h}(k+1) = \boldsymbol{h}(k) - \frac{1}{2}\mu\nabla_k.$$

The LMS algorithm is described by the recursion

$$\boldsymbol{h}(k+1) = \boldsymbol{h}(k) - \frac{1}{2}\mu\hat{\nabla}_k \tag{9.4.1}$$

where $\hat{\nabla}_k$ is called a *stochastic gradient*, *i.e.*, an approximation to the true gradient, ∇_k. We have seen that the true gradient is given by

$$\nabla_k = \frac{\partial J}{\partial \boldsymbol{h}(k)} = -2\boldsymbol{R}\boldsymbol{h} - 2\boldsymbol{p}.$$

Suppose we make the crude approximations

$$\boldsymbol{R} \approx \boldsymbol{x}(k)\boldsymbol{x}^T(k)$$

and

$$\boldsymbol{p} \approx \boldsymbol{d}(k)\boldsymbol{x}(k),$$

namely, we ignore the expectation operators. The stochastic gradient $\hat{\nabla}_k$ is then given by

$$\hat{\nabla}_k = 2(\boldsymbol{x}(k)\boldsymbol{x}^T(k))\boldsymbol{h}(k) - 2d(k)\boldsymbol{x}(k) \tag{9.4.2}$$

Equation 9.4.1 then becomes

$$\boldsymbol{h}(k+1) = \boldsymbol{h}(k) - \mu[\boldsymbol{x}(k)\boldsymbol{x}^T(k)\boldsymbol{h}(k) - d(k)\boldsymbol{x}(k)]. \tag{9.4.3}$$

This equation gives the tap-weight recursion which defines the LMS algorithm. The LMS algorithm can be put in an alternate form if we recognize that

$$e(k) = d(k) - \boldsymbol{x}(k)\boldsymbol{h}^T(k)$$

in which case Eq. 9.4.3 can be expressed as

$$\boldsymbol{h}(k+1) = \boldsymbol{h}(k) - \mu e(k)\boldsymbol{x}(k). \tag{9.4.4}$$

As with any adaptive algorithm, we need to examine the convergence properties of the LMS. It is desired that the algorithm should converge to the Wiener solution, which is the optimum tap-weight $\boldsymbol{h}_o$ which minimizes the mean-squared value of the error signal. It is relatively simple to show convergence in the mean of the LMS algorithm. Taking the expectation of both sides of Eq. 9.4.3, we get

$$\mathcal{E}[\boldsymbol{h}(k+1)] = \mathcal{E}[\boldsymbol{h}(k)] - \mu\mathcal{E}[\boldsymbol{x}(k)\boldsymbol{x}^T(k)\boldsymbol{h}(k)] + \mathcal{E}[d(k)\boldsymbol{x}(k)]. \tag{9.4.5}$$

A standard assumption which is made at this point is that the tap-weight $\boldsymbol{h}(k)$ and the input vector $\boldsymbol{x}(k)$ are independent [WS85]. This assumption is partially justified by the fact that $\boldsymbol{h}(k)$ is determined only by $\boldsymbol{x}(k-1), \boldsymbol{x}(k-2), \ldots$. In this case, Eq. 9.4.5 becomes

$$\mathcal{E}[\boldsymbol{h}(k+1)] = \mathcal{E}[\boldsymbol{h}(k)] - \mu\mathcal{E}[\boldsymbol{x}(k)\boldsymbol{x}^T(k)]\mathcal{E}[\boldsymbol{h}(k)] + \mathcal{E}[d(k)\boldsymbol{x}(k)]. \tag{9.4.6}$$

Recognizing the quantities on the right-hand side of Eq. 9.4.6, we get

$$\mathcal{E}[\boldsymbol{h}(k+1)] = [\boldsymbol{I} - \mu\boldsymbol{R}]\mathcal{E}[\boldsymbol{h}(k)] + \mu\boldsymbol{p}. \tag{9.4.7}$$

This is of the same form as the steepest descent algorithm, which was shown to converge to $\boldsymbol{h}_o$ if

$$0 < \mu < \frac{2}{\lambda_{max}}$$

where λ_{max} is the largest eigenvalue of the correlation matrix $\boldsymbol{R}$. Therefore, we conclude that the LMS algorithm converges in the mean to $\boldsymbol{h}_o$ if the same bounds are met. That is,

$$\lim_{k\to\infty} \mathcal{E}[\boldsymbol{h}(k)] = \boldsymbol{h}_o$$

if

$$0 < \mu < \frac{2}{\lambda_{max}}.$$

Recall that the sum of the eigenvalues of a matrix is equal to its trace. Because all of the eigenvalues of $\boldsymbol{R}$ are nonnegative, it follows that

$$\lambda_{max} \le tr(\boldsymbol{R}) = (N+1)r(0) = (N+1)\sigma_x^2.$$

Thus, a conservative bound for μ to guarantee convergence in the mean is

$$0 < \mu < \frac{2}{(N+1)\sigma_x^2}. \tag{9.4.8}$$

As with the method of steepest descent, the rate of convergence in the mean depends on μ. Larger values of μ will yield faster convergence in the mean.

Convergence in the mean of the LMS algorithm is similar to the type of convergence exhibited by the steepest descent algorithm: it is dependent on the modes of the matrix $(\boldsymbol{I} - \mu\boldsymbol{R})$. As with the steepest descent algorithm, the *same* parameter μ governs the rate of convergence in the direction of each eigenvector of $\boldsymbol{R}$. Therefore, the LMS algorithm also suffers from sensitivity to eigenvalue spread.

Proving convergence in the mean of the tap-weight vector is but a first step in examining the behavior of the LMS algorithm. Just because $\boldsymbol{h}(k)$ converges in the mean to $\boldsymbol{h}_o$ does not guarantee that the algorithm actually works, since the variance might diverge. Also, the mean-squared error behavior is a quadratic function of $\boldsymbol{h}(k)$ so that knowing $\boldsymbol{h}(k)$ converges in the mean to $\boldsymbol{h}_0$ does not actually guarantee that J converges to J_{min}.

To this end, we write the stochastic gradient $\hat{\nabla}_k$ as the sum of the true gradient ∇_k plus a noise term, $\boldsymbol{N}(k)$. That is,

$$\hat{\nabla}_k = \nabla_k + N(k) = 2\boldsymbol{R}\boldsymbol{h}(k) - 2\boldsymbol{p} + \boldsymbol{N}(k). \tag{9.4.9}$$

The LMS algorithm is then written as

$$\boldsymbol{h}(k+1) = \boldsymbol{h}(k) - \mu\boldsymbol{R}\boldsymbol{h}(k) + \mu\boldsymbol{p} - \frac{1}{2}\mu\boldsymbol{N}(k). \tag{9.4.10}$$

We again use the decomposition

$$\boldsymbol{R} = \boldsymbol{Q}\boldsymbol{\Lambda}\boldsymbol{Q}^H$$

to define the change of coordinates

$$\boldsymbol{z}(k) = \boldsymbol{Q}^H(\boldsymbol{h}(k) - \boldsymbol{h}_0),$$

which in turn implies that

$$h(k) = \boldsymbol{Q}\boldsymbol{z}(k) + \boldsymbol{h}_o.$$

Therefore, Eq. 9.4.10 becomes

$$\boldsymbol{Q}\boldsymbol{z}(k+1) + \boldsymbol{h}_o = \boldsymbol{Q}\boldsymbol{z}(k) + \boldsymbol{h}_o - \mu\boldsymbol{R}(\boldsymbol{Q}\boldsymbol{z}(k) + \boldsymbol{h}_o) + \mu\boldsymbol{p} - \frac{1}{2}\mu\boldsymbol{N}(k). \tag{9.4.11}$$

Collecting terms and recognizing that $\boldsymbol{R}\boldsymbol{h}_o = \boldsymbol{p}$, we get

$$\boldsymbol{Q}\boldsymbol{z}(k+1) = [\boldsymbol{I} - \mu\boldsymbol{R}\boldsymbol{Q}]\boldsymbol{z}(k) - \frac{1}{2}\mu\boldsymbol{N}(k). \tag{9.4.12}$$

Finally, pre-multiplying both sides of Eq. 9.4.12 by $\boldsymbol{Q}^H$ gives

$$\boldsymbol{z}(k+1) = [\boldsymbol{I} - \mu\boldsymbol{\Lambda}]\boldsymbol{z}(k) - \frac{1}{2}\boldsymbol{Q}^H\boldsymbol{N}(k). \tag{9.4.13}$$

This equation describes the evolution of the tap-weight vector in the transformed weight-space, where the optimal weight $\boldsymbol{h}_o$ corresponds to the origin. Recall that we have already showed convergence in the mean to $\boldsymbol{h}_o$, which means that $\boldsymbol{z}(k)$ converges in the mean to $\mathbf{0}$. Thus, to prove that the covariance of $\boldsymbol{h}(k)$ is bounded, we can show that

$$\lim_{k\to} \mathcal{E}[\boldsymbol{z}(k)\boldsymbol{z}^T(k)] < M$$

where M is some finite bound to be determined.

Let's take a closer look at Eq. 9.4.13. This equation represents a state variable system which is driven by a N-dimensional noise input, $\boldsymbol{N}(k)$. Recall the following result on the asymptotic stationarity of state variable systems: we are given the system

$$\boldsymbol{x}(k+1) = \boldsymbol{A}\boldsymbol{x}(k) + \boldsymbol{B}\boldsymbol{u}(k).$$

Assuming that the matrix $\boldsymbol{A}$ is stable and $\boldsymbol{u}(k)$ is a white noise input with zero mean and correlation matrix $\boldsymbol{\Sigma}$, we showed that $\boldsymbol{x}(k)$ is asymptotically stationary with zero mean and correlation matrix $\boldsymbol{K}$, where $\boldsymbol{K}$ is the solution to the Lyapunov matrix equation

$$\boldsymbol{K} = \boldsymbol{A}\boldsymbol{K}\boldsymbol{A}^T + \boldsymbol{B}\boldsymbol{\Sigma}\boldsymbol{B}^T. \tag{9.4.14}$$

Referring to Eq. 9.4.13, we make the identification

$$\boldsymbol{A} = \boldsymbol{I} - \mu\boldsymbol{\Lambda}$$

and

$$\boldsymbol{B} = -\frac{1}{2}\boldsymbol{Q}^H.$$

Since μ is confined to the range

$$0 < \mu \frac{2}{\lambda_{max}},$$

to guarantee convergence in the mean, the matrix $(\boldsymbol{I} - \mu\boldsymbol{\Lambda})$ is stable. At this point, we make the assumption that the noise vector $\boldsymbol{N}(k)$ is white, which is a standard assumption for this sort of analysis. Therefore, $\boldsymbol{z}(k)$ will be asymptotically stationary with zero mean and correlation matrix

$$\mathcal{E}[\boldsymbol{z}(k)\boldsymbol{z}^T(k)] = \boldsymbol{K}$$

where $\boldsymbol{K}$ is the solution to

$$\boldsymbol{K} = (\boldsymbol{I} - \mu\boldsymbol{\Lambda})\boldsymbol{K}(\boldsymbol{I} - \mu\boldsymbol{\Lambda}) + \frac{\mu^2}{4}\boldsymbol{Q}^H\mathcal{E}[\boldsymbol{N}(k)\boldsymbol{N}^T(k)]\boldsymbol{Q}. \tag{9.4.15}$$

We must now find an expression for the correlation matrix of $\boldsymbol{N}(k)$. Assume that the LMS algorithm is in a condition of near-convergence. Recall that

$$\hat{\nabla}_k = \nabla_k + \boldsymbol{N}(k).$$

Since we are near the optimal solution,

$$\nabla_k \approx \boldsymbol{0}$$

and thus

$$\boldsymbol{N}(k) \approx \hat{\nabla}_k.$$

We defined $\hat{\nabla}_k$ by

$$\hat{\nabla}_k = 2\boldsymbol{x}(k)\boldsymbol{x}^T(k)\boldsymbol{h}(k) - 2\boldsymbol{x}(k)d(k)$$

so that

$$\hat{\nabla}_k = 2\boldsymbol{x}(k)[\boldsymbol{x}^T(k)\boldsymbol{h}(k) - d(k)] = -2e(k)\boldsymbol{x}(k).$$

Therefore,

$$\boldsymbol{N}(k) \approx -2e(k)\boldsymbol{x}(k).$$

Now, the correlation matrix for $\boldsymbol{N}(k)$ is given by

$$\mathcal{E}[\boldsymbol{N}(k)\boldsymbol{N}^T(k)] \approx 4\mathcal{E}[e^2(k)\boldsymbol{x}(k)\boldsymbol{x}^T(k)]. \tag{9.4.16}$$

Recall from the principle of orthogonality that at convergence, we have

$$\mathcal{E}[e(k)\boldsymbol{x}(k)] = \boldsymbol{0}.$$

We need to make one final approximation. The Gaussian moment factoring theorem [Mil74] states that if x_1, x_2, x_3, x_4 are samples from a zero-mean Gaussian process, then

$$\mathcal{E}[x_1x_2x_3x_4] = \mathcal{E}[x_1x_2]\mathcal{E}[x_3x_4] + \mathcal{E}[x_1x_3]\mathcal{E}[x_2x_4] + \mathcal{E}[x_1x_4]\mathcal{E}[x_2x_3].$$

Assuming $e(k)$ and $\boldsymbol{x}(k)$ to be Gaussian, invoking the Gaussian moment factoring theorem, and using the principle of orthogonality, Eq. 9.4.16 becomes

$$\mathcal{E}[\boldsymbol{N}(k)\boldsymbol{N}^T(k)] \approx 4\mathcal{E}[e^2(k)]\mathcal{E}[\boldsymbol{x}(k)\boldsymbol{x}^T(k)]. \tag{9.4.17}$$

Again, since we are near convergence,

$$\mathcal{E}[e^2(k)] \approx J_{min}$$

and thus Eq. 9.4.17 can be simplified to

$$\mathcal{E}[\boldsymbol{N}(k)\boldsymbol{N}^T(k)] \approx 4J_{min}\boldsymbol{R}. \tag{9.4.18}$$

Now that we have an expression for the noise correlation matrix, Eq. 9.4.15 becomes

$$\boldsymbol{K} = (\boldsymbol{I} - \mu\boldsymbol{\Lambda})\boldsymbol{K}(\boldsymbol{I} - \mu\boldsymbol{\Lambda}) + \mu^2\boldsymbol{Q}^H\boldsymbol{R}\boldsymbol{Q}. \tag{9.4.19}$$

Since $Q^H\boldsymbol{R}\boldsymbol{Q} = \boldsymbol{\Lambda}$, we are left with the matrix Lyapunov equation

$$\boldsymbol{K} = (\boldsymbol{I} - \mu\boldsymbol{\Lambda})\boldsymbol{K}(\boldsymbol{I} - \mu\boldsymbol{\Lambda}) + \mu^2 J_{min}\boldsymbol{\Lambda} \tag{9.4.20}$$

In general, the solution to this equation is not obvious. Recall, however, that

$$\boldsymbol{K} = \lim_{k\to\infty} \mathcal{E}[\boldsymbol{z}(k)\boldsymbol{z}^T(k)].$$

Therefore, the diagonal elements of $\boldsymbol{K}$ give the variance of the elements of the zero-mean transformed weights, z_i. Namely, we have

$$K_{ii} = \lim_{k\to\infty} \mathcal{E}[z_i^2(k)].$$

Since all of the matrices in Eq. 9.4.20 are diagonal, it is simple to write the equation for K_{ii}. We have

$$K_{ii} = (1 - \mu\lambda_i)^2 K_{ii} + \mu^2 J_{min}\lambda_i. \tag{9.4.21}$$

The solution to this equation is

$$K_{ii} = \frac{\mu J_{min}}{2 - \mu\lambda_i}. \tag{9.4.22}$$

It can be seen that for small μ, the variance of z_i can be made small. In fact, for small μ, we can make the approximation

$$K_{ii} \approx \frac{\mu}{2} J_{min}.$$

Let's examine the mean-squared error behavior. The *excess mean-squared error* is defined as the average distance of the MSE from J_{min}. Recall that we can express the MSE as

$$J = J_{min} + \boldsymbol{z}^T\boldsymbol{\Lambda}\boldsymbol{z} = J_{min} + \sum_{i=1}^{N} \lambda_i z_i^2.$$

Thus,

$$\mathcal{E}[J - J_{min}] = \sum_{i=1}^{N} \lambda_i \mathcal{E}[z_i^2] = \sum_{i=1}^{N} \lambda_i K_i i.$$

Using the expression in Eq. 9.4.22, the excess MSE is given by

$$\mathcal{E}[J - J_{min}] = \mu J_{min} \sum_{i=1}^{N} \frac{\lambda_i}{2 - \mu\lambda_i}. \tag{9.4.23}$$

Again, for small μ, this can be approximated by

$$\mathcal{E}[J - J_{min}] = \frac{\mu J_{min}}{2} \sum_{i=1}^{N} \lambda_i = \frac{\mu J_{min} N}{2} \sigma_x^2. \tag{9.4.24}$$

Either of Eqs. 9.4.23 or 9.4.24 show that the excess MSE is proportional to μ. This should be contrasted with the rate of convergence in the mean. Larger values of μ will cause the convergence in the mean to be faster than small values of μ. The penalty paid, however, is larger excess MSE. This is the classic tradeoff of the LMS algorithm. If we have a situation which allows slow adaptation, the quality of adaptation will be better (*i.e.*, smaller excess MSE). However, if the signal statistics are changing with time, we can not always tolerate slow adaptation. In this case, we will suffer from excess mean as a result of using a large μ to speed convergence in the mean.

The *misadjustment*, M, is defined as the ratio of the excess MSE to J_{min}. It follows immediately from Eq. 9.4.23 that

$$M = \mu \sum_{i=1}^{N} \frac{\lambda_i}{2 - \mu\lambda_i}, \tag{9.4.25}$$

and for small μ, this can be approximated by

$$M = \frac{\mu}{2} \sum_{i=1}^{N} \lambda_i = \frac{\mu N}{2} \sigma_x^2. \tag{9.4.26}$$

Example 9.3

We will examine the behavior of the LMS algorithm with concern to the effect of eigenvalue spread applied to the problem of adaptive prediction for the AR(2) process

$$x(k) + ax(k-1) + bx(k-2) = v(k)$$

where $v(k)$ is zero mean white-noise with power

$$\sigma_v^2 = 1.$$

Let's try to parameterize the eigenvalue spread as a function of a and b. The Yule-Walker equations for the AR process are given by

$$\begin{bmatrix} r(0) & r(1) \\ r(1) & r(0) \end{bmatrix} \begin{bmatrix} -a \\ -b \end{bmatrix} = \begin{bmatrix} r(1) \\ r(2) \end{bmatrix}.$$

Also, the first three autocorrelation lags satisfy

$$r(0) + ar(1) + br(2) = \sigma_v^2 = 1.$$

Taken together, these two equations can be combined to give

$$\begin{bmatrix} 1 & a & b \\ -a & -(b+1) & 0 \\ -b & -a & -1 \end{bmatrix} \begin{bmatrix} r(0) \\ r(1) \\ r(2) \end{bmatrix} = \begin{bmatrix} 1 \\ 0 \\ 0 \end{bmatrix}. \tag{9.4.27}$$

The 2×2 correlation matrix $\boldsymbol{R}$ for the AR process depends only on the first two autocorrelation lags, $r(0)$ and $r(1)$. Equation 9.4.27 can be solved for $r(0)$ and $r(1)$ using Cramer's rule. Specifically,

$$r(0) = \frac{1}{\Delta} \begin{vmatrix} 1 & a & b \\ 0 & -(b+1) & 0 \\ 0 & -a & -1 \end{vmatrix}$$

and

$$r(1) = \frac{1}{\Delta} \begin{vmatrix} 1 & 1 & b \\ -a & 0 & 0 \\ -b & 0 & -1 \end{vmatrix}$$

where

$$\Delta = \begin{vmatrix} 1 & a & b \\ -a & -(b+1) & 0 \\ -b & -a & -1 \end{vmatrix}.$$

Evaluating the indicated determinants, we find that

$$r(0) = \frac{b+1}{\Delta} \quad \text{and} \quad r(1) = -\frac{a}{\Delta}. \tag{9.4.28}$$

The correlation matrix is thus given by

$$\boldsymbol{R} = \frac{1}{\Delta} \begin{bmatrix} b+1 & -a \\ -a & b+1 \end{bmatrix}.$$

The eigenvalues of $\Delta \boldsymbol{R}$ are equal to Δ times the eigenvalues of $\boldsymbol{R}$ and we are concerned only with the *ratio* of the eigenvalues, so the constant Δ is unimportant. Proceeding, the eigenvalues of $\Delta \boldsymbol{R}$ are found by evaluating the determinant

$$\begin{vmatrix} \lambda - (b+1) & a \\ a & \lambda - (b+1) \end{vmatrix} = \lambda^2 - 2(b+1)\lambda + [(b+1)^2 - a^2],$$

which has roots

$$\lambda = (b+1) \pm a.$$

Therefore, the ratio of eigenvalues is given by

$$\chi(\boldsymbol{R}) = \frac{b+1+a}{b+1-a}. \tag{9.4.29}$$

Because the process is AR(2), the Wiener solution for the predictor is given by

$$\boldsymbol{h}_0 = \begin{bmatrix} -a \\ -b \end{bmatrix}.$$

We now examine the behavior of the LMS algorithm for two different pairs of a, b.

First, let $a = -3/4$ and $b = -1/8$. According to Eq. 9.4.28, the signal power is computed to be $r(0) = 3.83$ and Eq. 9.4.29 gives the eigenvalue spread as $\chi(\boldsymbol{R}) = 13$. The LMS algorithm as described by Eq. 9.4.4 becomes

$$\begin{bmatrix} h_1(k+1) \\ h_2(k+1) \end{bmatrix} = \begin{bmatrix} h_1(k) \\ h_2(k) \end{bmatrix} + \mu \begin{bmatrix} x(k) \\ x(k-1) \end{bmatrix}.$$

The allowable range for μ is given by Eq. 9.4.8 as

$$0 < \mu < \frac{2}{2r(0)} = 0.26.$$

In practice, we usually find that μ should be chosen much smaller than the theoretical limit. Accordingly, we first examine the behavior with $\mu = 0.005$. Suppose we start with the initial weight

$$\boldsymbol{h}(0) = \begin{bmatrix} 0 \\ 0 \end{bmatrix}.$$

The behavior of $h_1(k)$ and $h_2(k)$ is shown in Fig. 9.4.1a. Notice that both weights approach their optimal values but their is some amount of "chattering" about the Wiener solution. This is due to the misadjustment which, according to Eq. 9.4.26, has a value of

$$M = \mu\sigma_x^2.$$

This illustrates the tradeoff between the speed of adaptation and the misadjustment. Suppose we instead use $\mu = 0.001$. The weight tracks are shown in Fig. 9.4.1b. Notice that the speed of adaptation is somewhat slower but that the weights settle closer to the Wiener solution than before.

Next, let $a = -0.5$ and $b = 0.9$. The power is then found to be equal to $r(0) = 5.65$ and the eigenvalue spread is $\chi(\boldsymbol{R}) = 1.71$. Intuitively, we should expect the rate of convergence to be better than before due to the smaller eigenvalue spread. The value of μ is bounded by

$$0 < \mu \frac{2}{2r(0)} = 0.17.$$

Let's again take $\mu = 0.001$ and examine the performance of the LMS algorithm. Fig. 9.4.1c shows that the convergence is more rapid than for the previous choices of a and b.

Another useful visualization of the convergence process is to examine the evolution of the prediction error filter zeros in the complex plane. Figure 9.4.2 shows the migration of the prediction error filter zeros to the locations determined by the Wiener prediction error filter for the process given by $a = -0.5, b = 0.9$. The optimal zero locations occur at

$$z = \frac{0.5 \pm \sqrt{0.5^2 - 4 \cdot 0.9}}{-2 \cdot 0.5} = 0.25 \pm 0.915j.$$

We can see that the prediction error filter zeros approach the optimal zeros as the filter coefficients evolve toward the optimal predictor coefficients.

Another useful visualization involves the projection of the filter coefficients onto the contours of constant error. While the steepest descent algorithm was a gradient descent from the initial weight to the bottom of the quadratic performance surface, the LMS algorithm gives a "noisy" descent to the minimum. Figure 9.4.3 shows the path taken for $a = -3/4, b = -1/8$ and $\mu = 0.001$. Qualitatively, we can see that a path is indeed followed to the minimum, but that the path is not orthogonal to the error contours and the minimum is never actually reached permanently. There is some "chatter" which keeps the weights fluctuating at the bottom of the error surface. This is where the misadjustment comes from.

The previous example clearly illustrated the tradeoff between speed of convergence and misadjustment. Obviously, if we have the luxury of allowing the filter to adapt slowly, the misadjustment can be made small. There are certain situations where this is not tolerable, however. For example, if we need to equalize a channel in real time for high speed digital communications, we must be able to track changes in the channel. This corresponds to the case where the input signal is no longer stationary. If the signal statistics are varying with time, we the filter must be able to respond to these statistics as they change. Thus, the gain μ must be chosen so that the time constant of the LMS algorithm is not longer than the period over which the signal can be regarded as stationary.

Example 9.4

Suppose we need to identify the parameters of the simple second-order moving average model

$$d(k) = au(k) + bu(k-1)$$

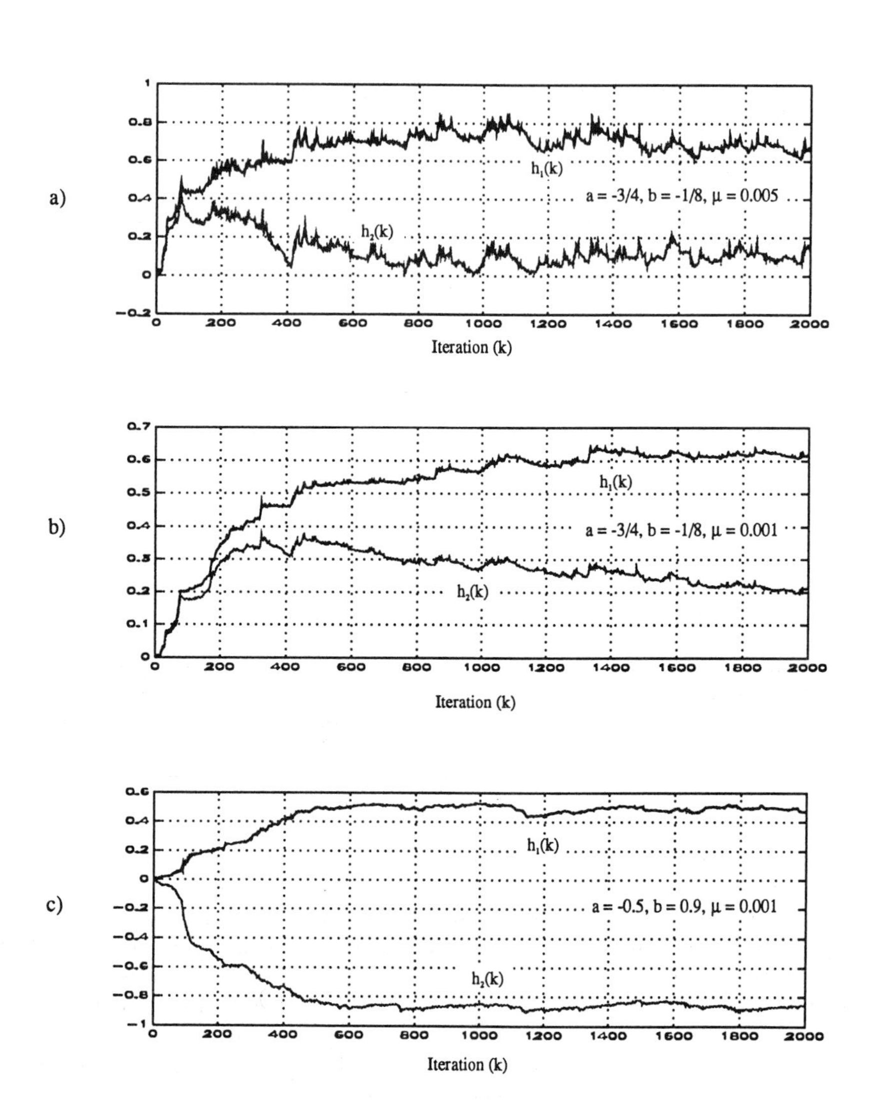

Figure 9.4.1: Behavior of the LMS algorithm for Example 9.3: (a) Tap weights for $a = -3/4, b = -1/8$ and $\mu = 0.005$; (b) tap weights for $a = -3/4, b = -1/8$ and $\mu = 0.001$; (c) tap weights for $a = -0.5, b = 0.9$ and $\mu = 0.001$.

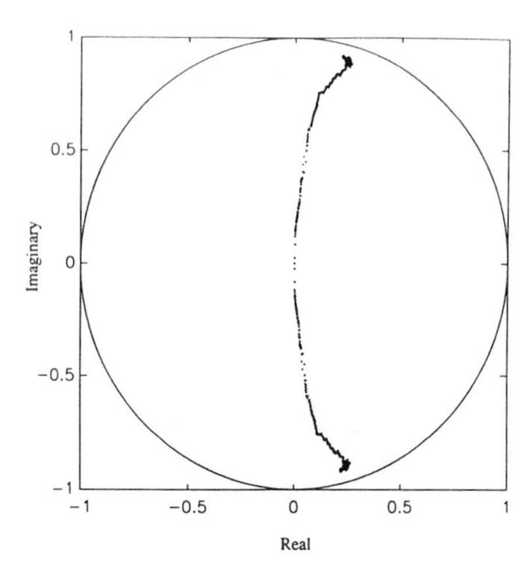

Figure 9.4.2: Convergence of the prediction error filter zeros $a = -0.5, b = 0.9, \mu = .001$.

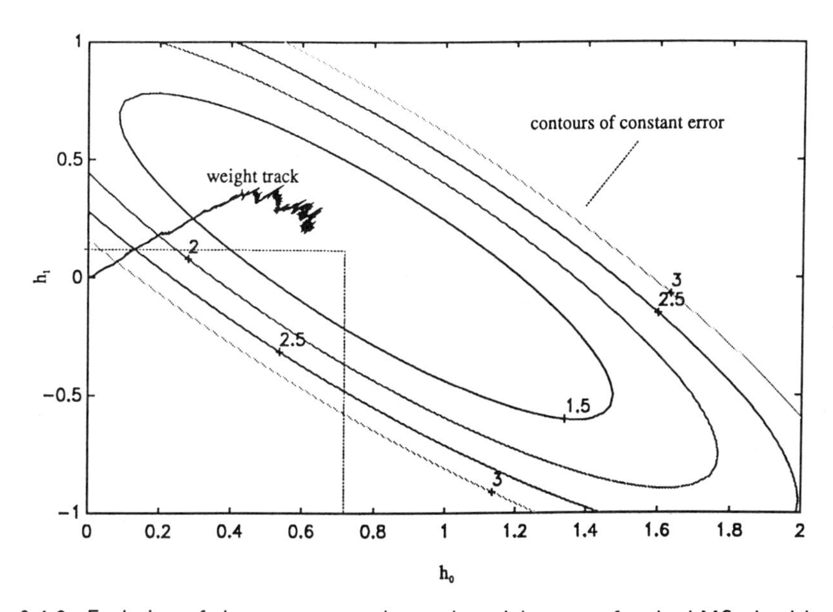

Figure 9.4.3: Evolution of the mean-squared error in weight space for the LMS algorithm with $a = -3/4, b = -1/8$ and $\mu = 0.001$.

where the parameters a and b can change their values during the identification process. The identification can be set up as shown in Fig. 9.4.4. The unknown system is driven with white noise and the output of the unknown system serves as a reference signal. The same white noise is used to drive our model which is used for identification. The output of the model is subtracted from the output of the actual system and the error is used to update the filter weights. Accordingly, the input signal $u(k)$ is unit variance white noise and the reference is $d(k)$. Therefore,

$$r(0) = 1, \quad r(1) = 0$$

and

$$p(0) = \mathcal{E}[d(k)u(k)] = \mathcal{E}[(au(k) + bu(k-1))u(k)] = a$$

and

$$p(1) = \mathcal{E}[d(k)u(k-1)] = \mathcal{E}[(au(k) + bu(k-1))u(k-1)] = b.$$

The Wiener solution is given by

$$\boldsymbol{h} = \boldsymbol{R}^{-1}\boldsymbol{p} = \begin{bmatrix} a \\ b \end{bmatrix},$$

as we would expect.

With $a = b = 1$, let's perform the identification using the LMS algorithm. Since $\sigma_u^2 = 1$, we must have $\mu < 1$. Let's try $\mu = 0.01$ for 2000 iterations. The convergence of the weights is shown in Fig. 9.4.5a. Observe that the coefficients converge to the Wiener solution.

Suppose, however, that the parameter b reverses polarity midway through the identification. Let's study the effect of μ on the ability of the LMS algorithm to track the polarity reversal. We choose $a = b = 1$ and perform the identification for 2000 iterations. Figure 9.4.5b shows the weights for $\mu = 0.01$. Notice that the coefficients converge to $a = 1, b = 1$ initially. At the thousandth iteration, the polarity reversal occurs and the coefficients this time head to $a = 1, b = -1$. The change takes nearly 500 iterations to complete.

This time, let's take case $\mu = 0.1$. The coefficients are shown in Fig. 9.4.5c. Notice that the tracking ability of the LMS algorithm is better in this case. The misadjustment is not very noticeable, but it can be seen that the polarity reversal is followed much more quickly.

The next example will illustrate the effect of eigenvalue spread on the convergence of the LMS algorithm.

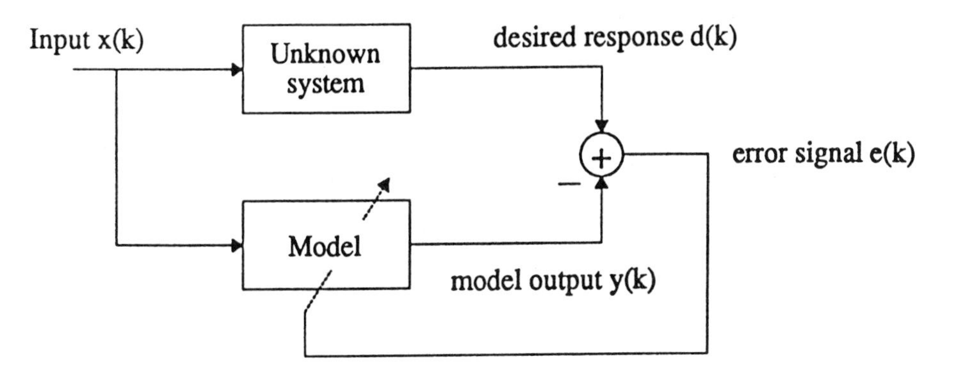

Figure 9.4.4: System identification.

Example 9.5

Consider again the problem of identifying the MA parameters of a given system. Suppose the system is of order nine and has an impulse response (MA parameters) given by

$$\{h(k)\} = \{0, 0.25, 0.5, 0.75, 1, 0.75, 0.5, 0.25, 0\}.$$

Instead of driving the system with white a white noise process, we instead use a colored noise process which is generated as the output of narrowband bandpass filter. The input $\{x(k)\}$ is generated by feeding the bandpass filter $G(z)$ with unit-variance white noise. Because $G(z)$ is narrowband and the power spectral density of $\{x(k)\}$ is given by

$$P_{xx}(\theta) = |G(e^{j\theta})|^2,$$

the ratio of maximum to minimum power spectral density will be large. We saw that this corresponds to a large eigenvalue spread for a correlation matrix of sufficiently large order, which means that the input signal is highly correlated. The evolution of the first three parameters is shown in Fig. 9.4.6a. Observe that the parameters do not converge even after 2000 iterations. Next, we perform the same identification problem with an input signal $\{x(k)\}$ which is simply white noise. With the same value of μ as before, the convergence of the same parameters is shown in Fig. 9.4.6b. Clearly, the convergence is much more well-behaved than for the highly correlated input signal.

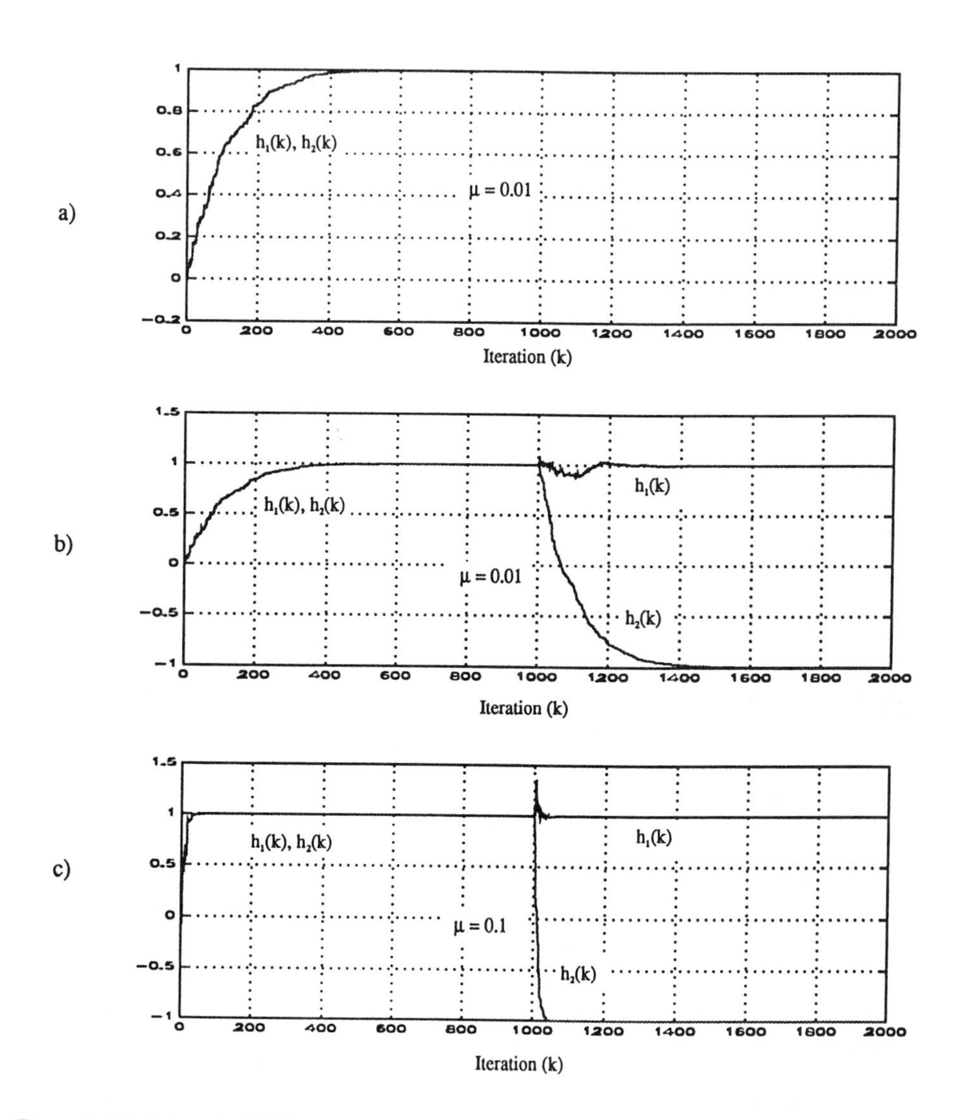

Figure 9.4.5: Using the LMS algorithm for parameter identification: (a) No polarity reversal and $\mu = 0.01$; (b) polarity reversal and $\mu = 0.01$; (c) polarity reversal and $\mu = 0.1$.

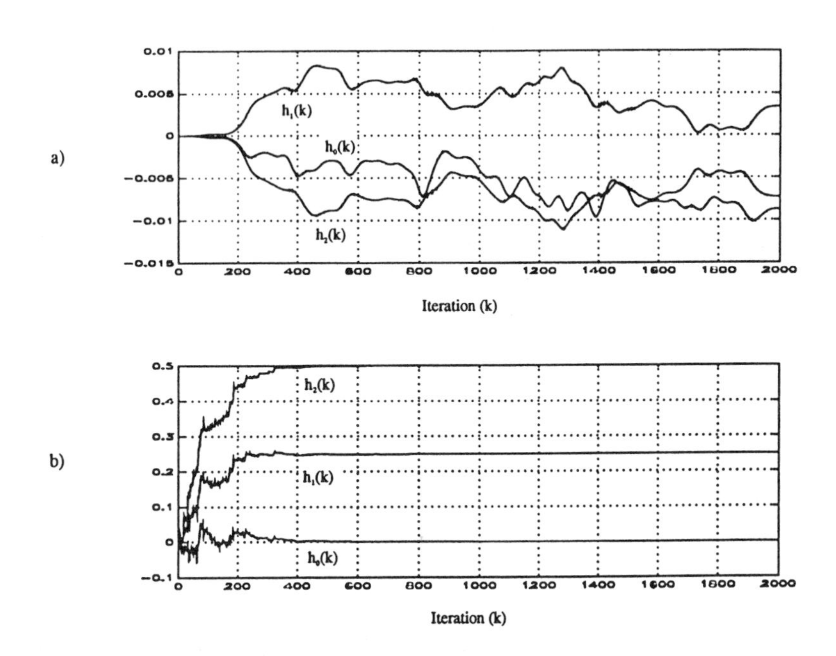

Figure 9.4.6: (a) Convergence of first three MA parameters for MA identification problem with highly correlated input signal; (b) convergence of same parameters with white noise input signal.

9.5 An LMS Lattice Algorithm

Recall that an N stage lattice predictor was described at each stage by the pair of equations

$$\begin{aligned} f_m(k) &= f_{m-1}(k) + \kappa_m b_{m-1}(k-1) \\ b_m(k) &= \kappa_m f_{m-1}(k) + b_{m-1}(k-1) \end{aligned} \tag{9.5.1}$$

with the initialization

$$f_0(k) = b_0(k) = x(k).$$

We can develop an LMS-type algorithm for the lattice predictor [Gri78] which has slightly higher computational complexity than the LMS algorithm for the transversal filter structure, but has better convergence properties.

Define the performance index for the m-th lattice stage by

$$J_m = \mathcal{E}[f_m^2(k) + b_m^2(k)].$$

We wish to develop a gradient descent algorithm for the m-th lattice stage. Taking the gradient of J_m with respect to κ_m, we get

$$\nabla J_m = \frac{\partial J_m}{\partial \kappa_m} = \mathcal{E}\left[2 f_m(k) \frac{\partial f_m(k)}{\partial \kappa_m} + 2 b_m(k) \frac{\partial b_m(k)}{\partial \kappa_m}\right].$$

Using Eq. 9.5.1, we have after some simplification

$$\nabla J = 2\mathcal{E}[f_m(k) b_{m-1}(k-1) + b_m(k) f_{m-1}(k)]. \tag{9.5.2}$$

At this point, we use the instantaneous estimates

$$\mathcal{E}[f_m(k) b_{m-1}(k-1)] \approx f_m(k) b_m(k-1)$$

and

$$\mathcal{E}[b_m(k) f_{m-1}(k)] \approx b_m(k) f_{m-1}(k).$$

This leads to the stochastic gradient estimate

$$\hat{\nabla}_m = 2 f_m(k) b_{m-1}(k-1) + 2 b_m(k) f_{m-1}(k). \tag{9.5.3}$$

We can now formulate a stochastic gradient algorithm for the reflection coefficient κ_m. As usual, we will proceed in the negative gradient direction using the iterative algorithm

$$\kappa_m(k+1) = \kappa_m(k) - \mu_m \hat{\nabla}_m \tag{9.5.4}$$

where $\hat{\nabla}$ is as given in Eq. 9.5.3 and the parameter μ_m controls the rate of convergence for the m-th lattice stage.

A consequence of the decoupling property of the lattice structure is that different values of μ_m can be used for *each* lattice stage. Consequently, the sensitivity of the gradient descent to eigenvalue spread in the input autocorrelation matrix is eliminated. This comes, of course, at the expense of increased computational complexity.

We have not yet given stability bounds for the gain parameters μ_m. In practice, a slight modification can be made to the algorithm in Eq. 9.5.4. Satorius and Alexander suggested [SA79] that μ_m can be allowed to vary with time such that it is normalized to the input signal power. The algorithm then assumes the form

$$\kappa_m(k+1) = \kappa_m(k) - \mu_m(k) \hat{\nabla}_m \tag{9.5.5}$$

and the time-varying gain $\mu_m(k)$ is given by

$$\mu_m(k) = p_m^{-1}(k)$$

where $p_m(k)$ is an estimate of the prediction error power. Therefore,

$$\kappa_m(k+1) = \kappa_m(k) - p_m^{-1}(k)\hat{\nabla}_m. \tag{9.5.6}$$

In practice, $p_m(k)$ can be computed as

$$p_m(k) = (1-\alpha)p_m(k-1) + f_m^2(k) + b_m^2(k)$$

where $\alpha << 1$. Heuristically, it is simple to understand what is occurring in Eq. 9.5.6. It can be seen that $p_m(k)$ will decrease for small prediction errors. Because $p_m(k)$ acts inversely in Eq. 9.5.6, the adaptation gain will be large. This is desirable for the following reason. Small prediction error correspond to a situation where the reflection coefficients have been estimated accurately. Therefore, a sudden increase in the prediction errors means that the model parameters have changed, and the large gain $p_m^{-1}(k)$ will allow the lattice to converge to the new model parameters rapidly. Similarly, suppose the adaptive lattice is operating in a noisy environment where the signal level is small compared to the noise background. In this case, the prediction error will be fairly large and the adaptation gain small. Although the speed of convergence of the lattice will now be slower, the reflection coefficients will be less responsive to the sudden "jumps" caused by large prediction errors which are due to the noise background.

Chapter 10

ADAPTIVE FILTERING: RECURSIVE LEAST SQUARES

10.1 Introduction

The recursive least squares (RLS) approach to adaptive filtering is distinctly different than the methods we have discussed thusfar. The Wiener filtering-based approaches were concerned with minimizing a mean-squared error criterion, which was dependent on the statistics of the relevant signals. Instead, the RLS approach to adaptive filtering is concerned with providing an *exact* solution to a minimization problem which is independent of the signal statistics.

The RLS technique is a generalization of the least squares method of estimation, which we will discuss next. The standard least squares problem seeks the multiple regression vector which minimizes the sum-of-squared-errors between the output of the multiple regression model and the desired response. The objective of *recursive* least squares is to include sequentially more observations and update the multiple regression model in a *recursive* fashion, *i.e.*, without having to explicitly solve the normal equations as each new observation is added.

It will be shown that the RLS techniques possess distinct advantages in both speed of convergence and misadjustment over the LMS-type algorithms. The only penalty paid is in computational complexity. Whereas the LMS algorithms have a complexity which is typically close to N multiplies per weight vector update (where N is the filter order), direct RLS techniques have a complexity which is proportional to N^2. Fortunately, there exists a collection of fast least-squares (FLS) algorithms which can be used to implement recursive least squares with a complexity proportional to N. These algorithms are somewhat sensitive to arithmetic errors and choices of initial conditions, however, and we will point out when these problems are likely to occur and how they can be avoided.

10.2 The Least Squares Method

The least squares (LS) method is a deterministic counterpart to the Wiener filtering method. Whereas the Wiener filtering method was based on ensemble averages of WSS stochastic processes, the LS method uses time averages and will result in a different optimum filter for each realization of the stochastic process.

The framework for the linear LS problem is as follows. We are given L ***observations*** $\{x(i)\}$ and a collection of L desired responses, $\{d(i)\}$. The observations $\{x(i)\}$ are regarded as *inputs* and the desired responses $\{d(i)\}$ are regarded as *outputs*. We hypothesize a *linear* relationship between the inputs and outputs. That is, we assume that each $d(i)$ can be expressed as

$$d(i) = \sum_{k=0}^{N-1} h_{ok} x(i-k) + e_o(i)$$

where N is the order of the model and $e_o(i)$ is some error term. The goal of the LS method is to *estimate* the parameters $\{h_{ok}\}$ of the model given the observations $\{x(i)\}$ and the desired response $\{d(i)\}$. For the LS problem, the observations $\{x(i)\}$ are regarded as *known* data. The error $e_o(i)$ can be regarded as a measurement error which accounts for the discrepancy between the output of the model and the desired response. A standard assumption of the LS method is that the error sequence is zero-mean and white, *i.e.*,

$$\mathcal{E}[e_o(i)] = 0$$

and

$$\mathcal{E}[e_o(i)e_o(j)] = \sigma^2 \delta(i-j).$$

Because the values of $x(i)$ are known, we have

$$\mathcal{E}[d(i)] = \sum_{k=0}^{N-1} h_{ok} x(i-k).$$

Consider the linear transversal filter of order N with tap weights $\{h_k\}$, as shown in Fig. 10.2.1. The input to the filter is $\{x(i)\}$ and the desired response is $\{d(i)\}$. With the output of the filter given by $y(i)$, where

$$y(i) = \sum_{k=0}^{N-1} h_k x(i-k),$$

the error between the output and the desired response is given by

$$e(i) = d(i) - \sum_{k=0}^{N-1} h_k x(i-k).$$

Recall that we are trying to *estimate* the hypothesized model parameters $\{h_{ok}\}$ from the input and the desired response. In other words, we wish to determine a *fixed* set of model parameters which "explain" the desired responses for *all* time indices over which the observations are made. The objective of the LS method is to determine the model parameters $\{h_k\}$ which minimize the sum of squared errors. Consequently, the parameters $\{h_k\}$ are *fixed* at some constant values and we wish to minimize the LS performance index

$$J(\boldsymbol{h}) = \sum_{i=i_a}^{i_b} e^2(i).$$

Notice that the starting and stopping indices i_a and i_b for the performance index have not yet been specified. This is because different choices of i_a and i_b lead to distinctly different performance criteria. If the available measurements are $x(1), x(2), \ldots, x(L)$, the taps of the transversal filter will be "covered" with measured data for the first time at $i = N$. Consequently, minimizing J with $i_a \leq N$ requires that we make assumptions (typically, "the data points are all zero) about the sequence $\{x(i)\}$ before measurements are actually available. Similarly, $i = L$ is the last time the filter taps will be "covered" with measured data so that minimizing J with $i_b \geq L$ also requires assumptions to be made about values of $\{x(i)\}$ which are unavailable. Therefore, we will take $i_a = N$ and $i_b = L$ so that

$$J = \sum_{i=N}^{L} e^2(i).$$

This performance index does not require us to make any assumptions about the data before $i = 1$ or after $i = L$.

10.3 Solution of the LS Problem

Let the vector of tap inputs to the transversal filter be denoted by $\boldsymbol{x}(i)$ where

$$\boldsymbol{x}(i) = [x(i), x(i-1), \ldots, x(i-N+1)]^T$$

and denote the vector of tap-weights by $\boldsymbol{h}$ where

$$\boldsymbol{h} = [h_0, h_1, \ldots, h_{N-1}]^T.$$

It follows that the output of the transversal is given by

$$y(i) = \boldsymbol{h}^T \boldsymbol{x}(i) = \boldsymbol{x}^T(i) \boldsymbol{h}$$

and the error is given by

$$e(i) = d(i) - y(i) = d(i) - \boldsymbol{h}^T \boldsymbol{x}(i). \tag{10.3.1}$$

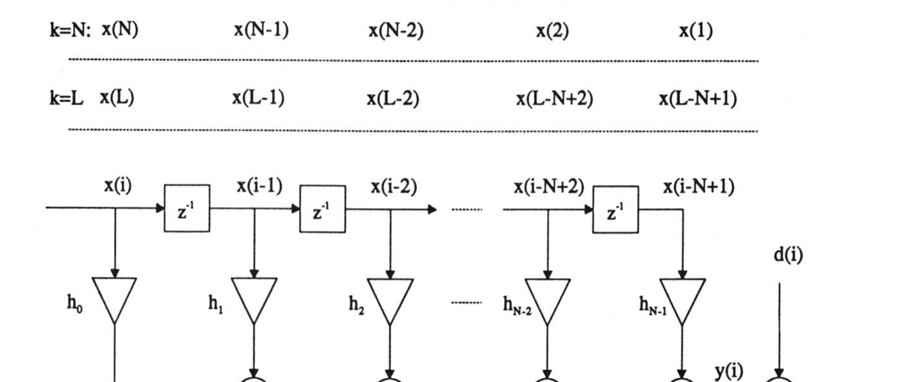

Figure 10.2.1: Linear transversal filter for the linear least-squares problem.

The LS performance index is

$$J(\boldsymbol{h}) = \sum_{i=N}^{L} e^2(i) = \sum_{i=N}^{L} (d(i) - \boldsymbol{h}^T \boldsymbol{x}(i))^2 \tag{10.3.2}$$

where the $J(\boldsymbol{h})$ now indicates the explicit dependence of J on the tap-weight vector, $\boldsymbol{h}$. Using Eq. 10.3.1 and recalling that $\boldsymbol{h}$ is held constant over the minimization interval, Eq. 10.3.2 becomes

$$J(\boldsymbol{h}) = \sum_{i=N}^{L} d^2(i) - 2\boldsymbol{h}^T \sum_{i=N}^{L} d(i)\boldsymbol{x}(i) + \boldsymbol{h}^T \left[\sum_{i=N}^{L} \boldsymbol{x}(i)\boldsymbol{x}^T(i) \right] \boldsymbol{h}. \tag{10.3.3}$$

Let us denote by $\hat{\boldsymbol{p}}$ the sum

$$\hat{\boldsymbol{p}} = \sum_{i=N}^{L} d(i)\boldsymbol{x}(i)$$

and denote by $\hat{\boldsymbol{R}}$ the sum

$$\hat{\boldsymbol{R}} = \sum_{i=N}^{L} \boldsymbol{x}(i)\boldsymbol{x}^T(i).$$

Equation 10.3.3 then becomes

$$J(\boldsymbol{h}) = \sum_{i=N}^{L} d^2(i) - 2\boldsymbol{h}^T \hat{\boldsymbol{p}} + \boldsymbol{h}^T \hat{\boldsymbol{R}} \boldsymbol{h}. \tag{10.3.4}$$

At this point, minimization of J should be a familiar procedure. We need to solve $\nabla(J) = \mathbf{0}$, where

$$\nabla(J) = \frac{\partial J}{\partial \boldsymbol{h}} = -2\hat{\boldsymbol{p}} + 2\hat{\boldsymbol{R}}\boldsymbol{h}.$$

Therefore, the optimal value of $\boldsymbol{h}$ is given by solving the system of equations

$$\hat{\boldsymbol{R}}\boldsymbol{h} = \hat{\boldsymbol{p}}$$

in which case

$$J_{min} = \sum_{i=N}^{L} d^2(i) - \boldsymbol{h}^T\hat{\boldsymbol{p}}.$$

Notice the similarity of this solution to the Wiener filtering problem. The quantities in this case, however, correspond to time averages rather than ensemble averages. Before exploring this idea further, it will help if we can put the LS problem in a geometric setting.

Let $\boldsymbol{d}$ denote the vector of desired responses,

$$\boldsymbol{d} = [d(N), d(N+1), \ldots, d(L)]^T.$$

The output of the linear model was given by

$$y(i) = \boldsymbol{x}^T(i)\boldsymbol{h}, \quad i = N, N+1, \ldots, L$$

where

$$\boldsymbol{x}^T(i) = [x(i), x(i-1), \ldots, x(i-N+1)].$$

Let the *data matrix* $\boldsymbol{X}$ be given by

$$\boldsymbol{X} = \begin{bmatrix} x(N) & x(N-1) & \cdots & x(1) \\ x(N+1) & x(N) & \cdots & x(2) \\ \vdots & \vdots & \vdots & \vdots \\ x(L) & x(L-1) & \cdots & x(L-N+1) \end{bmatrix}.$$

If we define the vector of outputs $\boldsymbol{y}$ by

$$\boldsymbol{y} = [y(N), y(N+1), \ldots, y(L)]^T,$$

it follows that we can express $\boldsymbol{y}$ as

$$\boldsymbol{y} = \boldsymbol{X}\boldsymbol{h}.$$

Similarly, define the vector of errors $\boldsymbol{e}$ by

$$\boldsymbol{e} = [e(N), e(N+1), \ldots, e(L)]^T.$$

Thus, we have

$$\boldsymbol{e} = \boldsymbol{d} - \boldsymbol{y} = \boldsymbol{d} - \boldsymbol{X}\boldsymbol{h}.$$

The performance index J is seen to be the euclidean norm of the error vector $\boldsymbol{e}$,

$$J = \boldsymbol{e}^T\boldsymbol{e} = (\boldsymbol{d} - \boldsymbol{X}\boldsymbol{h})^T(\boldsymbol{d} - \boldsymbol{X}\boldsymbol{h})$$

so that

$$J = \boldsymbol{d}^T\boldsymbol{d} - 2\boldsymbol{h}^T\boldsymbol{X}^T\boldsymbol{d} + \boldsymbol{h}^T\boldsymbol{X}^T\boldsymbol{X}\boldsymbol{h}.$$

The value of $\boldsymbol{h}$ which minimizes J is given by the solution to the system of equations

$$\boldsymbol{X}^T\boldsymbol{X}\boldsymbol{h} = \boldsymbol{X}^T\boldsymbol{d},$$

and if $\boldsymbol{X}^T\boldsymbol{X}$ is invertible, this solution is given by

$$\boldsymbol{h} = (\boldsymbol{X}^T\boldsymbol{X})^{-1}\boldsymbol{X}^T\boldsymbol{d} \tag{10.3.5}$$

and we have

$$J_{min} = \boldsymbol{d}^H\boldsymbol{d} - \boldsymbol{d}^H\boldsymbol{X}(\boldsymbol{X}^T\boldsymbol{X})^{-1}\boldsymbol{X}^T\boldsymbol{d}.$$

More formally, the LS problem can be viewed as follows. We have an $(L-N+1) \times N$ matrix $\boldsymbol{X}$ and an $(L-N+1) \times 1$ vector $\boldsymbol{d}$. The matrix $\boldsymbol{X}$ can be regarded as a mapping from the vector space R^N to the vector space $R^{(L-N+1)}$. We seek the vector $\boldsymbol{h}$ in R^N which is mapped by $\boldsymbol{X}$ to produce the vector $\boldsymbol{y}$ which is closest (in the Euclidean sense) to the vector $\boldsymbol{d}$ in $R^{(L-N+1)}$. According to Eq. 10.3.5 the solution $\boldsymbol{h}$ is given by

$$\boldsymbol{h} = (\boldsymbol{X}^T\boldsymbol{X})^{-1}\boldsymbol{X}^T\boldsymbol{d}.$$

With $\boldsymbol{h}$ so chosen, we get the vector of outputs

$$\boldsymbol{y} = \boldsymbol{X}\boldsymbol{h} = \boldsymbol{X}(\boldsymbol{X}^T\boldsymbol{X})^{-1}\boldsymbol{X}^T\boldsymbol{d}.$$

Define the matrix $\boldsymbol{P}$ by

$$\boldsymbol{P} = \boldsymbol{X}(\boldsymbol{X}^T\boldsymbol{X})^{-1}\boldsymbol{X}^T$$

so that

$$y = Pd.$$

The matrix P may be viewed as a *projection operator* which maps vectors in $R^{(L-N+1)}$ to the space spanned by the columns of X. Consider the relationship

$$PX = X(X^T X)^{-1} X^T X = X.$$

It is thus clear that P maps any column of X to itself, which is to be expected since P maps $R^{(L-N+1)}$ to the space spanned by the columns of X. Furthermore, it is easy to see that

$$P^2 = I$$

so that vectors which already lie in the space spanned by the columns of X are unaffected by P.

Next, consider the matrix Q defined by

$$Q = I - P = I - X(X^T X)^{-1} X^T.$$

Since

$$e = d - y = d - Pd,$$

it follows that the error vector can be expressed by

$$e = Qd.$$

The rows of P are shown to be orthogonal to the columns of Q by the relationship

$$P^T Q = X(X^T X)^{-1} X^T - X(X^T X)^{-1} X^T X (X^T X)^{-1} X^T = O.$$

What this means is that the matrix Q may be viewed as an operator which projects vectors in $R^{(L-N+1)}$ onto the *orthogonal complement* of the space spanned by the columns of X. Therefore,

$$y^T e = d^T P^T Q d = 0.$$

This shows that the error vector and the output vector are orthogonal.

The matrices P and Q represent a pair of projections. The projection P maps d onto the space spanned by the columns of X and the projection Q maps d onto the orthogonal complement of the space spanned by the columns of X. Because Q was defined by

$$Q = I - P,$$

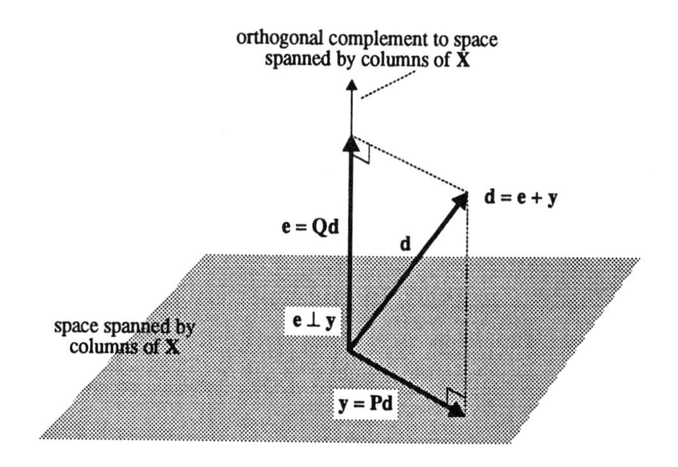

Figure 10.3.1: Geometrical depiction of the LS problem.

it follows that

$$\boldsymbol{P} + \boldsymbol{Q} = \boldsymbol{I}.$$

Thus,

$$\boldsymbol{y} + \boldsymbol{e} = (\boldsymbol{P} + \boldsymbol{Q})\boldsymbol{d} = \boldsymbol{d}.$$

Let's summarize what we have developed thusfar. We are given a desired response vector $\boldsymbol{d}$ and a data matrix $\boldsymbol{X}$. The problem was to determine the vector $\boldsymbol{h}$ which minimizes the distance $\boldsymbol{e}$ between the output vector $\boldsymbol{y} = \boldsymbol{X}\boldsymbol{h}$ and the desired response $\boldsymbol{d}$. The output $\boldsymbol{y}$ is regarded as the best approximation to $\boldsymbol{d}$ (in the LS sense) and is given by *orthogonally projecting* $\boldsymbol{d}$ onto the space spanned by the columns of $\boldsymbol{X}$. In this case, the error $\boldsymbol{e}$ is *orthogonal* to the best approximation $\boldsymbol{y}$. This is depicted in Fig. 10.3.1.

Example 10.1

Suppose

$$\boldsymbol{X} = \begin{bmatrix} 1 & 0 \\ 0 & 1 \\ 0 & 0 \end{bmatrix}$$

and

$$\boldsymbol{d} = \begin{bmatrix} d_1 \\ d_2 \\ d_3 \end{bmatrix}.$$

We wish to find the vector $\boldsymbol{y}$ which lies in the space spanned by the columns of $\boldsymbol{X}$ which is closest to $\boldsymbol{d}$. Let's first use intuition to solve the problem. The columns of $\boldsymbol{X}$ span a two-dimensional subspace of $\boldsymbol{R}^3$ which can be viewed as the plane defined by $z = 0$. Geometrically, we can see that the orthogonal projection of $\boldsymbol{d}$ onto this plane is simply

$$\boldsymbol{y} = \begin{bmatrix} d_1 \\ d_2 \\ 0 \end{bmatrix}$$

which results in the error vector

$$\boldsymbol{e} = \boldsymbol{d} - \boldsymbol{y} = \begin{bmatrix} 0 \\ 0 \\ d_3 \end{bmatrix}.$$

Using the theory we have developed, we find that

$$\boldsymbol{P} = \boldsymbol{X}(\boldsymbol{X}^T\boldsymbol{X})^{-1}\boldsymbol{X}^T = \begin{bmatrix} 1 & 0 & 0 \\ 0 & 0 & 1 \\ 0 & 0 & 0 \end{bmatrix}$$

and

$$\boldsymbol{Q} = \boldsymbol{I} - \boldsymbol{P} = \begin{bmatrix} 0 & 0 & 0 \\ 0 & 0 & 0 \\ 0 & 0 & 1 \end{bmatrix}.$$

Using the relationships $\boldsymbol{y} = \boldsymbol{P}\boldsymbol{d}$ and $\boldsymbol{e} = \boldsymbol{Q}\boldsymbol{d}$, we indeed confirm what we suspected by intuition. Furthermore, it is clear that

$$\boldsymbol{d} = \boldsymbol{y} + \boldsymbol{e}.$$

Finally, the optimal weight vector $\boldsymbol{h}$ is given by

$$\boldsymbol{h} = (\boldsymbol{X}^T\boldsymbol{X})^{-1}\boldsymbol{X}^T\boldsymbol{d} = \begin{bmatrix} d_1 \\ d_2 \end{bmatrix}.$$

This example is depicted in Fig. 10.3.2

Until now, we have implicitly assumed that the matrix $\boldsymbol{X}^T\boldsymbol{X}$ is invertible in order to solve the LS problem. This is not a necessary condition for the LS problem to have a solution. However, it *is* necessary that $\boldsymbol{X}^T\boldsymbol{X}$ be invertible for the solution to the LS problem to be *unique*. To best understand this, we must appeal to the *singular value decomposition* (SVD).

The essence of our problem is to find the vector $\boldsymbol{h}$ which gives

$$\min_{\boldsymbol{h}} ||\boldsymbol{d} - \boldsymbol{X}\boldsymbol{h}||^2.$$

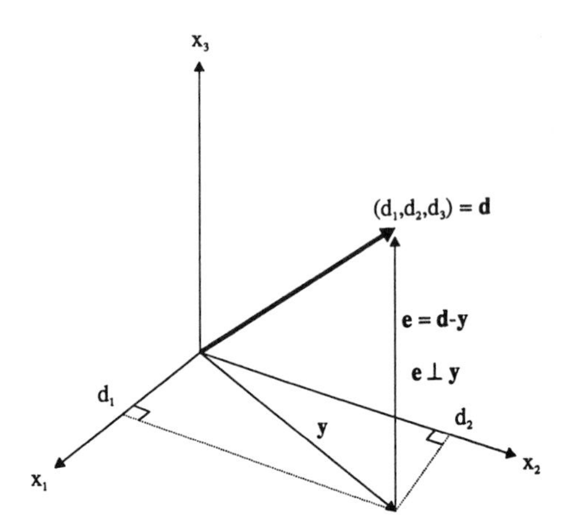

Figure 10.3.2: Geometric depiction of LS problem for Example 10.1.

We have shown that $\boldsymbol{h}$ can be found by solving the system of equations

$$\boldsymbol{X}^T\boldsymbol{X}\boldsymbol{h} = \boldsymbol{X}^T\boldsymbol{d}.$$

When $\boldsymbol{X}^T\boldsymbol{X}$ is invertible, this solution is given by

$$\boldsymbol{h} = (\boldsymbol{X}^T\boldsymbol{X})^{-1}\boldsymbol{X}^T\boldsymbol{d}.$$

What are the conditions that $\boldsymbol{X}^T\boldsymbol{X}$ be invertible? For our purposes, the matrix $\boldsymbol{X}$ will always have more rows than columns, in which case it is necessary and sufficient that the columns of $\boldsymbol{X}$ be *linearly independent.* If the columns of $\boldsymbol{X}$ are *not* linearly independent, we must use the SVD.

Thus, assume that $\boldsymbol{X}$ has only W linearly independent columns, which means that it has rank W. Referring to Appendix A, we have the following important result:

Theorem 7 *Suppose $\boldsymbol{X}$ is of rank W. Then there exist unitary matrices $\boldsymbol{U}$ and $\boldsymbol{V}$ such that*

$$\boldsymbol{U}^H\boldsymbol{A}\boldsymbol{V} = \begin{bmatrix} \boldsymbol{\Sigma} & \boldsymbol{O} \\ \boldsymbol{O} & \boldsymbol{O} \end{bmatrix}$$

where

$$\boldsymbol{\Sigma} = diag(\sigma_1, \sigma_2, \ldots, \sigma_W)$$

and

$$\sigma_1 \geq \sigma_2 \geq \cdots \geq \sigma_W > 0.$$

The *singular values* $\sigma_1, \sigma_2, \ldots, \sigma_W$ are the positive square roots of the nonzero eigenvalues of $\boldsymbol{X}^T\boldsymbol{X}$ (there are W of them since $\boldsymbol{X}^T\boldsymbol{X}$ has rank W). The matrix $\boldsymbol{V}$ has columns which are the eigenvectors of $\boldsymbol{X}^T\boldsymbol{X}$. Because $\boldsymbol{X}^T\boldsymbol{X}$ is symmetric, these eigenvectors are orthogonal so that $\boldsymbol{V}$ is unitary.

Because of the above theorem, we can express $\boldsymbol{X}$ as

$$\boldsymbol{X} = \boldsymbol{U}\begin{bmatrix} \Sigma & O \\ O & O \end{bmatrix}\boldsymbol{V}^H.$$

The *pseudoinverse* of $\boldsymbol{X}$ is denoted by $\boldsymbol{X}^\#$ where

$$\boldsymbol{X}^\# = \boldsymbol{V}\begin{bmatrix} \Sigma^{-1} & O \\ O & O \end{bmatrix}\boldsymbol{U}^H.$$

For the special case where $\boldsymbol{X}$ has linearly independent columns, the pseudoinverse reduces to

$$\boldsymbol{X}^\# = (\boldsymbol{X}^T\boldsymbol{X})^{-1}\boldsymbol{X}^T.$$

In general, the solution to the LS problem can be expressed as

$$\boldsymbol{h} = \boldsymbol{X}^\#\boldsymbol{d}. \tag{10.3.6}$$

As we have already stated, when $\boldsymbol{X}$ has linearly independent columns, this solution is the *unique* to the LS problem. If the columns of $\boldsymbol{X}$ are linearly *dependent*, the solution given by Eq. 10.3.6 is *not* a unique solution to the LS problem. This solution does, however, have an important property: it is the minimum norm solution (see Appendix A). That is, if another vector, $\hat{\boldsymbol{h}}$ solves the LS problem, it must be that

$$||\hat{\boldsymbol{h}}|| \geq ||\boldsymbol{h}||.$$

10.3.1 The Principle of Orthogonality for LS Filters

The solution to the linear LS problem has some properties which are analogous to the orthogonality properties for Wiener filters. Let's begin with the orthogonality of the output and the error vectors. Recall that when the filter is optimized in the LS sense, we had

$$\boldsymbol{y}^T\boldsymbol{e} = 0.$$

This means that

$$\sum_{i=N}^{L} y(i)e(i) = 0.$$

The summation above can be regarded as a time-average of the cross-correlation between the time series $\{e(i)\}$ and $\{y(i)\}$ and tells us that when the LS filter is optimized, the output and error sequences are orthogonal.

Next, consider the matrix-vector product $\boldsymbol{X}^T\boldsymbol{e}$. We have

$$\boldsymbol{X}^T\boldsymbol{e} = \boldsymbol{X}^T\boldsymbol{Q}\boldsymbol{d}.$$

Because $\boldsymbol{Q}$ was given by

$$\boldsymbol{Q} = \boldsymbol{I} - \boldsymbol{X}(\boldsymbol{X}^T\boldsymbol{X})^{-1}\boldsymbol{X}^T,$$

it follows that

$$\boldsymbol{X}^T\boldsymbol{Q} = \boldsymbol{X}^T - \boldsymbol{X}^T\boldsymbol{X}(\boldsymbol{X}^T\boldsymbol{X})^{-1}\boldsymbol{X}^T = \boldsymbol{O}.$$

Therefore,

$$\boldsymbol{X}^T\boldsymbol{e} = \boldsymbol{0}.$$

The scalar version of this equation is

$$\sum_{i=N}^{L} e(i)x(i-k) = 0, \quad k = 0, 1, \ldots, N-1.$$

For a fixed k, this equation represents a time average of the cross-correlation between the error sequence and the k-th filter tap. Thus, when the filter is optimized in the LS sense, the error time series $\{e(i)\}$ and the k-th filter tap time series $\{x(i-k)\}$ are orthogonal for $k = 0, 1, \ldots, N-1$.

10.3.2 Properties of the LS Solution

Let's return to the normal equations for the LS problem. Recall that we had the system of equations

$$\boldsymbol{X}^T\boldsymbol{X}\boldsymbol{h} = \boldsymbol{X}^T\boldsymbol{d}.$$

The solution is given by

$$\boldsymbol{h} = (\boldsymbol{X}^T\boldsymbol{X})^{-1}\boldsymbol{X}^T\boldsymbol{d}.$$

The matrix $\boldsymbol{X}^T\boldsymbol{X}$ can be expressed as

$$\boldsymbol{X}^T\boldsymbol{X} = \sum_{i=N}^{L} \boldsymbol{x}(i)\boldsymbol{x}^T(i). \tag{10.3.7}$$

As such, $\boldsymbol{X}^T\boldsymbol{X}$ is a time-average of the autocorrelation matrix for the time series $\{x(i)\}$. Clearly, $\boldsymbol{X}^T\boldsymbol{X}$ is symmetric. Because $\boldsymbol{X}^T\boldsymbol{X}$ is formed according to Eq. 10.3.7 and each outer product $\boldsymbol{x}(i)\boldsymbol{x}^T(i)$ is positive semidefinite, it follows that $\boldsymbol{X}^T\boldsymbol{X}$ is also positive semidefinite. If $\{x(i)\}$ is WSS, we have for large L

$$\boldsymbol{X}^T\boldsymbol{X} = \sum_{i=N}^{L} \boldsymbol{x}(i)\boldsymbol{x}^T(i) \approx (L - N + 1)\boldsymbol{R}.$$

Similarly, consider the vector $\boldsymbol{X}^T\boldsymbol{d}$. We have

$$\boldsymbol{X}^T\boldsymbol{d} = \sum_{i=N}^{L} d(i)\boldsymbol{x}(i),$$

which is a time-average of the cross-correlation between $x(i)$ and $d(i)$. Thus, if $\{x(i)\}$ and $\{d(i)\}$ are jointly WSS,

$$\boldsymbol{X}^T\boldsymbol{d} \approx (L - N + 1)\boldsymbol{p}.$$

Therefore, for WSS time series and large L, we have

$$\boldsymbol{h} \approx \boldsymbol{R}^{-1}\boldsymbol{p},$$

which corresponds to the Wiener solution.

Let's examine the statistical properties of the LS solution $\boldsymbol{h}$. Originally, we hypothesized that the underlying model for the desired response was

$$d(i) = \sum_{k=0}^{N-1} h_{ok}x(i-k) + e_o(k).$$

In vector notation, this can be expressed by

$$\boldsymbol{d} = \boldsymbol{y}_o + \boldsymbol{e} = \boldsymbol{X}\boldsymbol{h}_o + \boldsymbol{e}_o$$

The LS solution was shown to be given by

$$\boldsymbol{h} = (\boldsymbol{X}^T\boldsymbol{X})^{-1}\boldsymbol{X}^T\boldsymbol{d}.$$

Thus, it follows that

$$\boldsymbol{h} = (\boldsymbol{X}^T\boldsymbol{X})^{-1}\boldsymbol{X}^T\boldsymbol{X}\boldsymbol{h}_o + (\boldsymbol{X}^T\boldsymbol{X})^{-1}\boldsymbol{X}^T\boldsymbol{e}_o.$$

Thus,

$$\boldsymbol{h} = \boldsymbol{h}_o + (\boldsymbol{X}^T\boldsymbol{X})^{-1}\boldsymbol{X}^T\boldsymbol{e}_o. \qquad (10.3.8)$$

By assumption, the error time series $\{e_o(i)\}$ was assumed to be zero-mean. Thus,

$$\mathcal{E}[\boldsymbol{h}] = \boldsymbol{h}_o,$$

which means that the LS estimate is an unbiased estimate of $\boldsymbol{h}_o$. Let's compute the covariance of the LS estimate. We have

$$cov[\boldsymbol{h}] = \mathcal{E}[(\boldsymbol{h} - \boldsymbol{h}_o)(\boldsymbol{h} - \boldsymbol{h}_o)^T],$$

which by Eq. 10.3.8 can be expressed as

$$cov[\boldsymbol{h}] = \mathcal{E}[(\boldsymbol{X}^T\boldsymbol{X})^{-1}\boldsymbol{X}^T\boldsymbol{e}_o\boldsymbol{e}_o^T\boldsymbol{X}(\boldsymbol{X}^T\boldsymbol{X})^{-1}]$$

so that

$$cov[\boldsymbol{h}] = (\boldsymbol{X}^T\boldsymbol{X})^{-1}\boldsymbol{X}^T\mathcal{E}[\boldsymbol{e}_o\boldsymbol{e}_o^T]\boldsymbol{X}(\boldsymbol{X}^T\boldsymbol{X})^{-1}.$$

Since we assumed that the error time series $\{e_o(i)\}$ was white with variance σ^2, we have

$$\mathcal{E}[\boldsymbol{e}_o\boldsymbol{e}_o^T] = \sigma^2\boldsymbol{I}$$

which gives

$$cov[\boldsymbol{h}] = \sigma^2(\boldsymbol{X}^T\boldsymbol{X})^{-1}.$$

Thus, we have shown that the LS estimate is unbiased and has a covariance matrix given by $\sigma^2(\boldsymbol{X}^T\boldsymbol{X})^{-1}$ where σ^2 is the power of the error process.

An important property of the LS estimate is that it is the *best linear unbiased estimator* of the vector $\boldsymbol{h}_o$ [Hay86]. That is, if we produce another estimate of the form

$$\hat{\boldsymbol{h}} = \boldsymbol{E}\boldsymbol{d}$$

which is unbiased, this estimate will have a covariance matrix which satisfies

$$cov[\hat{\boldsymbol{h}}] \geq cov[\boldsymbol{h}].$$

Perhaps even more significantly, the LS estimate achieves the Cramer-Rao lower bound for unbiased estimates (we will make this notion precise in the chapter on spectral estimation).

10.4 The Recursive LS Problem

The recursive least squares (RLS) problem is an extension of the ordinary least squares problem we studied in the previous sections. The problem is simply stated as follows. At time k, we have observations $x(1), x(2), \ldots, x(k)$ and desired responses $d(1), d(2), \ldots, d(k)$. Assume that the weight vector which solves the LS problem for the available observations and desired responses has been computed. As we obtain a new measurement $x(k+1)$ and a new desired response $d(k+1)$, we would like to *update* the *previous* LS solution using the new data rather than *recomputing* the LS solution from scratch.

Assume we have an N-tap transversal filter with tap-weight vector $\boldsymbol{h}(k)$, where

$$\boldsymbol{h}(k) = [h_0(k), h_1(k), \ldots, h_{N-1}(k)]^T.$$

The input $\boldsymbol{x}(i)$ to the transversal filter consists of the N most recent samples,

$$\boldsymbol{x}(i) = [x(i), x(i-1), \ldots, x(i-N+1)]^T.$$

The desired response at time i is denoted by $d(i)$ and the error between the output of the filter and the desired response is given by

$$e(i) = d(i) - \boldsymbol{h}^T(k)\boldsymbol{x}(i) = d(i) - \boldsymbol{x}^T(i)\boldsymbol{h}(k). \tag{10.4.1}$$

At this point, it should be made clear why we are using k for the tap-weight index and i for the input and desired response. This is due to the nature of the RLS objective: at each instant k, we wish to perform a sort of multiple regression on the inputs and desired responses *up to* time k. That is, $h(k)$ is dependent on $\boldsymbol{x}(i)$ and $d(i)$ for $i = 1, 2, \ldots, k$.

Formally, we wish to determine the weight vector $\boldsymbol{h}(k)$ which minimizes the performance index given by

$$E(k) = \sum_{i=1}^{k} W^{k-i} e^2(i). \tag{10.4.2}$$

The constant W in Eq. 10.4.2 is restricted to lie in the range

$$0 < W \leq 1$$

and is sometimes known as a "forgetting factor." This is because W allows us to weight more recent errors (those closer to time k) more heavily than errors in the distant past. This is an important feature when the filter must operate in an environment where the signal statistics are varying with time.

Minimizing $E(k)$ is fairly straightforward. If Eq. 10.4.1 is substituted into Eq. 10.4.2, we have

$$E(k) = \sum_{i=1}^{k} W^{k-i}[d(i) - \boldsymbol{h}^T(k)\boldsymbol{x}(i)]^2 \tag{10.4.3}$$

which can be expanded to give

$$E(k) = E_d(k) - 2\boldsymbol{h}^T(k)\sum_{i=1}^{k} W^{k-i}d(i)\boldsymbol{x}(i) + \boldsymbol{h}^T(k)\left[\sum_{i=1}^{k} W^{k-i}\boldsymbol{x}(i)\boldsymbol{x}^T(i)\right]\boldsymbol{h}(k) \tag{10.4.4}$$

where $E_d(k)$ is defined as the quantity

$$E_d(k) = \sum_{i=1}^{k} W^{k-i}d^2(i),$$

which can be viewed as a weighted desired response energy. Similarly, let

$$\boldsymbol{p}(k) = \sum_{i=1}^{k} W^{k-i}d(i)\boldsymbol{x}(i)$$

and

$$\boldsymbol{R}(k) = \sum_{i=1}^{k} W^{k-i}\boldsymbol{x}(i)\boldsymbol{x}^T(i).$$

The vector $\boldsymbol{p}(k)$ can be regarded as a crosscorrelation estimate and the matrix $\boldsymbol{R}(k)$ an autocorrelation estimate. Equation 10.4.4 then becomes

$$E(k) = E_d(k) - 2\boldsymbol{h}^T(k)\boldsymbol{p}(k) + \boldsymbol{h}^T(k)\boldsymbol{R}(k)\boldsymbol{h}(k). \tag{10.4.5}$$

We can now minimize $E(k)$ by setting the gradient equal to zero, where

$$\nabla \boldsymbol{E}(k) = \frac{\partial E(k)}{\partial \boldsymbol{h}(k)} = -2\boldsymbol{p}(k) + 2\boldsymbol{R}(k)\boldsymbol{h}(k). \tag{10.4.6}$$

Setting the gradient equal to zero, we get the least squares (LS) normal equation

$$\boldsymbol{R}(k)\boldsymbol{h}(k) = \boldsymbol{p}(k)$$

which has the solution

$$\boldsymbol{h}(k) = \boldsymbol{R}^{-1}(k)\boldsymbol{p}(k). \tag{10.4.7}$$

When the weight vector assumes the optimal value as given by Eq. 10.4.7, the error energy $E(k)$ is minimized, and Eq. 10.4.5 becomes

$$E(k) = E_d(k) - \boldsymbol{h}^T(k)\boldsymbol{p}(k). \tag{10.4.8}$$

Recursive solution of the LS normal equation

From the definitions, it is clear that we can express $\boldsymbol{R}(k)$ and $\boldsymbol{p}(k)$ as

$$\boldsymbol{R}(k) = W\boldsymbol{R}(k-1) + \boldsymbol{x}(k)\boldsymbol{x}^T(k) \tag{10.4.9}$$

and

$$\boldsymbol{p}(k) = W\boldsymbol{p}(k-1) + d(k)\boldsymbol{x}(k). \tag{10.4.10}$$

What we would like to do is find an expression for $\boldsymbol{R}^{-1}(k)$ in terms of $\boldsymbol{R}^{-1}(k-1)$ so that the normal equation can be solved at each step without having to invert $\boldsymbol{R}(k)$ each time. To accomplish this, we can make use of the following.

Lemma 2 (Matrix Inversion Lemma) *Suppose the matrix* $\boldsymbol{A}$ *is given by*

$$\boldsymbol{A} = \boldsymbol{B}^{-1} + \boldsymbol{C}\boldsymbol{D}\boldsymbol{C}^T.$$

Then A^{-1} *is given by*

$$\boldsymbol{A}^{-1} = \boldsymbol{B} - \boldsymbol{B}\boldsymbol{C}[\boldsymbol{D} + \boldsymbol{C}^T\boldsymbol{B}\boldsymbol{C}]^{-1}\boldsymbol{C}^T\boldsymbol{B}.$$

To apply the matrix inversion lemma to our problem, refer to Eq. 10.4.9 and make the identifications

$$\boldsymbol{A} = \boldsymbol{R}(k), \quad \boldsymbol{B}^{-1} = W\boldsymbol{R}(k-1), \quad \boldsymbol{C} = \boldsymbol{x}(k), \quad \boldsymbol{D}^{-1} = 1.$$

The matrix inversion lemma then gives

$$\boldsymbol{R}^{-1}(k) = W^{-1}\boldsymbol{R}^{-1}(k-1) - \frac{W^{-1}\boldsymbol{R}^{-1}(k-1)\boldsymbol{x}(k)\boldsymbol{x}^T(k)\boldsymbol{R}^{-1}(k-1)}{W + \boldsymbol{x}^T(k)\boldsymbol{R}^{-1}(k-1)\boldsymbol{x}(k)}. \tag{10.4.11}$$

Equation 10.4.11 shows that the inverse of $\boldsymbol{R}$ at time k can be computed directly from the inverse of $\boldsymbol{R}$ at time $k-1$. This is the result we have been seeking. All we need is an initial value $\boldsymbol{R}^{-1}(0)$ from which to start the recursion. This is a subject which needs to be examined carefully. For now, we can simply let $\boldsymbol{R}(0) = \delta\boldsymbol{I}$ where δ is a small constant, in which case

$$\boldsymbol{R}^{-1}(0) = \delta^{-1}\boldsymbol{I}.$$

Let the vector $\boldsymbol{g}(k)$ be given by

$$\boldsymbol{g}(k) = \frac{\boldsymbol{R}^{-1}(k-1)\boldsymbol{x}(k)}{W + \boldsymbol{x}^T(k)\boldsymbol{R}^{-1}(k-1)\boldsymbol{x}(k)}. \tag{10.4.12}$$

Then Eq. 10.4.11 becomes

$$\boldsymbol{R}^{-1}(k) = W^{-1}\boldsymbol{R}^{-1}(k-1) - W^{-1}\boldsymbol{g}(k)\boldsymbol{x}^T(k)\boldsymbol{R}^{-1}(k-1). \tag{10.4.13}$$

Equation 10.4.12 can be rearranged to give

$$\boldsymbol{g}(k) = W^{-1}[\boldsymbol{R}^{-1}(k-1) - \boldsymbol{g}(k)\boldsymbol{x}^T(k)\boldsymbol{R}^{-1}(k-1)]\boldsymbol{x}(k),$$

and substituting the recursion for $\boldsymbol{R}(k)$ given by Eq. 10.4.13 into the above gives the following important relationship:

$$\boldsymbol{g}(k) = \boldsymbol{R}^{-1}(k)\boldsymbol{x}(k). \tag{10.4.14}$$

The vector $\boldsymbol{g}(k)$ is known as the *adaptation gain* and Eq. 10.4.14 should be remembered as the defining relationship for $\boldsymbol{g}(k)$. The adaptation gain plays a very important role in recursive least squares and will be a fundamental quantity in our derivation of the fast least-squares algorithms.

Weight vector update equation

Now that we have a recursive method for computing $\boldsymbol{R}^{-1}(k)$, we need to develop a recursion for the weight vector $\boldsymbol{h}(k)$ which gives the RLS weight vector at time k in terms of the optimal solution at time $k-1$. Recall that $\boldsymbol{h}(k)$ is defined by

$$\boldsymbol{h}(k) = \boldsymbol{R}^{-1}(k)\boldsymbol{p}(k).$$

Using Eq. 10.4.10 for the updating of $\boldsymbol{p}(k)$, we get

$$\boldsymbol{h}(k) = W\boldsymbol{R}^{-1}(k)\boldsymbol{p}(k-1) + \boldsymbol{R}^{-1}(k)\boldsymbol{x}(k)\boldsymbol{d}(k),$$

and substituting Eq. 10.4.13 for $\boldsymbol{R}^{-1}(k)$ in the above, we have

$$\boldsymbol{h}(k) = \boldsymbol{R}^{-1}(k-1)\boldsymbol{p}(k-1) - \boldsymbol{g}(k)\boldsymbol{x}^T(k)\boldsymbol{R}^{-1}(k-1)\boldsymbol{p}(k-1) + \boldsymbol{R}^{-1}(k)\boldsymbol{x}(k)d(k). \tag{10.4.15}$$

Making use of the defining relationship for $\boldsymbol{g}(k)$ as given by Eq. 10.4.14, Eq. 10.4.15 becomes

$$\boldsymbol{h}(k) = \boldsymbol{h}(k-1) + \boldsymbol{g}(k)[d(k) - \boldsymbol{h}^T(k-1)\boldsymbol{x}(k)]. \tag{10.4.16}$$

The quantity in brackets in Eq. 10.4.16 is called the *a priori estimation error* since it gives the error between the desired response and the output of the transversal filter *before* the weight is updated from $\boldsymbol{h}(k-1)$ to $\boldsymbol{h}(k)$. We denote the a priori estimation error by $\alpha(k)$, where

$$\alpha(k) = d(k) - \boldsymbol{h}^T(k-1)\boldsymbol{x}(k).$$

Substituting this relationship into Eq. 10.4.16, we finally obtain the weight vector update equation,

$$\boldsymbol{h}(k) = \boldsymbol{h}(k-1) + \boldsymbol{g}(k)\alpha(k). \tag{10.4.17}$$

Once the weight vector is updated, the *a posterior estimation error*, $e(k)$, can then be computed as

$$e(k) = d(k) - \boldsymbol{h}^T(k)\boldsymbol{x}(k).$$

Updating the error energy

So far, we have obtained recursive relationships for the autocorrelation matrix and the weight vector. It will also prove useful to have a recursion for the minimum error energy. Recall from Eq. 10.4.8 that the minimum error energy is given by

$$E(k) = E_d(k) - \boldsymbol{p}^T(k)\boldsymbol{h}(k) \tag{10.4.18}$$

where $\boldsymbol{h}(k)$ is the least-squares solution. From the definition, we can see that

$$E_d(k) = WE_d(k-1) + d^2(k). \tag{10.4.19}$$

Recall also that $\boldsymbol{p}(k)$ can be expressed as

$$\boldsymbol{p}(k) = W\boldsymbol{p}(k-1) + d(k)\boldsymbol{x}(k) \tag{10.4.20}$$

and that the weight vector is updated according to

$$\boldsymbol{h}(k) = \boldsymbol{h}(k-1) + \boldsymbol{g}(k)\alpha(k) \tag{10.4.21}$$

where $\boldsymbol{g}(k)$ is the adaptation gain and $\alpha(k)$ is the a priori estimation error. Substituting Eqs. 10.4.19, 10.4.20, and 10.4.21 into Eq. 10.4.18 gives

$$\begin{aligned} E(k) \;=\; & WE_d(k-1) + d^2(k) - W\boldsymbol{p}(k-1)\boldsymbol{h}(k-1) - W\boldsymbol{p}^T(k-1)\boldsymbol{g}(k)\alpha(k) \\ & - d(k)\boldsymbol{x}^T(k)\boldsymbol{h}(k-1) - d(k)\boldsymbol{x}^T(k)\boldsymbol{g}(k)\alpha(k). \end{aligned} \tag{10.4.22}$$

But

$$E_d(k-1) - \boldsymbol{p}^T(k-1)\boldsymbol{h}(k-1) = E(k-1) \tag{10.4.23}$$

and

$$d(k) - \boldsymbol{x}^T(k)\boldsymbol{h}(k-1) = \alpha(k) \tag{10.4.24}$$

so that, using Eq. 10.4.20, we can rewrite Eq. 10.4.22 as

$$E(k) = WE(k-1) + [d(k) - \boldsymbol{p}^T(k)\boldsymbol{g}(k)]\alpha(k). \tag{10.4.25}$$

Now, we make use of the relationships

$$\boldsymbol{R}(k)\boldsymbol{h}(k) = \boldsymbol{p}(k)$$

and

$$\boldsymbol{g}(k) = \boldsymbol{R}^{-1}(k)\boldsymbol{x}(k)$$

to determine that

$$\boldsymbol{p}^T(k)\boldsymbol{g}(k) = \boldsymbol{h}^T(k)\boldsymbol{x}(k). \tag{10.4.26}$$

Therefore, Eq. 10.4.25 becomes

$$E(k) = WE(k-1) + [d(k) - \boldsymbol{h}^T(k)\boldsymbol{x}(k)]\alpha(k).$$

The term in brackets is recognized as the a posteriori estimation error, $e(k)$, and we can finally write

$$E(k) = WE(k-1) + \alpha(k)e(k). \tag{10.4.27}$$

Equation 10.4.27 will be used frequently in subsequent discussions.

Summary

The RLS algorithm is summarized as follows. $\boldsymbol{R}^{-1}(0)$ is specified by $\boldsymbol{R}^{-1}(0) = \delta^{-1}\boldsymbol{I}$. Next, we perform the following recursion:

$$\boldsymbol{g}(k) = \frac{\boldsymbol{R}^{-1}(k-1)\boldsymbol{x}(k)}{W + \boldsymbol{x}^T(k)\boldsymbol{R}^{-1}(k-1)\boldsymbol{x}(k)}$$

$$\alpha(k) = d(k) - \boldsymbol{h}^T(k-1)\boldsymbol{x}(k)$$

$$\boldsymbol{h}(k) = \boldsymbol{h}(k-1) + \boldsymbol{g}(k)\alpha(k)$$

$$\boldsymbol{R}^{-1}(k) = W^{-1}[\boldsymbol{R}^{-1}(k-1) - \boldsymbol{g}(k)\boldsymbol{x}^T(k)\boldsymbol{R}^{-1}(k-1)]$$

The a posteriori estimation error is computed as

$$e(k) = d(k) - \boldsymbol{h}^T(k)\boldsymbol{x}(k)$$

The minimum error energy can be updated according to

$$E(k) = WE(k-1) + \alpha(k)e(k)$$

Because of the matrix multiplication used in the update equation for $\boldsymbol{R}^{-1}(k)$, the RLS algorithm as expressed by the summary requires roughly N^2 multiplications per iteration. For even modest filter orders, this can represent a major computational bottleneck which can make real-time implementation impossible. We will dedicate the latter part of this chapter to the development of fast least squares algorithms which can implement the recursive LS computations with a complexity which is proportional to N.

10.5 Linear Prediction

One important application of recursive least squares is linear prediction. In addition to being an application in its own right, however, linear prediction also plays an important part in the development of several fast least squares algorithms. Namely, the algorithms will use both forward and backward linear prediction as a part of determining the adaptation gain, $\boldsymbol{g}(k)$. What follows is a detailed description of both forward and backward linear prediction.

10.5.1 Forward Linear Prediction

The set-up for RLS forward linear prediction is identical to that used in the Wiener filtering approach to forward linear prediction. The input vector consists of the N most recent samples of the input, and is denoted by $\boldsymbol{x}_N(i-1)$ where

$$\boldsymbol{x}_N(i-1) = [x(i-1), x(i-2), \ldots, x(i-N)]^T.$$

The desired response is the input at time i, *i.e.*,

$$d(i) = x(i).$$

The tap-weight vector is given the symbol $\boldsymbol{h}_N^f(k)$ where

$$\boldsymbol{h}_N^f(k) = [h_1(k), h_2(k), \ldots, h_N(k)]^T$$

where the superscript "f" indicates forward prediction and the subscript N indicates the order. This is a convention we will follow for prediction. The error between the output of the predictor and the desired response is given by

$$e_N^f(i) = x(i) - \boldsymbol{h}_N^{fT}(k)\boldsymbol{x}_N(i-1).$$

The objective of RLS forward prediction is to minimize at each k the forward prediction error energy,

$$E_N^f(k) = \sum_{i=1}^{k} W^{k-i}[e_N^f(i)]^2.$$

The solution to the forward prediction problem is simple. making the appropriate identifications with the general LS solution we discussed, the input correlation matrix is given by

$$\boldsymbol{R}_N(k-1) = \sum_{i=1}^{k} W^{k-i}\boldsymbol{x}_N(i-1)\boldsymbol{x}_N^T(i-1). \tag{10.5.1}$$

Notice that the input correlation matrix is denoted by $\boldsymbol{R}_N(i-1)$. This is consistent with the fact that the input is $\boldsymbol{x}_N(i-1)$. The crosscorrelation matrix is given by

$$\boldsymbol{p}_N^f(k) = \sum_{i=1}^{k} W^{k-i} x(i)\boldsymbol{x}_N(i-1). \tag{10.5.2}$$

The optimal forward predictor is then given by

$$\boldsymbol{h}_N^f = \boldsymbol{R}_N^{-1}(k-1)\boldsymbol{p}_N^f(k). \tag{10.5.3}$$

When the forward predictor is optimized, the forward prediction error energy is given by (see Eq. 10.4.8)

$$E_N^f(k) = \sigma_f^2(k) - \boldsymbol{p}_N^{fT}(k)\boldsymbol{h}_N^f(k) \tag{10.5.4}$$

where

$$\sigma_f^2(k) = \sum_{i=1}^{k} W^{k-i} x^2(i).$$

We define the *forward prediction error filter* $\boldsymbol{a}_N(k)$ by

$$\boldsymbol{a}_N(k) = \begin{bmatrix} 1 \\ -\boldsymbol{h}_N^f(k) \end{bmatrix}.$$

Let the vector $\boldsymbol{x}_{N+1}(i)$ indicate the vector of $N+1$ most recent samples, which we can partition as

$$\boldsymbol{x}_{N+1}(i) = \begin{bmatrix} x(i) \\ x_N(i-1) \end{bmatrix}.$$

Then the forward prediction error can be expressed as

$$e_N^f(i) = \boldsymbol{a}_N^T(k)\boldsymbol{x}_{N+1}(i). \tag{10.5.5}$$

Consider the correlation matrix for the input $\boldsymbol{x}_{N+1}(i)$. We have

$$\boldsymbol{R}_{N+1}(k) = \sum_{i=1}^{k} W^{k-i} \boldsymbol{x}_{N+1}(i)\boldsymbol{x}_{N+1}^T(i). \tag{10.5.6}$$

Using the previous expression for $\boldsymbol{x}_{N+1}(i)$, the outer product $\boldsymbol{x}_{N+1}(i)\boldsymbol{x}_{N+1}^T(i)$ can be seen to equal

$$\begin{bmatrix} x^2(i) & x(i)\boldsymbol{x}_N^T(i-1) \\ x(i)\boldsymbol{x}_N(i-1) & \boldsymbol{x}_N(i-1)\boldsymbol{x}_N^T(i-1) \end{bmatrix}$$

so that Eq. 10.5.6 becomes

$$\boldsymbol{R}_{N+1}(k) = \begin{bmatrix} \sigma_f^2(k) & \boldsymbol{p}_N^{fT}(k) \\ \boldsymbol{p}_N^f(k) & \boldsymbol{R}_N(k-1) \end{bmatrix}. \tag{10.5.7}$$

In a manner analogous to the Wiener filtering approach to forward prediction, we can develop augmented normal equations for the LS forward predictor. Using Eq. 10.5.7, it follows that

$$\boldsymbol{R}_{N+1}(k)\boldsymbol{a}_N(k) = \begin{bmatrix} \sigma_f^2(k) - \boldsymbol{p}_N^{fT}\boldsymbol{h}_N^f(k) \\ \boldsymbol{p}_N^f(k) - \boldsymbol{R}_N(k-1)\boldsymbol{h}_N^f(k) \end{bmatrix},$$

which, according to Eqs. 10.5.3 and 10.5.4, reduces to

$$\boldsymbol{R}_{N+1}(k)\boldsymbol{a}_N(k) = \begin{bmatrix} E_N^f(k) \\ \boldsymbol{0} \end{bmatrix}. \tag{10.5.8}$$

Equation 10.5.8 is known as the *augmented normal equation* for forward LS prediction.

With regard to the RLS parameters for forward prediction, we have as the a priori forward prediction error

$$\alpha_N^f(k) = x(k) - \boldsymbol{h}_N^{fT}(k-1)\boldsymbol{x}_N(k-1)$$

which we can express using the forward prediction error filter as

$$\alpha_N^f(k) = \boldsymbol{a}_N^T(k-1)\boldsymbol{x}_{N+1}(k). \tag{10.5.9}$$

Referring to the definition of the adaptation gain, $\boldsymbol{g}(k)$ as given by Eq. 10.4.14, the adaptation gain for RLS forward prediction is given by

$$\boldsymbol{g}_N(k-1) = \boldsymbol{R}_N^{-1}(k-1)\boldsymbol{x}_N(k-1). \tag{10.5.10}$$

Notice that the adaptation gain for the forward predictor has index $N-1$. This is again consistent with the fact that the input is $\boldsymbol{x}_N(k-1)$.

Once the adaptation gain and a priori forward prediction error have been computed, we can update the forward predictor in analogy with Eq. 10.4.17 as

$$\boldsymbol{h}_N^f(k) = \boldsymbol{h}_N^f(k-1) + \boldsymbol{g}_N(k-1)\alpha_N^f(k). \tag{10.5.11}$$

It is obvious that the forward prediction error filter can be similarly updated as

$$\boldsymbol{a}_N(k) = \boldsymbol{a}_N(k-1) - \begin{bmatrix} 0 \\ \boldsymbol{g}_N(k-1) \end{bmatrix}\alpha_N^f(k). \tag{10.5.12}$$

The a posteriori forward prediction error $e_N^f(k)$ is then computed according to

$$e_N^f(k) = x(k) - \boldsymbol{h}_N^{fT}(k)\boldsymbol{x}_N(k-1) = \boldsymbol{a}_N^T(k)\boldsymbol{x}_{N+1}(k). \tag{10.5.13}$$

Finally, referring to Eq. 10.4.27, we can update the forward prediction error energy by the recursion

$$E_N^f(k) = WE_N^f(k-1) + \alpha_N^f(k)e_N^f(k). \tag{10.5.14}$$

10.5.2 Backward Linear Prediction

The set-up for RLS backward linear prediction is identical to that used in the Wiener filtering approach to forward linear prediction. The input vector consists of the N most recent samples of the input, and is denoted by $\boldsymbol{x}_N(i)$ where

$$\boldsymbol{x}_N(i) = [x(i), x(i-1), \ldots, x(i-N+1)]^T.$$

The desired response is the input at time $i-N$, *i.e.*,

$$d(i) = x(i-N).$$

The tap-weight vector is denoted by $\boldsymbol{h}_N^b(k)$ where

$$\boldsymbol{h}_N^b(k) = [h_0(k), h_1(k), \ldots, h_{N-1}(k)]^T.$$

The error between the output of the predictor and the desired response is given by

$$e_N^b(i) = x(i) - \boldsymbol{h}_N^{bT}(k)\boldsymbol{x}_N(i).$$

The objective of RLS backward prediction is to minimize at each k the backward prediction error energy,

$$E_N^b(k) = \sum_{i=1}^{k} W^{k-i}[e_N^b(i)]^2.$$

The solution to the backward prediction problem is nearly identical to the forward prediction problem. The input correlation matrix is given by

$$\boldsymbol{R}_N(k) = \sum_{i=1}^{k} W^{k-i}\boldsymbol{x}_N(i)x_N^T(i). \tag{10.5.15}$$

The crosscorrelation matrix is given by

$$\boldsymbol{p}_N^b(k) = \sum_{i=1}^{k} W^{k-i}x(i-N)\boldsymbol{x}_N(i). \tag{10.5.16}$$

The optimal backward predictor is then given by

$$\boldsymbol{h}_N^b = \boldsymbol{R}_N^{-1}(k)\boldsymbol{p}_N^b(k). \tag{10.5.17}$$

When the backward predictor is optimized, the backward prediction error energy is given by

$$E_N^b(k) = \sigma_b^2(k) - \boldsymbol{p}_N^{bT}(k)\boldsymbol{h}_N^b(k) \tag{10.5.18}$$

where

$$\sigma_b^2(k) = \sum_{i=1}^{k} W^{k-i}x^2(i-N).$$

We define the *backward prediction error filter* $\boldsymbol{b}_N(k)$ by

$$\boldsymbol{b}_N(k) = \begin{bmatrix} -\boldsymbol{h}_N^b(k) \\ 1 \end{bmatrix}.$$

Let the vector $\boldsymbol{x}_{N+1}(i)$ indicate the vector of $N+1$ most recent samples, which we can partition as

$$\boldsymbol{x}_{N+1}(i) = \begin{bmatrix} \boldsymbol{x}_N(i) \\ x(i-N) \end{bmatrix}.$$

Then the backward prediction error can be expressed as

$$e_N^b(i) = \boldsymbol{b}_N^T(k)\boldsymbol{x}_{N+1}(i). \tag{10.5.19}$$

Consider the correlation matrix for the input $\boldsymbol{x}_{N+1}(i)$. We have

$$\boldsymbol{R}_{N+1}(k) = \sum_{i=1}^{k} W^{k-i}\boldsymbol{x}_{N+1}(i)\boldsymbol{x}_{N+1}^T(i). \tag{10.5.20}$$

Using the above partition for $\boldsymbol{x}_{N+1}(i)$, the outer product $\boldsymbol{x}_{N+1}(i)\boldsymbol{x}_{N+1}^T(i)$ can be seen to equal

$$\begin{bmatrix} \boldsymbol{X}_N(i)\boldsymbol{x}_N^T(i) & \boldsymbol{x}_N(i)x(i-N) \\ \boldsymbol{x}_N^T(i)x(i-N) & x^2(i-N) \end{bmatrix}$$

so that Eq. 10.5.20 becomes

$$\boldsymbol{R}_{N+1}(k) = \begin{bmatrix} \boldsymbol{R}_N(k) & \boldsymbol{p}_N^b(k) \\ \boldsymbol{p}_N^{bT}(k) & \sigma_b^2(k) \end{bmatrix}. \tag{10.5.21}$$

To develop the augmented normal equations for the LS backward predictor, we use Eq. 10.5.21, giving

$$\boldsymbol{R}_{N+1}(k)\boldsymbol{b}_N(k) = \begin{bmatrix} \boldsymbol{p}_N^b(k) - \boldsymbol{R}_N(k)\boldsymbol{h}_N^b(k) \\ \sigma_b^2(k) - \boldsymbol{p}_N^{bT}\boldsymbol{h}_N^b(k) \end{bmatrix},$$

which, according to Eqs. 10.5.17 and 10.5.18, reduces to

$$\boldsymbol{R}_{N+1}(k)\boldsymbol{b}_N(k) = \begin{bmatrix} \mathbf{0} \\ E_N^b(k) \end{bmatrix}. \tag{10.5.22}$$

Equation 10.5.22 is known as the *augmented normal equation* for backward LS prediction.

With regard to the RLS parameters for forward prediction, we have as the a priori forward prediction error

$$\alpha_N^b(k) = x(k-N) - \boldsymbol{h}_N^{bT}(k-1)\boldsymbol{x}_N(k)$$

which we can express using the backward prediction error filter as

$$\alpha_N^b(k) = \boldsymbol{a}_b^T(k-1)\boldsymbol{x}_{N+1}(k). \tag{10.5.23}$$

Referring to the definition of the adaptation gain, $\boldsymbol{g}(k)$ as given by Eq. 10.4.14, the adaptation gain for RLS backward prediction is given by

$$\boldsymbol{g}_N(k) = \boldsymbol{R}_N^{-1}(k)\boldsymbol{x}_N(k). \tag{10.5.24}$$

Once the adaptation gain and a priori backward prediction error have been computed, we can update the backward predictor in analogy with Eq. 10.4.17 as

$$\boldsymbol{h}_N^b(k) = \boldsymbol{h}_N^b(k-1) + \boldsymbol{g}_N(k)\alpha_N^b(k). \tag{10.5.25}$$

It is obvious that the backward prediction error filter can be similarly updated as

$$\boldsymbol{b}_N(k) = \boldsymbol{b}_N(k-1) - \begin{bmatrix} \boldsymbol{g}_N(k-1) \\ 0 \end{bmatrix} \alpha_N^b(k). \tag{10.5.26}$$

The a posteriori backward prediction error $e_N^b(k)$ is then computed according to

$$e_N^b(k) = x(k-N) - \boldsymbol{h}_N^{bT}(k)\boldsymbol{x}_N(k) = \boldsymbol{b}_N^T(k)\boldsymbol{x}_{N+1}(k). \tag{10.5.27}$$

Finally, referring to Eq. 10.4.27, we can update the backward prediction error energy by the recursion

$$E_N^b(k) = WE_N^b(k-1) + \alpha_N^b(k)e_N^b(k).$$

10.6 Adaptation Gain Relationships

The key quantity in the recursive least squares algorithm is the adaptation gain, $\boldsymbol{g}(k)$. Once the adaptation gain is available, the LS weight vector can be updated according to

$$\boldsymbol{h}(k) = \boldsymbol{h}(k-1) + \boldsymbol{g}(k)\alpha(k).$$

Most fast algorithms for recursive least squares are based on tricks which compute the adaptation gain via the use of prediction parameters rather than explicit inversion of the autocorrelation matrix, $\boldsymbol{R}(k)$. We will see that the relationship between the gains for filters of orders N and $N+1$ plays a central role in the development of these fast algorithms. This section will concentrate on establishing these relationships.

A posteriori adaptation gain relationships

The adaptation gain $\boldsymbol{g}_N(k)$ was shown to satisfy

$$\boldsymbol{R}_N(k)\boldsymbol{g}_N(k) = \boldsymbol{x}_N(k). \tag{10.6.1}$$

Because this expression involves $\boldsymbol{R}_N(k)$, $\boldsymbol{g}_N(k)$ is called the *a posteriori adaptation gain.* It follows from Eq. 10.6.1 that

$$\boldsymbol{g}_N(k) = \boldsymbol{R}_N^{-1}(k)\boldsymbol{x}_N(k).$$

Suppose the order is now increased to $N+1$. The a posteriori adaptation gain for order $N+1$ then satisfies

$$\boldsymbol{g}_{N+1}(k) = \boldsymbol{R}_{N+1}^{-1}(k)\boldsymbol{x}_{N+1}(k). \tag{10.6.2}$$

We need to establish a relationship between the gains for orders N and $N+1$. To this end, consider the autocorrelation matrices. Recall that $\boldsymbol{R}_{N+1}(k)$ can be partitioned as

$$E_N^f(k) = \sigma_f^2(k) - \boldsymbol{p}_N^{fT}(k)\boldsymbol{h}_N^f(k) \tag{10.6.3}$$

We claim that $\boldsymbol{R}_{N+1}^{-1}(k)$ can be expressed as

$$\boldsymbol{R}_{N+1}^{-1}(k) = \begin{bmatrix} 0 & \boldsymbol{0} \\ \boldsymbol{0} & \boldsymbol{R}_N^{-1}(k-1) \end{bmatrix} + \frac{1}{E_N^f(k)}\boldsymbol{a}_N(k)\boldsymbol{a}_N^T(k). \tag{10.6.4}$$

To verify this, premultiply Eq. 10.6.4 by $\boldsymbol{R}_{N+1}(k)$ as given by Eq. 10.5.7, resulting in

$$\begin{bmatrix} 0 & \boldsymbol{R}_N(k-1)\boldsymbol{p}_N^f(k) \\ \boldsymbol{0} & \boldsymbol{I}_N \end{bmatrix} + \frac{1}{E_N^f(k)}\boldsymbol{R}_{N+1}(k)\boldsymbol{a}_N(k)\boldsymbol{a}_N^T(k). \tag{10.6.5}$$

We have already seen that

$$\boldsymbol{R}_{N+1}\boldsymbol{a}_N(k) = \begin{bmatrix} E_N^f(k) \\ \boldsymbol{0} \end{bmatrix}$$

and

$$\boldsymbol{R}_N(k-1)\boldsymbol{p}_N^f(k) = \boldsymbol{h}_N^f(k)$$

so that Eq. 10.6.5 becomes

$$\begin{bmatrix} 0 & \boldsymbol{h}_N^f(k) \\ \boldsymbol{0} & \boldsymbol{I}_N \end{bmatrix} + \begin{bmatrix} 1 \\ \boldsymbol{0} \end{bmatrix} \boldsymbol{a}_N^T(k) = \boldsymbol{I}_{N+1},$$

thus verifying Eq. 10.6.4. In terms of backward predictors, we can similarly show that

$$\boldsymbol{R}_{N+1}^{-1}(k) = \begin{bmatrix} \boldsymbol{R}_N(k) & \boldsymbol{0} \\ \boldsymbol{0} & 0 \end{bmatrix} + \frac{1}{E_N^b(k)}\boldsymbol{b}_N(k)\boldsymbol{b}_N^T(k). \tag{10.6.6}$$

We can now express $\boldsymbol{g}_{N+1}$ in terms of $\boldsymbol{g}_N$. Partition $\boldsymbol{x}_{N+1}(k)$ as

$$\boldsymbol{x}_{N+1}(k) = \begin{bmatrix} x(k) \\ \boldsymbol{x}_N(k-1) \end{bmatrix}$$

By definition,

$$\boldsymbol{g}_{N+1}(k) = \boldsymbol{R}_{N+1}^{-1}(k)\boldsymbol{x}_{N+1}(k).$$

We multiply by $\boldsymbol{R}_{N+1}^{-1}(k)$ as given by Eq. 10.6.4, which yields

$$\boldsymbol{g}_{N+1}(k) = \begin{bmatrix} 0 \\ \boldsymbol{R}_N^{-1}(k-1)\boldsymbol{x}_N(k-1) \end{bmatrix} + \frac{\boldsymbol{a}_N(k)\boldsymbol{a}_N^T(k)\boldsymbol{x}_{N+1}(k)}{E_N^f(k)}. \tag{10.6.7}$$

By definition,

$$\boldsymbol{R}_N^{-1}(k-1)\boldsymbol{x}_N(k-1) = \boldsymbol{g}_N(k-1)$$

and

$$\boldsymbol{a}_N^T(k)\boldsymbol{x}_{N+1}(k) = e_N^f(k)$$

so that Eq. 10.6.7 becomes

$$\boldsymbol{g}_{N+1}(k) = \begin{bmatrix} 0 \\ \boldsymbol{g}_N(k-1) \end{bmatrix} + \frac{e_N^f(k)}{E_N^f(k)}\boldsymbol{a}_N(k). \tag{10.6.8}$$

This is the relationship we have been seeking. Similarly, if we use the backward prediction parameters, we obtain

$$\boldsymbol{g}_{N+1}(k) = \begin{bmatrix} \boldsymbol{g}_N(k) \\ 0 \end{bmatrix} + \frac{e_N^b(k)}{E_N^b(k)} \boldsymbol{b}_N(k). \tag{10.6.9}$$

Notice that Eq. 10.6.8 involves both time and order updates whereas Eq. 10.6.9 involves only an order update.

A priori adaptation gain relationships

The adaptation gain $\boldsymbol{g}_N(k)$ was called the a posteriori adaptation gain because it involved the matrix $\boldsymbol{R}_N(k)$. We define the *a priori adaptation gain* $\boldsymbol{t}_N(k)$ as the gain vector which satisfies

$$\boldsymbol{R}_N(k-1)\boldsymbol{t}_N(k) = \boldsymbol{x}_N(k) \tag{10.6.10}$$

so that

$$\boldsymbol{t}_N(k) = \boldsymbol{R}_N^{-1}(k-1)\boldsymbol{x}_N(k).$$

As with the a posteriori adaptation gain, we can derive useful order relationships for the a priori adaptation gain. The gain $\boldsymbol{t}_N(k)$ is a crucial quantity in the development of several FLS algorithms.

It follows immediately from Eqs. 10.6.4 and 10.6.6 that we can express $\boldsymbol{R}_N^{-1}(k-1)$ as

$$\boldsymbol{R}_{N+1}^{-1}(k-1) = \begin{bmatrix} 0 & \boldsymbol{0} \\ \boldsymbol{0} & \boldsymbol{R}_N^{-1}(k-2) \end{bmatrix} + \frac{1}{E_N^f(k-1)} \boldsymbol{a}_N(k-1)\boldsymbol{a}_N^T(k-1) \tag{10.6.11}$$

or

$$\boldsymbol{R}_{N+1}^{-1}(k-1) = \begin{bmatrix} \boldsymbol{R}_N(k-1) & \boldsymbol{0} \\ \boldsymbol{0} & 0 \end{bmatrix} + \frac{1}{E_N^b(k-1)} \boldsymbol{b}_N(k-1)\boldsymbol{b}_N^T(k-1). \tag{10.6.12}$$

By definition,

$$\boldsymbol{t}_{N+1}(k) = \boldsymbol{R}_{N+1}^{-1}(k-1)\boldsymbol{x}_{N+1}(k).$$

If we multiply $\boldsymbol{x}_{N+1}(k)$ by $\boldsymbol{R}_{N+1}^{-1}(k-1)$ as given by Eq. 10.6.11, we get

$$\boldsymbol{t}_{N+1}(k) = \begin{bmatrix} 0 \\ \boldsymbol{R}_N^{-1}(k-2)\boldsymbol{x}_N(k-1) \end{bmatrix} + \frac{\boldsymbol{a}_N(k-1)\boldsymbol{a}_N^T(k-1)\boldsymbol{x}_{N+1}(k)}{E_N^f(k-1)}. \tag{10.6.13}$$

According to Eq. 10.6.10,

$$\boldsymbol{R}_N^{-1}(k-2)\boldsymbol{x}_N(k-1) = \boldsymbol{t}_N(k-1)$$

and by definition,

$$\boldsymbol{a}_N^T(k)\boldsymbol{x}_{N+1}(k) = \alpha_N^f(k).$$

Thus, Eq. 10.6.13 becomes

$$\boldsymbol{t}_{N+1}(k) = \begin{bmatrix} 0 \\ \boldsymbol{t}_N(k-1) \end{bmatrix} + \frac{\alpha_N^f(k)}{E_N^f(k-1)}\boldsymbol{a}_N(k-1). \tag{10.6.14}$$

Using backward prediction parameters, we can similarly show that

$$\boldsymbol{t}_{N+1}(k) = \begin{bmatrix} \boldsymbol{t}_N(k) \\ 0 \end{bmatrix} + \frac{\alpha_N^b(k)}{E_N^b(k-1)}\boldsymbol{b}_N(k-1). \tag{10.6.15}$$

Let's establish the relationship between $\boldsymbol{t}_N(k)$ and $\boldsymbol{g}_N(k)$. Using Eqs. 10.6.1 and 10.6.10, it immediately follows that

$$\boldsymbol{t}_N(k) = \boldsymbol{R}_N^{-1}(k-1)\boldsymbol{R}_N(k)\boldsymbol{g}_N(k). \tag{10.6.16}$$

Recall that

$$\boldsymbol{R}_N(k) = W\boldsymbol{R}_N(k-1) + \boldsymbol{x}_N(k)\boldsymbol{x}_N^T(k).$$

Therefore, Eq. 10.6.16 becomes

$$\boldsymbol{t}_N(k) = \boldsymbol{R}_N^{-1}(k-1)[W\boldsymbol{R}_N(k-1) + \boldsymbol{x}_N(k)\boldsymbol{x}_N^T(k)]\boldsymbol{g}_N(k).$$

Recognizing that

$$\boldsymbol{R}_N^{-1}(k-1)\boldsymbol{x}_N(k) = \boldsymbol{t}_N(k),$$

we obtain

$$\boldsymbol{t}_N(k) = W\boldsymbol{g}_N(k) + \boldsymbol{t}_N(k)\boldsymbol{x}_N^T(k)\boldsymbol{g}_N(k).$$

Solving for $\boldsymbol{t}_N(k)$, we get

$$\boldsymbol{t}_N(k) = \frac{W}{1 - \boldsymbol{g}_N^T(k)\boldsymbol{x}_N(k)}\boldsymbol{g}_N(k). \tag{10.6.17}$$

Error ratios

Another important quantity in recursive least squares is the ratio of a posteriori and a priori estimation errors. In general, we define $\varphi(k)$ as

$$\varphi(k) = \frac{e(k)}{\alpha(k)} \tag{10.6.18}$$

where $\alpha(k)$ is the a priori estimation error, given by

$$\alpha(k) = d(k) - \boldsymbol{h}^T(k-1)\boldsymbol{x}(k) \tag{10.6.19}$$

and $e(k)$ is the a posteriori estimation error, given by

$$e(k) = d(k) - \boldsymbol{h}^T(k)\boldsymbol{x}(k). \tag{10.6.20}$$

In order to obtain a useful expression for $\varphi(k)$, recall that the LS weight vector is updated according to

$$\boldsymbol{h}(k) = \boldsymbol{h}(k-1) + \boldsymbol{g}(k)\alpha(k). \tag{10.6.21}$$

Substituting Eq. 10.6.21 into Eq. 10.6.20, we get

$$e(k) = [d(k) - \boldsymbol{h}^T(k-1)\boldsymbol{x}(k)] - \boldsymbol{g}^T(k)\boldsymbol{x}(k)\alpha(k).$$

The term in brackets is recognized as $\alpha(k)$ so that

$$e(k) = \alpha(k) - \boldsymbol{g}^T(k)\boldsymbol{x}(k)\alpha(k).$$

Therefore,

$$\varphi(k) = \frac{e(k)}{\alpha(k)} = 1 - \boldsymbol{g}^T(k)\boldsymbol{x}(k). \tag{10.6.22}$$

An alternate expression can be obtained if we use the relationship

$$\boldsymbol{g}(k) = \boldsymbol{R}^{-1}(k)\boldsymbol{x}(k),$$

which gives

$$\varphi(k) = 1 - \boldsymbol{x}^T(k)\boldsymbol{R}^{-1}(k)\boldsymbol{x}(k). \tag{10.6.23}$$

Because $\varphi(k)$ is a ratio of estimation errors, it is sometimes called a *conversion factor*. That is, if we know the a priori estimation error and the conversion factor, the a posteriori estimation error can be obtained as

$$e(k) = \varphi(k)\alpha(k).$$

For the forward prediction problem, we have according to Eq. 10.6.22

$$\frac{e_N^f(k)}{\alpha_N^f(k)} = 1 - \boldsymbol{g}_N^T(k-1)\boldsymbol{x}_N(k-1), \tag{10.6.24}$$

which we denote by the symbol $\varphi_N(k-1)$, *i.e.*,

$$\varphi_N(k-1) = \frac{e_N^f(k)}{\alpha_N^f(k)}.$$

For backward prediction, we have according to Eq. 10.6.22

$$\frac{e_N^b(k)}{\alpha_N^b(k)} = 1 - \boldsymbol{g}_N^T(k)\boldsymbol{x}_N(k), \tag{10.6.25}$$

which we denote by $\varphi_N(k)$, *i.e.*,

$$\varphi_N(k) = \frac{e_N^b(k)}{\alpha_N^b(k)}.$$

Using either of Eq. 10.6.24 or 10.6.25, we can relate the a priori adaptation gain $\boldsymbol{t}_N(k)$ to the a posteriori adaptation gain $\boldsymbol{g}_N(k)$. From Eq. 10.6.17, recall that

$$\boldsymbol{t}_N(k) = \frac{W}{1 - \boldsymbol{g}_N^T(k)\boldsymbol{x}_N(k)}\boldsymbol{g}_N(k).$$

It immediately follows that

$$\boldsymbol{t}_N(k) = \frac{W}{\varphi_N(k)}\boldsymbol{g}_N(k) \tag{10.6.26}$$

or

$$\boldsymbol{g}_N(k) = \frac{\varphi_N(k)}{W}\boldsymbol{t}_N(k). \tag{10.6.27}$$

Error ratio updating

We can obtain useful equations for updating the prediction error ratios when the filter order is increased by one. From Eqs. 10.6.22 and 10.6.24, we have

$$\varphi_{N+1}(k) = \frac{e_{N+1}^f(k+1)}{\alpha_{N+1}^f(k+1)} = 1 - \boldsymbol{g}_{N+1}^T(k)\boldsymbol{x}_{N+1}(k).$$

According to Eq. 10.6.8, $\boldsymbol{g}_{N+1}$ is obtained from $\boldsymbol{g}_N$ by

$$\boldsymbol{g}_{N+1}(k) = \begin{bmatrix} 0 \\ \boldsymbol{g}_N(k-1) \end{bmatrix} + \frac{e_N^f(k)}{E_N^f(k)} \boldsymbol{a}_N(k).$$

Using the partition

$$\boldsymbol{x}_{N+1}(k) = \begin{bmatrix} x(k) \\ \boldsymbol{x}_N(k-1) \end{bmatrix},$$

it follows that

$$1 - \boldsymbol{g}_{N+1}(k)\boldsymbol{x}_{N+1}(k) = [1 - \boldsymbol{g}_N^T(k-1)\boldsymbol{x}_N(k-1)] - \frac{e_N^f(k)}{E_N^f(k)} \boldsymbol{a}_N^T(k)\boldsymbol{x}_{N+1}(k).$$

The term in brackets is recognized as $\varphi_N(k-1)$, and remembering that

$$\boldsymbol{a}_N(k)\boldsymbol{x}_{N+1}(k) = e_N^f(k),$$

we get

$$\varphi_{N+1}(k) = \varphi_N(k-1) - \frac{(e_N^f(k))^2}{E_N^f(k)}. \tag{10.6.28}$$

Similarly, if backward prediction parameters are used, we get

$$\varphi_{N+1}(k) = \varphi_N(k) - \frac{(e_N^b(k))^2}{E_N^b(k)}. \tag{10.6.29}$$

The prediction error ratio can also be updated via the use of the a priori adaptation gain $\boldsymbol{t}_N(k)$. For this case, it will be more convenient to use the *inverse* ratio,

$$\frac{1}{\varphi_N(k)} = \frac{\alpha_N^f(k)}{e_N^f(k)}.$$

Recall that

$$\varphi_N(k) = 1 - \boldsymbol{g}_N^T(k)\boldsymbol{x}_N(k).$$

In terms of $\boldsymbol{t}_N(k)$, we use Eq. 10.6.27 in the above equation, which gives

$$\varphi_N(k) = 1 - W^{-1}\varphi_N(k)\boldsymbol{t}_N^T(k)\boldsymbol{x}_N(k),$$

so that

$$\frac{1}{\varphi_N(k)} = 1 + W^{-1}\boldsymbol{t}_N^T(k)\boldsymbol{x}_N(k). \tag{10.6.30}$$

To obtain the order update, we use Eq. 10.6.30, which states that

$$\frac{1}{\varphi_{N+1}(k)} = 1 + W^{-1}\boldsymbol{t}_{N+1}^T(k)\boldsymbol{x}_{N+1}(k). \tag{10.6.31}$$

According to Eq. 10.6.14, $\boldsymbol{t}_{N+1}$ can be obtained from $\boldsymbol{t}_N$ according to

$$\boldsymbol{t}_{N+1}(k) = \begin{bmatrix} 0 \\ \boldsymbol{t}_N(k-1) \end{bmatrix} + \frac{\alpha_N^f(k)}{E_N^f(k-1)}\boldsymbol{a}_N(k-1).$$

Therefore, Eq. 10.6.31 becomes

$$\frac{1}{\varphi_{N+1}(k)} = [1 + W^{-1}\boldsymbol{t}_N^T(k-1)\boldsymbol{x}_N(k-1)] + W^{-1}\frac{\alpha_N^f(k)}{E_N^f(k-1)}\boldsymbol{a}_N^T(k-1)\boldsymbol{x}_{N+1}(k).$$

The term in brackets is equal to $1/\varphi_N(k-1)$ and we also have

$$\boldsymbol{a}_N^T(k-1)\boldsymbol{x}_{N+1}(k) = \alpha_N^f(k).$$

Therefore,

$$\frac{1}{\varphi_{N+1}(k)} = \frac{1}{\varphi_N(k-1)} + \frac{W^{-1}(\alpha_N^f(k))^2}{E_N^f(k-1)}. \tag{10.6.32}$$

Similarly, using backward prediction parameters, we obtain

$$\frac{1}{\varphi_{N+1}(k)} = \frac{1}{\varphi_N(k)} + \frac{W^{-1}(\alpha_N^b(k))^2}{E_N^b(k-1)}. \tag{10.6.33}$$

10.7 Fast Least Squares

10.7.1 The Fast Kalman Algorithm

The first fast algorithm for recursive least squares we will discuss is known as the *fast Kalman* algorithm [FL78].

We begin with the forward prediction error filter $\boldsymbol{a}_N(k-1)$. The forward a priori prediction error is given by

$$\alpha_N^f(k) = \boldsymbol{a}_N^T(k-1)\boldsymbol{x}_{N+1}(k). \tag{10.7.1}$$

The backward a priori prediction error is similarly computed by

$$\alpha_N^b(k) = \boldsymbol{b}_N^T(k-1)\boldsymbol{x}_{N+1}(k). \tag{10.7.2}$$

Now that we have $\alpha_N^f(k)$, the forward prediction error filter can be updated according to

$$\boldsymbol{a}_N(k) = \boldsymbol{a}_N(k-1) + \begin{bmatrix} 0 \\ \boldsymbol{g}_N(k-1) \end{bmatrix} \alpha_N^f(k). \tag{10.7.3}$$

Once the forward prediction error filter has been updated, the a posteriori prediction error is computed by

$$e_N^f(k) = \boldsymbol{a}_N^T(k)\boldsymbol{x}_{N+1}(k) \tag{10.7.4}$$

and the forward prediction error energy can be updated according to

$$E_N^f(k) = WE_N^f(k-1) + \alpha_N^f(k)e_N^f(k). \tag{10.7.5}$$

The a priori adaptation gain for order $N+1$ is next updated using

$$\boldsymbol{g}_{N+1}(k) = \begin{bmatrix} 0 \\ \boldsymbol{g}_N(k-1) \end{bmatrix} + \frac{e_N^f(k)}{E_N^f(k)}\boldsymbol{a}_N(k), \tag{10.7.6}$$

which we partition as

$$\boldsymbol{g}_{N+1}(k) = \begin{bmatrix} \boldsymbol{Q}(k) \\ q(k) \end{bmatrix}. \tag{10.7.7}$$

It should be noted that $\boldsymbol{Q}(k)$ is an $N \times 1$ vector and $q(k)$ is a scalar which, by definition, is equal to the last element of $\boldsymbol{g}_{N+1}(k)$.

The quantities $\boldsymbol{Q}(k)$ and $q(k)$ are important for the order N adaptation gain updating. Let's look at the backward prediction equation for $\boldsymbol{g}_{N+1}(k)$. We have

$$\boldsymbol{g}_{N+1}(k) = \begin{bmatrix} \boldsymbol{Q}(k) \\ q(k) \end{bmatrix} = \begin{bmatrix} \boldsymbol{g}_N(k) \\ 0 \end{bmatrix} + \frac{e_N^b(k)}{E_N^b(k)}\boldsymbol{b}_N(k). \tag{10.7.8}$$

Because $\boldsymbol{b}_N(k)$ is given by

$$\boldsymbol{b}_N(k) = \begin{bmatrix} -\boldsymbol{h}_N^b(k) \\ 1 \end{bmatrix},$$

it can be seen from Eq. 10.7.8 that

$$q(k) = \frac{e_N^b(k)}{E_N^b(k)}$$

and that $\boldsymbol{Q}(k)$ can be expressed by

$$\boldsymbol{Q}(k) = \boldsymbol{g}_N(k) - q(k)\boldsymbol{h}_N^b(k). \tag{10.7.9}$$

Rearranging Eq. 10.7.9 to solve for $\boldsymbol{g}_N(k)$, we have

$$\boldsymbol{g}_N(k) = \boldsymbol{Q}(k) + q(k)\boldsymbol{h}_N^b(k). \tag{10.7.10}$$

The vector $\boldsymbol{Q}(k)$ and the scalar $q(k)$ have already been computed in Eq. 10.7.6. The only unknown quantity in Eq. 10.7.10 is $\boldsymbol{h}_N^b(k)$. Recall that we have

$$\boldsymbol{h}_N^b(k) = \boldsymbol{h}_N^b(k-1) + \boldsymbol{g}_N(k)\alpha_N^b(k). \tag{10.7.11}$$

But $\boldsymbol{g}_N(k)$ is not yet available. We can, however, substitute Eq. 10.7.11 into Eq. 10.7.10 which gives

$$\boldsymbol{g}_N(k) = \boldsymbol{Q}(k) + q(k)\boldsymbol{h}_N^b(k-1) + q(k)\boldsymbol{g}_N(k)\alpha_N^b(k). \tag{10.7.12}$$

Simplifying, we have

$$\boldsymbol{g}_N(k) = \frac{\boldsymbol{Q}(k) + q(k)\boldsymbol{h}_N^b(k-1)}{1 - q(k)\alpha_N^b(k)}. \tag{10.7.13}$$

Now that $\boldsymbol{g}_N(k)$ is available, the backward prediction error filter can be updated by

$$\boldsymbol{b}_N(k) = \boldsymbol{b}_N(k-1) + \begin{bmatrix} \boldsymbol{g}_N(k) \\ 0 \end{bmatrix} \alpha_N^b(k). \tag{10.7.14}$$

The determination of the adaptation gain $\boldsymbol{g}_N(k)$ is the crucial computation of this algorithm. This is because $\boldsymbol{g}_N(k)$ is not only the adaptation gain for the predictors; it is also the adaptation gain for the LS filter. This is immediately apparent from the definition:

$$\boldsymbol{g}_N(k) = \boldsymbol{R}_N^{-1}(k)\boldsymbol{x}_N(k).$$

For the LS filter, $\boldsymbol{x}(k) = \boldsymbol{x}_N(k)$ and $\boldsymbol{R}(k) = \boldsymbol{R}_N(k)$. Thus, $\boldsymbol{g}_N(k)$ is the same as the $\boldsymbol{g}(k)$ in Eq. 10.4.14.

Now that $\boldsymbol{g}_N(k)$ is available, we can perform the LS filtering and updating. We compute the a priori estimation error by

$$\alpha(k) = d(k) - \boldsymbol{h}^T(k-1)\boldsymbol{x}(k) \tag{10.7.15}$$

and then update the LS weight vector by

$$\boldsymbol{h}(k) = \boldsymbol{h}(k-1) + \boldsymbol{g}_N(k)\alpha(k). \tag{10.7.16}$$

Summary

Summary of the fast Kalman algorithm. The algorithm is begun with $E_N^f(0)$, $\boldsymbol{a}_N(0)$, $\boldsymbol{b}_N(0)$, $\boldsymbol{h}(0)$. At each instant k, the following are available:

$$\boldsymbol{a}_N(k-1),\ \boldsymbol{b}_N(k-1),\ \boldsymbol{g}_N(k-1),\ E_N^f(k-1).$$

The following steps are then performed:

Prediction and adaptation gain updating

$$\alpha_N^f(k) = \boldsymbol{a}_N^T(k-1)\boldsymbol{x}_{N+1}(k)$$

$$\alpha_N^b(k) = \boldsymbol{b}_N^T(k-1)\boldsymbol{x}_{N+1}(k)$$

$$\boldsymbol{a}_N(k) = \boldsymbol{a}_N(k-1) - \begin{bmatrix} 0 \\ \boldsymbol{g}_N(k-1) \end{bmatrix} \alpha_N^f(k)$$

$$e_N^f(k) = \boldsymbol{a}_N^T(k)\boldsymbol{x}_{N+1}(k)$$

$$E_N^f(k) = WE_N^f(k-1) + \alpha_N^f(k)e_N^f(k)$$

$$\begin{bmatrix} \boldsymbol{Q}(k) \\ q(k) \end{bmatrix} = \begin{bmatrix} 0 \\ \boldsymbol{g}_N(k-1) \end{bmatrix} + \frac{e_N^f(k)}{E_N^f(k)}\boldsymbol{a}_N(k)$$

$$\boldsymbol{g}_N(k) = \frac{\boldsymbol{Q}(k) + q(k)\boldsymbol{h}_N^b(k-1)}{1 - q(k)\alpha_N^b(k)}$$

$$\boldsymbol{b}_N(k) = \boldsymbol{b}_N(k-1) - \begin{bmatrix} \boldsymbol{g}_N(k) \\ 0 \end{bmatrix} \alpha_N^b(k)$$

Filtering

$$\alpha(k) = d(k) - \boldsymbol{h}^T(k-1)\boldsymbol{x}(k)$$

$$\boldsymbol{h}(k) = \boldsymbol{h}(k-1) + \boldsymbol{g}_N(k)\alpha(k)$$

From the summary, it can be seen that the Fast Kalman algorithm requires roughly $8N$ multiplications for the adaptation gain computation and $2N$ multiplications for the filtering computation. This represents a substantial improvement over the N^2 multiplications required by direct application of the RLS algorithm.

10.7.2 The FAEST Algorithm

The fast Kalman algorithm primarily used a priori prediction errors for the adaptation gain computations. If a posteriori prediction errors are used, it is possible to reduce the number of multiplications even further. This is the idea behind the next FLS algorithm, which is known as the *fast a priori error sequential technique* (FAEST) [CMK83].

The FAEST algorithm is based on the a priori adaptation gain $\boldsymbol{t}_N(k)$ rather than the a posteriori gain $\boldsymbol{g}_N(k)$. We begin by computing the a priori forward and backward prediction errors,

$$\alpha_N^f(k) = \boldsymbol{a}_N^T(k-1)\boldsymbol{x}_{N+1}(k) \tag{10.7.17}$$

and

$$\alpha_N^b(k) = \boldsymbol{b}_N^T(k-1)\boldsymbol{x}_{N+1}(k). \tag{10.7.18}$$

Recall from Eq. 10.6.27 that $\boldsymbol{g}_N(k)$ is related to $\boldsymbol{t}_N(k)$ through

$$\boldsymbol{g}_N(k) = W^{-1}\varphi_N(k)\boldsymbol{t}_N(k).$$

Therefore,

$$\boldsymbol{g}_N(k-1) = W^{-1}\varphi_N(k-1)\boldsymbol{t}_N(k-1)$$

and the forward prediction error filter update equation (Eq. 10.5.12) becomes

$$\boldsymbol{a}_N(k) = \boldsymbol{a}_N(k-1) - \begin{bmatrix} 0 \\ \boldsymbol{t}_N(k-1) \end{bmatrix} W^{-1}\varphi_N(k-1)\alpha_N^f(k). \tag{10.7.19}$$

The adaptation gain for order $N+1$ is next updated according to

$$\boldsymbol{t}_{N+1}(k) = \begin{bmatrix} 0 \\ \boldsymbol{t}_N(k-1) \end{bmatrix} + \frac{\alpha_N^f(k)}{E_N^f(k-1)}\boldsymbol{a}_N(k-1), \tag{10.7.20}$$

which we partition as

$$\boldsymbol{t}_{N+1}(k) = \begin{bmatrix} \boldsymbol{Q}(k) \\ q(k) \end{bmatrix}.$$

Again, note that $\boldsymbol{Q}(k)$ is an $N \times 1$ vector and $q(k)$ is a scalar which is equal to the last element of $\boldsymbol{t}_{N+1}(k)$.

As with the fast Kalman algorithm, $\boldsymbol{Q}(k)$ and $q(k)$ are important for the order N adaptation gain updating. Let's look at the backward prediction equation for $\boldsymbol{t}_{N+1}(k)$.

$$\boldsymbol{t}_{N+1}(k) = \begin{bmatrix} \boldsymbol{t}_N(k) \\ 0 \end{bmatrix} + \frac{\alpha_N^b(k)}{E_N^b(k-1)} \boldsymbol{b}_N(k-1). \tag{10.7.21}$$

From the last row of Eq. 10.7.21, it can be seen that

$$q(k) = \frac{\alpha_N^b(k)}{E_N^b(k-1)} \tag{10.7.22}$$

and the first N rows of Eq. 10.7.21 give

$$\boldsymbol{t}_N(k) - q(k)\boldsymbol{h}_N^b(k-1) = \boldsymbol{Q}(k)$$

so that

$$\boldsymbol{t}_N(k) = \boldsymbol{Q}(k) + q(k)\boldsymbol{h}_N^b(k-1). \tag{10.7.23}$$

Thus, $\boldsymbol{t}_N(k)$ can be computed since $\boldsymbol{Q}(k)$ and $q(k)$ were already obtained in Eq. 10.7.20.

Next, the forward prediction error energy is updated. Recall that

$$E_N^f(k) = WE_N^f(k-1) + \alpha_N^f(k)e_N^f(k). \tag{10.7.24}$$

We have not yet computed $e_N^f(k)$, however. We showed that

$$\varphi_N(k-1) = \frac{e_N^f(k-1)}{\alpha_N^f(k-1)} \tag{10.7.25}$$

so that

$$e_N^f(k) = \varphi_N(k-1)\alpha_N^f(k).$$

Hence, Eq. 10.7.24 becomes

$$E_N^f(k) = WE_N^f(k-1) + \varphi_N(k-1)[\alpha_N^f(k)]^2. \tag{10.7.26}$$

The next important step is updating the conversion factor $\varphi_N(k)$. This must be done indirectly by first order-updating the inverse error ratio. Recall that

$$\frac{1}{\varphi_{N+1}(k)} = \frac{1}{\varphi_N(k-1)} + \frac{W^{-1}(\alpha_N^f(k))^2}{E_N^f(k-1)}, \tag{10.7.27}$$

which can be computed from the available quantities. We can now obtain $\varphi_N(k)$ from $\varphi_{N+1}(k)$. Using backward prediction parameters, we also had the order update given by

$$\frac{1}{\varphi_{N+1}(k)} = \frac{1}{\varphi_N(k)} + \frac{W^{-1}(\alpha_N^b(k))^2}{E_N^b(k-1)}. \tag{10.7.28}$$

Using Eq. 10.7.22 for $q(k)$, we get

$$\frac{1}{\varphi_{N+1}(k)} = \frac{1}{\varphi_N(k)} + W^{-1}q(k)\alpha_N^b(k). \tag{10.7.29}$$

Thus, $\varphi_N(k)$ can be obtained by

$$\frac{1}{\varphi_N(k)} = \frac{1}{\varphi_{N+1}(k)} - W^{-1}q(k)\alpha_N^b(k). \tag{10.7.30}$$

Finally, the backward prediction error filter is updated according to

$$\boldsymbol{b}_N(k) = \boldsymbol{b}_N(k-1) - \begin{bmatrix} \boldsymbol{t}_N(k) \\ 0 \end{bmatrix} W^{-1}\varphi_N(k)\alpha_N^b(k). \tag{10.7.31}$$

This completes the prediction section of the algorithm.

Now that $\boldsymbol{t}_N(k)$ is available, we can perform the LS filtering and updating. We compute the a priori estimation error by

$$\alpha(k) = d(k) - \boldsymbol{h}^T(k-1)\boldsymbol{x}(k). \tag{10.7.32}$$

The LS weight vector is updated through $\boldsymbol{g}_N(k)$ by

$$\boldsymbol{h}(k) = \boldsymbol{h}(k-1) + \boldsymbol{g}_N(k)\alpha(k). \tag{10.7.33}$$

Since we are using the a priori adaptation gain, $\boldsymbol{t}_N(k)$, we have the following LS weight vector update equation:

$$\boldsymbol{h}(k) = \boldsymbol{h}(k-1) + W^{-1}\varphi_N(k)\boldsymbol{t}_N(k)\alpha(k) \tag{10.7.34}$$

and this completes the algorithm.

Summary

Summary of the FAEST algorithm:

The algorithm is begun with $E_N^f(0)$, $\boldsymbol{a}_N(0)$, $\boldsymbol{b}_N(0)$, $\boldsymbol{h}(0)$. At each instant k, the following are available:

$$\boldsymbol{a}_N(k-1),\ \boldsymbol{b}_N(k-1),\ \boldsymbol{t}_N(k-1),\ E_N^f(k-1).$$

The following steps are then performed:

Prediction and adaptation gain updating

$$\alpha_N^f(k) = \boldsymbol{a}_N^T(k-1)\boldsymbol{x}_{N+1}(k)$$

$$\alpha_N^b(k) = \boldsymbol{b}_N^T(k-1)\boldsymbol{x}_{N+1}(k)$$

$$\boldsymbol{a}_N(k) = \boldsymbol{a}_N(k-1) - \begin{bmatrix} 0 \\ \boldsymbol{t}_N(k-1) \end{bmatrix} W^{-1}\varphi_N(k-1)\alpha_N^f(k)$$

$$\begin{bmatrix} \boldsymbol{Q}(k) \\ q(k) \end{bmatrix} = \begin{bmatrix} 0 \\ \boldsymbol{t}_N(k-1) \end{bmatrix} + \frac{\alpha_N^f(k)}{E_N^f(k-1)}\boldsymbol{a}_N(k-1)$$

$$\boldsymbol{t}_N(k) = \boldsymbol{Q}(k) + q(k)\boldsymbol{h}_N^b(k-1)$$

$$E_N^f(k) = WE_N^f(k-1) + \varphi_N(k-1)[\alpha_N^f(k)]^2$$

$$\frac{1}{\varphi_{N+1}(k)} = \frac{1}{\varphi_N(k-1)} + \frac{W^{-1}(\alpha_N^f(k))^2}{E_N^f(k-1)}$$

$$\frac{1}{\varphi_N(k)} = \frac{1}{\varphi_{N+1}(k)} - W^{-1}q(k)\alpha_N^b(k)$$

$$\boldsymbol{b}_N(k) = \boldsymbol{b}_N(k-1) - \begin{bmatrix} \boldsymbol{t}_N(k) \\ 0 \end{bmatrix} W^{-1}\varphi_N(k)\alpha_N^b(k)$$

Filtering

$$\alpha(k) = d(k) - \boldsymbol{h}^T(k-1)\boldsymbol{x}(k)$$

$$\boldsymbol{h}(k) = \boldsymbol{h}(k-1) + W^{-1}\varphi_N(k)\boldsymbol{t}_N(k)\alpha(k)$$

The computational complexity of the FAEST algorithm is roughly $6N$ multiplies for the adaptation gain updating and another $2N$ multiplies for the filtering operation. This represents nearly a 20% reduction in complexity over the fast Kalman algorithm.

10.7.3 The Fast Transversal Filters Algorithm

The fast transversal filters (FTF) [CK84] algorithm is nearly identical in structure to the FAEST algorithm, with one important difference: the way in which the conversion factor $\varphi_N(k)$ is updated.

We have shown that the conversion factor can be order-updated using forward prediction parameters according to

$$\varphi_{N+1}(k) = \varphi_N(k-1) - \frac{[e_N^f(k)]^2}{E_N^f(k)}. \tag{10.7.35}$$

From Eq. 10.6.24, we saw that

$$\varphi_N(k-1) = \frac{e_N^f(k)}{\alpha_N^f(k)} \tag{10.7.36}$$

and Eq. 10.5.14 showed that the forward prediction error energy could be updated by

$$E_N^f(k) = WE_N^f(k-1) + \alpha_N^f(k)e_N^f(k). \tag{10.7.37}$$

Substituting Eq. 10.7.36 in Eq. 10.7.35, after a little simplification we have

$$\varphi_{N+1}(k) = \varphi_N(k-1)\left[\frac{E_N^f(k) - \alpha_N^f(k)e_N^f(k)}{E_N^f(k)}\right],$$

which, after using Eq. 10.7.37, becomes

$$\varphi_{N+1}(k) = \frac{WE_N^f(k-1)}{E_N^f(k)}\varphi_N(k-1). \tag{10.7.38}$$

In a similar fashion, we can use backward prediction parameters to show that

$$\varphi_{N+1}(k) = \frac{WE_N^b(k-1)}{E_N^b(k)}\varphi_N(k). \tag{10.7.39}$$

Now, the FTF algorithm begins exactly like the FAEST algorithm until the point where we have the pair of equations

$$\frac{1}{\varphi_{N+1}(k)} = \frac{1}{\varphi_N(k-1)} + \frac{W^{-1}(\alpha_N^f(k))^2}{E_N^f(k-1)} \tag{10.7.40}$$

and

$$\frac{1}{\varphi_N(k)} = \frac{1}{\varphi_{N+1}(k)} - W^{-1}q(k)\alpha_N^b(k). \tag{10.7.41}$$

Instead of using Eq. 10.7.40 to order-update $1/\varphi_{N+1}(k)$, we use Eq. 10.7.38:

$$\varphi_{N+1}(k) = \frac{WE_N^f(k-1)}{E_N^f(k)}\varphi_N(k-1). \tag{10.7.42}$$

Now that we have $\varphi_{N+1}(k)$, we wish to obtain $\varphi_N(k)$. Using Eq. 10.7.39, we can write

$$\varphi_N(k) = \frac{E_N^b(k)}{WE_N^b(k-1)}\varphi_{N+1}(k). \tag{10.7.43}$$

We can use the backward prediction error energy update equation,

$$E_N^b(k) = WE_N^b(k-1) + \alpha_N^b(k)e_N^b(k)$$

in Eq. 10.7.43, which gives

$$\varphi_N(k) = \varphi_{N+1}(k)\left[1 + \frac{\alpha_N^b(k)e_N^b(k)}{WE_N^b(k-1)}\right]. \tag{10.7.44}$$

Now, recall that we had the scalar parameter $q(k)$ which was given by

$$q(k) = \frac{\alpha_N^b(k)}{E_N^b(k-1)}.$$

Also, the a posteriori backward prediction error is related to the a priori backward prediction error through the conversion factor according to

$$e_N^b(k) = \varphi_N(k)\alpha_N^b(k).$$

Thus, Eq. 10.7.44 becomes

$$\varphi_N(k) = \varphi_{N+1}(k) + W^{-1}\varphi_{N+1}(k)\alpha_N^b(k)q(k)\varphi_N(k),$$

which gives

$$\varphi_N(k) = \frac{\varphi_{N+1}(k)}{1 - W^{-1}q(k)\varphi_{N+1}(k)\alpha_N^b(k)}. \tag{10.7.45}$$

Equations 10.7.42 and 10.7.45 are the pair of equations used by the FTF algorithm for conversion factor updating. The rest of the algorithm proceeds exactly as the FAEST algorithm, and the computational complexities of the two algorithms are nearly identical.

Summary

Summary of the FTF algorithm:

The algorithm is begun with $E_N^f(0)$, $\boldsymbol{a}_N(0)$, $\boldsymbol{b}_N(0)$, $\boldsymbol{h}(0)$. At each instant k, the following are available:

$$\boldsymbol{a}_N(k-1),\ \boldsymbol{b}_N(k-1),\ \boldsymbol{t}_N(k-1),\ E_N^f(k-1).$$

The following steps are then performed:

Prediction and adaptation gain updating

$$\alpha_N^f(k) = \boldsymbol{a}_N^T(k-1)\boldsymbol{x}_{N+1}(k)$$

$$\alpha_N^b(k) = \boldsymbol{b}_N^T(k-1)\boldsymbol{x}_{N+1}(k)$$

$$\boldsymbol{a}_N(k) = \boldsymbol{a}_N(k-1) - \begin{bmatrix} 0 \\ \boldsymbol{t}_N(k-1) \end{bmatrix} W^{-1}\varphi_N(k-1)\alpha_N^f(k)$$

$$\begin{bmatrix} \boldsymbol{Q}(k) \\ q(k) \end{bmatrix} = \begin{bmatrix} 0 \\ \boldsymbol{t}_N(k-1) \end{bmatrix} + \frac{\alpha_N^f(k)}{E_N^f(k-1)}\boldsymbol{a}_N(k-1)$$

$$\boldsymbol{t}_N(k) = \boldsymbol{Q}(k) + q(k)\boldsymbol{h}_N^b(k-1)$$

$$E_N^f(k) = WE_N^f(k-1) + \varphi_N(k-1)[\alpha_N^f(k)]^2$$

$$\varphi_{N+1}(k) = \frac{WE_N^f(k-1)}{E_N^f(k)}\varphi_N(k-1)$$

$$\varphi_N(k) = \frac{\varphi_{N+1}(k)}{1 - W^{-1}q(k)\varphi_{N+1}(k)\alpha_N^b(k)}$$

$$\boldsymbol{b}_N(k) = \boldsymbol{b}_N(k-1) - \begin{bmatrix} \boldsymbol{t}_N(k) \\ 0 \end{bmatrix} W^{-1}\varphi_N(k)\alpha_N^b(k)$$

Filtering

$$\alpha(k) = d(k) - \boldsymbol{h}^T(k-1)\boldsymbol{x}(k)$$

$$\boldsymbol{h}(k) = \boldsymbol{h}(k-1) + W^{-1}\varphi_N(k)\boldsymbol{t}_N(k)\alpha(k)$$

The computational complexity of the FTF algorithm is essentially identical to the FAEST algorithm: roughly $8N$ multiplies for the adaptation gain updating and $2N$ multiplies for the filtering operation.

10.8 Performance of RLS Algorithms

At each instant k, we can express the sequence of a priori estimation errors as

$$\begin{bmatrix} \alpha(1) \\ \alpha(2) \\ \vdots \\ \alpha(N) \\ \vdots \\ \alpha(k) \end{bmatrix} = \begin{bmatrix} d(1) \\ d(2) \\ \vdots \\ d(N) \\ \vdots \\ d(k) \end{bmatrix} - \begin{bmatrix} x(1) & 0 & 0 & \cdots & 0 \\ x(2) & x(1) & 0 & \cdots & 0 \\ \vdots & \vdots & \vdots & \vdots & \vdots \\ x(N) & x(N-1) & \cdots & \cdots & x(1) \\ \vdots & \vdots & \vdots & \vdots & \vdots \\ x(k) & x(k-1) & \cdots & \cdots & x(k-N+1) \end{bmatrix} \begin{bmatrix} h_0(k) \\ h_1(k) \\ \vdots \\ h_{N-1}(k) \end{bmatrix}.$$

At each k, the $\{h_i(k)\}$ are computed so as to minimize the sum of error squares. Clearly, for $k \leq N$, the errors can be made identically zero since the system of equations is underdetermined. At $k = N + 1$, the system of equations becomes overdetermined and the LS procedure begins.

Let's analyze the behavior of the RLS algorithm for the case of LS parameter estimation. It is assumed for this case that the desired response is given by

$$d(k) = \boldsymbol{h}_o^T \boldsymbol{x}(k) + e_o(k) \tag{10.8.1}$$

where $\boldsymbol{h}_o$ is the vector of true parameters and the sequence of measurement errors $\{e_o(i)\}$ is zero-mean, white, and uncorrelated with the measurements $\{x(i)\}$. Recall that the RLS solution to the estimation problem is given by

$$h(k) = \boldsymbol{R}_N^{-1}(k)\boldsymbol{p}(k) \tag{10.8.2}$$

where

$$\boldsymbol{R}_N(k) = \sum_{i=1}^{k} W^{k-i} \boldsymbol{x}(i)\boldsymbol{x}^T(i)$$

and

$$\boldsymbol{p}(k) = \sum_{i=1}^{k} W^{k-i} d(i)\boldsymbol{x}(i).$$

With the relationship expressed by Eq. 10.8.1, the RLS solution given by Eq. 10.8.2 becomes

$$\boldsymbol{h}(k) = \boldsymbol{R}_N^{-1}(k) \left[\sum_{i=1}^{k} W^{k-i} \boldsymbol{x}(i)\boldsymbol{x}^T(i) \right] \boldsymbol{h}_o + \boldsymbol{R}_N^{-1}(k) \sum_{i=1}^{k} \boldsymbol{x}(i)e_o(i).$$

Therefore,

$$\boldsymbol{h}(k) = \boldsymbol{h}_o + \boldsymbol{R}_N^{-1}(k)\sum_{i=1}^{k}\boldsymbol{x}(i)e_o(i). \tag{10.8.3}$$

Taking the expectation and invoking the assumptions about the measurement error sequence, we have

$$\mathcal{E}[\boldsymbol{h}(k)] = \boldsymbol{h}_o$$

so that the exact RLS method yields an unbiased estimate of the vector $\boldsymbol{h}_o$. In actuality, we are not using the true matrix $\boldsymbol{R}_N(k)$ because of the initialization $\boldsymbol{R}_N(0) = \boldsymbol{I}$. It can be shown that this leads to an estimate $\boldsymbol{h}(k)$ which satisfies

$$\mathcal{E}[\boldsymbol{h}(k)] = \boldsymbol{h}_o + \frac{1}{k}\boldsymbol{R}_N^{-1}\boldsymbol{h}_o$$

which is *asymptotically unbiased.* In the long run, this distinction is not important.

Define the *weight deviation* $\Delta\boldsymbol{h}(k)$ by

$$\Delta\boldsymbol{h}(k) = \boldsymbol{h}(k) - \boldsymbol{h}_o.$$

Using Eq. 10.8.3, we have

$$\Delta\boldsymbol{h}(k) = \boldsymbol{R}_N^{-1}(k)\sum_{i=1}^{k}\boldsymbol{x}(i)e_o(i). \tag{10.8.4}$$

The covariance of $\Delta\boldsymbol{h}(k)$ is given by

$$\mathcal{E}[\Delta\boldsymbol{h}(k)(\Delta\boldsymbol{h}(k))^T] = \boldsymbol{R}_N^{-1}(k)\mathcal{E}\left[\sum_{i=1}^{k}\sum_{j=1}^{k}W^{k-i}W^{k-j}\boldsymbol{x}(i)\boldsymbol{x}^T(j)e_o(i)e_o(j)\right]\boldsymbol{R}_N^{-1}(k). \tag{10.8.5}$$

The double summation can be simplified because $\{e_o(i)\}$ is assumed to be white with power σ^2, giving

$$\mathcal{E}[\Delta\boldsymbol{h}(k)(\Delta\boldsymbol{h}(k))^T] = \boldsymbol{R}_N^{-1}(k)\left[\sum_{i=1}^{k}W^{2(k-i)}\boldsymbol{x}(i)\boldsymbol{x}^T(i)\right]\boldsymbol{R}_N^{-1}(k). \tag{10.8.6}$$

For the case $W = 1$, Eq. 10.8.6 becomes

$$\mathcal{E}[\Delta\boldsymbol{h}(k)(\Delta\boldsymbol{h}(k))^T] = \sigma^2\boldsymbol{R}_N^{-1}(k)\boldsymbol{R}_N(k)\boldsymbol{R}_N^{-1}(k).$$

Thus,

$$\mathcal{E}[\Delta \boldsymbol{h}(k)(\Delta \boldsymbol{h}(k))^T] = \sigma^2 \boldsymbol{R}_N^{-1}(k). \tag{10.8.7}$$

Next, recall that the a priori estimation error is given by

$$\alpha(k) = d(k) - \boldsymbol{h}^T(k-1)\boldsymbol{x}(k).$$

Using Eq. 10.8.1, we can write

$$\alpha(k) = e_o(k) - \boldsymbol{x}^T(k)\Delta \boldsymbol{h}(k-1).$$

Invoking again the assumptions on the measurement error sequence, we have

$$\mathcal{E}[\alpha^2(k)] = \sigma^2 + \boldsymbol{x}^T(k)\mathcal{E}[\Delta \boldsymbol{h}(k-1)(\Delta \boldsymbol{h}(k-1))^T]\boldsymbol{x}(k),$$

which, using Eq. 10.8.7, becomes

$$\mathcal{E}[\alpha^2(k)] = \sigma^2 + \sigma^2 \boldsymbol{x}^T(k)\boldsymbol{R}_N^{-1}(k-1)\boldsymbol{x}(k). \tag{10.8.8}$$

At this point, we need to make some approximations. If $\{x(k)\}$ is WSS, the time-averaged autocorrelation matrix is approximately equal to the ensemble-averaged autocorrelation matrix so that

$$\boldsymbol{R}_N(k) \approx k\boldsymbol{R}.$$

Thus,

$$\boldsymbol{R}_N^{-1}(k-1) \approx \frac{1}{k-1}\boldsymbol{R}^{-1}. \tag{10.8.9}$$

Next, because the trace of a scalar is identical to a scalar, we have

$$\boldsymbol{x}^T(k)\boldsymbol{R}_N^{-1}(k-1)\boldsymbol{x}(k) = trace[\boldsymbol{x}^T(k)\boldsymbol{R}_N^{-1}(k-1)\boldsymbol{x}(k)].$$

Using the fact that $trace(\boldsymbol{AB}) = trace(\boldsymbol{BA})$, it follows that

$$trace[\boldsymbol{x}^T(k)\boldsymbol{R}_N^{-1}(k-1)\boldsymbol{x}(k)] = trace[\boldsymbol{R}_N^{-1}(k-1)\boldsymbol{x}(k)\boldsymbol{x}^T(k)].$$

Combining this with Eq. 10.8.9, Eq. 10.8.9 becomes

$$\mathcal{E}[\alpha^2(k)] = \sigma^2 + \frac{\sigma^2}{k-1} trace[\boldsymbol{R}^{-1}\boldsymbol{x}(k)\boldsymbol{x}^T(k)]. \tag{10.8.10}$$

Finally, ensemble-averaging over all realizations of $\{x(k)\}$ gives us the *mean residual error*

$$E_R(k) = \sigma^2 + \frac{\sigma^2}{k-1} trace[\boldsymbol{I}] = \sigma^2 \left[1 + \frac{N}{k-1}\right]. \tag{10.8.11}$$

Equation 10.8.11 shows that as k approaches infinity,

$$E_R(\infty) = \sigma^2,$$

which is the minimum MSE for the parameter estimation problem. Thus, in theory, the RLS algorithm produces *zero misadjustment.* Furthermore, we see from Eq. 10.8.11 that the convergence of the MSE is *independent* of the eigenvalue spread. Recall that the steepest descent (and similarly, the LMS algorithm) had a MSE time constant approximately equal to $1/(2\mu\lambda_{min})$. The convergence of the MSE for the RLS algorithm is roughly an order of magnitude faster and does not depend on eigenvalue spread of the input signal. This comes, of course, at the cost of extra computational complexity.

For the case where a nonunity weighting factor is used, we can derive the mean residual error if we recognize that

$$\boldsymbol{R}_N(k) = \sum_{i=1}^{k} W^{k-i} \boldsymbol{x}(i)\boldsymbol{x}^T(i) \approx \frac{1-W^k}{1-W}\boldsymbol{R}.$$

Following the same derivation as before, we get

$$E_R(k) = \sigma^2 \left[1 + N\frac{1-W}{1+W}\frac{1+W^k}{1-W^k}\right]. \tag{10.8.12}$$

As k approaches infinity, we have

$$E_R(\infty) = \sigma^2 \left[1 + N\frac{1-W}{1+W}\right].$$

Thus, the misadjustment is given by

$$M = \frac{E_R(\infty) - E_{min}}{E_{min}} = N\frac{1-W}{1+W}.$$

The weight W is chosen as a "forgetting factor" to account for time-varying signal statistics. It can be shown that for large k, the weight $\boldsymbol{h}(k)$ converges to $\boldsymbol{h}_o$ with a time constant roughly equal to $(1-W)^{-1}$. Thus, W close to unity will give a large time constant for the adaptation, but small misadjustment. The speed of adaptation is still considerably better than the LMS algorithm. If, however, the signal statistics are varying with time, we need to make the time constant smaller to be able to "track" the signal statistics. This will have the effect of increasing the misadjustment proportional to $1-W$.

It should be noted that RLS is in general superior to the LMS algorithm in both the initial rate of convergence and in misadjustment. It has been shown, however, that the tracking properties of the LMS algorithm are better than those of RLS [EF86]. The user should carefully measure the tradeoffs between computational complexity and the required performance of the adaptive filter. If the ability to track rapidly varying signal statistics is the objective, an RLS-based solution may not be effective. If, however, initial speed of adaptation and misadjustment are critical, an RLS solution may be the only logical choice.

The recursive least squares algorithms require an initialization of the variables which are used in the computations. Since we have assumed knowledge of the signal only after time $k = 0$, it is reasonable to assume that the signal is equal to zero before this time. Consequently, the predictor coefficients can all be set to zero initially. However, the forward prediction error energy must be initialized to some small positive value δ. For the LS computations to proceed along the right track, it is important that the filter be started from initial conditions which correspond to a least-squares configuration. With the predictor coefficients and adaptation gain all equal to zero, this positive prediction error energy can be regarded as being due to a signal which satisfies

$$\begin{aligned} x(-N) &= (W^{-N}\delta)^{1/2} \\ x(k) &= 0, \qquad k = -N+1, -N+2, \ldots, 0. \end{aligned}$$

Consequently, the backward prediction error energy has an initial value given by

$$E_N^b(0) = x^2(-N) = W^{-N}\delta.$$

The magnitude of δ is related to the initial bias in the weight vector. In practice, δ can not be chosen arbitrarily small due to limitations of computational precision (which can be experienced even with floating-point arithmetic). Experience has shown that an initial value of

$$\delta \geq 0.01\sigma_x^2$$

is often satisfactory [Hay86].

Example 10.2

This example illustrates the superior performance of the RLS, even when the input signal has a large eigenvalue spread. Consider again the MA identification problem. We assume that the unknown system is driven with a colored noise process $\{x(k)\}$ which is generated as the output of a narrow bandpass filter. The MA parameters are given by

$$\{h(k)\} = \{0, 0.25, 0.5, 0.75, 1, 0.75, 0.5, 0.25, 0\}.$$

The RLS identification problem is configured as in the LMS identification problem, with the signal $\{x(k)\}$ fed both to the adaptive system and to the unknown system. The evolution of the first three coefficients is shown in Fig. 10.8.1a. These plots correspond to a weight $W = 0.999$ and an initial prediction error energy of $0.01\sigma_x^2$. Notice that the RLS algorithm is capable of identifying the MA parameters quite rapidly, whereas the LMS algorithm failed to do so. To examine the impact of the choice of the initial prediction error energy, Fig. 10.8.1b shows the evolution of the same coefficients corresponding to an initial prediction error energy of $0.1\sigma_x^2$. Observe that the coefficients adapt more slowly than before.

Example 10.3

Consider again the problem of linear prediction for the AR(2) process

$$x(k) + ax(k-1) + b(k-2) = v(k)$$

from the previous chapter. The choice $a = -3/4, b = -1/8$ led to an eigenvalue spread of $\chi(\boldsymbol{R}) = 13$ and the choice $a = -0.5, b = 0.9$ led to an eigenvalue spread of $\chi(\boldsymbol{R}) = 1.71$. For the purposes of comparison, the RLS weight tracks are shown in Fig. 10.8.2 where $W = 0.999$ and the initial prediction error energy has been taken as $0.1\sigma_x^2$. Notice that the rate of convergence is more or less independent of the eigenvalue spread.

In closing, it should be mentioned that most of the fast algorithms for recursive least square which we have discussed up to this point are extremely sensitive to finite-wordlength effects [FL78], [CK84]. This is typically due to the indirect manner in which the adaptation is updated through the use of auxiliary variables and the accumulation of roundoff error. For this reason, high precision is required for most of the transversal FLS algorithms. Usually, floating-point arithmetic will suffice, but in some special circumstances, the finite precision on the mantissa will cause even a floating-point implementation to fail. This has prompted the development of QR-rotation algorithms [Hay86], which we will not discuss here, and lattice algorithms, which are the topic of the next section.

10.9 RLS Lattice Filters

We have seen that there are several algorithms for performing the recursive least-squares computations for the transversal filter structure. Recursive least squares can also be performed with a lattice structure. Whereas the FLS algorithms for transversal structures were based on time recursions, the lattice structures require the use of time and order recursions. The recursive least-squares lattice algorithms require more computations than their transversal counterparts, but result in better numerical behavior and generate adaptive filters of all intermediate orders, which is useful when the proper order is not known ahead of time.

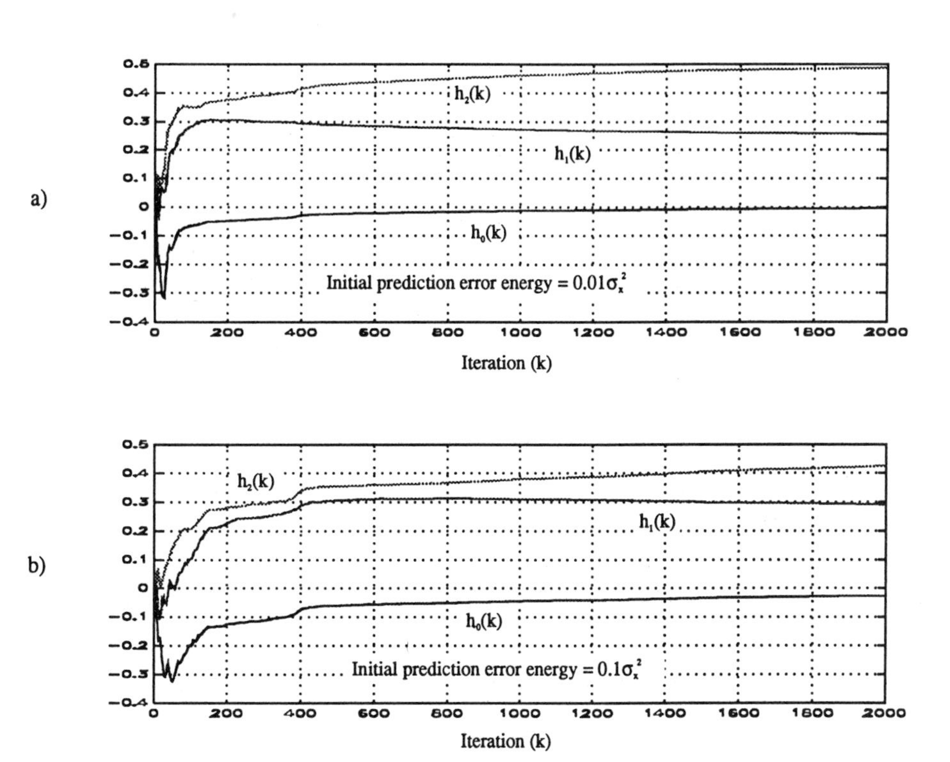

Figure 10.8.1: (a) Evolution of MA coefficients with an initial prediction error energy of $0.01\sigma_x^2$; (b) evolution of MA coefficients with an initial prediction error energy of $0.1\sigma_x^2$.

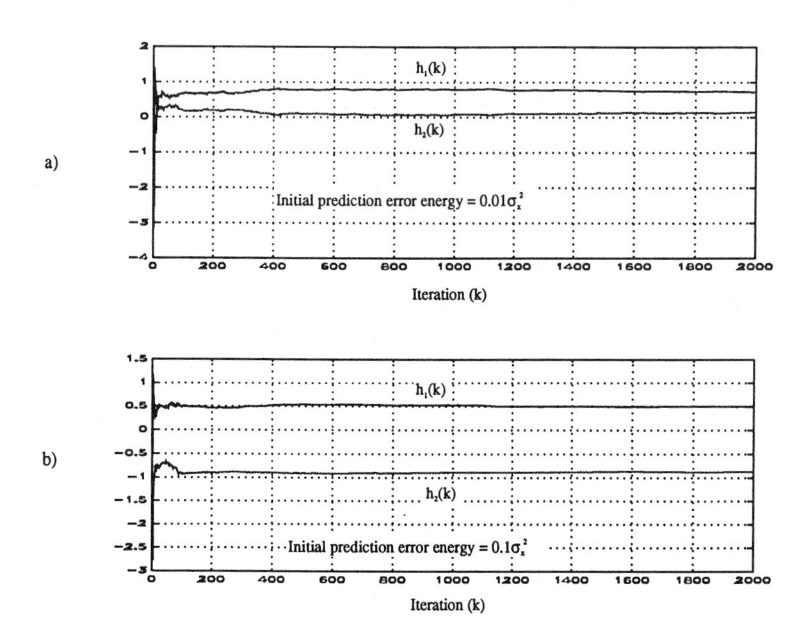

Figure 10.8.2: (a) Convergence of the tap weights for $a = -3/4, b = -1/8$; (b) convergence of the tap weights for $a = -0.5, b = 0.9$.

The RLS lattice algorithms are is similar in form to the Levinson-Durbin algorithm for the lattice Wiener filter, but are based on time averages rather than ensemble averaged quantities. We begin with the order recursions for the predictor coefficients. Recall the augmented normal equations for forward and backward prediction were given by

$$\boldsymbol{R}_N(k)\boldsymbol{a}_{N-1}(k) = \begin{bmatrix} E^f_{N-1}(k) \\ \mathbf{0} \end{bmatrix}$$

and

$$\boldsymbol{R}_N(k)\boldsymbol{b}_{N-1}(k) = \begin{bmatrix} \mathbf{0} \\ E^b_{N-1}(k) \end{bmatrix},$$

respectively. The RLS lattice algorithms are based on both time and order recursions. We saw that the correlation matrix $\boldsymbol{R}_N(k)$ can be updated according to either

$$\boldsymbol{R}_{N+1}(k) = \begin{bmatrix} \sigma^2_f(k) & \boldsymbol{p}^{fT}_N(k) \\ \boldsymbol{p}^f_N(k) & \boldsymbol{R}_N(k-1) \end{bmatrix} \tag{10.9.1}$$

or

$$\boldsymbol{R}_{N+1}(k) = \begin{bmatrix} \boldsymbol{R}_N(k) & \boldsymbol{p}_N^b(k) \\ \boldsymbol{p}_N^{bT}(k) & \sigma_b^2(k) \end{bmatrix} \tag{10.9.2}$$

As with the Wiener filter, we claim that the forward prediction error filter can be order-updated according to

$$\boldsymbol{a}_N(k) = \begin{bmatrix} \boldsymbol{a}_{N-1}(k) \\ 0 \end{bmatrix} + \Gamma_N^f(k) \begin{bmatrix} 0 \\ \boldsymbol{b}_N(k-1) \end{bmatrix}. \tag{10.9.3}$$

To show that this is true, we use Eq. 10.9.2 to compute

$$\boldsymbol{R}_{N+1} \begin{bmatrix} \boldsymbol{a}_{N-1}(k) \\ 0 \end{bmatrix} = \begin{bmatrix} \boldsymbol{R}_N(k)\boldsymbol{a}_{N-1}(k) \\ \boldsymbol{p}_N^{bT}(k)\boldsymbol{a}_{N-1}(k) \end{bmatrix}.$$

But $\boldsymbol{R}_N(k)\boldsymbol{a}_{N-1}(k)$ is easily computed using the augmented normal equation for order $N-1$ so that

$$\boldsymbol{R}_{N+1} \begin{bmatrix} \boldsymbol{a}_{N-1}(k) \\ 0 \end{bmatrix} = \begin{bmatrix} E_{N-1}^f(k) \\ \boldsymbol{0} \\ \boldsymbol{p}_N^{bT}(k)\boldsymbol{a}_{N-1}(k) \end{bmatrix}. \tag{10.9.4}$$

Similarly, we find that

$$\boldsymbol{R}_{N+1} \begin{bmatrix} 0 \\ \boldsymbol{b}_{N-1}(k-1) \end{bmatrix} = \begin{bmatrix} \boldsymbol{p}_N^{fT}(k)\boldsymbol{b}_{N-1}(k-1 \\ \boldsymbol{0} \\ E_{N-1}^b(k-1) \end{bmatrix}. \tag{10.9.5}$$

Define $\Gamma_N^f(k)$ by

$$\Gamma_N^f(k) = -\frac{\boldsymbol{p}_N^{bT}(k)\boldsymbol{a}_{N-1}(k)}{E_{N-1}^b(k-1)}. \tag{10.9.6}$$

It follows from Eqs. 10.9.4, 10.9.5, and 10.9.6 that with $\boldsymbol{a}_N(k)$ given by Eq. 10.9.3 and $\Gamma_N^f(k)$ as above that

$$\boldsymbol{R}_{N+1}(k)\boldsymbol{a}_N(k) = \begin{bmatrix} E_{N-1}^f(k) + \Gamma_N^f(k)\boldsymbol{p}_N^{fT}(k)\boldsymbol{b}_{N-1}(k-1) \\ \boldsymbol{0} \end{bmatrix}. \tag{10.9.7}$$

This is easily recognized as the augmented normal equation for order-N forward prediction and shows that Eq. 10.9.3 can be used to order-update the forward predictor. From the right-hand side of Eq. 10.9.7, we see that the forward prediction error energy is order-updated according to

$$E_N^f(k) = E_{N-1}^f(k) + \Gamma_N^f(k)\boldsymbol{p}_N^{fT}(k)\boldsymbol{b}_{N-1}(k-1). \tag{10.9.8}$$

Note the similarity between these equations and the Levinson recursions.

Next, we derive the order-update equation for backward prediction. Assume that we can update the backward predictor by

$$\boldsymbol{b}_N(k) = \begin{bmatrix} 0 \\ \boldsymbol{b}_{N-1}(k-1) \end{bmatrix} + \Gamma_N^b(k) \begin{bmatrix} \boldsymbol{a}_N(k) \\ 0 \end{bmatrix}. \tag{10.9.9}$$

Let

$$\Gamma_N^b(k) = -\frac{\boldsymbol{p}_N^{fT}(k)\boldsymbol{b}_{N-1}(k)}{\boldsymbol{E}_{N-1}^f(k)}. \tag{10.9.10}$$

Using Eqs. 10.9.4, 10.9.5, and 10.9.10, we have

$$\boldsymbol{R}_{N+1}(k)\boldsymbol{b}_N(k) = \begin{bmatrix} \boldsymbol{0} \\ E_{N-1}^b(k-1) + \Gamma_N^b(k)\boldsymbol{p}_N^{bT}(k)\boldsymbol{a}_{N-1}(k) \end{bmatrix}. \tag{10.9.11}$$

This is easily recognized as the augmented normal equation for order-N backward prediction and shows that Eq. 10.9.10 can be used to order-update the backward predictor. From the right-hand side of Eq. 10.9.3, we see that the backward prediction error energy is order-updated according to

$$E_N^b(k) = E_{N-1}^b(k-1) + \Gamma_N^b(k)\boldsymbol{p}_N^{bT}(k)\boldsymbol{a}_{N-1}(k) \tag{10.9.12}$$

Again, note the similarity between these equations and the Levinson recursions for the lattice Wiener predictor.

Using Eq. 10.9.4, we see that

$$\begin{bmatrix} 0 & \boldsymbol{b}_{N-1}^T(k-1) \end{bmatrix} \boldsymbol{R}_{N+1}(k) \begin{bmatrix} \boldsymbol{a}_{N-1}(k) \\ 0 \end{bmatrix} = \boldsymbol{p}_N^{bT}(k)\boldsymbol{a}_{N-1}(k) \tag{10.9.13}$$

because the last element of $\boldsymbol{b}_{N-1}(k-1)$ equals one. Similarly, using Eq. 10.9.5, we see that

$$\begin{bmatrix} 0 & \boldsymbol{b}_{N-1}^T(k-1) \end{bmatrix} \boldsymbol{R}_{N+1}(k) \begin{bmatrix} \boldsymbol{a}_{N-1}(k) \\ 0 \end{bmatrix} = \boldsymbol{p}_N^{fT}(k)\boldsymbol{b}_{N-1}(k-1) \tag{10.9.14}$$

Thus, comparing Eqs. 10.9.13 and 10.9.14, we see that

$$\boldsymbol{p}_N^{bT}(k)\boldsymbol{a}_{N-1}(k) = \boldsymbol{p}_N^{fT}(k)\boldsymbol{b}_{N-1}(k-1).$$

Let us denote these quantities by $\Delta_N(k)$, *i.e.*,

$$\Delta_N(k) = \boldsymbol{p}_N^{bT}(k)\boldsymbol{a}_{N-1}(k) = \boldsymbol{p}_N^{fT}(k)\boldsymbol{b}_{N-1}(k-1).$$

Referring to Eqs. 10.9.6 and 10.9.10, we have

$$\Gamma_N^f(k) = -\frac{\Delta_N(k)}{E_{N-1}^b(k-1)} \tag{10.9.15}$$

and

$$\Gamma_N^b(k) = -\frac{\Delta_N(k)}{E_{N-1}^f(k)}. \tag{10.9.16}$$

We can see at this point that $\Gamma_N^f(k)$ and $\Gamma_N^b(k)$ are time-averaged estimates of the reflection coefficients.

The error energy update equations then become

$$E_N^f(k) = E_{N-1}^f(k) - \frac{\Delta_N^2(k)}{E_{N-1}^b(k-1)} \tag{10.9.17}$$

and

$$E_N^b(k) = E_{N-1}^b(k) - \frac{\Delta_N^2(k)}{E_{N-1}^f(k)} \tag{10.9.18}$$

The equations for the prediction error filter order updates can be used to derive a lattice structure for the computations. We repeat these equations for convenience. For forward prediction, we have

$$\boldsymbol{a}_N(k) = \begin{bmatrix} \boldsymbol{a}_{N-1}(k) \\ 0 \end{bmatrix} + \Gamma_N^f(k) \begin{bmatrix} 0 \\ \boldsymbol{b}_N(k-1) \end{bmatrix} \tag{10.9.19}$$

and for backward prediction,

$$\boldsymbol{b}_N(k) = \begin{bmatrix} 0 \\ \boldsymbol{b}_{N-1}(k-1) \end{bmatrix} + \Gamma_N^b(k) \begin{bmatrix} \boldsymbol{a}_N(k) \\ 0 \end{bmatrix}. \tag{10.9.20}$$

Recall that we can partition the vector $\boldsymbol{x}_{N+1}(k)$ as either

$$\boldsymbol{x}_{N+1}(k) = \begin{bmatrix} x(k) \\ \boldsymbol{x}_N(k-1) \end{bmatrix} \tag{10.9.21}$$

or

$$\boldsymbol{x}_{N+1}(k) = \begin{bmatrix} \boldsymbol{x}_N(k) \\ x(k-N) \end{bmatrix} \tag{10.9.22}$$

The order-N forward a posteriori prediction error is given by

$$e_N^f(k) = \boldsymbol{a}_N^T(k)\boldsymbol{x}_{N+1}(k).$$

Using Eqs. 10.9.19, 10.9.21, and 10.9.22, we have

$$e_N^f(k) = \boldsymbol{a}_{N-1}^T(k)\boldsymbol{x}_N(k) + \Gamma_N^f(k)\boldsymbol{b}_{N-1}^T(k-1)\boldsymbol{x}_N(k-1)$$

so that

$$e_N^f(k) = e_{N-1}^f(k) + \Gamma_N^f(k)e_{N-1}^b(k-1). \tag{10.9.23}$$

The order-N backward a posteriori prediction error is given by

$$e_N^b(k) = \boldsymbol{b}_N^T(k)\boldsymbol{x}_{N+1}(k).$$

Using Eqs. 10.9.20, 10.9.21, and 10.9.22, we have

$$e_N^b(k) = \boldsymbol{b}_{N-1}^T(k-1)\boldsymbol{x}_N(k-1) + \Gamma_N^b(k)\boldsymbol{a}_{N-1}^T(k)\boldsymbol{x}_N(k)$$

so that

$$e_N^b(k) = e_{N-1}^b(k-1) + \Gamma_N^b(k)e_{N-1}^f(k). \tag{10.9.24}$$

Equations 10.9.23 and 10.9.24 have a signal flow graph as shown in Fig. 10.9.1. Using the relations for a priori estimation errors, we can show in an identical manner that

$$\alpha_N^f(k) = \alpha_{N-1}^f(k) + \Gamma_N^f(k-1)\alpha_{N-1}^b(k-1). \tag{10.9.25}$$

and

$$\alpha_N^b(k) = \alpha_{N-1}^b(k-1) + \Gamma_N^b(k-1)\alpha_{N-1}^f(k). \tag{10.9.26}$$

The predictor coefficients are indirectly order-updated through the quantity $\Delta_N(k)$. In order to provide time-updates for the predictor coefficients, it is important that we develop a time update equation for $\Delta_N(k)$. According to Eqs. 10.9.5 and 10.9.14,

$$\begin{bmatrix} \Delta_N(k) & \mathbf{0} & E_{N-1}^b(k-1) \end{bmatrix} = \begin{bmatrix} \mathbf{0} & \boldsymbol{b}_{N-1}^T(k-1) \end{bmatrix} \boldsymbol{R}_{N+1}(k). \tag{10.9.27}$$

Therefore,

$$\Delta_N(k) = \begin{bmatrix} \mathbf{0} & \boldsymbol{b}_{N-1}^T(k-1) \end{bmatrix} \boldsymbol{R}_{N+1}(k) \begin{bmatrix} \boldsymbol{a}_{N-1}(k-1) \\ 0 \end{bmatrix} \tag{10.9.28}$$

since the leading element of $\boldsymbol{a}_{N-1}(k-1)$ is equal to one. Now, recall that the correlation matrix can be time-updated by

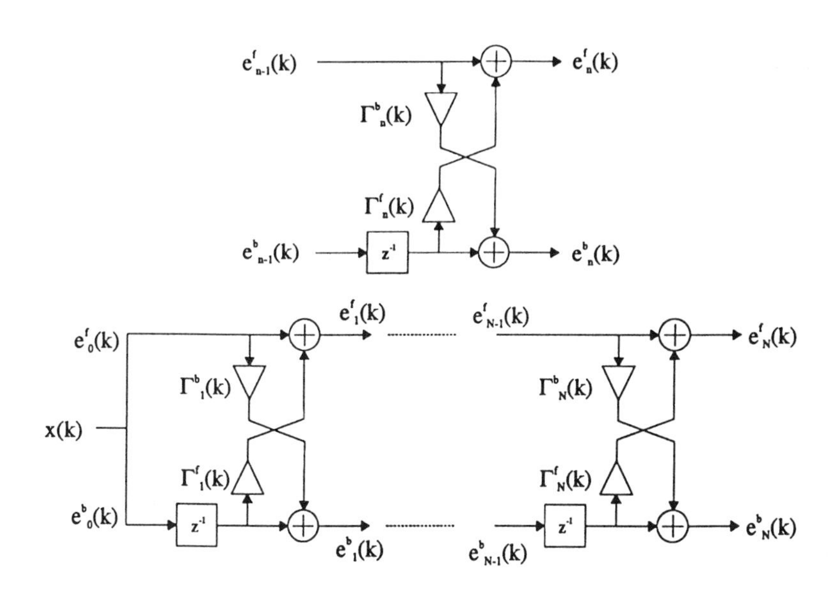

Figure 10.9.1: (a) RLS lattice section; (b) complete RLS lattice predictor.

$$\boldsymbol{R}_{N+1}(k) = W\boldsymbol{R}_{N+1}(k-1) + \boldsymbol{x}_{N+1}(k)\boldsymbol{x}^T_{N+1}(k). \tag{10.9.29}$$

Substituting Eq. 10.9.29 into Eq. 10.9.28, and depending on how we partition $\boldsymbol{x}_{N+1}(k)$, we obtain a pair of time recursions for $\Delta_N(k)$:

$$\Delta_N(k) = W\Delta_N(k-1) + \alpha^f_{N-1}(k)e^b_{N-1}(k-1) \tag{10.9.30}$$

and

$$\Delta_N(k) = W\Delta_N(k-1) + e^f_{N-1}(k)\alpha^b_{N-1}(k-1). \tag{10.9.31}$$

It is clear from either of these equations that $\Delta_N(k)$ is a time-averaged estimate of the crosscorrelation between the forward and delayed backward prediction errors.

10.9.1 Joint Process Estimation

So far, we have developed the equations for the RLS lattice predictor. If the lattice structure is to be used for joint process estimation (*i.e.*, a reference signal is present), we need to incorporate additional parameters into the structure.

The a priori error for the order N RLS filter is given by

$$\alpha_N(k) = d(k) - \boldsymbol{h}_N^T(k-1)\boldsymbol{x}_N(k)$$

where $\boldsymbol{h}_N(k)$ is given by

$$\boldsymbol{R}_N(k)\boldsymbol{h}_N(k) = \boldsymbol{p}_N(k)$$

and

$$\boldsymbol{p}_N(k) = \sum_{i=1}^{k} W^{k-i} d(i)\boldsymbol{x}_N(i).$$

For the filter of order $N+1$, we have

$$\alpha_{N+1}(k) = d(k) - \boldsymbol{h}_{N+1}^T(k-1)\boldsymbol{x}_{N+1}(k)$$

where

$$\boldsymbol{R}_{N+1}(k)\boldsymbol{h}_{N+1}(k+1) = \boldsymbol{p}_{N+1}(k) \tag{10.9.32}$$

and

$$\boldsymbol{p}_{N+1}(k) = \sum_{i=1}^{k} W^{k-i} d(i)\boldsymbol{x}_{N+1}(i).$$

Using the partition

$$\boldsymbol{x}_{N+1}(i) = \begin{bmatrix} \boldsymbol{x}_N(i) \\ x(i-N) \end{bmatrix},$$

it follows that

$$\boldsymbol{p}_{N+1}(k) = \begin{bmatrix} \boldsymbol{p}_N(k) \\ \sum_{i=1}^{k} W^{k-i} d(i)x(i-N) \end{bmatrix}. \tag{10.9.33}$$

We wish to derive an order-update relationship between $\boldsymbol{h}_{N+1}(k)$ and $\boldsymbol{h}_N(k)$ which is similar to either of Eqs. 10.9.3 or 10.9.9. Using the partition of $\boldsymbol{R}_{N+1}(k)$ from Eq. 10.9.2, we can write

$$\boldsymbol{R}_{N+1}(k)\begin{bmatrix} \boldsymbol{h}_N(k) \\ 0 \end{bmatrix} = \begin{bmatrix} \boldsymbol{R}_N(k)\boldsymbol{h}_N(k) \\ \boldsymbol{p}_N^{bT}(k)\boldsymbol{h}_N(k) \end{bmatrix}. \tag{10.9.34}$$

We know that

$$\boldsymbol{R}_N(k)\boldsymbol{h}_N(k) = \boldsymbol{p}_N(k) \tag{10.9.35}$$

Also,

$$\boldsymbol{p}_N^{bT}(k)\boldsymbol{h}_N(k) = \boldsymbol{p}_N^{bT}(k)\boldsymbol{R}_N^{-1}(k)\boldsymbol{p}_N(k),$$

which, using the relationship

$$\boldsymbol{R}_N^{-1}(k)\boldsymbol{p}_N^b(k) = \boldsymbol{h}_N^b(k)$$

becomes

$$\boldsymbol{p}_N^{bT}(k)\boldsymbol{h}_N(k) = \boldsymbol{h}_N^{bT}(k)\boldsymbol{p}_N(k). \tag{10.9.36}$$

Substituting Eqs. 10.9.35 and 10.9.36 into Eq. 10.9.34 yields

$$\boldsymbol{R}_{N+1}(k)\begin{bmatrix} \boldsymbol{h}_N(k) \\ 0 \end{bmatrix} = \begin{bmatrix} \boldsymbol{p}_N(k) \\ \boldsymbol{h}_N^{bT}(k)\boldsymbol{p}_N(k) \end{bmatrix}. \tag{10.9.37}$$

Now, if we subtract Eq. 10.9.37 from Eq. 10.9.32 and use the expression for $\boldsymbol{p}_{N+1}(k)$ in Eq. 10.9.33, we get

$$\boldsymbol{R}_{N+1}(k)\left(\boldsymbol{h}_{N+1}(k) - \begin{bmatrix} \boldsymbol{h}_N(k) \\ 0 \end{bmatrix}\right) = \begin{bmatrix} \boldsymbol{0} \\ K_N^f(k) \end{bmatrix} \tag{10.9.38}$$

where

$$K_N^f(k) = \sum_{i=1}^{k} d(i)x(i-N) - \boldsymbol{h}_N^{bT}(k)\boldsymbol{p}_N(k).$$

It is fairly simple to show using the definition of $\boldsymbol{p}_N(k)$ that $K_N^f(k)$ can also be expressed as

$$K_N^f(k) = \sum_{i=1}^{k} W^{k-i}d(i)[x(i-N) - \boldsymbol{h}_N^{bT}(k)\boldsymbol{x}_N(i)].. \tag{10.9.39}$$

It can be seen from this equation that $K_N^f(k)$ is a time-averaged estimate of the cross correlation between the reference $d(k)$ and the backward prediction error.

Equation 10.9.38 is very similar to the augmented normal equation for backward prediction. In fact, if we multiply both sides of Eq. 10.9.38 by $E_N^b(k)/K_N^f(k)$, we get

$$\boldsymbol{R}_{N+1}(k)\left(\boldsymbol{h}_{N+1}(k) - \begin{bmatrix} \boldsymbol{h}_N(k) \\ 0 \end{bmatrix}\right)\frac{E_N^b(k)}{K_N^f(k)} = \begin{bmatrix} \boldsymbol{0} \\ E_N^b(k) \end{bmatrix} \tag{10.9.40}$$

Equation 10.9.40 is the augmented normal equation for backward prediction, and it follows that

$$\boldsymbol{b}_N(k) = \left(\boldsymbol{h}_{N+1}(k) - \begin{bmatrix} \boldsymbol{h}_N(k) \\ 0 \end{bmatrix}\right)\frac{E_N^b(k)}{K_N^f(k)}$$

so that

$$\boldsymbol{h}_{N+1}(k) = \begin{bmatrix} \boldsymbol{h}_N(k) \\ 0 \end{bmatrix} + \frac{K_N^f(k)}{E_N^b(k)} \boldsymbol{b}_N(k). \tag{10.9.41}$$

In Eqs. 10.9.23–10.9.26, we gave order update equations for the a priori and a posterior prediction errors. When the RLS lattice is used for joint process estimation, we need to provide order recursions for the *filter* a priori and a posteriori estimation errors. The a priori estimation error for order $N+1$ is given by

$$\alpha_{N+1}(k) = d(k) - \boldsymbol{h}_{N+1}^T(k-1)\boldsymbol{x}_{N+1}(k). \tag{10.9.42}$$

Using Eq. 10.9.21 for $\boldsymbol{x}_{N+1}(k)$ and Eq. 10.9.41 for $\boldsymbol{h}_{N+1}(k-1)$, we get

$$\boldsymbol{h}_{N+1}^T(k-1)\boldsymbol{x}_{N+1}(k) = \boldsymbol{h}_N^T(k-1)\boldsymbol{x}_N(k) + \frac{K_N^f(k-1)}{E_N^b(k-1)} \boldsymbol{b}_N^T(k-1)\boldsymbol{x}_{N+1}(k)$$

so that Eq. 10.9.42 becomes

$$\alpha_{N+1}(k) = \alpha_N(k) - \frac{K_N^f(k-1)}{E_N^b(k-1)} \alpha_N^b(k). \tag{10.9.43}$$

The a posteriori estimation of order $N+1$ is given by

$$e_{N+1}(k) = d(k) - \boldsymbol{h}_{N+1}^T(k)\boldsymbol{x}_{N+1}(k),$$

which, in a manner similar to the a priori estimation error, can be expressed as

$$e_{N+1}(k) = e_N(k) - \frac{K_N^f(k)}{E_N^b(k)} e_N^b(k). \tag{10.9.44}$$

Define the quantity $c_N(k)$ by

$$c_N(k) = \frac{K_N^f(k)}{E_N^b(k)}.$$

Then we can rewrite Eqs. 10.9.43 and 10.9.44 respectively as

$$\alpha_{N+1}(k) = \alpha_N(k) - c_N(k-1)\alpha_N^b(k) \tag{10.9.45}$$

and

$$e_{N+1}(k) = e_N(k) - c_N(k)e_N^b(k). \tag{10.9.46}$$

The estimation error energy can also be order-updated. Recall that the RLS estimation error energy can computed according to

$$E_N(k) = \sigma_d^2 - \boldsymbol{h}_N^T(k)\boldsymbol{R}_N(k)\ h_N(k) = \sigma_d^2 - \boldsymbol{h}_N^T(k)\boldsymbol{p}_N(k). \tag{10.9.47}$$

Thus, for order $N+1$, we have

$$E_{N+1}(k) = \sigma_d^2 - \boldsymbol{h}_{N+1}^T(k)\boldsymbol{R}_{N+1}(k)\boldsymbol{h}_{N+1}(k). \tag{10.9.48}$$

Using Eqs. 10.9.41 and 10.9.2, we have

$$\boldsymbol{R}_{N+1}(k)\boldsymbol{h}_{N+1}(k) = \begin{bmatrix} \boldsymbol{p}_N(k) \\ \boldsymbol{p}_N^{bT}(k)\boldsymbol{h}_N(k) \end{bmatrix} + \frac{K_N^f(k)}{E_N^b(k)} \begin{bmatrix} \boldsymbol{0} \\ E_N^b(k) \end{bmatrix}. \tag{10.9.49}$$

Next, premultiplying Eq. 10.9.49 by $\boldsymbol{h}_{N+1}^T(k)$ as given by Eq. 10.9.41 yields, after some simplification

$$\boldsymbol{h}_{N+1}^T(k)\boldsymbol{R}_{N+1}(k)\boldsymbol{h}_{N+1}(k) = \boldsymbol{h}_N^T(k)\boldsymbol{p}_N(k) + \frac{(K_N^f(k))^2}{E_N^b(k)}. \tag{10.9.50}$$

Therefore, Eq. 10.9.48 becomes

$$E_{N+1}(k) = \sigma_d^2(k) - \boldsymbol{h}_N^T(k)\boldsymbol{p}_N(k) + \frac{(K_N^f(k))^2}{E_N^b(k)}.$$

Using Eq. 10.9.47, this becomes

$$E_{N+1}(k) = E_N(k) - \frac{(K_N^f(k))^2}{E_N^b(k)}. \tag{10.9.51}$$

Equation 10.9.51 gives us the relationship we seek: the estimation error energy for order $N+1$ as a function of the estimation error energy for order N.

The *conversion factor* $\varphi_N(k)$ is an important quantity in the RLS lattice filter since it allows a posteriori errors to be computed from a priori errors. We showed that the conversion factor could be computed from the adaptation gain according to

$$\varphi_N(k) = \frac{e_N(k)}{\alpha_N(k)} = 1 - \boldsymbol{g}_N^T(k)\boldsymbol{x}_N(k). \tag{10.9.52}$$

We also saw that the adaptation gain could be order-updated by

$$\boldsymbol{g}_N(k) = \begin{bmatrix} \boldsymbol{g}_{N-1}(k) \\ 0 \end{bmatrix} + \frac{e_{N-1}^b(k)}{E_{N-1}^b(k)}\boldsymbol{b}_{N-1}(k). \tag{10.9.53}$$

Partitioning $\boldsymbol{x}_N(k)$ as

$$\boldsymbol{x}_N(k) = \begin{bmatrix} \boldsymbol{x}_{N-1}(k) \\ x(k-N+1) \end{bmatrix},$$

we can use Eq. 10.9.53 to yield

$$1 - \boldsymbol{g}_N^T(k)\boldsymbol{x}_N(k) = 1 - \boldsymbol{g}_{N-1}^T(k)\boldsymbol{x}_{N-1}(k) - \frac{e_{N-1}^b(k)}{E_{N-1}^b(k)}\boldsymbol{b}_{N-1}^T(k)\boldsymbol{x}_N(k). \tag{10.9.54}$$

Recognizing that

$$\boldsymbol{b}_{N-1}^T(k)\boldsymbol{x}_N(k) = e_{N-1}^b(k)$$

and applying the relationship in Eq. 10.9.52 to both sides of Eq. 10.9.54 immediately gives

$$\varphi_N(k) = \varphi_{N-1}(k) - \frac{(e_{N-1}^b(k))^2}{E_{N-1}^b(k)}. \tag{10.9.55}$$

This recursion for $\varphi_N(k)$ is order-initialized according to

$$\varphi_0(k) = \frac{\alpha_0(k)}{e_0(k)} = 1.$$

10.9.2 RLS Lattice Properties

Recall that the lattice Wiener filter had the property of *uncorrelated* backward prediction errors. The backward prediction errors in the RLS lattice are also uncorrelated, but in a time-averaged sense. To show this, we denote by $\boldsymbol{B}(i)$ the vector of a posteriori backward prediction errors,

$$\boldsymbol{B}(i) = \begin{bmatrix} e_0^b(i) \\ e_1^b(i) \\ \vdots \\ e_N^b(i) \end{bmatrix}.$$

It follows immediately that $B(i)$ can be formed from the input vector $\boldsymbol{x}_{N+1}(i)$ according to

$$\boldsymbol{B}(i) = \boldsymbol{L}(k)\boldsymbol{x}_{N+1}(i) \tag{10.9.56}$$

where $\boldsymbol{L}(k)$ is a matrix which consists of the backward prediction filters of all intermediate orders. That is,

$$L(k) = \begin{bmatrix} 1 & 0 & \cdots & 0 \\ -h^b_{1,1}(k) & 1 & \cdots & 0 \\ \vdots & \vdots & \ddots & \vdots \\ -h^b_{N,1}(k) & -h^b_{N,2}(k) & \cdots & 1 \end{bmatrix}. \tag{10.9.57}$$

The time-averaged correlation matrix for $\boldsymbol{B}(k)$ is given by

$$\boldsymbol{Q}(k) = \sum_{i=1}^{k} W^{k-i} \boldsymbol{B}(i)\boldsymbol{B}^T(i),$$

and using the relationship in Eq. 10.9.57, we get

$$\boldsymbol{Q}(k) = \boldsymbol{L}(k)\boldsymbol{R}_{N+1}(k)\boldsymbol{L}^T(k). \tag{10.9.58}$$

Consider the product of $\boldsymbol{R}_{N+1}(k)$ and $\boldsymbol{L}^T(k)$. The m-th principal minor of $\boldsymbol{R}_{N+1}(k)$ is $\boldsymbol{R}_m(k)$ and the m-th column of $\boldsymbol{L}^T(k)$ is $\boldsymbol{b}_{m-1}(k)$. Therefore, the product of $\boldsymbol{R}_{N+1}(k)$ and the m-th column of $\boldsymbol{L}^T(k)$ contains the augmented normal equation for order-m backward prediction. Overall, we find that

$$\boldsymbol{R}_{N+1}(k)\boldsymbol{L}^T(k) = \begin{bmatrix} E^b_0(k) & 0 & 0 & \cdots & 0 \\ \times & E^b_1(k) & 0 & \cdots & 0 \\ \times & \times & E^b_2(k) & \cdots & 0 \\ \vdots & \vdots & \vdots & \ddots & \vdots \\ \times & \times & \times & \cdots & E^b_N(k) \end{bmatrix} \tag{10.9.59}$$

where $\times$ indicates "don't care." Next, taking the product of $\boldsymbol{L}(k)$ as given by Eq. 10.9.57 and $\boldsymbol{R}_{N+1}(k)\boldsymbol{L}^T(k)$ as given by Eq. 10.9.59, we have

$$\boldsymbol{Q}(k) = \boldsymbol{L}(k)\boldsymbol{R}_{N+1}(k)\boldsymbol{L}^T(k) = \begin{bmatrix} E^b_0(k) & 0 & 0 & \cdots & 0 \\ 0 & E^b_1(k) & 0 & \cdots & 0 \\ 0 & 0 & E^b_2(k) & \cdots & 0 \\ \vdots & \vdots & \vdots & \ddots & \vdots \\ 0 & 0 & 0 & \cdots & E^b_N(k) \end{bmatrix} \tag{10.9.60}$$

This shows that the backward a posteriori prediction errors are uncorrelated. In particular, since $e^b_o(k) = x(k)$, the backward prediction errors are also uncorrelated with the input.

Next, we can establish a connection between the ladder parameters $c_i(k)$ and the solution to the transversal RLS problem. Recall that the transversal RLS solution $\boldsymbol{h}_{N+1}(k)$ satisfies

$$\boldsymbol{R}_{N+1}\boldsymbol{h}_{N+1}(k) = \boldsymbol{p}_{N+1}(k). \tag{10.9.61}$$

Let $\boldsymbol{c}_N(k)$ denote the vector of ladder parameters,

$$\boldsymbol{c}_(k) = \begin{bmatrix} c_o(k) \\ c_1(k) \\ \vdots \\ c_N(k) \end{bmatrix}.$$

The $c_i(k)$ are chosen to weight the backward a posteriori prediction errors in such a manner that the performance index

$$J(k) = \sum_{i=1}^{k} W^{k-i}[d(i) - \boldsymbol{c}_N^T(k)\boldsymbol{B}(i)]^2$$

is minimized at each instant k. In direct analogy with the transversal RLS problem, the vector is found by solving

$$\left[\sum_{i=1}^{k} W^{k-i}\boldsymbol{B}(i)\boldsymbol{B}^T(i)\right] \boldsymbol{c}_N(k) = \sum_{i=1}^{k} W^{k-i}d(i)\boldsymbol{B}(i). \tag{10.9.62}$$

The summation on the left is immediately recognized as $\boldsymbol{Q}(k)$. Using Eq. 10.9.56, we can write the summation on the right-hand side of Eq. 10.9.62 as

$$\sum_{i=1}^{k} W^{k-i}d(i)\boldsymbol{B}(i) = \boldsymbol{L}(k)\sum_{i=1}^{k} W^{k-i}d(i)\boldsymbol{x}_{N+1}(i) = \boldsymbol{L}(k)\boldsymbol{p}_{N+1}(k).$$

Thus, Eq. 10.9.62 becomes

$$\boldsymbol{Q}(k)\boldsymbol{c}_N(k) = \boldsymbol{L}(k)\boldsymbol{p}_{N+1}(k)$$

which has the solution

$$\boldsymbol{c}_N(k) = \boldsymbol{Q}^{-1}(k)\boldsymbol{L}(k)\boldsymbol{p}_{N+1}(k). \tag{10.9.63}$$

Using Eq. 10.9.60, we can rewrite Eq. 10.9.63 as

$$\boldsymbol{c}_N(k) = [L(k)\boldsymbol{R}_{N+1}(k)\boldsymbol{L}^T(k)]^{-1}\boldsymbol{L}(k)\boldsymbol{p}_{N+1}(k).$$

The matrix $\boldsymbol{L}(k)$ is surely invertible since it has a determinant which is equal to one. Therefore, we get

$$\boldsymbol{c}_N(k) = (\boldsymbol{L}^T(k))^{-1}\boldsymbol{R}_{N+1}^{-1}(k)\boldsymbol{p}_{N+1}(k)$$

which is equivalent to

$$\boldsymbol{c}_N(k) = (\boldsymbol{L}^T(k))^{-1}\boldsymbol{h}_{N+1}(k). \tag{10.9.64}$$

This relationship further implies that the transversal solution can be computed from the ladder parameters according to

$$\boldsymbol{h}_{N+1}(k) = \boldsymbol{L}^T(k)\boldsymbol{c}_N(k). \tag{10.9.65}$$

We can also derive a time recursion for $K_N^f(k)$. Recall from Eq. 10.9.39 that

$$\boldsymbol{K}_N^f(k) = \sum_{i=1}^{k} W^{k-i} d(i)[x(i-N) - \boldsymbol{h}_N^{bT}(k)\boldsymbol{x}_N(i)]. \tag{10.9.66}$$

We know that the backward predictor is updated according to

$$\boldsymbol{h}_N^b(k) = \boldsymbol{h}_N^b(k-1) + \boldsymbol{g}_N(k)\alpha_N^b(k)$$

so that after some manipulation, Eq. 10.9.66 becomes

$$K_N^f(k) = WK_N^f(k-1) + \alpha_N^b(k)[d(k) - \boldsymbol{g}_N^T(k)\boldsymbol{p}_N(k)]. \tag{10.9.67}$$

Using the fact that $\boldsymbol{g}_N(k) = \boldsymbol{R}_N^{-1}(k)\boldsymbol{p}_N(k)$, we have

$$d(k) - \boldsymbol{g}_N^T(k)\boldsymbol{p}_N(k) = d(k) - \boldsymbol{x}_N^T(k)\boldsymbol{h}_N(k) = e_N(k)$$

which means that

$$K_N^f(k) = WK_N^f(k-1) + e_N(k)\alpha_N^b(k). \tag{10.9.68}$$

According to Eq. 10.9.68, $K_N^f(k)$ is a time-averaged estimate of the crosscorrelation between the filter output error and the backward prediction error. Earlier, we showed that $K_N^f(k)$ is an estimate of the crosscorrelation between the reference and the backward prediction error. The compatibility between these two interpretations lies in the fact that the backward prediction errors are uncorrelated with the input in a time-averaged sense.

At this point, we can now describe the least squares lattice algorithm based on a posteriori errors [ML78]. It is important to recall that a posteriori error can be obtained from a priori errors through the relationships

$$\varphi_N(k-1) = \frac{e_N^f(k-1)}{\alpha_N^f(k-1)}, \quad \varphi_N(k) = \frac{e_N^b(k)}{\alpha_N^b(k)}, \quad \varphi_N(k) = \frac{e_N(k)}{\alpha_N(k)}.$$

The variables for this algorithm must be initialized in both time and in order. We can begin with the reflection and ladder coefficients all equal to zero for each lattice stage. That is,

$$\Gamma_i^f(0) = \Gamma_i^b(0) = c_i(0) = 0.$$

Furthermore, the prediction error energies are set to a small constant,

$$E_i^f(0) = E_i^b(0) = \delta,$$

where again the exact choice of δ is unimportant in the long run. Also, the initial conversion factor is chosen as

$$\varphi_0(0) = 1.$$

This completes the order initializations. For the time recursions, the zeroth-order a priori prediction errors are initialized as

$$\alpha_0^f(k) = \alpha_0^b(k) = x(k)$$

and the zeroth-order filter a priori error is initialized as

$$\alpha_0(k) = d(k).$$

The zeroth-order prediction error energies are set equal to the running average of the input signal power according to

$$E_0^f(k) = E_0^b(k) = WE_0^f(k-1) + x^2(k)$$

and the zeroth-order conversion factor is given by

$$\varphi_0(k) = 1.$$

Summary

Recursive LSL algorithm based on a posteriori errors

Prediction section: for $i = 1, 2, \ldots, N$

$$\Delta_i(k) = W\Delta_i(k-1) + \frac{e_{i-1}^f(k)e_{i-1}^b(k-1)}{\varphi_{i-1}(k-1)}$$

$$\Gamma_i^f(k) = -\frac{\Delta_i(k)}{E_{i-1}^b(k-1)}$$

$$\Gamma_i^b(k) = -\frac{\Delta_i(k)}{E_{i-1}^f(k)}$$

$$e_i^f(k) = e_{i-1}^f(k) + \Gamma_i^f(k)e_{i-1}^b(k-1)$$

$$e_i^b(k) = e_{i-1}^b(k-1) + \Gamma_i^b(k)e_{i-1}^f(k)$$

$$E_i^f(k) = E_{i-1}^f(k) - \frac{\Delta_i^2(k)}{E_{i-1}^b(k-1)}$$

$$E_i^b(k) = E_{i-1}^b(k) - \frac{\Delta_i^2(k)}{E_{i-1}^f(k)}$$

$$\varphi_i(k) = \varphi_{i-1}(k) - \frac{(e_{i-1}^b(k))^2}{E_{i-1}^b(k)}$$

Filtering section: for $i = 1, 2, \ldots, N$

$$K_i^f(k) = WK_i^f(k-1) + \frac{e_i(k)e_i^b(k)}{\varphi_i(k)}$$

$$c_i(k) = \frac{K_i^f(k)}{E_i^b(k)}$$

$$e_{i+1}(k) = e_i(k) - c_i(k)e_i^b(k)$$

Initializations:

$$\Gamma_i^f(0) = \Gamma_i^b(0) = c_i(0) = 0.$$

$$E_i^f(0) = E_i^b(0) = \delta,$$

$$\varphi_0(0) = 1.$$

$$\alpha_0^f(k) = \alpha_0^b(k) = x(k)$$

$$\alpha_0(k) = d(k).$$

$$E_0^f(k) = E_0^b(k) = WE_0^f(k-1) + x^2(k)$$

$$\varphi_0(k) = 1.$$

$$e_0(k) = d(k)$$

The lattice filter which performs joint process estimation based on a posteriori errors is shown in Fig. 10.9.2. There is also an algorithm for the lattice structure which is based on a priori errors rather than a posteriori errors [LMP85]. The algorithm is described by the following summary.

Summary

Recursive LSL algorithm based on a priori errors

Prediction section: for $i = 1, 2, \ldots, N$

$$\alpha_i^f(k) = \alpha_{i-1}^f(k) + \Gamma_i^f(k-1)\alpha_{i-1}^b(k-1)$$

$$\alpha_i^b(k) = \alpha_{i-1}^b(k-1) + \Gamma_i^b(k-1)\alpha_{i-1}^f(k)$$

$$\Delta_i(k) = W\Delta_i(k-1) + \alpha_{i-1}^f(k)\varphi_{i-1}(k-1)\alpha_{i-1}^b(k-1)$$

$$\Gamma_i^f(k) = -\frac{\Delta_i(k)}{E_{i-1}^b(k-1)}$$

$$E_{i-1}^b(k) = WE_{i-1}^b(k-1) + \varphi_{i-1}(k)[\alpha_i^b(k)]^2$$

$$E_{i-1}^f(k) = WE_{i-1}^f(k-1) + \varphi_{i-1}(k-1)[\alpha_{i-1}^f(k)]^2$$

$$\Gamma_i^b(k) = -\frac{\Delta_i(k)}{E_{i-1}^f(k)}$$

$$\varphi_i(k) = \varphi_{i-1}(k) - \frac{[\varphi_{i-1}(k)\alpha_{i-1}^b(k)]^2}{E_{i-1}^b(k)}$$

Filtering section: for $i = 1, 2, \ldots, N$

$$K_i^f(k) = WK_i^f(k-1) + \varphi_i(k)\alpha_i^b(k)\alpha_i(k)$$

$$\alpha_{i+1}(k) = \alpha_i(k) - c_i(k-1)\alpha_i^b(k)$$

$$E_i^b(k) = E_{i-1}^b(k) - \frac{\Delta_i^2(k)}{E_{i-1}^f(k)}$$

$$c_i(k) = \frac{K_i^f(k)}{E_i^b(k)}$$

Initializations:

$$\Gamma_i^f(0) = \Gamma_i^b(0) = c_i(0) = 0.$$

$$E_i^f(0) = E_i^b(0) = \delta,$$

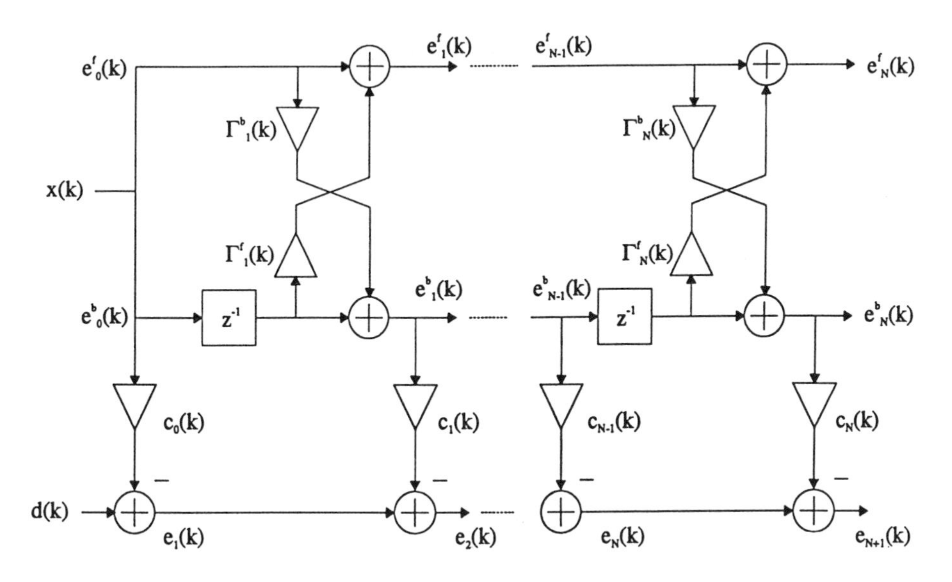

Figure 10.9.2: Lattice structure based on a posteriori errors.

$$\varphi_0(0) = 1.$$

$$\alpha_0^f(k) = \alpha_0^b(k) = x(k)$$

$$\alpha_0(k) = d(k).$$

$$E_0^f(k) = E_0^b(k) = WE_0^f(k-1) + x^2(k)$$

$$\varphi_0(k) = 1.$$

The RLS lattice filter using a priori errors is shown in Fig. 10.9.3.

The RLS lattice algorithms using a priori and a posteriori errors are sensitive to numerical error. One reason for this is that the reflection coefficients and ladder parameters are updated indirectly through $\Delta_N(k)$ and $K_N^f(k)$. A more well-behaved algorithm results if we can update these parameters directly. The resulting algorithm is called the least-squares lattice algorithm based on a priori errors with error feedback [LMP85], for reasons which will soon become apparent.

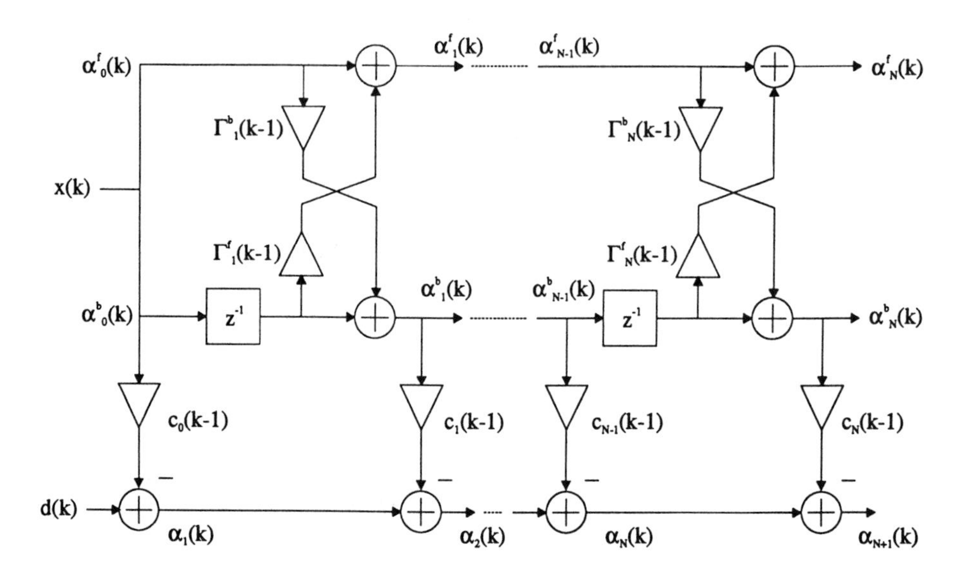

Figure 10.9.3: Lattice structure based on a priori errors.

We wish to derive time recursions for the reflection coefficients. We defined $\Gamma^f_N(k)$ by

$$\Gamma^f_N(k) = -\frac{\Delta_N(k)}{E^b_{N-1}(k-1)}.$$

Therefore,

$$E^b_{N-1}(k-1)\Gamma^f_N(k) = -\Delta_N(k). \tag{10.9.69}$$

Using Eq. 10.9.30 for time $k+1$, we have

$$\Delta_N(k+1) = W\Delta_N(k) + e^b_{N-1}(k)\alpha^f_{N-1}(k+1)$$

which means that

$$\Delta_N(k) = W^{-1}[\Delta_N(k+1) - e^b_{N-1}(k)\alpha^f_{N-1}(k+1)]. \tag{10.9.70}$$

Recall that the backward prediction error energy can be time-updated by the recursion

$$E^b_{N-1}(k) = WE^b_{N-1}(k-1) + e^b_{N-1}(k)\alpha^b_{N-1}(k)$$

so that

$$E^b_{N-1}(k-1) = W^{-1}[E^b_{N-1}(k) - e^b_{N-1}(k)\alpha^b_{N-1}(k)]. \tag{10.9.71}$$

Substituting Eqs. 10.9.70 and 10.9.71 into Eq. 10.9.69 gives

$$[E^b_{N-1}(k-1) - e^b_{N-1}(k)\alpha^b_{N-1}(k)]\Gamma^f_N(k) = -\Delta_N(k+1) + e^b_{N-1}(k)\alpha^f_{N-1}(k+1). \tag{10.9.72}$$

By definition, we have

$$\Gamma^f_N(k+1) = -\frac{\Delta_N(k+1)}{E^b_{N-1}(k)},$$

and after some simplification, Eq. 10.9.72 becomes

$$\Gamma^f_N(k+1) = \Gamma^f_N(k) - \frac{e^b_{N-1}(k)}{E^b_{N-1}(k)}[\alpha^f_{N-1}(k+1) + \Gamma^f_N(k)\alpha^b_{N-1}(k)]. \tag{10.9.73}$$

According to Eq. 10.9.25,

$$\alpha^f_N(k+1) = \alpha^f_{N-1}(k+1) + \Gamma^f_N(k)\alpha^b_{N-1}(k)$$

and Eq. 10.9.73 reduces to

$$\Gamma^f_N(k+1) = \Gamma^f_N(k) - \frac{e^b_{N-1}(k)\alpha^f_N(k+1)}{E^b_{N-1}(k)}. \tag{10.9.74}$$

In a similar manner, we can show that the time-update for the backward reflection coefficients is

$$\Gamma^b_N(k+1) = \Gamma^b_N(k) - \frac{e^f_{N-1}(k+1)\alpha^b_N(k+1)}{E^f_{N-1}(k+1)}. \tag{10.9.75}$$

Equations 10.9.74 and 10.9.75 can be written for time k as

$$\Gamma^f_N(k) = \Gamma^f_N(k-1) - \frac{e^b_{N-1}(k-1)\alpha^f_N(k)}{E^b_{N-1}(k-1)}. \tag{10.9.76}$$

and

$$\Gamma^b_N(k) = \Gamma^b_N(k-1) - \frac{e^f_{N-1}(k)\alpha^b_N(k)}{E^f_{N-1}(k)}. \tag{10.9.77}$$

Finally, we wish to derive time-recursions for the output section of the lattice. Define the quantity $c_N(k)$ by

$$c_N(k) = \frac{K_N^f(k)}{E_N^b(k)}. \tag{10.9.78}$$

Therefore,

$$E_N^b(k-1)c_N(k-1) = K_N^f(k-1). \tag{10.9.79}$$

Equation 10.9.68 can be rearranged to give

$$K_N^f(k-1) = W^{-1}[K_N^f(k) - e_N(k)\alpha_N^b(k)] \tag{10.9.80}$$

and the backward prediction error energy updating equation can be rearranged to give

$$E_N^b(k-1) = W^{-1}[E_N^b(k) - e_N^b(k)\alpha_N^b(k)]. \tag{10.9.81}$$

Substituting Eqs. 10.9.81 and 10.9.80 into Eq. 10.9.79, we have

$$[E_N^b(k) - e_N^b(k)\alpha_N^b(k)]c_N(k-1) = K_N^f(k) - e_N(k)\alpha_N^b(k)$$

which means that

$$K_N^f(k) = [E_N^b(k) - e_N^b(k)\alpha_N^b(k)]c_N(k-1) + e_N(k)\alpha_N^b(k). \tag{10.9.82}$$

Using Eq. 10.9.78, both sides of Eq. 10.9.82 are divided by $E_N^b(k)$ giving

$$c_N(k) = c_N(k-1) + \frac{\alpha_N^b(k)}{E_N^b(k)}[e_N(k) - c_N(k-1)e_N^b(k)]. \tag{10.9.83}$$

Using the conversion factor $\varphi_N(k)$, can be expressed as

$$e_N(k) - c_N(k-1)e_N^b(k) = \varphi_N(k)\left[\alpha_N(k) - c_N(k-1)\alpha_N^b(k)\right].$$

Equation 10.9.43 says that

$$\alpha_{N+1}(k) = \alpha_N(k) - c_N(k-1)\alpha_N^b(k)$$

so that

$$e_N(k) - c_N(k-1)e_N^b(k) = \varphi\alpha_{N+1}(k).$$

Therefore, Eq. 10.9.83 becomes

$$c_N(k) = c_N(k-1) + \frac{\varphi_N(k)\alpha_N^b(k)\alpha_{N+1}(k)}{E_N^b(k)}. \tag{10.9.84}$$

The reason we use the term *error feedback* in the description of the algorithm is that the a priori errors (prediction and filtering) are fed back in order to time-update the reflection and ladder coefficients.

Summary

Recursive LSL algorithm based on a priori errors with error feedback

Prediction section: for $i = 1, 2, \ldots, N$ where N is the order of the lattice, compute

$$\alpha_i^f(k) = \alpha_{i-1}^f(k) + \Gamma_i^f(k-1)\alpha_{i-1}^b(k-1)$$

$$\alpha_i^b(k) = \alpha_{i-1}^b(k-1) + \Gamma_i^b(k-1)\alpha_{i-1}^f(k)$$

$$\Gamma_i^f(k) = \Gamma_i^f(k-1) - \frac{\varphi_{i-1}(k)\alpha_{i-1}^b(k-1)\alpha_i^f(k)}{E_{i-1}^b(k-1)}$$

$$E_{i-1}^f(k) = WE_{i-1}^f(k-1) + \varphi_{i-1}(k-1)[\alpha_{i-1}^f(k)]^2$$

$$E_{i-1}^b(k) = WE_{i-1}^b(k-1) + \varphi_{i-1}(k)[\alpha_i^b(k)]^2$$

$$\Gamma_i^b(k) = \Gamma_i^b(k-1) - \frac{\varphi_{i-1}(k-1)\alpha_{i-1}^f(k)\alpha_i^b(k)}{E_{i-1}^f(k)}$$

$$\varphi_i(k) = \varphi_{i-1}(k) - \frac{[\varphi_{i-1}(k)\alpha_{i-1}^b(k)]^2}{E_{i-1}^b(k)}$$

Filtering section: for $i = 1, 2, \ldots, N$

$$\alpha_{i+1}(k) = \alpha_i(k) - \mathbf{c}_i(k-1)\alpha_i^b(k)$$

$$c_i(k) = c_i(k-1) + \frac{\varphi_i(k)\alpha_i^b(k)\alpha_{i+1}(k)}{E_i^b(k)}$$

Initializations:

$$\Gamma_i^f(0) = \Gamma_i^b(0) = c_i(0) = 0.$$

$$E_i^f(0) = E_i^b(0) = \delta,$$

$$\varphi_0(0) = 1.$$

$$\alpha_0^f(k) = \alpha_0^b(k) = x(k)$$

$$\alpha_0(k) = d(k).$$

$$E_0^f(k) = E_0^b(k) = WE_0^f(k-1) + x^2(k)$$

$$\varphi_0(k) = 1.$$

As a note to the user, the computational complexity of the various lattice-ladder algorithms we have discussed is between $15N$ and $20N$. For even modest filter orders N, this is considerably better than the order N^2 complexity of direct RLS implementation, but not quite as good as some of the transversal FLS algorithms we highlighted. Experience will show that the choice of which algorithm or structure to use is situation-dependent. Typically, the demands of real-time will dictate that direct RLS is an impossibility and that some fast algorithm must be used. If a fixed-point processor is used, most of the transversal FLS algorithms will be too sensitive to finite-precision effects, unless a large wordwidth or multiple precision arithmetic can be used. Floating-point arithmetic can not always be looked upon as a cure-all either; it too suffers from finite precision effects (the mantissa is usually 24 bits in most DSP processors) and some of the transversal FLS algorithms may still fail. Therefore, the RLS lattice-ladder algorithms serve an important purpose; they are numerically robust algorithms for recursive least squares adaptation with fairly low computational complexity.

Chapter 11

POWER SPECTRUM ESTIMATION

11.1 Introduction

Many of the important results in Wiener and adaptive filtering assume that the power spectrum, or equivalently, the autocorrelation sequence, is known. In practice, these quantities need to be estimated. The power spectrum is a quantity which depends on the *ensemble* characteristics of a stochastic process; it depends on the ensemble of realizations. In practice, an estimate of the power spectrum must be made from a finite number of realizations of the process, or in the extreme case, a *single* measured time series of the process.

There are a number of techniques for spectral estimation. These techniques can be grouped, more or less, into two categories: nonparametric and parametric. Nonparametric techniques make no assumption about the underlying model for the stochastic process and instead estimate the power spectrum directly from the observed data. We will see that the nonparametric techniques tend to provide a spectral estimate which is not as good as that obtained using parametric techniques, which *do* make assumptions about the underlying model.

We will study a number of nonparametric and parametric spectral estimators. While we make no claim of thoroughness, the techniques we cover are the ones which are most commonly found in use in practice. In particular, we will examine periodogram techniques, which are popular nonparametric spectral estimators, and autoregressive techniques, which are powerful parametric spectral estimators. The chapter will conclude with a brief look at some *high resolution* spectral estimation techniques which are based on the singular value decomposition (SVD). SVD methods have shown great promise in array signal processing and have been a topic of much study in recent years.

Concisely stated, the problem is as follows. It is assumed that $\{x(k)\}$ is a WSS stochastic process with autocorrelation sequence $\{r_{xx}(k)\}$ where

$$r_{xx}(k) = \mathcal{E}[x(n)x(n+k)].$$

and power spectrum given by

$$P_{xx}(\theta) = \sum_{k=-\infty}^{\infty} r_{xx}(k)e^{-jk\theta}. \tag{11.1.1}$$

Given a finite collection

$$\{x_1(k)\}, \{x_2(k)\}, \ldots, \{x_R(k)\}$$

of realizations of $\{x(k)\}$, we would like to form an estimate $\hat{P}_{xx}(\theta)$ of the true power spectrum $P_{xx}(\theta)$.

The power spectrum may be expressed in the convenient form

$$P_{xx}(\theta) = \lim_{M\to\infty} \mathcal{E}\left[\frac{1}{2M+1}\left|\sum_{k=-M}^{M} x(k)e^{-jk\theta}\right|^2\right]. \tag{11.1.2}$$

That this is so may be demonstrated by writing

$$\left|\sum_{k=-M}^{M} x(k)e^{-jk\theta}\right|^2 = \sum_{k=-M}^{M}\sum_{l=-M}^{M} x(k)x(l)e^{-j(k-l)\theta}.$$

Thus,

$$\mathcal{E}\left[\left|\sum_{k=-M}^{M} x(k)e^{-jk\theta}\right|^2\right] = \sum_{k=-M}^{M}\sum_{l=-M}^{M} r_{xx}(k-l)e^{-j(k-l)\theta},$$

which we can express equivalently as

$$\mathcal{E}\left[\left|\sum_{k=-M}^{M} x(k)e^{-jk\theta}\right|^2\right] = \sum_{m=-2M}^{2M} (2M+1-|m|)r_{xx}(m)e^{-jm\theta}. \tag{11.1.3}$$

Substituting Eq. 11.1.3 into Eq. 11.1.2, we get

$$\lim_{M\to\infty} \mathcal{E}\left[\frac{1}{2M+1}\left|\sum_{k=-M}^{M} x(k)e^{-jk\theta}\right|^2\right] = \lim_{M\to\infty}\sum_{m=-2M}^{2M}\left[1-\frac{|m|}{2M+1}\right] r_{xx}(m)e^{-jm\theta}. \tag{11.1.4}$$

If the autocorrelation sequence satisfies

$$\lim_{M\to\infty}\sum_{m=-2M}^{2M} |m| r_{xx}(m) = 0, \tag{11.1.5}$$

then Eq. 11.1.2 becomes

$$\lim_{M\to\infty} \mathcal{E}\left[\frac{1}{2M+1}\left|\sum_{k=-M}^{M} x(k)e^{-jk\theta}\right|^2\right] = \sum_{m=-\infty}^{\infty} r_{xx}(m)e^{-jm\theta} = P_{xx}(\theta),$$

proving the validity of Eq. 11.1.2. The condition in Eq. 11.1.5 means that the autocorrelation sequence has a "sufficient" rate of decay. This condition is typically met by stochastic processes with zero mean and no sinusoidal components. If this is not true, the definition of power spectrum can be broadened to include Dirac delta functions.

11.2 Estimators

Let $x(k)$ be a sequence of observations given by

$$x(k) = \theta + n(k) \tag{11.2.1}$$

where θ is a constant and $\{n(k)\}$ is a zero-mean white noise process with power σ_n^2. We would like to *estimate* θ from a collection of N observations of $\{x(k)\}$. Define the *estimator* $\hat{\theta}_N$ by

$$\hat{\theta}_N = \frac{1}{N}\sum_{k=0}^{N-1} x(k). \tag{11.2.2}$$

It should be noted that $\hat{\theta}$ is a random variable because of the randomness of each $x(k)$. The expected value of $\hat{\theta}_N$ is given by

$$\mathcal{E}[\hat{\theta}_N] = \frac{1}{N}\sum_{i=0}^{N-1} \mathcal{E}[\theta + n(k)] = \theta$$

because of the zero-mean assumption imposed on $\{n(k)\}$. The estimator $\hat{\theta}_N$ is called *unbiased* because

$$\mathcal{E}[\hat{\theta}_N] = \theta,$$

i.e., the expected value of the estimator is equal to the parameter it is trying to estimate. In general, we define the *bias* of an estimator $\hat{\theta}$ as

$$B(\hat{\theta}) = \theta - \mathcal{E}[\hat{\theta}]. \tag{11.2.3}$$

Clearly, then, an unbiased estimator satisfies

$$B(\hat{\theta}) = 0.$$

The variance of an estimator gives a measure of its spread about its mean. For the estimator to be useful, we expect intuitively that its variance should be small. By definition,

$$var(\hat{\theta}) = \mathcal{E}[(\hat{\theta} - \mathcal{E}[\hat{\theta}])^2]. \tag{11.2.4}$$

The variance of the estimator merely expresses the dispersion of the estimator about *its* mean, not about the true parameter θ. For unbiased estimators, the variance also measures the dispersion of the estimator about the parameter θ since the variance reduces to

$$var(\hat{\theta}) = \mathcal{E}[(\hat{\theta} - \theta)^2]. \tag{11.2.5}$$

We define the *mean-squared error*, $M(\hat{\theta})$, by

$$M(\hat{\theta}) = \mathcal{E}[(\hat{\theta} - \theta)^2]. \tag{11.2.6}$$

For unbiased estimators, the mean-squared error and the variance are identical. For biased estimators, it is simple to show from Eqs. 11.2.4, 11.2.6, and 11.2.3 that

$$M(\hat{\theta}) = var(\hat{\theta}) + B^2(\hat{\theta}).$$

Let's look at the variance of our estimator $\hat{\theta}_N$ from Eq. 11.2.2. Since $\hat{\theta}_N$ is unbiased, we have from Eq. 11.2.5

$$var(\hat{\theta}_N) = \mathcal{E}[(\hat{\theta}_N - \theta)^2].$$

According to Eqs. 11.2.1 and 11.2.2,

$$(\hat{\theta}_N - \theta)^2 = \left(\frac{1}{N}\sum_{k=0}^{N-1} x(k) - \theta\right)^2 = \frac{1}{N^2}\sum_{k=0}^{N-1}\sum_{l=0}^{N-1} n(k)n(l). \tag{11.2.7}$$

By assumption, the $n(k)$ are uncorrelated with variance σ_n^2 so that

$$\mathcal{E}[n(k)n(l)] = \sigma_n^2\delta(k-l)$$

in which case Eq. 11.2.7 becomes

$$\mathcal{E}[(\hat{\theta}_N - \theta)^2] = \frac{1}{N^2}\sigma_n^2.$$

Thus,

$$var(\hat{\theta}_N) = \frac{\sigma_n^2}{N}.$$

In general, an estimator $\hat{\theta}$ is called *consistent* if

$$\lim_{N\to\infty} var(\hat{\theta}) = 0.$$

Clearly, our estimator $\hat{\theta}_N$ is consistent since

$$\lim_{N\to\infty} \frac{\sigma_n^2}{N} = 0.$$

Consistency means that if enough samples are used in the computation of $\hat{\theta}$, we can be reasonably sure that $\hat{\theta}$ is close to θ.

An important concept is the tradeoff between bias and variance. This is a problem which we must consider often when performing spectral estimation. A simple example will illustrate. Suppose we are trying to estimate some parameter θ and we have an unbiased estimator $\hat{\theta}$, *i.e.*,

$$B(\hat{\theta}) = 0.$$

Let $|c| < 1$ and define the new estimator $\bar{\theta}$ by

$$\bar{\theta} = c\hat{\theta}.$$

It follows that

$$\mathcal{E}[\bar{\theta}] = c\mathcal{E}[\hat{\theta}],$$

and because $\hat{\theta}$ is unbiased,

$$\mathcal{E}[\bar{\theta}] = c\theta$$

so that $\bar{\theta}$ is biased with bias

$$B(\bar{\theta}) = \theta - c\theta = (1-c)\theta.$$

The variance of $\bar{\theta}$ is then given by

$$var(\bar{\theta}) = c^2 var(\hat{\theta}).$$

Thus, we are able to achieve a reduction in variance at the expense of an increase in bias.

11.3 Maximum Likelihood Estimation

The principle behind maximum likelihood estimation (MLE) is very simple and intuitively pleasing. Suppose a vector $\boldsymbol{x}_o$ of observations $x(1), x(2), \ldots, x(N)$ has a PDF which depends on some parameter vector $\boldsymbol{\theta}$. The problem is to estimate the vector of parameters $\boldsymbol{\theta}$ from the observations $\boldsymbol{x}_o$. The MLE estimator of $\boldsymbol{\theta}$ is given by

$$\hat{\boldsymbol{\theta}} = \max_{\boldsymbol{\theta}} p(\boldsymbol{x}; \boldsymbol{\theta})$$

when the observations $\boldsymbol{x}_o$ are substituted for $\boldsymbol{x}$. The reasoning behind the MLE approach is that by maximizing $p(\boldsymbol{x}_o, \boldsymbol{\theta})$ over $\boldsymbol{\theta}$, we obtain the value of $\boldsymbol{\theta}$ which gives the highest probability of $\boldsymbol{x}_o$ being observed. Since we observed $\boldsymbol{x}_o$, this choice of $\boldsymbol{\theta}$ is reasonable. The MLE estimator has many desirable properties. In particular, It can be shown to be asymptotically unbiased and asymptotically efficient (we will explain efficiency shortly).

If we define the *log-likelihood function* $L(\boldsymbol{x}, \boldsymbol{\theta})$ by

$$L(\boldsymbol{\theta}) = \ln p(\boldsymbol{x}, \boldsymbol{\theta}),$$

the MLE estimator can also be found by

$$\hat{\boldsymbol{\theta}} = \max_{\boldsymbol{\theta}} L(\boldsymbol{\theta}).$$

This is sometimes useful when dealing with Gaussian distributions.

Example 11.1

Suppose we have N observations of a Gaussian white noise process with mean m_x and variance σ_x^2. The observation vector $\boldsymbol{x}_o$ has a PDF which is parameterized by the vector

$$\boldsymbol{\theta} = \begin{bmatrix} m_x \\ \sigma_x^2 \end{bmatrix}.$$

The PDF for $\boldsymbol{x}$ is given by

$$p(\boldsymbol{x}, \boldsymbol{\theta}) = \frac{1}{(2\pi\sigma_x^2)^{N/2}} \exp\left[-\frac{1}{2\sigma_x^2}\sum_{i=1}^{N}[x(i) - m_x]^2\right].$$

Accordingly,

$$L(\boldsymbol{x}, \boldsymbol{\theta}) = -\frac{N}{2}\ln(2\pi\sigma_x^2) + -\frac{1}{2\sigma_x^2}\sum_{i=1}^{N}[x(i) - m_x]^2.$$

By solving

$$\frac{\partial L(\boldsymbol{x}, \boldsymbol{\theta})}{\partial \boldsymbol{\theta}} = \mathbf{0},$$

we can show that the MLE estimates of m_x and σ_x^2 are given by

$$\hat{m_x} = \frac{1}{N} \sum_{i=1}^{N} x(i)$$

and

$$\hat{\sigma_x}^2 = \frac{1}{N} \sum_{i=1}^{N} [x(i) - \hat{m_x}]^2.$$

That is, the MLE estimates are the sample mean and variance. This is not a general property, but we have at least shown that it holds for Gaussian distributions.

Another interesting example is given by the least squares estimation problem. Assume we have two sets of L observations, $\{d(i)\}$ and $\{x(i)\}$. It is further assumed that there is a linear relationship between each $d(k)$ and the N most recent samples $x(k), x(k-1), \ldots, x(k-N+1)$ which is obscured by the presence of some measurement error, $e_o(k)$, which is Gaussian and white with zero mean and variance σ^2. That is, we have

$$d(i) = w_0 x(i) + w_1 x(i-1) + \cdots + W_{N-1} x(i-N+1) + e_o(i).$$

The problem is to estimate the vector of parameters

$$\boldsymbol{\theta} = \begin{bmatrix} w_0 \\ w_1 \\ \vdots \\ w_{N-1} \end{bmatrix}$$

from the observation vector $\boldsymbol{d}$. In vector form, we can write

$$\boldsymbol{d}_o = \boldsymbol{X}\boldsymbol{\theta} + \boldsymbol{e}_o$$

where

$$\boldsymbol{X} = \begin{bmatrix} x(1) & 0 & 0 & \cdots & 0 \\ x(2) & x(1) & 0 & \cdots & 0 \\ \vdots & \vdots & \vdots & \ddots & \vdots \\ x(N) & x(N-1) & x(N-2) & \cdots & x(1) \\ \vdots & \vdots & \vdots & \vdots & \vdots \\ x(L) & x(L-1) & x(L-2) & \cdots & x(L-N+1) \end{bmatrix}.$$

Since the covariance matrix of $\boldsymbol{e}$ is equal to $\sigma^2\boldsymbol{I}$, the vector $\boldsymbol{d}_o$ will be Gaussian distributed with mean $\boldsymbol{X\theta}$ and covariance $\sigma^2\boldsymbol{I}$. Thus,

$$p(\boldsymbol{d},\boldsymbol{\theta}) = \frac{1}{(2\pi\sigma^2)^{N/2}} \exp\left[-\frac{1}{2\sigma^2}(\boldsymbol{d}-\boldsymbol{X\theta})^T(\boldsymbol{d}-\boldsymbol{X\theta})\right].$$

Maximizing $p(\boldsymbol{d\theta})$ when $\boldsymbol{d} = \boldsymbol{d}_o$ is seen to be equivalent to minimizing the inner product

$$(\boldsymbol{d}_o - \boldsymbol{X\theta})^T(\boldsymbol{d}_o - \boldsymbol{X\theta}) = ||\boldsymbol{d}_o - \boldsymbol{X\theta}||_2^2.$$

We have already seen that this is accomplished by choosing

$$\hat{\boldsymbol{\theta}} = (\boldsymbol{X}^T\boldsymbol{X})^{-1}\boldsymbol{X}^T\boldsymbol{d}_o.$$

Thus, the maximum likelihood estimate of the linear regression parameters is given by the least squares solution to the parameter estimation problem. Again, this holds for the *particular* case where the measurement error is Gaussian and white.

The Cramer-Rao bound

Given an unbiased estimator $\hat{\boldsymbol{\theta}}$ of a L-dimensional parameter vector $\boldsymbol{\theta}$, what is the minimum variance which can be achieved? This question is answered by the Cramer-Rao bound for unbiased estimators. Suppose first that θ is a scalar parameter and the PDF is given by $p(\boldsymbol{x};\theta)$. The Cramer-Rao bound for the unbiased estimator $\hat{\theta}$ is given by

$$var[\hat{\theta}] \geq \frac{1}{\mathcal{E}[(\partial \ln p(\boldsymbol{x};\theta)/\partial\theta)^2]}. \tag{11.3.1}$$

That is, if $\hat{\theta}$ is an unbiased estimator of θ, the variance of the estimator will always be bounded from below by the relationship in Eq. 11.3.1. In practice, it is sometimes useful to make use of the relationship

$$\mathcal{E}\left[\left(\frac{\partial \ln p(\boldsymbol{x};\theta)}{\partial\theta}\right)^2\right] = -\mathcal{E}\left[\frac{\partial^2 \ln p(\boldsymbol{x};\theta)}{\partial\theta}^2\right]. \tag{11.3.2}$$

An estimator which meets the Cramer-Rao lower bound is said to be an *efficient* estimator.

If $\boldsymbol{\theta}$ is a vector of parameters, the Cramer-Rao bound assumes a slightly different form. Define the *Fisher information matrix* $\boldsymbol{J}$ by

$$\mathcal{E}\left[\frac{\partial \ln p(\boldsymbol{x};\boldsymbol{\theta})}{\partial\boldsymbol{\theta}}\left(\frac{\partial \ln p(\boldsymbol{x};\boldsymbol{\theta})}{\partial\boldsymbol{\theta}}\right)^T\right]. \tag{11.3.3}$$

The matrix $\boldsymbol{J}$ has i, j-the element given by

$$[\boldsymbol{J}]_{i,j} = -\mathcal{E}\left[\frac{\partial^2 \ln p(\boldsymbol{x};\boldsymbol{\theta})}{\partial\theta_i\,\partial\theta_j}\right]. \tag{11.3.4}$$

The Cramer-Rao bound for unbiased estimators of a vector parameter $\boldsymbol{\theta}$ is then given by

$$cov(\boldsymbol{\theta}) \geq \boldsymbol{J}^{-1}, \tag{11.3.5}$$

which means that the matrix $cov(\boldsymbol{\theta}) - \boldsymbol{J}^{-1}$ is positive semidefinite. In particular, this means that the individual elements of $\boldsymbol{\theta}$ have variances bounded by

$$var(\theta_i) \geq [\boldsymbol{J}^{-1}]_{i,i}. \tag{11.3.6}$$

11.4 Estimation of the Autocorrelation Sequence

Given a finite number of samples

$$x(0), x(1), x(2), \ldots, x(N-1)$$

of a stochastic process $\{x(k)\}$, we would like to estimate the autocorrelation sequence $\{r_{xx}(k)\}$. Consider the estimate

$$\hat{r}_{xx}(k) = \frac{1}{N-|k|}\sum_{n=0}^{N-|k|-1} x(n)x(n+|k|). \tag{11.4.1}$$

The mean of this estimator is

$$\mathcal{E}[\hat{r}_{xx}(k)] = \frac{1}{N-|k|}\sum_{n=0}^{N-|k|-1} \mathcal{E}[x(n)x(n+|k|)] = r_{xx}(k)$$

so that $\hat{r}_{xx}(k)$ is an unbiased estimate of $r_{xx}(k)$. The variance of this estimator is somewhat more difficult to compute. It can be shown that

$$var(\hat{r}_{xx}(k)) \approx \frac{N}{(N-|k|)^2}\sum_{n=-\infty}^{\infty} [r_{xx}^2(n) + r_{xx}(k-n)r_{xx}(k+n).$$

if the lag k is much less than the number of samples N. For large N, we then have

$$\lim_{N\to\infty} var(\hat{r}_{xx}(k)) = 0$$

so that the estimator $\hat{r}_{xx}(k)$ is consistent. Notice that for fixed N, the variance of $\hat{r}_{xx}(k)$ increases with the lag index k. This is simple to understand. For larger k, fewer data points enter the computation of $\hat{r}_{xx}(k)$, hence the higher variability. At the extreme case, for $k = N - 1$, only one data point enters into the computation.

The situation can be remedied somewhat by using the autocorrelation estimate

$$\bar{r}_{xx}(k) = \frac{1}{N} \sum_{n=0}^{N-|k|-1} x(n)x(n+|k|). \tag{11.4.2}$$

Notice that this estimator is related to the estimator $\hat{r}_{xx}(k)$ by

$$\bar{r}_{xx}(k) = \left(1 - \frac{|k|}{N}\right) \hat{r}_{xx}(k).$$

Therefore,

$$\mathcal{E}[\bar{r}_{xx}(k)] = \left(1 - \frac{|k|}{N}\right) r_{xx}(k)$$

so that the estimate $\bar{r}_{xx}(k)$ is biased. We do have the property that

$$\lim_{N\to\infty} \bar{r}_{xx}(k) = r_{xx}(k)$$

so that the estimator is asymptotically unbiased. More importantly,

$$var(\bar{r}_{xx}(k)) = \left(1 - \frac{|k|}{N}\right)^2 var(\hat{r}_{xx}(k))$$

so that the variance of the estimator $\bar{r}_{xx}(k)$ is smaller than the variance of the estimator $\hat{r}_{xx}(k)$. The estimator $\bar{r}_{xx}(k)$ is also consistent in that

$$\lim_{N\to\infty} var(\bar{r}_{xx}(k)) = 0.$$

The estimator $\hat{r}_{xx}(k)$ can be shown in some cases to lead to estimated autocorrelation sequences which are not positive semidefinite, which will sometimes cause problems with spectral estimation algorithms. Thus, the biased estimator $\bar{r}_{xx}(k)$ is often preferred.

11.5 Nonparametric Spectral Estimators

11.5.1 The Periodogram Methods

Recall that we can define the power spectrum by

$$P_{xx}(\theta) = \lim_{M\to\infty} \mathcal{E}\left[\frac{1}{2M+1}\left|\sum_{k=-M}^{M} x(k)e^{-jk\theta}\right|^2\right]. \tag{11.5.1}$$

Given samples $x(0), x(1), \ldots, x(N-1)$, the periodogram [JW68] is obtained by neglecting the expectation operator, giving

$$P_{PER}(\theta) = \frac{1}{N}\left|\sum_{k=0}^{N-1} e^{-jk\theta}\right|^2. \tag{11.5.2}$$

The spectral estimate given by the periodogram at a particular frequency θ_0 can be regarded as the output of a bandpass filter which is centered at θ_0. To see this, let

$$h(k) = \begin{cases} \frac{1}{N}e^{j\theta_0 k}, & k = -(N-1), -(N-2), \ldots, 0 \\ 0, & \text{otherwise} \end{cases}.$$

It then follows that we can rewrite Eq. 11.5.2 as

$$P_{PER}(\theta_0) = \left[N\left|\sum_{n=0}^{N-1} x(n)h(k-n)\right|^2\right] \quad \text{at} \quad k=0. \tag{11.5.3}$$

The frequency response of $\{h(k)\}$ is given by

$$H(e^{j\theta}) = e^{j(\theta-\theta_0)(N-1)/2}\frac{\sin(\frac{N}{2}(\theta-\theta_0))}{N\sin((\theta-\theta_0)/2)}$$

which is a bandpass response centered at $\theta = \theta_0$. The 3 dB bandwidth of this filter can be shown to be approximately equal to $1/N$. According to Eq. 11.5.3, $P_{PER}(\theta_0)$ is computed by filtering $\{x(k)\}$ through $H(e^{j\theta})$ and taking the magnitude squared at $k = 0$.

Let's look at the spectral estimate produced by the periodogram for a unit variance Gaussian noise process. Fig. 11.5.1 shows the results for $N = 128$, $N = 256$, and $N = 1024$. We would hope for a spectral estimate which is flat across all frequencies. Observe that the periodogram fluctuates wildly and does not seem to improve for larger N. The reason for this is fairly simple to understand. Using Eq. 11.5.2, an alternative expression for the periodogram is given by

$$P_{PER}(\theta) = \sum_{k=-(N-1)}^{N-1} \bar{r}_{xx}(k)e^{-jk\theta}$$

where $\bar{r}_{xx}(k)$ is the biased autocorrelation estimate given in Eq. 11.4.2. Consequently,

$$\mathcal{E}[P_{PER}(\theta)] = \sum_{k=-(N-1)}^{N-1} \mathcal{E}[\hat{r}_{xx}(k)]e^{-jk\theta}.$$

We have seen that

$$\mathcal{E}[\hat{r}_{xx}(k)] = \left(1 - \frac{|k|}{N}\right) r_{xx}(k),$$

which is a triangular-windowed version of the true autocorrelation sequence $r_{xx}(k)$. Therefore,

$$\mathcal{E}[P_{PER}(\theta)] = \sum_{k=-\infty}^{\infty} r_{xx}(k) w_T(k) e^{-jk\theta}$$

where $w_T(k)$ is a triangular window with width $2N+1$. In the frequency domain, this can be expressed using the convolution theorem, giving

$$\mathcal{E}[P_{PER}(\theta)] = \frac{1}{2\pi} \int_{-\pi}^{\pi} P_{xx}(\varphi) W_T(\theta - \varphi)\, d\varphi. \tag{11.5.4}$$

Equation 11.5.4 shows that the expected value of the periodogram is obtained by "blurring" the true power spectrum with the Fourier transform of the triangular window. Thus, the mean of the estimate is degraded by the finite length of the window, and hence by the leakage due to the sidelobes. It is fairly simple to see, however, that

$$\lim_{N\to\infty} \mathcal{E}[P_{PER}(\theta)] = P_{xx}(\theta)$$

so that the periodogram is asymptotically unbiased.

The Fourier transform of the triangular window is given by

$$W_T(e^{j\theta}) = \frac{1}{N} \frac{\sin^2 N\theta/2}{\sin^2 \theta/2}.$$

In order to avoid blurring the spectral detail in the power spectrum, the window length N (*i.e.*, the number of points used for the estimator) should be chosen so that the window main lobe width is considerably less than the width of the spectral peaks in $P_{xx}(\theta)$. Because the main lobe has a 3 dB bandwidth of roughly $2\pi/N$, the periodogram will not be able to resolve details in the spectrum which have width less than $2\pi/N$.

The variance is somewhat more difficult to compute, and depends on the process being analyzed. It can be shown that for Gaussian white noise,

$$var[P_{PER}(\theta)] = P_{xx}^2(\theta) \left[1 + \frac{\sin^2 N\theta}{N^2 \sin^2 \theta}\right],$$

which in the limit as N goes to infinity becomes

$$\lim_{N\to\infty} var[P_{PER}(\theta)] = P_{xx}^2(\theta).$$

Thus, the periodogram is not a consistent estimator of the power spectrum. In fact, even as we collect an infinite number of samples, the variance is equal to the square of the quantity we are trying to analyze. This explains the fluctuations in the periodogram estimates in Fig. 11.5.1, even for large N.

11.5.2 The Averaged Periodogram Method

What, then can be done to decrease the variance of the periodogram? Assume we have K sets of uncorrelated measurements $\{x_i(k)\}$ of the process $\{x(k)\}$. Let the length of each set of measurements be M and compute the periodogram of each set as

$$P_{PER}^i(\theta) = \frac{1}{M}\left|\sum_{k=0}^{M-1} x_i(k)e^{-jk\theta}\right|^2, \quad i = 0, 1, \ldots, K-1.$$

Finally, we obtain the *averaged periodogram* spectral estimator by averaging the $P_{PER}^i(\theta)$, giving

$$P_{AV}(\theta) = \frac{1}{K}\sum_{i=0}^{K-1} P_{PER}^i(\theta). \tag{11.5.5}$$

What has been gained by this approach? We are trying to approximate the expectation operator in Eq. 11.5.1. The mean of the averaged periodogram is given by

$$\mathcal{E}[P_{AV}(\theta)] = \frac{1}{K}\sum_{i=0}^{K-1} \mathcal{E}[P_{PER}^i(\theta)]$$

and since the sets of measurements were uncorrelated with one another, we have

$$\mathcal{E}[P_{AV}(\theta)] = \mathcal{E}[P_{PER}^i(\theta)]$$

so that the averaged periodogram is still an asymptotically unbiased estimator of the power spectrum. However, each $P_{PER}^i(\theta)$ was computed using M points which means that its mean is obtained by "blurring" the true spectrum with a triangular window which has a wider mainlobe in the frequency domain, introducing more leakage, and hence, bias. Thus, the spectral resolution has been reduced to $2\pi/M$.

The variance, however, decreases by K. To show this, since the sequences $\{x_i(k)\}$ were uncorrelated with one another, the variance is given by

$$var[P_{AV}(\theta)] = \frac{1}{K^2}\sum_{i=1}^{K} var[P_{PER}^i(\theta)],$$

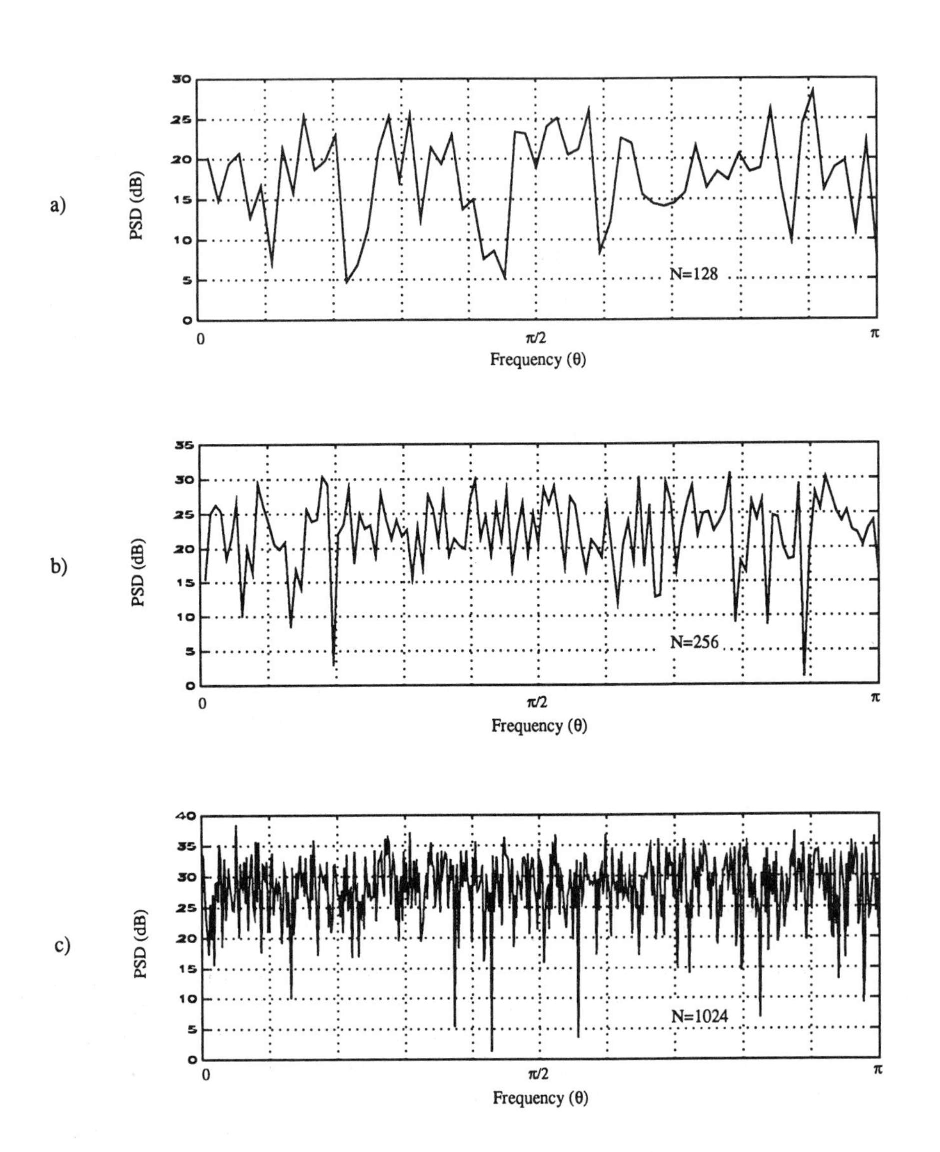

Figure 11.5.1: Periodogram spectral estimates for zero-mean Gaussian noise with unit variance: (a) $N = 128$; (b) $N = 256$; (c) $N = 1024$.

and again using the independence of the individual periodograms,

$$var[P_{AV}(\theta) = \frac{1}{K} var[P^i_{PER}(\theta)].$$

For the case of Gaussian noise, we have

$$var[P_{AV}(\theta)] = \frac{1}{K} P^2_{xx}(\theta) \left[1 + \frac{\sin^2 M\theta}{M^2 \sin^2 \theta}\right].$$

Consequently,

$$\lim_{M \to \infty} var[P_{AV}(\theta)] = \frac{1}{K} P^2_{xx}(\theta)$$

which is K times smaller than the variance of the ordinary periodogram.

To summarize, the averaged periodogram has a variance which is reduced by $1/K$ at the expense of decreasing the spectral resolution to $2\pi/M$ from $2\pi/N$. This is yet another illustration of the tradeoff between bias and variance.

In practice, we may not have access to several sets of measurements. In this case, we may segment N-point sequence $\{x(k)\}$ into K nonoverlapping subsequences $\{x_i(k)\}$ of M points each where

$$x_i(k) = x(k + iM), \quad i = 0, 1, \ldots, K - 1: \quad k = 0, 1, \ldots M - 1.$$

The sets of measurements are no longer uncorrelated since they are taken from a contiguous segment of $\{x(k)\}$. In fact, the only stochastic process for which the subsequences $\{x_i(k)\}$ are independent is white noise. If the autocorrelation sequence of the process dies of rapidly (as is the case for most processes which do not contain a sinusoidal component), the subsequences are approximately uncorrelated and the the averaged periodogram will still perform considerably than the ordinary periodogram.

Figure 11.5.2 shows the results of applying the averaged periodogram method the the estimation of the power spectrum of a 2048-point Gaussian white noise sequence which is divided into $K = 8$ segments of $M = 256$ segments each. Notice that the fluctuations in this spectral estimator are smaller than the ordinary periodogram. This is due to the decrease in variance by $1/K$.

11.5.3 The Welch Method

A slight modification of the averaged periodogram spectral estimator results in the Welch method. The Welch method [Wel67] segments the sequence $\{x(k)\}$ into L possibly overlapping length-M subsequences $\{x_i(k)\}$ where

$$x_i(k) = x(k + iD), \quad k = 0, 1, \ldots, M - 1: \quad i = 0, 1, \ldots, L - 1.$$

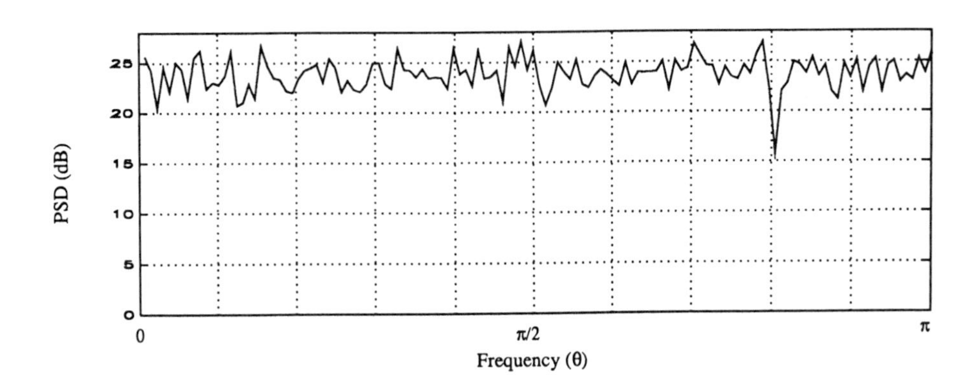

Figure 11.5.2: Averaged periodogram spectral estimate of Gaussian white noise with $N = 2048$, $K = 8$, $M = 256$.

The parameter D determines the overlap; $D = M$ corresponds to no overlap and $D = M/2$ corresponds to 50% overlap. Next, we compute a modified periodogram estimate with each sequence $\{x_i(k)\}$ given by

$$P_W^i(\theta) = \frac{1}{MR}\left|\sum_{k=0}^{M-1} x_i(k)w(k)e^{-jk\theta}\right|^2, \quad i = 0, 1, \ldots, L-1$$

where $w(k)$ is some window function and R is given by

$$R = \frac{1}{M}\sum_{k=0}^{M-1} w^2(k).$$

The constant R serves to normalize the power contribution due to the window. The Welch estimator is then given by

$$P_W(\theta) = \frac{1}{L}\sum_{i=0}^{L-1} P_W^i(\theta).$$

Making the same assumptions we made for the analysis of the averaged periodogram estimator, it follows that

$$\mathcal{E}[P_W(\theta)] \approx \mathcal{E}[P_W^i(\theta)].$$

It can be shown that

$$\mathcal{E}[P_W^i(\theta)] = \frac{1}{2\pi}\int_{-\pi}^{\pi} P_{xx}(\varphi)\Psi(e^{j(\theta-\varphi)})\, d\varphi$$

where $\Psi(e^{j\theta})$ is proportional to the squared Fourier transform of the window $w(k)$. Specifically,

$$\Psi(e^{j\theta}) = \frac{1}{MR}W^2(e^{j\theta}).$$

Again, we can see that the window function serves to blur the power spectrum, thus introducing bias in the estimate and hence decreasing the resolution.

The variance of the Welch estimator is difficult to compute. For the case of zero overlap between segments, Welch showed that

$$var[P_W(\theta)] \approx \frac{1}{L}P_{xx}^2(\theta).$$

For 50% overlap and $w(k)$ equal to a triangular window, the variance is given by

$$var[P_W(\theta)] \approx \frac{9}{8L}P_{xx}^2(\theta).$$

Thus, at the expense of increasing bias, the variance is reduced.

11.5.4 The Blackman-Tukey Method

Another popular nonparametric spectral estimator is the Blackman-Tukey (BT) estimator [BT58]. Recall that the periodogram can be expressed as

$$P_{PER}(\theta) = \sum_{k=-(N-1)}^{N-1} \bar{r}_{xx}(k)e^{-jk\theta}$$

where $\bar{r}_{xx}(k)$ is the biased autocorrelation estimate given by

$$\bar{r}_{xx}(k) = \frac{1}{N}\sum_{n=0}^{N-|k|-1} x(n)x(n+|k|).$$

The large variance of the periodogram spectral estimator is due in large part to the large variance of the estimator $\bar{r}_{xx}(k)$. Notice that at the extreme edges of the sequence $\{\bar{r}_{xx}(k)\}$, very few terms enter into the computation of the estimate. In fact, for $k = N-1$, we have

$$\bar{r}_{xx}(N-1) = \frac{1}{N}x(0)x(N-1)$$

so that only one product term is used; hence the high variance. This uncertainty enters into the computation of the periodogram. One possible solution to this problem is to compute a periodogram where the autocorrelation estimates for large lag indices are weighted less heavily. Specifically, the BT spectral estimator is defined by

$$P_{BT}(\theta) = \sum_{k=-(N-1)}^{N-1} \bar{r}_{xx}(k)w(k)e^{-jk\theta} \tag{11.5.6}$$

where $w(k)$ is some window of width M where M is less than or equal to $2N+1$ and is centered at the origin. We must be careful when choosing the window function since some windows will lead to power spectrum estimates which are negative at some frequencies. It is known that both the Hamming and the Hann window can cause this phenomenon to occur. The triangular window is a "safe" window which will not cause this problem to occur.

As a consequence of decreasing the variance, we should expect the BT estimator to have a larger bias than the periodogram. To see that this is so, according to Eq. 11.5.6, $P_{BT}(\theta)$ is the Fourier transform of the weighted, estimated sequence $w(k)\bar{r}_{xx}(k)$. Thus, we use the convolution theorem to give

$$P_{BT}(\theta) = \frac{1}{2\pi}\int_{-\pi}^{\pi} P_{PER}(\varphi)W(e^{j(\theta-\varphi)})\,d\varphi$$

and therefore,

$$\mathcal{E}[P_{BT}(\theta)] = \frac{1}{2\pi}\int_{-\pi}^{\pi} \mathcal{E}[P_{PER}(\varphi)]W(e^{j(\theta-\varphi)})\,d\varphi.$$

For large data lengths N, since $P_{PER}(\theta)$ is asymptotically biased we have

$$\mathcal{E}[P_{PER}(\theta)] \approx P_{xx}(\theta)$$

so that

$$\mathcal{E}[P_{BT}(\theta)] \approx \frac{1}{2\pi}\int_{-\pi}^{\pi} P_{xx}(\varphi)W(e^{j(\theta-\varphi)})\,d\varphi. \tag{11.5.7}$$

Again, we see that the mean of BT estimator is a blurred version of the true power spectrum. If we assume that the main lobe of $W(e^{j\theta})$ is narrow compared to $P_{xx}(\theta)$, it can be shown that

$$var[P_{BT}(\theta) \approx \frac{P_{xx}^2(\theta)}{2\pi N}\int_{-\pi}^{\pi} W^2(e^{j\theta})\,d\theta$$

which, using Parseval's theorem, becomes

$$var[P_{BT}(\theta) \approx \frac{P_{xx}^2(\theta)}{N}\sum_{k=-(M-1)}^{M-1} w^2(k).$$

If $w(k)$ is a triangular window, the variance is given by

$$var[P_{BT}(\theta)] \approx \frac{2M}{3N} P_{xx}^2(\theta). \tag{11.5.8}$$

This illustrates again the tradeoff between bias and variance. According to Eq. 11.5.8, the variance can be made small by choosing the window length M small. From Eq. 11.5.7, however, we see that making the window length small will make the window main lobe width larger and thus blur the power spectrum more.

11.5.5 The Capon Method

Recall that the periodogram method measured the power spectrum at a frequency θ_0 by passing $\{x(k)\}$ through a bandpass filter $H(e^{j\theta})$ which is centered at θ_0, and $H(e^{j\theta_0}) = 1$ with 3 dB bandwidth equal to approximately $1/N$. For each value of θ_0, the bandwidth of the filter was identical and the magnitude of the sidelobes was fairly high. Thus, the periodogram suffers from leakage outside the band of interest. For a good spectral estimate, the output power of the filter $H(e^{j\theta})$ should only be due to the power spectrum near θ_0. The Capon method uses a set of filters which adjust their sidelobes to minimize the power at the filter outputs due to power outside a narrow band centered at θ_0. In other words, we wish to determine the filter $H(e^{j\theta})$ which minimizes the output power

$$P = \frac{1}{2\pi} \int_{-\pi}^{\pi} |H(e^{j\theta})|^2 P_{xx}(\theta)\, d\theta$$

subject to the constraint

$$H(e^{j\theta_0}) = 1.$$

This is a constrained minimization problem which can be solved simply. Recalling that

$$H(e^{j\theta}) = \sum_{k=-(N-1)}^{0} h(k) e^{-jk\theta},$$

the output power P can be expressed as

$$P = \frac{1}{2\pi} \int_{-\pi}^{\pi} \sum_{k=-(N-1)}^{0} \sum_{l=-(N-1)}^{0} h(k) h^*(l) e^{-j(k-l)\theta} P_{xx}(\theta)\, d\theta.$$

Reversing the order of summation and integration, we have

$$P = \sum_{k=-(N-1)}^{0} \sum_{l=-(N-1)}^{0} h(k) h^*(l) \frac{1}{2\pi} \int_{-\pi}^{\pi} P_{xx}(\theta) e^{-j(k-l)\theta}\, d\theta.$$

The integral is recognized as the autocorrelation sequence for lag $k-l$. Thus,

$$P = \sum_{k=-(N-1)}^{0} \sum_{l=-(N-1)}^{0} h(k)h^*(l)r_{xx}(k-l).$$

Denoting by $\boldsymbol{h}$ the vector

$$\boldsymbol{h} = \begin{bmatrix} h(0) \\ h(-1) \\ \vdots \\ h(-(N-1)) \end{bmatrix},$$

we can express P as the quadratic form

$$P = \boldsymbol{h}^H \boldsymbol{R}_{xx} \boldsymbol{h}$$

where $\boldsymbol{R}_{xx}$ is the $N \times N$ autocorrelation matrix for the process $\{x(k)\}$. The constraint $H(e^{j\theta_0}) = 1$ can be expressed as

$$\boldsymbol{h}^H \boldsymbol{e} = 1$$

where $\boldsymbol{e}$ is the vector given by

$$\boldsymbol{e} = \begin{bmatrix} 1 \\ e^{j\theta_0} \\ \vdots \\ e^{j(N-1)\theta_0} \end{bmatrix}.$$

Thus, our constrained minimization can be stated as

$$\text{minimize} \quad \boldsymbol{h}^H \boldsymbol{R}_{xx} \boldsymbol{h} \quad \text{subject to} \quad \boldsymbol{h}^H \boldsymbol{e} = 1.$$

We show in Appendix A that the solution to this problem is given by

$$\boldsymbol{h} = \frac{\boldsymbol{R}_{xx}^{-1} \boldsymbol{e}}{\boldsymbol{e}^H \boldsymbol{R}_{xx} \boldsymbol{e}}$$

which results in the minimum output power equal to

$$P = \frac{1}{\boldsymbol{e}^H \boldsymbol{R}_{xx}^{-1} \boldsymbol{e}}.$$

The Capon estimator [Cap69] is sometimes referred to as the *minimum variance estimator* or the *maximum likelihood estimator*. These names are not accurate, but reflect the origins of the method. In practice, we do not know the optimal order for the filter $\boldsymbol{h}$ and define the Capon estimator by

$$P_C(\theta) = \frac{1}{\boldsymbol{e}^H(\theta)\hat{\boldsymbol{R}}_{xx}^L \boldsymbol{e}(\theta)} \tag{11.5.9}$$

where $\hat{\boldsymbol{R}}_{xx}^L$ is an estimate of the $L \times L$ autocorrelation matrix for $\{x(k)\}$. The entries of $\hat{\boldsymbol{R}}_{xx}^L$ can be computed by any of our standard autocorrelation estimators, but L should be chosen considerably smaller than the data length N to avoid using estimates of the autocorrelation with too large a lag.

It has been shown that the Capon estimator has higher resolution than the periodogram-based methods. The tradeoff between bias and variance still exists, however. If a larger autocorrelation matrix is estimated, the bandpass filters will be narrow, giving better resolution. The price paid, however, will be an increase in variance due to the greater uncertainty in the autocorrelation matrix estimate $\hat{\boldsymbol{R}}_{xx}^L$.

11.6 Parametric Spectral Estimators

The fundamental problem with nonparametric spectral estimation techniques is due to the fact that they implicitly window the autocorrelation sequence, resulting in a blurred spectral estimate. This is necessary since it is not possible to get accurate estimates (or *any* estimates) of the autocorrelation sequence for large lags. If we have some a priori informations about the stochastic process, we may be able to hypothesize a model for the process and base a spectral estimate on the model parameters which are estimated from the data. This is the essence of parametric spectral estimation.

The most popular parametric spectral estimation methods are autoregressive techniques. There are several reasons for this, not the least of which is computational simplicity. We have seen that the AR parameters can be obtained as the solution to a linear system of equations, whereas MA and ARMA methods require the solution of nonlinear equations. Furthermore, an AR model can often be used as a reasonable approximation to other power spectra. For these reasons, we will emphasize the AR spectral estimation techniques.

11.6.1 AR Process Properties

In our discussion of Wiener filtering, we highlighted the connection between the linear prediction problem and the Yule-Walker equation for AR processes. To repeat, the forward prediction problem sought the tap weight vector $\boldsymbol{h}_N^f$ which minimized the mean-squared value of the forward prediction error which was given by

$$e_N^f(k) = x(k) - \sum_{i=1}^{N} h_{N,i}^f x(k-i).$$

With the forward prediction error $\boldsymbol{a}_N$ filter defined by

$$\boldsymbol{a}_N = \begin{bmatrix} 1 \\ -\boldsymbol{h}_N^f \end{bmatrix},$$

we saw that the forward prediction error filter coefficients of the Wiener filter assumed the values of the AR parameters. Furthermore, the prediction error power P_N was shown to be equal to σ_v^2, which is the power of the white noise which drives the AR model, and the forward prediction error filter was minimum-phase. It is important to note that the order-N Wiener forward prediction error filter acts as an *inverse filter* when the input is indeed an AR(N) process. The forward prediction error is then equal to the white noise which drives the AR model, and for this reason, the forward prediction error filter is also known as a *whitening filter.*

The backward linear prediction problem sought the tap weight vector $\boldsymbol{h}_N^b$ which minimized the mean-squared value of the backward prediction error which was given by

$$e_N^b(k) = x(k-N) - \sum_{i=0}^{N-1} h_{N,i}^b x(k-i).$$

With the backward prediction error filter defined by

$$\boldsymbol{b}_N = \begin{bmatrix} -\boldsymbol{h}_N^b \\ 1 \end{bmatrix},$$

we saw that the backward prediction error filter was obtained by reversing the coefficients of the forward prediction error filter and that the backward prediction error power was equal to the forward prediction error power. Also, we showed that the backward prediction error filter was maximum-phase.

The Levinson-Durbin algorithm provides an efficient solution to the normal equations for the linear predictor. This algorithm allowed forward and backward predictors of all intermediate orders $1 \leq m \leq N$ to be generated. Repeating the algorithm for convenience, we define the vector $\boldsymbol{r}_m$ by

$$\boldsymbol{r}_m = \mathcal{E}[\boldsymbol{x}_m(k-1)x(k)]$$

where $\boldsymbol{x}_m(k-1)$ is the vector of m most recent samples of $\{x(k)\}$,

$$\boldsymbol{x}_m(k-1) = \begin{bmatrix} x(k-1) \\ x(k-2) \\ \vdots \\ x(k-m) \end{bmatrix}$$

so that

$$\boldsymbol{r}_m = \begin{bmatrix} r(1) \\ r(2) \\ \vdots \\ r(m) \end{bmatrix}.$$

The Levinson-Durbin algorithm is then summarized by the following.

Summary

The zeroth order forward and backward prediction error filters are defined by $\boldsymbol{a}^{(0)} = \boldsymbol{b}^{(0)} = 1$. We begin the algorithm with $P_0 = r(0)$ and $\Delta_0 = r(1)$. For $m = 1, 2, \ldots, N$, we perform the following:

$$\Delta_{m-1} = \boldsymbol{r}_m^T \boldsymbol{b}^{(m-1)}$$

$$\kappa_m = -\frac{\Delta_{m-1}}{P_{m-1}}$$

$$\boldsymbol{a}^{(m)} = \begin{bmatrix} \boldsymbol{a}^{(m-1)} \\ 0 \end{bmatrix} + \kappa_m \begin{bmatrix} 0 \\ \boldsymbol{b}^{(m-1)} \end{bmatrix}$$

$$\boldsymbol{b}^{(m)} = \boldsymbol{a}^{(m)B}.$$

$$P_m = (1 - \kappa_m^2) P_{m-1}$$

The Levinson-Durbin algorithm successively generates the prediction error filters for all orders $1, 2, \ldots, N$. The κ_m are called the *reflection coefficients* and we will show that each κ_m is bounded in magnitude by unity. This, in turn, can be used to show that the forward prediction error filter is minimum phase. Also, because

$$P_m = (1 - \kappa_m^2) P_{m-1},$$

the prediction error power will be monotonically decreasing and will reach a minimum at $m = N$ if $\{x(k)\}$ is an AR(N) process. This is a useful fact which can help in determining the appropriate model order if we do not know N a priori.

11.6.2 AR Spectral Estimators Based on ACS

One obvious approach to AR spectral estimation is to estimate the autocorrelation sequence directly, compute the AR parameters from the Yule-Walker equation, and form the AR spectral estimate from the AR parameters. Assuming that the stochastic process $\{x(k)\}$ is AR of order N, we can compute the first $N+1$ lags of the autocorrelation sequence using either the unbiased estimator

$$\hat{r}(k) = \frac{1}{N-|k|+1} \sum_{n=0}^{N-|k|+1} x(n)x(n+k), \quad k = 0, 1, \ldots, N$$

or the biased estimator

$$\bar{r}(k) = \frac{1}{N} \sum_{n=0}^{N-|k|+1} x(n)x(n+k), \quad k = 0, 1, \ldots, N.$$

Again, the biased estimator $\bar{r}(k)$ is usually preferable due to its smaller variance. Next, the AR parameters are estimated by the Yule-Walker equations according to

$$\begin{bmatrix} \bar{r}(0) & \bar{r}(1) & \cdots & \bar{r}(N-1) \\ \bar{r}(1) & \bar{r}(0) & \cdots & \bar{r}(N-2) \\ \vdots & \vdots & \ddots & \vdots \\ \bar{r}(N-1) & \bar{r}(N-2) & \cdots & \bar{r}(0) \end{bmatrix} \begin{bmatrix} \hat{a}_1 \\ \hat{a}_2 \\ \vdots \\ \hat{a}_N \end{bmatrix} = \begin{bmatrix} \bar{r}(1) \\ \bar{r}(2) \\ \vdots \\ \bar{r}(N) \end{bmatrix}. \tag{11.6.1}$$

The power of the white noise which drives the AR model is estimated by

$$\hat{P} = \bar{r}(0) + \sum_{k=1}^{p} \hat{a}_k \bar{r}(k).$$

Once $\hat{P}$ and the $\hat{a}_i$ are computed, the AR spectral estimate is given by

$$P_{AR}(\theta) = \frac{\hat{P}}{|1 + \sum_{k=1}^{N} \hat{a}_k e^{-jk\theta}|^2}. \tag{11.6.2}$$

This technique is known as the *autocorrelation method* [Mak75]. The difference between the autocorrelation method and the periodogram is the manner in which the estimated autocorrelation sequence is used. The periodogram method uses the estimated autocorrelation values to compute the spectral estimate

$$P_{PER}(\theta) = \sum_{k=-N}^{N} r(k)e^{-jk\theta}. \tag{11.6.3}$$

The poor resolution of the periodogram estimator is due to the implicit windowing of the true autocorrelation sequence (*i.e.*, the finite range for the summation in Eq. 11.6.3). The AR spectral estimate given by Eq. 11.6.2, however, is equivalent to

$$P_{AR}(\theta) = \sum_{k=-\infty}^{\infty} \bar{r}(k)e^{-jk\theta}$$

where the values of $\bar{r}(k)$ for k greater than N are implicitly generated by the recursion

$$\bar{r}(k) = -\sum_{m=1}^{N} \hat{a}_m \bar{r}(k-m), \quad k > N.$$

Thus, the AR spectral estimate contains an implied "autocorrelation extension" whereby the windowing of the autocorrelation sequence is eliminated. When $\{x(k)\}$ is actually an AR(N) process or is reasonably approximated by one, we can thus expect the AR spectral estimate to have higher resolution.

Example 11.2

Consider the AR(4) process whose power spectrum is shown in Fig. 11.6.1a. Because there are spectral peaks which are fairly narrow, we should expect that the periodogram would perform poorly. A periodogram estimate of the power spectrum which is based on 512 samples is shown in Fig. 11.6.1b. Next, consider the AR(4) spectral estimate based on the same number of points in Fig. 11.6.1c. Notice that the AR estimate gives a much more accurate picture of the true power spectrum.

An interesting property of the autocorrelation spectral estimator is called the *maximum entropy* property. Given the autocorrelation values $r(0), r(1), \ldots, r(N)$, there are an infinite number of extensions of the autocorrelation sequence which result in a positive semidefinite autocorrelation sequence. Burg proposed that the sequence should be extended so as to maximize the entropy of the time series which corresponds to the autocorrelation sequence. The reason for this is that the time series which produced the autocorrelation sequence would be the most random one which matches $r(0), r(1), \ldots, r(N)$. For Gaussian random processes, the entropy is proportional to

$$\int_{-\pi}^{\pi} \ln P(\theta)\, d\theta$$

where $P(\theta)$ is the power spectrum of the process. If $P(\theta)$ is maximized subject to the constraints

$$\frac{1}{2\pi}\int_{-\pi}^{\pi} P(\theta)e^{jk\theta}\, d\theta = r(k), \quad k = 0, 1, \ldots, N$$

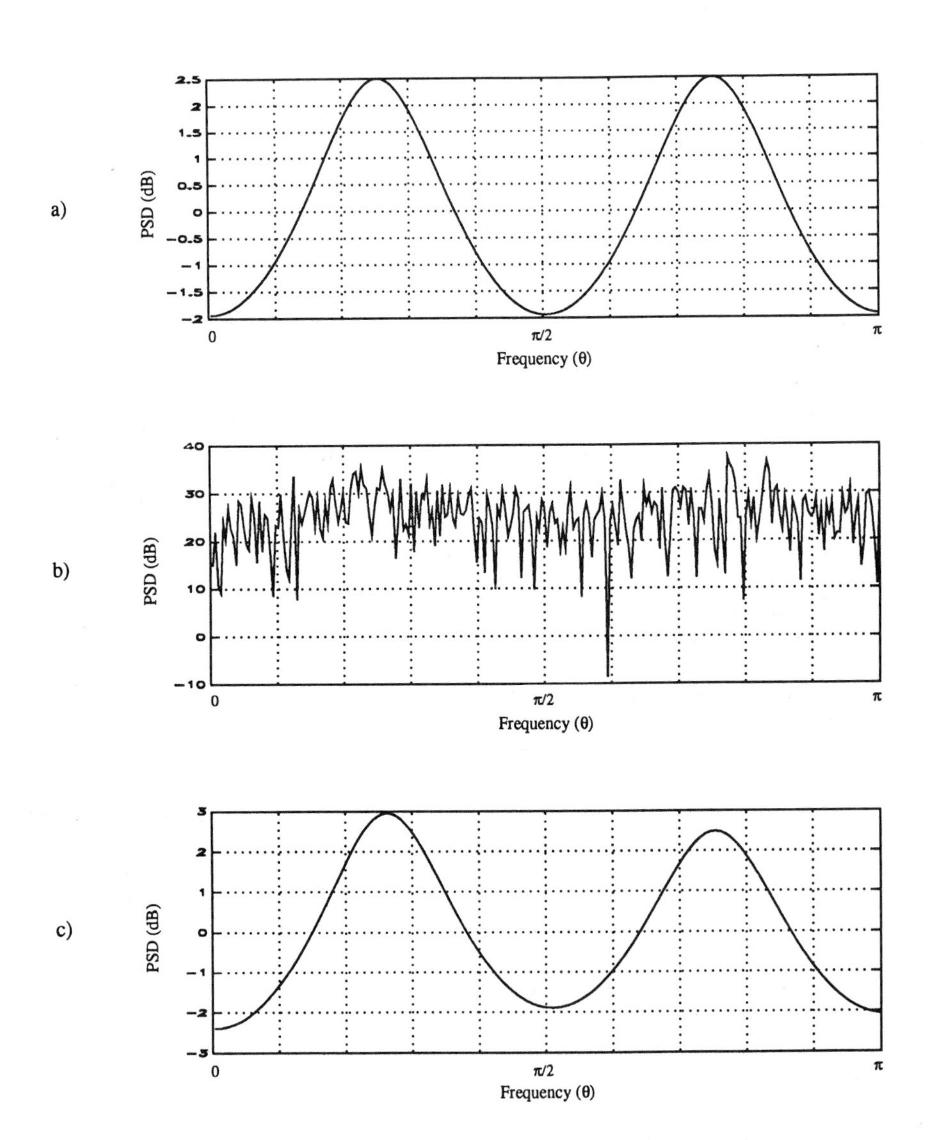

Figure 11.6.1: (a) AR(4) power spectrum; (b) 512-point periodogram estimate; (c) 512-point AR(4) estimate.

we find that

$$P(\theta) = \frac{\hat{P}}{1 + \sum_{k=1}^{N} \hat{a}_k e^{-jk\theta}}$$

where $\hat{P}$ and $\{\hat{a}_i\}$ are found via the autocorrelation method. Therefore, the autocorrelation method and maximum entropy estimation are equivalent for Gaussian random processes [Kay88]. This is not true for other processes, however.

The autocorrelation method may be viewed as the solution to a least-squares prediction problem. Given L observations of $\{x(k)\}$, we wish to find the forward predictor coefficients $\{h_{N,i}^f\}$ which minimizes the sum of squared prediction errors over the index range from 1 to $L+N$. The forward prediction estimate of $x(k)$ is given by

$$\hat{x}^f(k) = \sum_{i=1}^{N} h_{N,i}^f x(k-i)$$

and the forward prediction error is given by

$$e_N^f(k) = x(k) - \sum_{i=1}^{N} h_{N,i}^f x(k-i). \tag{11.6.4}$$

The problem is to find the $h_{N,i}^f$ such that the sum of squared errors

$$\sum_{i=1}^{L+N} [e_N^f(i)]^2$$

is minimized. In matrix form, we would like to find the least-squares solution of the system

$$\begin{bmatrix} x(1) \\ x(2) \\ \vdots \\ x(L-1) \\ \vdots \\ 0 \end{bmatrix} = \begin{bmatrix} x(0) & 0 & \cdots & 0 \\ x(1) & x(0) & \cdots & 0 \\ \vdots & \vdots & \ddots & \vdots \\ x(N-1) & x(N-2) & \cdots & x(1) \\ \vdots & \vdots & \ddots & \vdots \\ x(L-1) & x(L-2) & \cdots & x(L-N) \\ 0 & x(L-1) & \cdots & x(L-N+1) \\ \vdots & \vdots & \ddots & \vdots \\ 0 & 0 & \cdots & x(L-1) \end{bmatrix} \begin{bmatrix} h_{N,1}^f \\ h_{N,2}^f \\ \vdots \\ h_{N,N}^f \end{bmatrix}. \tag{11.6.5}$$

In other words, we keep track of the prediction error for the whole time the data is "in the filter." We seek the coefficients $\{h_{N,i}^f\}$ which minimize Euclidean norm of vector of prediction errors. With the data matrix denoted by $\boldsymbol{X}$ and the vector of predictions denoted by $\hat{\boldsymbol{x}}$, we have

$$\hat{\boldsymbol{x}} = \boldsymbol{X}\boldsymbol{h}_N^f.$$

The vector of prediction errors is then given by

$$\boldsymbol{e}^f = \boldsymbol{x} - \hat{\boldsymbol{x}} = \boldsymbol{x} - \boldsymbol{X}\boldsymbol{h}_N^f.$$

Therefore,

$$||\boldsymbol{e}^f||_2 = ||\boldsymbol{x} - \boldsymbol{X}\boldsymbol{h}_N^f||_2.$$

Thus, the problem is to find the vector $\boldsymbol{h}_N^f$ such that $\boldsymbol{X}\boldsymbol{h}_N^f$ is closest to $\boldsymbol{x}$ in the Euclidean sense. We have seen that the solution to this problem is given by solving the normal equations

$$(\boldsymbol{X}^T\boldsymbol{X})\boldsymbol{h}_N^f = \boldsymbol{X}^T\boldsymbol{x}.$$

Examining the expression for $\boldsymbol{X}$, we can see that the i,j-th element of $\boldsymbol{X}^T\boldsymbol{X}$ is equal to $L\bar{r}(i-j)$ where $\bar{r}(k)$ is the biased autocorrelation estimate. Similarly, the i-th element of $\boldsymbol{X}^T\boldsymbol{x}$ can be seen to equal $\bar{r}(i+1)$. Thus, the least-squares solution $\boldsymbol{h}_N^f$ to the system equations is nearly identical to the Yule-Walker equations using the unbiased autocorrelation estimate. The only difference is in the sign of $\boldsymbol{X}^T\boldsymbol{x}$, which is explained by the fact that $\boldsymbol{a}_N = -\boldsymbol{h}_N^f$. For complex data, the normal equations are modified slightly to give

$$(\boldsymbol{X}^H\boldsymbol{X})\boldsymbol{h}_N^f = \boldsymbol{X}^H\boldsymbol{x}.$$

Examining Eq. 11.6.5, it can be seen that we needed to make the implicit assumption that the values of $\{x(k)\}$ for k outside the range $0 \leq k \leq L$ were equal to zero. The *covariance* method [Mak75] of AR spectral estimation makes no assumptions about the data outside this range. The first time that the taps of the forward predictor are filled with *known* data is at $k = N-1$ and the last time that the taps are filled with known data is at $k = L-1$. Therefore, the first useful forward prediction we can make is of $x(N)$ and the last useful forward prediction we can make is of $x(L)$. Since $x(L)$ is not known, we have no measure of the error for the prediction of $x(L)$ and hence we will only predict up to $x(L-1)$. Therefore, we seek the least-squares solution to the system of equations given by

$$\begin{bmatrix} x(N) \\ x(N+1) \\ \vdots \\ x(L-1) \end{bmatrix} = \begin{bmatrix} x(N-1) & x(N-2) & \cdots & x(0) \\ x(N) & x(N-1) & \cdots & x(1) \\ \vdots & \vdots & \ddots & \vdots \\ x(L-2) & x(L-3) & \cdots & x(L-N-1) \end{bmatrix} \begin{bmatrix} h_{N,1}^f \\ h_{N,2}^f \\ \vdots \\ h_{N,N}^f \end{bmatrix}. \tag{11.6.6}$$

This time, with the data matrix given by C, the least-squares solution is given by

$$(\boldsymbol{C}^T \boldsymbol{C})\boldsymbol{h}_n^f = \boldsymbol{C}^T \boldsymbol{x}.$$

This system of equations is slightly different than the equations used for the autocorrelation method. Specifically, the i, j-th element of $\boldsymbol{C}^T \boldsymbol{C}$ is given by

$$(L-N) \sum_{n=N}^{L-1} x(n-i)x(n-k)$$

and the i-th element of $\boldsymbol{C}^T \boldsymbol{x}$ is given by

$$(L-N) \sum_{n=N}^{L-1} x(n)x(n-i).$$

This is still a Yule-Walker type of equation, but with different estimates of the autocorrelation sequence.

The principal difference between the autocorrelation and covariance approaches to AR power spectrum estimation is in the manner in which the autocorrelation sequence is estimated. It can be shown that the autocorrelation method will always result in a stable AR model, while the covariance method may not. For large data records, the results of the autocorrelation and covariance methods are similar. One strength of the covariance method, however, is its ability to locate spectral peaks due to pure sinusoids, a feature which is not shared by the covariance method.

An extension of the covariance method, known as the *modified covariance method* [Nut76], minimizes the sum of squared forward *and* backward prediction errors. For this reason the modified covariance method is sometimes called the *forward-backward linear prediction* (FBLP) method. We wish to find the *single* predictor vector which minimizes the sum of the forward *and* backward prediction errors. Recall from our discussion of Wiener filtering that for WSS inputs, the forward and backward predictors were obtained from one another by reversing the entries. Thus, we reverse the tap weights for the backward predictor as depicted in Fig. 11.6.2. Furthermore, for the case of complex data, the predictor taps also need to be complex-conjugated to obtain the backward predictor. It is simple to set up the normal equations for the FBLP method. We simply concatenate the normal equations for forward and backward prediction using the covariance method. Again, we want to use *only* the available data.

The first time the backward predictor taps are filled with known data is at $k = N - 1$ and the last time the taps are filled with known data is at $k = L - 1$. Therefore, the first useful backward prediction we can make is of $x(-1)$ and the last useful backward prediction we can make is of $x(L - 1 - N)$. Since $x(-1)$ is not known, we have no measure of the

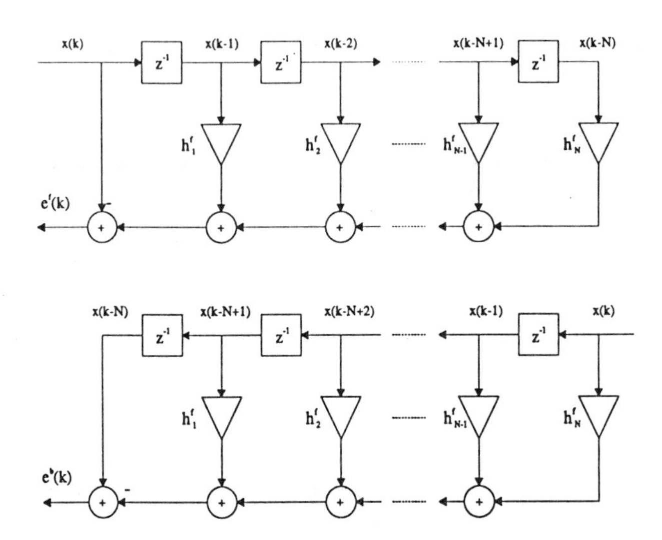

Figure 11.6.2: Using the same predictor for both forward and backward prediction.

prediction error. Therefore, we only predict $x(0)$ through $x(L-1-N)$. Thus, for the backward predictor, we seek the least-squares solution to the system of equations given by

$$\begin{bmatrix} x(0) \\ x(1) \\ \vdots \\ x(L-N-1) \end{bmatrix} = \begin{bmatrix} x(N) & x(N-1) & \cdots & x(1) \\ x(N+1) & x(N) & \cdots & x(2) \\ \vdots & \vdots & \ddots & \vdots \\ x(L-1) & x(L-2) & \cdots & x(L-N) \end{bmatrix} \begin{bmatrix} h^*_{N,N} \\ h^*_{N,N-1} \\ \vdots \\ h^*_{N,1} \end{bmatrix}. \quad (11.6.7)$$

This system of equations can be rewritten as

$$\begin{bmatrix} x(0) \\ x(1) \\ \vdots \\ x(L-N-1) \end{bmatrix} = \begin{bmatrix} x(1) & x(2) & \cdots & x(N) \\ x(2) & x(3) & \cdots & x(N+1) \\ \vdots & \vdots & \ddots & \vdots \\ x(L-N) & x(L-N+1) & \cdots & x(L-1) \end{bmatrix} \begin{bmatrix} h^*_{N,1} \\ h^*_{N,2} \\ \vdots \\ h^*_{N,N} \end{bmatrix}. \quad (11.6.8)$$

Next, we combine the forward and backward prediction equations Eqs. 11.6.6 and 11.6.8 into the single equation

$$\begin{bmatrix} x(N) \\ \vdots \\ x(L-1) \\ x^*(0) \\ \vdots \\ x^*(L-N-1) \end{bmatrix} = \begin{bmatrix} x(N-1) & x(N-2) & \cdots & x(0) \\ \vdots & \vdots & \ddots & \vdots \\ x(L-2) & x(L-3) & \cdots & x(L-N-1) \\ x^*(1) & x^*(2) & \cdots & x^*(N) \\ \vdots & \vdots & \ddots & \vdots \\ x^*(L-N) & x^*(L-N+1) & \cdots & x^*(L-1) \end{bmatrix} \begin{bmatrix} h^f_{N,1} \\ h^f_{N,2} \\ \vdots \\ h^f_{N,N} \end{bmatrix}$$

which we abbreviate by

$$\boldsymbol{C}\boldsymbol{h}_N = \boldsymbol{x} \tag{11.6.9}$$

where the meanings of C is the $2(L-N) \times N$ data matrix and x is a $2(L-N) \times 1$ vector. As usual, the least-squares solution is given by

$$(\boldsymbol{C}^H\boldsymbol{C})\boldsymbol{h}_N = \boldsymbol{C}^H\boldsymbol{x}.$$

The matrix $\boldsymbol{C}^T\boldsymbol{C}$ again provides an estimate of the ensemble-averaged autocorrelation matrix for $\{x(k)\}$, albeit a different estimate than those used by the covariance and autocorrelation methods. The normal equation is simply a different approximation of the Yule-Walker equation.

The FBLP method is extremely useful for extracting the frequencies of sinusoids, which is an important problem in spectral estimation. This problem has many applications, most notably in the area of array signal processing, where it is often necessary to determine the direction of arrival of a source which is impinging on a linear array of antennas. A typical test signal for spectral estimators of this class is a sinusoid in white noise. A good estimator should be able to locate the frequency of the sinusoid accurately and distinguish it from the white noise. Typical problems with sinusoid estimation are *frequency bias* and *line splitting.* Frequency bias refers to a displacement in the estimated frequency of the sinusoid from its true location and usually occurs as a consequence of the additive noise. Line splitting is a phenomenon where the estimated spectrum contains *two* closely spaced peaks when there should only be one. The FBLP method is known to be fairly insensitive to frequency bias [Swi79], and experimental evidence has suggested that the FBLP method does not suffer from line splitting [KM79]. Other AR spectral estimation techniques (such as the Burg algorithm, which we will soon discuss) can produce both frequency bias and line splitting.

An interesting interpretation of the FBLP method is provided by the singular value decomposition (SVD). Suppose the matrix $\boldsymbol{C}$ is of column rank M. Then $\boldsymbol{C}$ can be factored as

$$\boldsymbol{C} = \boldsymbol{U}\begin{bmatrix} \boldsymbol{\Sigma} & \boldsymbol{O} \\ \boldsymbol{O} & \boldsymbol{O} \end{bmatrix}\boldsymbol{V}^H$$

where

$$\boldsymbol{\Sigma} = diag(\sigma_1, \sigma_2, \ldots, \sigma_M)$$

and

$$\sigma_1 \geq \sigma_2 \geq \cdots \geq \sigma_M > 0.$$

The singular values σ_i are the eigenvalues of $\boldsymbol{C}^H\boldsymbol{C}$ and the columns of $\boldsymbol{V}$ are the eigenvectors of $\boldsymbol{C}^H\boldsymbol{C}$ corresponding to the σ_i. This allows us to write $\boldsymbol{C}$ in the form

$$\boldsymbol{C} = \sum_{i=1}^{M} \sigma_i \boldsymbol{u}_i \boldsymbol{v}_i^H,$$

meaning that the matrix $\boldsymbol{C}^H\boldsymbol{C}$, which is an approximation of the correlation matrix, can be expressed as

$$\boldsymbol{C}^H\boldsymbol{C} = \sum_{i=1}^{M} \sigma_i^2 \boldsymbol{v}_i \boldsymbol{v}_i^H.$$

Given the system of equations

$$\boldsymbol{C}\boldsymbol{h}_N = \boldsymbol{x},$$

the least-squares solution is given by

$$\boldsymbol{h}_N = \boldsymbol{C}^{\#}\boldsymbol{x}$$

where $\boldsymbol{C}^{\#}$ is the pseudoinverse of $\boldsymbol{C}$ and is given by

$$\boldsymbol{C}^{\#} = \boldsymbol{V} \begin{bmatrix} \boldsymbol{\Sigma}^{-1} & \boldsymbol{O} \\ \boldsymbol{O} & \boldsymbol{O} \end{bmatrix} \boldsymbol{U}^H.$$

This means that

$$\boldsymbol{C}^{\#} = \sum_{i=1}^{M} \sigma_i^{-1} \boldsymbol{v}_i \boldsymbol{u}_i^H.$$

Similarly, this will give

$$(\boldsymbol{C}^H\boldsymbol{C})^{-1} = \sum_{i=1}^{N} \sigma_i^{-2} \boldsymbol{v}_i \boldsymbol{v}_i^H.$$

Therefore,

$$\boldsymbol{h}_N = \boldsymbol{C}^{\#}\boldsymbol{x} = \sum_{i=1}^{N} \sigma_i^{-1} \boldsymbol{v}_i \boldsymbol{u}_i^H \boldsymbol{x}. \tag{11.6.10}$$

Consider the stochastic process which consists of R uncorrelated complex sinusoids in an uncorrelated white noise background. In other words,

$$x(k) = \sum_{i=1}^{R} A_i e^{j(k\theta_i + \varphi_i)} + v(k)$$

where the φ_i are are the phases, which are assumed to be random and uniformly distributed over $[0, 2\pi)$. We have already seen that the autocorrelation sequence of $\{x(k)\}$ is given by

$$r(k) = \sum_{i=1}^{R} A_i^2 e^{jk\theta_i} + \sigma_v^2 \delta(k)$$

where σ_v^2 is the power of the white noise, and that the $N \times N$ ensemble-averaged autocorrelation matrix for the process $\{x(k)\}$ is given by

$$\boldsymbol{R} = \boldsymbol{E}\boldsymbol{D}\boldsymbol{E}^H + \sigma^2 \boldsymbol{I} \tag{11.6.11}$$

where

$$\boldsymbol{E} = \begin{bmatrix} 1 & 1 & \cdots & 1 \\ e^{j\theta_1} & e^{j\theta_2} & \cdots & e^{j\theta_R} \\ \vdots & \vdots & \vdots & \vdots \\ e^{j(N-1)\theta_1} & e^{j(N-1)\theta_2} & \cdots & e^{j(N-1)\theta_R} \end{bmatrix}$$

and

$$\boldsymbol{D} = diag(A_1^2, A_2^2, \ldots, A_R^2).$$

Examining Eq. 11.6.11, it can be seen that the eigenvalues of $\boldsymbol{R}$ are given by

$$\lambda_i = \begin{cases} \sigma^2 + P_i, & i = 1, 2, \ldots, R \\ \sigma^2, & i = R+1, \ldots, N \end{cases}$$

where the P_i are the eigenvalues of $\boldsymbol{E}\boldsymbol{D}\boldsymbol{E}^H$. Thus, for the noise-free case there will be R nonzero eigenvalues and $N - R$ eigenvalues which are equal to zero. When noise is present at reasonable signal-to-noise ratios, there will be R large eigenvalues and $N - R$ small eigenvalues.

Let's consider the application of the FBLP method to the estimation of complex sinusoids in noise [KT83]. Suppose the signal consists of R uncorrelated sinusoids and white noise of power σ^2. In the zero-noise case, the data matrix $\boldsymbol{C}$ will be singular if the predictor order N is larger than the number of sinusoids R. Thus, there will be R nonzero singular values and $N - R$ singular values which are equal to zero. When there is additive noise, however, the matrix $\boldsymbol{C}$ can have full column rank and consequently, N nonzero singular values.

Using a predictor of order N, we form the data matrix $\boldsymbol{C}$ as in Eq. 11.6.9. Because $\boldsymbol{C}^H\boldsymbol{C}$ is an estimate of the $N \times N$ autocorrelation matrix for the signal, we should expect that $\boldsymbol{C}^H\boldsymbol{C}$ will have R large eigenvalues and $N - R$ small eigenvalues. Correspondingly, $\boldsymbol{C}$

will have R large singular values and $N - R$ small singular values. Direct application of the FBLP method yields the estimated AR parameter vector as

$$\boldsymbol{h}_N = \sum_{i=1}^{N} \sigma_i^{-1} \boldsymbol{v}_i \boldsymbol{u}_i^H \boldsymbol{x}. \tag{11.6.12}$$

We call the $\sigma_1, \sigma_2, \ldots, \sigma_R$ the *signal singular values* and $\sigma_{R+1}, \ldots, \sigma_N$ the *noise singular values.* Because the contribution of each singular value σ_i to the predictor vector $\boldsymbol{h}_N$ is proportional to σ_i^{-1}, the noise singular values can introduce a substantial amount of inaccuracy into its computation.

One remedy to this condition is *rank reduction.* The idea behind rank reduction is to replace the matrix $\boldsymbol{C}$ with a lower rank matrix which still preserves the salient features of the signal spectrum. What we can do is examine the singular values of $\boldsymbol{C}$ and separate them into two parts: large singular values and small singular values. The distinction between large and small is typically simple to make when the signal-to-noise ratio is not excessive. The large singular values are attributed to the sinusoids and the small singular values are attributed to the noise. Next, we compute the predictor as

$$\boldsymbol{h}_N = \sum_{i=1}^{R} \sigma_i^{-1} \boldsymbol{v}_i \boldsymbol{u}_i^H \boldsymbol{x} \tag{11.6.13}$$

where $\sigma_1, \ldots, \sigma_R$ are the large singular values. What we have done is equivalent to replacing the rank N matrix

$$\boldsymbol{C} = \sum_{i=1}^{N} \sigma_i \boldsymbol{u}_i \boldsymbol{v}_i^H$$

with the rank R matrix

$$\tilde{\boldsymbol{C}} = \sum_{i=1}^{R} \sigma_i \boldsymbol{u}_i \boldsymbol{v}_i^H.$$

The effect of this rank reduction is to reduce the contribution of the spurious nonzero singular values which are due to the noise.

For either the full-rank or reduced-rank FBLP method, once the predictor $\boldsymbol{h}_N$ is computed, the spectral estimate is produced according to

$$P_{FBLP}(\theta) = \frac{1}{|1 + \sum_{k=1}^{N} a_{N,i}^* e^{-jk\theta}|^2} \tag{11.6.14}$$

where

$$a_{N,k} = -h_{N,k}.$$

The choice of the predictor order N is nontrivial. If N is substantially larger than the number of sinusoids, the separation between signal and noise singular values becomes difficult, and consequently the spectral estimate will be degraded. Empirical studies have suggested that the optimal value of N is $3L/4$ where L is the number of data samples [Kum82].

Example 11.3

Consider the application of the FBLP method to the signal

$$x(k) = \exp[j(0.97\pi k + .124\pi)] + \exp[j(1.01\pi k - 0.615\pi)] + v(k)$$

where $\{v(k)\}$ is a white noise process with a power σ^2 which is 20 dB less than the power of either sinusoid. We will use a predictor of order $N = 12$. Given 25 samples of the signal, direct application of the DFT to $\{x(k)\}$ is shown in Fig. 11.6.3a. Notice that the sinusoids are indistinguishable. The singular values of the data matrix $\boldsymbol{C}$ are given by

$$\begin{aligned}
\sigma_1 &= 30.72 \\
\sigma_2 &= 3.39 \\
\sigma_3 &= 0.48 \\
\sigma_4 &= 0.46 \\
\sigma_5 &= 0.39 \\
\sigma_6 &= 0.35 \\
\sigma_7 &= 0.31 \\
\sigma_8 &= 0.30 \\
\sigma_9 &= 0.19 \\
\sigma_{10} &= 0.18 \\
\sigma_{11} &= 0.13 \\
\sigma_{12} &= 0.12
\end{aligned}$$

The full-rank spectral estimate is shown in Fig. 11.6.3b. Observe that the sinusoids can be located and are at the correct frequencies but that there is substantial spurious spectral content due to the noise singular values. At lower signal-to-noise ratios, these spurious peaks could possibly overwhelm the peaks which are due to the sinusoids. The reduced-rank spectral estimate is shown in Fig. 11.6.3c. Only the singular values σ_1 and σ_2 have been retained. Again, the sinusoids are easily recognized, but the spurious spectral peaks have been reduced greatly.

The FBLP method belongs to a class of spectral estimation techniques which are sometimes called *super-resolution* methods. Another such method is called the multiple signal classification (MUSIC) method [Sch83]. The MUSIC method is also based on the eigenstructure of the data matrix. Consider again the stochastic process

$$x(k) = \sum_{i=1}^{R} A_i e^{jk\theta_i + \varphi_i} + v(k).$$

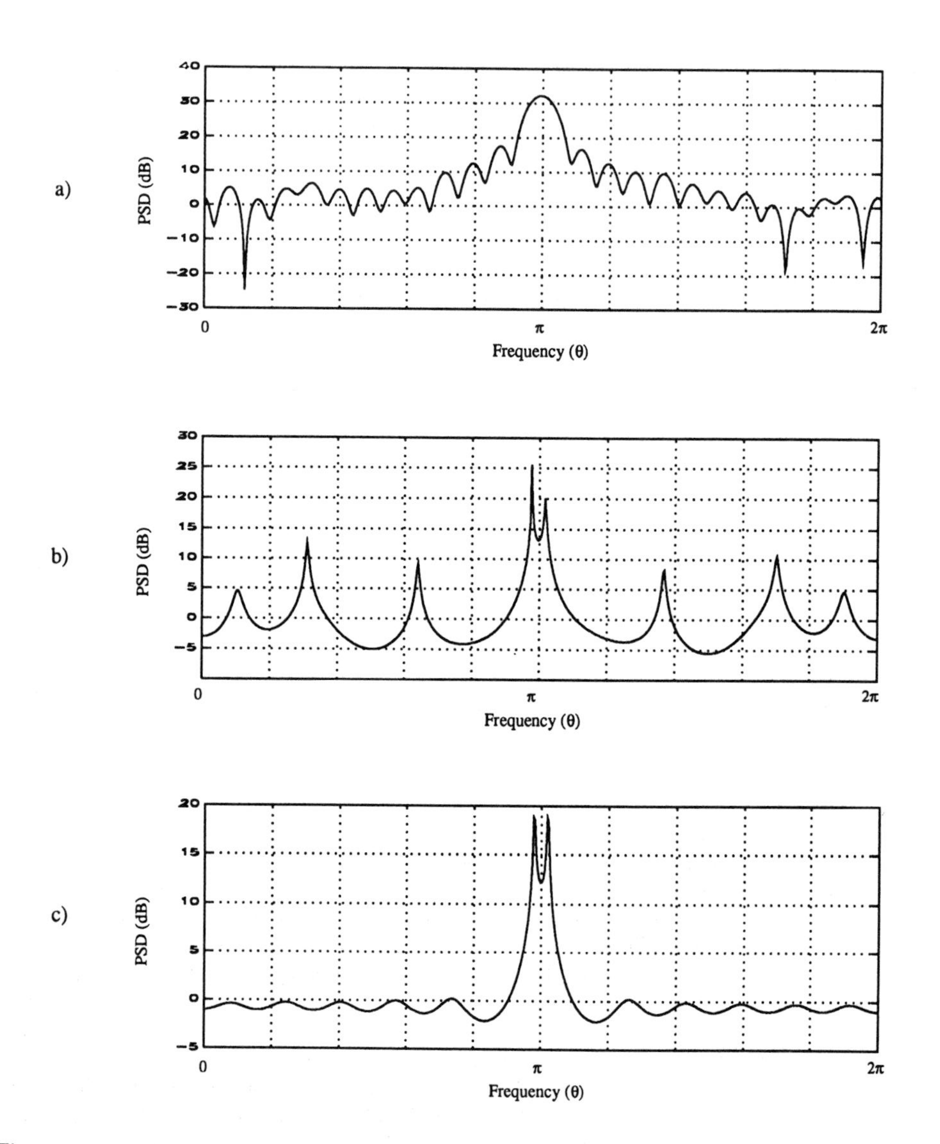

Figure 11.6.3: (a) DFT of two sinusoids in noise (25 samples); (b) full-rank FBLP spectral estimate; (c) reduced-rank spectral estimate.

Recall that the $N \times N$ ensemble-averaged autocorrelation matrix for $\{x(k)\}$ can be expressed as

$$\boldsymbol{R} = \boldsymbol{E}\boldsymbol{D}\boldsymbol{E}^H + \sigma^2 \boldsymbol{I}. \tag{11.6.15}$$

The eigenvalues of $\boldsymbol{R}$ are given by

$$\lambda_i = \begin{cases} \sigma^2 + P_i, & i = 1, 2, \ldots, R \\ \sigma^2, & i = R+1, \ldots, N \end{cases}$$

so that the eigenvectors $\boldsymbol{v}_i$ associated with the $N - R$ smallest eigenvalues of $\boldsymbol{R}$ satisfy

$$\boldsymbol{R}\boldsymbol{v}_i = \sigma^2 \boldsymbol{v}_i, \quad i = R+1, R+2, \ldots, N$$

which means that

$$(\boldsymbol{R} - \sigma^2 \boldsymbol{I})\boldsymbol{v}_i = \boldsymbol{0}, \quad i = R+1, R+2, \ldots, N. \tag{11.6.16}$$

Using the expression for $\boldsymbol{R}$ in Eq. 11.6.15, we can see that Eq. 11.6.16 implies that

$$\boldsymbol{E}\boldsymbol{D}\boldsymbol{E}^H \boldsymbol{v}_i = \boldsymbol{0}, \quad i = R+1, R+2, \ldots, N. \tag{11.6.17}$$

Since all of the sinusoids were assumed to have distinct frequencies, the columns of $\boldsymbol{E}$ are linearly independent. Therefore, Eq. 11.6.17 implies that

$$\boldsymbol{E}^H \boldsymbol{v}_i = \boldsymbol{0}, \quad i = R+1, R+2, \ldots, N. \tag{11.6.18}$$

What Eq. 11.6.18 means is that the eigenvectors of $\boldsymbol{R}$ which corresponds to the smallest singular values are *orthogonal* to the columns of $\boldsymbol{E}$. Let $\boldsymbol{e}_l$ denote the l-th column of $\boldsymbol{E}$, *i.e.*,

$$\boldsymbol{e}_l = \begin{bmatrix} 1 \\ e^{j\theta_l} \\ \vdots \\ e^{j(N-1)\theta_l} \end{bmatrix}.$$

The $\boldsymbol{e}_l$ are called the *signal vectors* since they correspond to the complex sinusoids which are present in the signal. The $\boldsymbol{v}_i$ corresponding to the eigenvalue σ^2 are called the *noise eigenvectors* since they are due to the presence of the white noise term. Then Eq. 11.6.18 means that

$$\boldsymbol{e}_l^H \boldsymbol{v}_i = 0, \quad l = 1, 2, \ldots, R, \quad i = R+1, R+2, \ldots, N \tag{11.6.19}$$

indicating that the noise eigenvectors are orthogonal to the signal vectors. Because $\boldsymbol{R}$ is symmetric, its eigenvectors are orthogonal. Because $\boldsymbol{v}_{R+1}, \boldsymbol{v}_{R+2}, \ldots, \boldsymbol{v}_N$ span a subspace which is orthogonal to the subspace spanned by the signal vectors, the remaining eigenvectors $\boldsymbol{v}_1, \boldsymbol{v}_2, \ldots, v_R$ must span the *same* subspace spanned by the signal vectors. Define the matrices $\boldsymbol{V}_S$ and $\boldsymbol{V}_N$ by

$$\boldsymbol{V}_S = \begin{bmatrix} \boldsymbol{v}_1 & \boldsymbol{v}_2 & \cdots & \boldsymbol{v}_R \end{bmatrix}$$

and

$$\boldsymbol{V}_N = \begin{bmatrix} \boldsymbol{v}_{R+1} & \boldsymbol{v}_{R+2} & \cdots & \boldsymbol{v}_N \end{bmatrix}$$

Then the columns of $\boldsymbol{V}_S$ span the signal subspace and the columns of $\boldsymbol{V}_N$ span the noise subspace. Furthermore, the signal vectors $\boldsymbol{e}_i$ are orthogonal to each column of $\boldsymbol{V}_N$ and the columns of $\boldsymbol{V}_N$ and $\boldsymbol{V}_S$ are orthogonal to each other, so that

$$\boldsymbol{e}_i^H \boldsymbol{V}_N = \mathbf{0}^T$$

and

$$\boldsymbol{V}_N^H \boldsymbol{V}_S = \boldsymbol{O}.$$

This suggests a procedure for extracting the frequencies of sinusoids in white noise.

Given the data matrix $\boldsymbol{C}$ from either the covariance or the FBLP method, we have seen that the matrix $\boldsymbol{C}^H\boldsymbol{C}$ is an approximation of the ensemble-averaged correlation matrix $\boldsymbol{R}$. Correspondingly, we would expect $\boldsymbol{C}^H\boldsymbol{C}$ to have an eigenstructure which is similar to that of $\boldsymbol{R}$. The singular values of $\boldsymbol{C}$ are the square roots of the eigenvalues of $\boldsymbol{C}^H\boldsymbol{C}$, so we should find that there are R large singular values corresponding to the signal and $N-R$ "small" singular values corresponding to the noise. Given the singular value decomposition

$$\boldsymbol{C} = \boldsymbol{U}\boldsymbol{\Sigma}\boldsymbol{V}^H,$$

let $\boldsymbol{v}_{R+1}, \boldsymbol{v}_{R+2}, \ldots, \boldsymbol{v}_N$ be the right singular vectors corresponding to the $N-R$ smallest singular values. We form the matrix $\hat{\boldsymbol{V}}_N$ as

$$\hat{\boldsymbol{V}}_N = \begin{bmatrix} \boldsymbol{v}_{R+1} & \boldsymbol{v}_{R+2} & \cdots & \boldsymbol{v}_N \end{bmatrix}$$

so that $\hat{\boldsymbol{V}}_N$ is an estimate of the noise subspace. Now, let $\boldsymbol{e}(\theta)$ be defined by

$$\boldsymbol{e}(\theta) = \begin{bmatrix} 1 \\ e^{j\theta} \\ \vdots \\ e^{j(N-1)\theta} \end{bmatrix}.$$

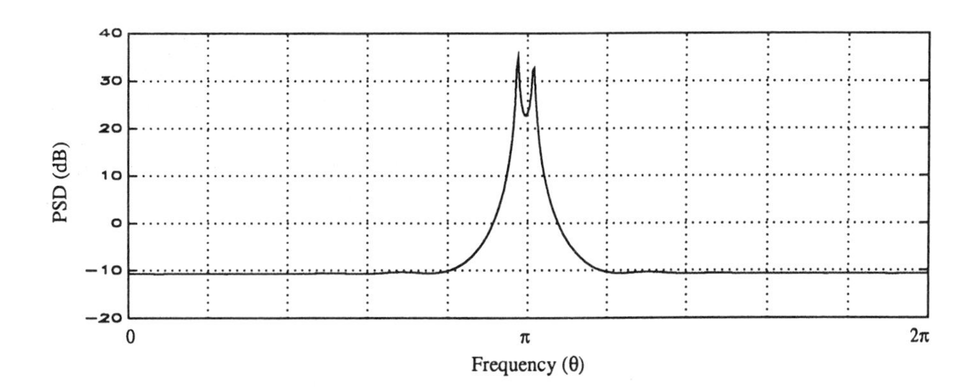

Figure 11.6.4: MUSIC spectral estimate for two complex sinusoids in white noise.

In the ensemble-averaged case, we know that the signal vectors $\boldsymbol{e}_i$ are orthogonal to the noise subspace. Because $\boldsymbol{C}^H\boldsymbol{C}$ is an approximation of $\boldsymbol{R}$, the $\boldsymbol{e}_i$ are only *approximately* orthogonal to the *estimated* noise subspace spanned by the columns of $\hat{\boldsymbol{V}}_N$. Consider the product

$$\boldsymbol{e}(\theta)^H\hat{\boldsymbol{V}}_N.$$

Because the frequencies of the sinusoids are unknown, we "sweep" theta from 0 to 2π. We would expect that as θ approaches the frequency of one of the sinusoids, then

$$\boldsymbol{e}(\theta_i)^H\hat{\boldsymbol{V}}_N \approx 0.$$

The MUSIC spectral estimate is given by

$$P_{MUSIC}(\theta) = \frac{1}{\boldsymbol{e}^H(\theta)\hat{\boldsymbol{V}}_N\hat{\boldsymbol{V}}_N\boldsymbol{e}(\theta)}. \tag{11.6.20}$$

Thus, the MUSIC spectrum should exhibit peaks at the frequencies of the sinusoids. The MUSIC method has been studied extensively and has been shown to provide reliable results for the location of sinusoids in noise. Fig. 11.6.4 shows the results of the MUSIC method applied to the same data as Example 11.3.

11.6.3 AR Spectral Estimators Based on Reflection Coefficients

We have seen the equivalent representations of prediction error filters via transversal structures and lattice structures. Namely, given a transversal prediction error filter of order N, we can compute reflection coefficients $\kappa_1, \kappa_2, \ldots, \kappa_N$ which parameterize the lattice and vice versa. Because of the connection between prediction error filters and the Yule-Walker equation for an AR process, we can compute an AR spectral estimate by first estimating the prediction coefficients. Thus, we would expect that if the reflection coefficients of a prediction error filter are estimated directly from the data, the equivalent transversal prediction error coefficients can be obtained and an AR spectral estimate then computed. This is the idea behind reflection coefficient-based AR spectral estimation techniques.

We have seen that the lattice structure is characterized by the pair of equations

$$\begin{aligned} e_m^f(k) &= e_{m-1}^f(k) + \kappa_m e_{m-1}^b(k-1) \\ e_m^b(k) &= \kappa_m e_{m-1}^f(k) + e_{m-1}^b(k-1) \end{aligned}$$

with the initializations

$$e_0^f(k) = e_0^b(k) = x(k).$$

There are several criteria for optimization of the lattice structure. We will discuss two of them.

The *Burg* [Bur75] method computes the reflection coefficient κ_m so as to minimize the sum of the forward and backward prediction error powers at the m-th lattice stage. We saw earlier that this value of κ_m is given by

$$\kappa_m = \frac{-2\mathcal{E}[e_{m-1}^f(k)e_{m-1}^b(k-1)]}{\mathcal{E}[(e_{m-1}^f(k))^2 + (e_{m-1}^b(k-1))^2]}. \tag{11.6.21}$$

Because we do not have access to the ensemble-averaged quantities, we must estimate the reflection coefficient from the available data. Assuming we have L samples of $\{x(k)\}$, the estimate used by the Burg method is

$$\hat{\kappa}_m = -\frac{\sum_{n=m+1}^{L} e_{m-1}^b(k-1)e_{m-1}^f(k)}{\sum_{n=m+1}^{L} [(e_{m-1}^f(k))^2 + (e_{m-1}^b(k-1))^2]}, \quad m = 1, 2, \ldots$$

with a block of data of length L. We begin with $e_0^b(k) = e_0^f(k) = x(k)$ and compute $\hat{\kappa}_1$. Once $\hat{\kappa}_1$ is available, the prediction errors at the second stage, and hence $\hat{\kappa}_2$, can be computed. The procedure continues until the final stage is reached. The reason for the choice of $n = m + 1$ as the lower limit on the summations is because this is the first time at which all input samples contribute to the prediction error outputs at the m-th stage. Once $\hat{\kappa}_1, \hat{\kappa}_2, \ldots, \hat{\kappa}_N$ are computed, the transversal prediction error filter parameters $\hat{a}_1, \hat{a}_2, \ldots, \hat{a}_N$ are computed using the inverse form of the Levinson-Durbin algorithm.

To determine the final prediction filter and the final prediction error power given the signal power P_0 and the reflection coefficients, recall from that the forward prediction error filter is order-updated according to

$$\boldsymbol{a}^{(m)} = \begin{bmatrix} \boldsymbol{a}^{(m-1))} \\ 0 \end{bmatrix} + \kappa_m \begin{bmatrix} 0 \\ \boldsymbol{b}^{(m-1))} \end{bmatrix}.$$

Because the last element of $\boldsymbol{b}^{(m-1)}$ is unity, it follows that the last element of $\boldsymbol{a}^{(m)}$ is equal to κ_m. That is,

$$a_m^{(m)} = \kappa_m.$$

Furthermore, we have seen that

$$\begin{aligned} A_m(z) &= A_{m-1}(z) + \kappa_m z^{-1} B_{m-1}(z) \\ B_m(z) &= \kappa_m A_m(z) + z^{-1} B_{m-1}(z). \end{aligned} \tag{11.6.22}$$

Remembering that the forward and backward predictors are the reverse of one another, it also follows that

$$B_m(z) = z^{-m} A_m(z^{-1}).$$

Therefore, we have

$$A_m(z) = A_{m-1}(z) + \kappa_m z^{-1} z^{-(m-1)} A_{m-1}(z^{-1}) \tag{11.6.23}$$

and the backward prediction error filter is obtained by reversing the coefficients of $A_m(z)$. Recall also that the prediction error power is updated according to

$$P_m = (1 - \kappa_m^2) P_{m-1}. \tag{11.6.24}$$

We can use Eqs. 11.6.23 and 11.6.24 iteratively to find the final prediction error filter and final prediction error power from the reflection coefficients and the input power.

Finally, the AR spectrum estimate is computed as

$$P_{BURG}(\theta) = \frac{\hat{P}}{|1 + \sum_{k=1}^{N} \hat{a}_k e^{-jk\theta}|^2} \tag{11.6.25}$$

where $\hat{P}$ can be computed from the $\hat{\kappa}_i$ using the Levinson recursions. We begin with

$$\hat{P}_0 = \frac{1}{L} \sum_{k=0}^{L-1} |x(k)|^2$$

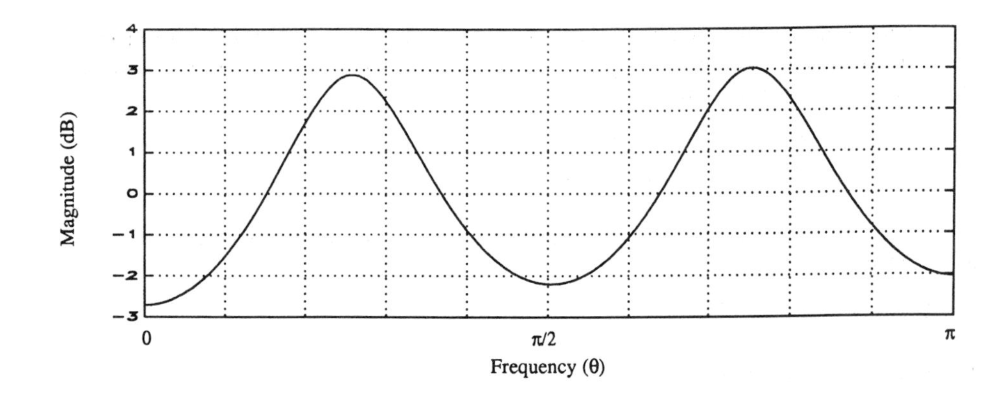

Figure 11.6.5: AR(4) estimate using the Burg method.

and update the power at each stage according to

$$\hat{P}_m = (1 - \hat{\kappa}_m^2)\hat{P}_{m-1}.$$

The Burg method is capable of fairly high resolution and can also be useful for estimating the frequencies of sinusoids in noise. It has been shown, however, that under some conditions the Burg method suffers from frequency bias which is related to the initial phase of the sinusoids and that the Burg method can also produce line splitting whereby to closely spaced peaks can arise when only one should be present [Kay88].

Consider the same AR(4) process whose power spectrum was shown in Fig. 11.6.1a. The AR(4) spectral estimate based on the Burg method is shown in Fig. 11.6.5.

11.6.4 Determining the Model Order

In general, the proper order of the AR model is not known a priori. Too low a model order can result in a smoothed spectrum and too high a model order can result in spurious peaks. This is yet another illustration of the tradeoff between bias and variance. It is important to have available some criterion of performance which provides some insight into the appropriate model order.

One plausible indicator of the appropriate model order is the prediction error. While this will help in determining an order which is *large enough*, it may actually overestimate the proper model order. This is because the prediction error power is typically a monotonically decreasing quantity as model order increases. Eventually, we will reach a point at which the prediction error power does not change with an increase in model order.

With the prediction error power for the order-N estimator given by $\hat{P}_N$, Akaike defined the *final prediction error* (FPE) criterion [Aka69] by

$$FPE(N) = \hat{P}_N \frac{L+N}{L-N}$$

where L is the number of data samples. This criterion is a product of two terms, one of which decreases with model order, the other of which increases with model order. The model order is chosen as the value of N which minimizes $FPE(N)$. The FPE criterion works well for processes which are actually AR, but tends to select too low a model order in practice.

Akaike also suggested another criterion which is known as the *Akaike information criterion* (AIC) [Aka74]. The AIC criterion is given by

$$AIC(N) = L \ln \hat{P}_N + 2N.$$

Again, the model order is chosen as the value of N which minimizes $AIC(N)$. It has been shown that the AIC criterion is asymptotically equivalent to the FPE criterion as the model order grows to infinity. The AIC is an inconsistent estimator of the model as the number of sample approaches infinity in that the probability of error in choosing the correct model order does not approach zero. For processes which are not actually AR, the AIC tends to underestimate the model order, while for AR processes, the model order will frequently be overestimated as the number of samples increases. Consequently, Rissanen proposed a modification of the AIC called the *minimum description length* (MDL) criterion [Ris78], which is given by

$$MDL(N) = L \ln \hat{P}_N + N \ln L.$$

The MDL criterion *is* a consistent estimator of the model order, and, as usual, the model order is chosen as the value of N which minimizes $MDL(N)$.

Appendix

MATHEMATICAL REVIEW

In this chapter, we will review some important results from linear algebra and probability theory. For more detailed coverage, an excellent source for matrix theory is [Nob69]. For probability theory and stochastic processes, the reader is referred to [Pap65].

A.1 Linear Algebra and Matrix Theory

Suppose $\boldsymbol{x}_1, \boldsymbol{x}_2, \ldots, \boldsymbol{x}_m$ are vectors in a vector space V over the real or the complex field. Then the collection of all vectors

$$\boldsymbol{x} = \alpha_1 \boldsymbol{x}_1 + \alpha_2 \boldsymbol{x}_2 + \cdots + \alpha_m \boldsymbol{x}_m$$

is known as the *span* of the vectors $\boldsymbol{x}_1, \boldsymbol{x}_2, \ldots, \boldsymbol{x}_m$ where the α_i are real or complex field, respectively.

Vectors $\boldsymbol{x}_1, \boldsymbol{x}_2, \ldots, \boldsymbol{x}_m$ are said to be *linearly independent* if the relation

$$\sum_{i=1}^{m} \alpha_i \boldsymbol{x}_i = 0 \tag{A.1.1}$$

implies that all of the α_i are equal to zero. If the set of vectors is not linearly independent, it is possible to write at least one of the vectors as a linear combination of the others. For example, suppose $\alpha_j \neq 0$. Then

$$\boldsymbol{x}_j = \sum_{i \neq j} (\alpha_i / \alpha_j) \boldsymbol{x}_i. \tag{A.1.2}$$

Consider an $m \times n$ matrix $\boldsymbol{A}$ with elements a_{ij}, $i = 1, 2, \ldots, m$ and $j = 1, 2, \ldots, n$. The elements of $\boldsymbol{A}$ are denoted using the notation

$$[\boldsymbol{A}]_{ij} = a_{ij}. \tag{A.1.3}$$

The elements a_{ij} can be either real or complex. When the a_{ij} are real, it is useful to view $\boldsymbol{A}$ as representing a linear mapping from R^n to R^m. When the a_{ij} are complex, $\boldsymbol{A}$ can be viewed as representing a linear mapping from C^n to C^m.

The principal operations on matrices are matrix addition, scalar multiplication, and matrix multiplication. Given $m \times n$ matrices $\boldsymbol{A}$ and $\boldsymbol{B}$, their sum is the $m \times n$ matrix $\boldsymbol{C}$ whose ij-th element is given by

$$c_{ij} = a_{ij} + b_{ij}. \tag{A.1.4}$$

Given a scalar, α, and an $m \times n$ matrix $\boldsymbol{A}$, the scalar product $\alpha\boldsymbol{A}$ of α and $\boldsymbol{A}$ is the $m \times n$ matrix whose ij-th element is given by

$$[\alpha\boldsymbol{A}]_{ij} = \alpha a_{ij}. \tag{A.1.5}$$

Finally, if $\boldsymbol{A}$ is $m \times n$ and $\boldsymbol{B}$ is $n \times p$, the product $\boldsymbol{C} = \boldsymbol{AB}$ is the $m \times p$ matrix whose ij-th element is given by

$$c_{ij} = \sum_{k=1}^{n} a_{ik} b_{kj}. \tag{A.1.6}$$

The term *conformable* is used to indicate that matrices have the proper dimensions for multiplication or addition, whichever the context indicates.

Two special matrices are the *null matrix*, $\boldsymbol{O}$, and the identity matrix, $\boldsymbol{I}$. The null matrix consists of all zeros, and the identity matrix is a square matrix with all non-diagonal elements equal to zero and ones on the diagonal. If $\boldsymbol{A}$ and $\boldsymbol{O}$ are conformable matrices, then

$$\boldsymbol{AO} = \boldsymbol{O} \quad \text{and} \quad \boldsymbol{A} + \boldsymbol{O} = \boldsymbol{A}$$

and

$$\boldsymbol{AI} = \boldsymbol{A}.$$

For any matrix $\boldsymbol{A}$, the *transpose* is defined as the matrix whose rows and columns are interchanged from $\boldsymbol{A}$'s. If $\boldsymbol{A}$ is $m \times n$, the transpose is $n \times m$ and is denoted by the symbol $\boldsymbol{A}^T$. Formally,

$$[\boldsymbol{A}^T]_{ji} = [\boldsymbol{A}]_{ij}. \tag{A.1.7}$$

For a matrix $\boldsymbol{A}$ with complex elements, the conjugate transpose is used and is denoted by $\boldsymbol{A}^H$ where

$$[\boldsymbol{A}^H]_{ji} = [\boldsymbol{A}]_{ij}^*. \tag{A.1.8}$$

If $\boldsymbol{A}$ and $\boldsymbol{B}$ are conformable matrices, then

$$(\boldsymbol{AB})^T = \boldsymbol{B}^T\boldsymbol{A}^T$$

and

$$(\boldsymbol{AB})^H = \boldsymbol{B}^H\boldsymbol{A}^H.$$

A matrix for which $\boldsymbol{A}^T = \boldsymbol{A}$ is known as a *symmetric* matrix. If $\boldsymbol{A}^H = \boldsymbol{A}$, then $\boldsymbol{A}$ is called *Hermitian.*

Let $\boldsymbol{A}$ be the 2×2 matrix given by

$$\begin{pmatrix} a_{11} & a_{12} \\ a_{21} & a_{22} \end{pmatrix}.$$

The *determinant* of $\boldsymbol{A}$ is defined by the scalar

$$|\boldsymbol{A}| = a_{11}a_{22} - a_{12}a_{21}. \tag{A.1.9}$$

For larger matrices, the determinant is defined recursively. If $\boldsymbol{A}$ is $n \times n$, $|\boldsymbol{A}|$ is defined by

$$|\boldsymbol{A}| = \sum_{i=1}^{n} a_{ij}A_{ij} \tag{A.1.10}$$

where A_{ij} is the *cofactor* of a_{ij}, defined by $(-1)^{i+j}$ times the determinant of the $(n-1)\times(n-1)$ matrix obtained by deleting the i-th row and j-th column from $\boldsymbol{A}$.

A square matrix $\boldsymbol{A}$ is said to be invertible (or *nonsingular*) if there exists a matrix $\boldsymbol{B}$ such that

$$\boldsymbol{AB} = \boldsymbol{BA} = \boldsymbol{I}.$$

The matrix $\boldsymbol{B}$ will be unique and the inverse is denoted by $\boldsymbol{B} = \boldsymbol{A}^{-1}$. If $\boldsymbol{A}$ and $\boldsymbol{B}$ are conformable matrices, then

$$(\boldsymbol{AB})^{-1} = \boldsymbol{B}^{-1}\boldsymbol{A}^{-1}$$

assuming the indicated inverses exist.

If $\boldsymbol{A}$ is invertible, there is a solution to the matrix equation

$$\boldsymbol{Ax} = \boldsymbol{b}$$

where $\boldsymbol{A}$ is $n \times n$, $\boldsymbol{b}$ is $n \times 1$, and $\boldsymbol{x}$ is an unknown $n \times 1$ vector. The solution is given simply by

$$\boldsymbol{x} = \boldsymbol{A}^{-1}\boldsymbol{b}.$$

A square matrix $\boldsymbol{A}$ is invertible if and only if its columns are linearly independent. A simple test for invertibility is to check the determinant. It can be shown that $\boldsymbol{A}$ is invertible if and only if $|\boldsymbol{A}| \neq 0$.

If $|\boldsymbol{A}| = 0$ (*i.e.*, $\boldsymbol{A}$ is not invertible) there are nonzero solutions to the matrix equation

$$\boldsymbol{A}\boldsymbol{x} = \boldsymbol{0}.$$

Such vectors $\boldsymbol{x}$ are said to lie in the *null space* of $\boldsymbol{A}$. Consequently, a matrix is nonsingular if and only if its null space consists of the vector $\boldsymbol{0}$ alone. The null space of $\boldsymbol{A}$ will be denoted by $\mathcal{N}(\boldsymbol{A})$.

The *column space* of a matrix $\boldsymbol{A}$ is defined as the space spanned by the columns of $\boldsymbol{A}$. Consequently, a square matrix $\boldsymbol{A}$ is nonsingular if its columns span the entire vector space. The number of linearly independent columns (the dimension of the column space) is referred to as the *rank* of the matrix. In general, the sum of the dimensions of the column space and the null space is equal to the number of columns.

A particularly simple closed-form expression for the inverse of a matrix $\boldsymbol{A}$ is given using determinants. The *adjoint* of $\boldsymbol{A}$ is the matrix given by

$$[adj(\boldsymbol{A})]_{ij} = [A_{ji}]^*. \tag{A.1.11}$$

In other words, $adj(\boldsymbol{A})$ is formed by first replacing the ij-th element of $\boldsymbol{A}$ by the determinant formed by striking the i-th row and j-th column of $\boldsymbol{A}$, and then complex transposing (which is equivalent to simple transposition in the case where $\boldsymbol{A}$ is real). If $\boldsymbol{A}$ is nonsingular, its inverse is then given by

$$\boldsymbol{A}^{-1} = \frac{adj(\boldsymbol{A})}{|\boldsymbol{A}|}. \tag{A.1.12}$$

A.1.1 Inner Product Spaces and Orthogonality

If V is a vector space over R or C, an *inner product* is a function $\langle \cdot, \cdot \rangle$ from V to either R or C which satisfies

1. $\langle \boldsymbol{x}, \boldsymbol{y} \rangle = (\langle \boldsymbol{y}, \boldsymbol{x} \rangle)^*$ for all $\boldsymbol{x}, \boldsymbol{y} \in V$.
2. $\langle a\boldsymbol{x} + b\boldsymbol{y}, \boldsymbol{z} \rangle = a^* \langle \boldsymbol{x}, \boldsymbol{z} \rangle + b^* \langle \boldsymbol{y}, \boldsymbol{z} \rangle$ for all $a, b \in F$, $\boldsymbol{x}, \boldsymbol{y}, \boldsymbol{z} \in V$.
3. $\langle \boldsymbol{x}, \boldsymbol{x} \rangle \geq 0$, with equality if and only if $\boldsymbol{x} = 0$.

An important inner product for vector spaces over R is given by

$$\langle \boldsymbol{x}, \boldsymbol{y} \rangle = \boldsymbol{x}^T \boldsymbol{y} = \sum_{i=1}^{n} x_i y_i.$$

Over C, the definition needs to be modified according to

$$\langle \boldsymbol{x}, \boldsymbol{y} \rangle = \boldsymbol{x}^H \boldsymbol{y} = \sum_{i=1}^{n} x_i^* y_i.$$

It is a simple matter to prove that these inner products satisfy the conditions of the definition. In Euclidean space, the length of a vector $\boldsymbol{x}$ is given by

$$||\boldsymbol{x}|| = \sqrt{\langle \boldsymbol{x}, \boldsymbol{x} \rangle}.$$

This idea can be generalized to more abstract vector spaces, instead referring to the length as the *norm.*

An *inner product space* is simply a vector space which is endowed with an inner product. Another important notion is the concept of *orthogonality.* Given an inner product space, two vectors are said to be orthogonal if

$$\langle \boldsymbol{x}, \boldsymbol{y} \rangle = 0.$$

In general, a set of vectors $\boldsymbol{x}_1, \boldsymbol{x}_2, \ldots, \boldsymbol{x}_m$ is called an *orthogonal set* if $\langle \boldsymbol{x}_i, \boldsymbol{x}_j \rangle = 0$ whenever $i \neq j$. Furthermore, if the vectors each satisfy $||\boldsymbol{x}_i||=1$, we call the set of vectors *orthonormal.* A simple but important consequence of orthogonality is that a set of nonzero orthogonal or orthonormal vectors is also linearly independent.

Suppose a matrix $\boldsymbol{U}$ has columns which form an orthonormal set. It is simple to see that

$$\boldsymbol{U}^H \boldsymbol{U} = \boldsymbol{U} \boldsymbol{U}^H = \boldsymbol{I}, \tag{A.1.13}$$

with complex transpose replaced by simple transpose for purely real matrices. A matrix with orthonormal columns is called *unitary.* It can be shown that the product of two unitary matrices is unitary.

A.1.2 Eigenanalysis

Let $\boldsymbol{A}$ be an $n \times n$ matrix. We wish to find *non-trivial* solutions to the equation

$$\boldsymbol{A}\boldsymbol{x} = \lambda \boldsymbol{x} \tag{A.1.14}$$

where λ is some scalar which is yet to be determined. To analyze Eq. A.1.14, rewrite it in the form

$$\lambda \boldsymbol{I}\boldsymbol{x} - \boldsymbol{A}\boldsymbol{x} = (\lambda \boldsymbol{I} - \boldsymbol{A})\boldsymbol{x} = 0. \tag{A.1.15}$$

Thus, we seek vectors $\boldsymbol{x}$ which lie in the null space of the matrix $(\lambda\boldsymbol{I} - \boldsymbol{A})$. This matrix has a nontrivial null space if and only if

$$|\lambda\boldsymbol{I} - \boldsymbol{A}| = 0. \qquad \text{(A.1.16)}$$

The determinant in Eq. A.1.16 yields a polynomial of degree n, expressed by

$$|\lambda\boldsymbol{I} - \boldsymbol{A}| = \lambda^n + a_{n-1}\lambda^{n-1} + \cdots + a_1\lambda + a_0 = p(\lambda). \qquad \text{(A.1.17)}$$

Values of λ for which $p(\lambda) = 0$ are known as *eigenvalues* and correspond to scalars for which the equation $\boldsymbol{A}\boldsymbol{x} = \lambda\boldsymbol{x}$ has a nontrivial solution. The polynomial $p(\lambda)$ is of degree n, and hence has n solutions $\lambda_1, \lambda_2, \ldots, \lambda_n$. Thus, a $n \times n$ matrix has n (not necessarily distinct) eigenvalues.

The polynomial $p(\lambda)$ is known as the *characteristic polynomial* for the matrix $\boldsymbol{A}$, and according to Eq. A.1.17, the roots of the characteristic polynomial of a matrix give the eigenvalues of the matrix. What we must do now is determine for each eigenvalue λ_i the corresponding vector $\boldsymbol{x}_i$ which satisfies $\boldsymbol{A}\boldsymbol{x}_i = \lambda_i\boldsymbol{x}_i$. The vector $\boldsymbol{x}_i$ is known as the *eigenvector* corresponding to the eigenvalue λ_i. The existence of a nonzero $\boldsymbol{x}_i$ is guaranteed by the nullity of the matrix $(\lambda_i\boldsymbol{I} - \boldsymbol{A})$.

One important fact which must be mentioned is that the eigenvectors corresponding to distinct eigenvalues are *linearly independent.* Even when the eigenvalues are not distinct, it is still possible to find a set of linearly independent eigenvectors.

A useful matrix decomposition is given using eigenvalues and eigenvectors. Let $\boldsymbol{A}$ be an $n \times n$ matrix with eigenvalues $\lambda_1, \lambda_2, \ldots, \lambda_n$ and corresponding eigenvectors $\boldsymbol{x}_1, \boldsymbol{x}_2, \ldots, \boldsymbol{x}_n$. For each i,

$$\boldsymbol{A}\boldsymbol{x}_i = \lambda_i\boldsymbol{x}_i \qquad \text{(A.1.18)}$$

so that

$$\boldsymbol{A}\begin{bmatrix} \boldsymbol{x}_1 & \boldsymbol{x}_2 & \cdots & \boldsymbol{x}_n \end{bmatrix} = \begin{bmatrix} \boldsymbol{x}_1 & \boldsymbol{x}_2 & \cdots & \boldsymbol{x}_n \end{bmatrix} \begin{pmatrix} \lambda_1 & 0 & 0 & \cdots & 0 \\ 0 & \lambda_2 & 0 & \cdots & 0 \\ \vdots & \vdots & \vdots & \ddots & \vdots \\ 0 & 0 & 0 & \cdots & \lambda_n \end{pmatrix}. \qquad \text{(A.1.19)}$$

If the diagonal matrix of eigenvalues is denoted by $\boldsymbol{\Lambda}$ and the matrix of eigenvectors by $\boldsymbol{T}$, Eq. A.1.19 can be written concisely as

$$\boldsymbol{A}\boldsymbol{T} = \boldsymbol{T}\boldsymbol{\Lambda}. \qquad \text{(A.1.20)}$$

Now, we have already stated that the eigenvectors of a matrix are linearly independent. Because the columns of $\boldsymbol{T}$ are the eigenvectors of $\boldsymbol{A}$, $\boldsymbol{T}$ has linearly independent columns and is thus invertible. This means that Eq. A.1.20 can be rearranged to give

$$\boldsymbol{A} = \boldsymbol{T}\boldsymbol{\Lambda}\boldsymbol{T}^{-1}. \qquad \text{(A.1.21)}$$

To see why Eq. A.1.21 is useful, consider computing powers of $\boldsymbol{A}$. We have

$$\boldsymbol{A}^2 = \boldsymbol{T}\boldsymbol{\Lambda}\boldsymbol{T}^{-1}\boldsymbol{T}\boldsymbol{\Lambda}\boldsymbol{T}^{-1} = \boldsymbol{T}\boldsymbol{\Lambda}^2\boldsymbol{T}^{-1}. \tag{A.1.22}$$

But $\boldsymbol{\Lambda}$ is a diagonal matrix so that $\boldsymbol{\Lambda}^p$ is also diagonal, with $[\boldsymbol{\Lambda}^p]_{ii} = \lambda_{ii}^p$. Successive powers of $\boldsymbol{A}$ can be computed from this relationship:

$$\boldsymbol{A}^3 = \boldsymbol{A}^2\boldsymbol{A} = \boldsymbol{T}\boldsymbol{\Lambda}^2\boldsymbol{T}^{-1}\boldsymbol{T}\boldsymbol{\Lambda}\boldsymbol{T}^{-1} = \boldsymbol{T}\boldsymbol{\Lambda}_3\boldsymbol{T}^{-1}, \tag{A.1.23}$$

and in general,

$$A^k = \boldsymbol{T}\boldsymbol{\Lambda}^k\boldsymbol{T}^{-1}. \tag{A.1.24}$$

A simple extension of this reasoning can be used to show that if $p(x)$ is any polynomial function, we can evaluate $p(\boldsymbol{A})$ by

$$p(\boldsymbol{A}) = \boldsymbol{T}p(\boldsymbol{\Lambda})\boldsymbol{T}^{-1}. \tag{A.1.25}$$

The matrix $p(\boldsymbol{\Lambda})$ is diagonal, with elements

$$[p(\boldsymbol{\Lambda})]_{ii} = p(\lambda_i). \tag{A.1.26}$$

If a matrix is Hermitian (or symmetric for real matrices), its eigenvalues are real and, if the eigenvalues are distinct, the eigenvectors form an orthogonal set. This means that the matrix $\boldsymbol{T}$ of eigenvectors is unitary and Eq. A.1.21 becomes

$$\boldsymbol{A}^{-1} = \boldsymbol{T}\boldsymbol{\Lambda}\boldsymbol{T}^H \tag{A.1.27}$$

Eq. A.1.24 becomes

$$A^k = \boldsymbol{T}\boldsymbol{\Lambda}^k\boldsymbol{T}^H \tag{A.1.28}$$

and

$$p(\boldsymbol{A}) = \boldsymbol{T}p(\boldsymbol{\Lambda})\boldsymbol{T}^H. \tag{A.1.29}$$

A useful *outer product* decomposition exists for a Hermitian matrix $\boldsymbol{A}$. If the orthonormal eigenvectors are given by $\boldsymbol{x}_1, \boldsymbol{x}_2, \ldots, \boldsymbol{x}_n$, Eq. A.1.27 becomes

$$\boldsymbol{A} = \sum_{i=1}^{n} \lambda_i \boldsymbol{x}_i \boldsymbol{x}_i^H. \tag{A.1.30}$$

Also, because $\boldsymbol{A} = \boldsymbol{T}\boldsymbol{\Lambda}\boldsymbol{T}^H$ and $\boldsymbol{T}$ is unitary,

$$\boldsymbol{A}^{-1} = \boldsymbol{T}\boldsymbol{\Lambda}^{-1}\boldsymbol{T}^H,$$

or

$$\boldsymbol{A}^{-1} = \sum_{i=1}^{n} \frac{1}{\lambda_i} \boldsymbol{x}_i \boldsymbol{x}_i^H. \tag{A.1.31}$$

A.1.3 Real Quadratic Forms

A function $V(x)$ of a scalar variable x is said to be *quadratic* if it is of the form

$$V(x) = p - 2qx + rx^2 \tag{A.1.32}$$

where p, q and r are constants. $V(x)$ has a unique extremum at $x_0 = q/r$ and we have

$$V(x_0) = p - q^2/r. \tag{A.1.33}$$

The geometry of the quadratic form is more evident if we complete the square and rewrite Eq. A.1.32 in the form

$$V(x) = V(x_0) + r(x - x_0)^2 \tag{A.1.34}$$

from which one can readily identify $V(x_0)$ as the extremum.

The notion of quadratic form can be extended to the vector case. Let

$$\boldsymbol{x} = \begin{pmatrix} x_1 \\ x_2 \\ \vdots \\ x_n \end{pmatrix},$$

and define the quadratic form $V(\boldsymbol{x})$ by

$$V(\boldsymbol{x}) = \boldsymbol{p} - 2\sum_{i=1}^{n} q_i x_i + \sum_{i=1}^{n}\sum_{j=1}^{n} r_{ij} x_i x_j \tag{A.1.35}$$

where $\boldsymbol{R}$ is an $n \times n$ matrix with $[\boldsymbol{R}]_{ij} = r_{ij}$ and $\boldsymbol{q}$ is an $n \times 1$ vector. Eq. A.1.35 can then be expressed as

$$V(\boldsymbol{x}) = p - 2\boldsymbol{q}^T\boldsymbol{x} + \boldsymbol{x}^T\boldsymbol{R}\boldsymbol{x} = \begin{pmatrix} 1 & \boldsymbol{x}^T \end{pmatrix} \begin{pmatrix} p & -\boldsymbol{q}^T \\ -\boldsymbol{q} & \boldsymbol{R} \end{pmatrix} \begin{pmatrix} 1 \\ \boldsymbol{x} \end{pmatrix}. \tag{A.1.36}$$

If $\boldsymbol{R}$ is nonsingular, we can complete the square for the vector quadratic form. The minimum of $V(\boldsymbol{x})$ is found by differentiating the quadratic form with respect to $\boldsymbol{x}$ and setting the result to zero:

$$\frac{\partial V}{\partial \boldsymbol{x}} = -2\boldsymbol{q} + 2\boldsymbol{R}\boldsymbol{x} = \boldsymbol{0}. \tag{A.1.37}$$

so that

$$\boldsymbol{x}_0 = \boldsymbol{R}^{-1}\boldsymbol{q}. \tag{A.1.38}$$

Then $V(\boldsymbol{x})$ can be rewritten as

$$V(\boldsymbol{x}) = V(\boldsymbol{x}_0) + (\boldsymbol{x} - \boldsymbol{x}_0)^T \boldsymbol{R}(\boldsymbol{x} - \boldsymbol{x}_0). \qquad \text{(A.1.39)}$$

In order to characterize the extremum as a minimum or a maximum, we need a condition which is analogous to the sign of r in the scalar quadratic form. To this end, a matrix $\boldsymbol{R}$ is said to be *positive definite* if for all real vectors $\boldsymbol{z}$,

$$\boldsymbol{z}^T \boldsymbol{R} \boldsymbol{z} \geq 0 \qquad \text{(A.1.40)}$$

with equality only when $\boldsymbol{z} = \boldsymbol{0}$ (for complex matrices, the transpose is replaced with the Hermitian transpose). The matrix $\boldsymbol{R}$ is *positive semidefinite* if $\boldsymbol{z}^T \boldsymbol{R} \boldsymbol{z} \geq \boldsymbol{0}$ with equality possible for nonzero $\boldsymbol{z}$. A simple test for definiteness is given by the eigenvalues of the matrix. If the eigenvalues are all positive, the matrix is positive definite. If the eigenvalues are all nonnegative, the matrix is positive semidefinite. It is simple to see that for *any* matrix $\boldsymbol{A}$, the matrix $\boldsymbol{A}^T \boldsymbol{A}$ is positive semidefinite, for let $\boldsymbol{z}$ be any vector. Then

$$\boldsymbol{z}^T \boldsymbol{A}^T \boldsymbol{A} \boldsymbol{z} = (\boldsymbol{A}\boldsymbol{z})^T (\boldsymbol{A}\boldsymbol{z})$$

and the length of $\boldsymbol{A}\boldsymbol{z}$ will always be greater than or equal to zero.

Returning to the quadratic form, it can be seen that if $\boldsymbol{R}$ is positive definite, $\boldsymbol{x}_0$ is a minimum and that

$$V(\boldsymbol{x}) > V(\boldsymbol{x}_0) \qquad \text{(A.1.41)}$$

for all $\boldsymbol{x} \neq \boldsymbol{x}_0$.

A.1.4 Matrix Calculus

Let $\boldsymbol{x}$ be a vector given by

$$\boldsymbol{x} = \begin{bmatrix} x_1 \\ x_2 \\ \vdots \\ x_N \end{bmatrix}.$$

We will frequently be interested in scalar functions of a vector $\boldsymbol{x}$. Suppose $f(\boldsymbol{x})$ is a function which returns a scalar value. Then the *gradient* of f with respect to $\boldsymbol{x}$ is a vector defined by

$$\nabla f(\boldsymbol{x}) = \begin{bmatrix} \partial f / \partial x_1 \\ \partial f / \partial x_2 \\ \vdots \\ \partial f / \partial x_2 \end{bmatrix}.$$

For example, suppose $\boldsymbol{x}$ and $\boldsymbol{a}$ are $\boldsymbol{n} \times 1$ vectors and let $f(\boldsymbol{x})$ be given by

$$f(\boldsymbol{x}) = \boldsymbol{a}^T\boldsymbol{x} = \boldsymbol{x}^T\boldsymbol{a}.$$

Writing the $f(\boldsymbol{x})$ as

$$f(\boldsymbol{x}) = \sum_{i=1}^{n} a_i x_i,$$

it can be seen that

$$\frac{\partial f}{\partial x_i} = a_i$$

so that the gradient is given by

$$\nabla(\boldsymbol{a}^T\boldsymbol{x}) = \boldsymbol{a}. \tag{A.1.42}$$

Next, consider the quadratic form $\boldsymbol{x}^T\boldsymbol{A}\boldsymbol{x}$ where $\boldsymbol{A}$ is a symmetric square matrix. Expanding the quadratic form as

$$\boldsymbol{x}^T\boldsymbol{A}\boldsymbol{x} = \sum_{i=1}^{n}\sum_{j=1}^{n} a_{ij}x_i x_j$$

and recognizing that $a_{ij} = a_{ji}$, it is fairly simple to show that

$$\nabla(\boldsymbol{x}^T\boldsymbol{A}\boldsymbol{x}) = 2\boldsymbol{A}\boldsymbol{x}. \tag{A.1.43}$$

Equations A.1.42 and A.1.43 are the fundamental gradient relations which will be needed for our purposes.

A.2 Least Squares Normal Equations

A important problem which frequently occurs is fitting a linear model to a set of observations which are assumed to correspond to a collection of data. To this end, suppose we have observations $y(n)$, $1 \le n \le N$ and sequences $x_1(n), x_2(n), \ldots, x_m(n)$, $1 \le n \le N$. We wish to approximate $y(n)$ by $\hat{y}(n)$ where $\hat{y}(n)$ is a linear combination of the $x_i(n)$. In other words, we seek the values of parameters w_i such that

$$\hat{y}(n) = w_1 x_1(n) + w_2 x_2(n) + \cdots + w_m x_m(n) \tag{A.2.1}$$

where $1 \le n \le N$. We further assume that $N > m$ so that there are more equations than unknowns.

What must be done first is to establish an appropriate criterion which measures how well the $\hat{y}(n)$ approximate the $y(n)$. A frequently used criterion is the sum of squared errors,

$$E = \sum_{n=1}^{n} |e(i)|^2 \tag{A.2.2}$$

where $e(n) = y(n) - \hat{y}(n)$. If $\boldsymbol{X}$ and $\boldsymbol{y}$ are defined by

$$\boldsymbol{X} = \begin{pmatrix} x_1(1) & x_2(1) & \cdots & x_m(1) \\ x_1(2) & x_2(2) & \cdots & x_m(2) \\ \vdots & \vdots & \ddots & \vdots \\ x_1(N) & x_2(N) & \cdots & x_m(N) \end{pmatrix}, \quad \boldsymbol{y} = \begin{pmatrix} y(1) \\ y(2) \\ \vdots \\ y(N) \end{pmatrix} \tag{A.2.3}$$

and $\boldsymbol{w}$ and $\boldsymbol{e}$ are defined by

$$\boldsymbol{w} = \begin{pmatrix} w_1 \\ w_2 \\ \vdots \\ w_m \end{pmatrix}, \boldsymbol{e} = \begin{pmatrix} e(1) \\ e(2) \\ \vdots \\ e(N) \end{pmatrix}, \tag{A.2.4}$$

the vector of errors can be written as

$$\boldsymbol{e} = \boldsymbol{y} - \boldsymbol{X}\boldsymbol{w}. \tag{A.2.5}$$

It then follows that the sum of squared errors is given by

$$E = \boldsymbol{e}^H\boldsymbol{e} = \boldsymbol{y}^H\boldsymbol{y} - \boldsymbol{y}^H\boldsymbol{X}\boldsymbol{w} - \boldsymbol{w}^H\boldsymbol{X}\boldsymbol{X}^H\boldsymbol{y} + \boldsymbol{w}^H\boldsymbol{X}^H X\boldsymbol{w}. \tag{A.2.6}$$

The optimal value of $\boldsymbol{w}$ is found by setting the partial derivative of E with respect to $\boldsymbol{w}$ equal to zero. That is,

$$\frac{\partial E}{\partial \boldsymbol{w}} = -\boldsymbol{X}^H\boldsymbol{y} - \boldsymbol{X}^H\boldsymbol{y} + 2\boldsymbol{X}^H\boldsymbol{X}\boldsymbol{w} = 0, \tag{A.2.7}$$

which means that

$$\boldsymbol{X}^H\boldsymbol{X}\boldsymbol{w} = \boldsymbol{X}^H\boldsymbol{y}. \tag{A.2.8}$$

Equation A.2.8 is known as the *normal* equation for the least squares problem. If the matrix $(\boldsymbol{X}^H\boldsymbol{X})$ is non-singular (*i.e.*, $\boldsymbol{X}$ is of full column rank), the solution to the least-squares problem is given by

$$\boldsymbol{w} = (\boldsymbol{X}^H\boldsymbol{X})^{-1}\boldsymbol{X}^H\boldsymbol{y}. \tag{A.2.9}$$

The minimum value of the sum of squared errors is obtained by substituting either of Eq. A.2.8 or A.2.9 into Eq. A.2.6, which gives

$$E_{min} = \boldsymbol{y}^H \boldsymbol{y} - \boldsymbol{y}^H \boldsymbol{X} \boldsymbol{w}. \tag{A.2.10}$$

Equation A.2.10 and A.2.8 can be combined into a single matrix equation to obtain

$$\begin{pmatrix} \boldsymbol{y}^H \boldsymbol{y} & \boldsymbol{y}^H \boldsymbol{X} \\ \boldsymbol{X}^H \boldsymbol{y} & \boldsymbol{X}^H \boldsymbol{X} \end{pmatrix} \begin{pmatrix} 1 \\ -\boldsymbol{w} \end{pmatrix} = \begin{pmatrix} E_{min} \\ O_m \end{pmatrix} \tag{A.2.11}$$

A.2.1 Singular Value Decomposition

The singular value decomposition (SVD) is an elegant matrix decomposition which gives quantitative information about the structure of a linear system of equations. In particular, we are interested in least-squares solutions to the equation

$$\boldsymbol{A}\boldsymbol{w} = \boldsymbol{b} \tag{A.2.12}$$

where $\boldsymbol{A}$ is a known $L \times M$ matrix, $\boldsymbol{b}$ is a known $L \times 1$ vector, and $\boldsymbol{w}$ represents an unknown $M \times 1$ parameter vector. We have already showed in the previous subsection how to deal with the case when $L > M$ and $\boldsymbol{A}$ is of full column rank. In this case, the least-squares solution is given by

$$\hat{\boldsymbol{w}} = (\boldsymbol{A}^H \boldsymbol{A})^{-1} \boldsymbol{A}^H \boldsymbol{b}. \tag{A.2.13}$$

The SVD will assist us in determining solutions to this equation even when $\boldsymbol{A}$ is not of full column rank.

Theorem 8 *Suppose $\boldsymbol{A}$ is of rank W. Then there exist unitary matrices $\boldsymbol{X}$ and $\boldsymbol{Y}$ such that*

$$\boldsymbol{Y}^H \boldsymbol{A} \boldsymbol{X} = \begin{pmatrix} \boldsymbol{\Sigma} & \boldsymbol{O} \\ \boldsymbol{O} & \boldsymbol{O} \end{pmatrix}$$

where

$$\boldsymbol{\Sigma} = diag(\sigma_1, \sigma_2, \ldots, \sigma_W)$$

and

$$\sigma_1 \geq \sigma_2 \geq \cdots \geq \sigma_W > 0.$$

A proof of the SVD is quite instructive and uses much of what we have developed thusfar. We will only prove the case where $L > M$, which corresponds to a set of overdetermined equations. By construction, the $M \times M$ matrix $\boldsymbol{A}^H\boldsymbol{A}$ is Hermitian and positive semidefinite so that its eigenvalues are all real and nonnegative. Thus, we can denote the eigenvalues of $\boldsymbol{A}^H\boldsymbol{A}$ as $\sigma_1^2, \sigma_2^2, \ldots, \sigma_M^2$. It is simple to impose the ordering

$$\sigma_1 \geq \sigma_2 \geq \cdots \geq \sigma_W \tag{A.2.14}$$

by a reordering of columns and because $\text{rank}(\boldsymbol{A}^H\boldsymbol{A}) = \text{rank}\boldsymbol{A} = W$, it furthermore follows that

$$\sigma_{W+1} = \sigma_{W+2} = \cdots = \sigma_M = 0. \tag{A.2.15}$$

Because $\boldsymbol{A}^H\boldsymbol{A}$ is Hermitian, its eigenvectors $\boldsymbol{x}_1, \boldsymbol{x}_2, \ldots, \boldsymbol{x}_M$ are orthonormal, with $\boldsymbol{x}_i$ corresponding to the eigenvalue σ_i^2. Denote by $\boldsymbol{X}$ the unitary matrix whose columns are the orthonormal eigenvectors, $\{\boldsymbol{x}_i\}$. It then follows that

$$\boldsymbol{X}^H\boldsymbol{A}^H\boldsymbol{A}\boldsymbol{X} = \begin{pmatrix} \boldsymbol{\Sigma}^2 & \boldsymbol{O} \\ \boldsymbol{O} & \boldsymbol{O} \end{pmatrix}. \tag{A.2.16}$$

Partition the columns of $\boldsymbol{X}$ according to

$$\boldsymbol{X} = [\boldsymbol{X}_1, \boldsymbol{X}_2] \tag{A.2.17}$$

where $\boldsymbol{X}_1$ is the $M \times W$ matrix given by

$$\boldsymbol{X}_1 = [\boldsymbol{x}_1, \boldsymbol{x}_2, \ldots, \boldsymbol{x}_W] \tag{A.2.18}$$

and $\boldsymbol{X}_2$ is the $M \times (M - W)$ matrix given by

$$\boldsymbol{X}_2 = [\boldsymbol{x}_{W+1}, \boldsymbol{x}_{W+2} \ldots, \boldsymbol{x}_M]. \tag{A.2.19}$$

Because the $\boldsymbol{x}_i$ are orthonormal, it follows that $\boldsymbol{X}_1^H\boldsymbol{X}_2 = \boldsymbol{O}$. Referring to Eq. A.2.16, it can be seen that

$$\boldsymbol{X}_1^H\boldsymbol{A}^H\boldsymbol{A}\boldsymbol{X}_1 = \boldsymbol{\Sigma}^2 \tag{A.2.20}$$

so that

$$\boldsymbol{\Sigma}^{-1}\boldsymbol{X}_1^H\boldsymbol{A}^H\boldsymbol{A}\boldsymbol{X}_1\boldsymbol{\Sigma}^{-1} = \boldsymbol{I}. \tag{A.2.21}$$

From Eq. A.2.16, it can also be seen that

$$\boldsymbol{X}_2^H\boldsymbol{A}^H\boldsymbol{A}\boldsymbol{X}_2 = (\boldsymbol{A}\boldsymbol{X}_2)^H(\boldsymbol{A}\boldsymbol{X}_2) = \boldsymbol{O}, \tag{A.2.22}$$

from which it immediately follows that

$$\boldsymbol{A}\boldsymbol{X}_2 = \boldsymbol{O}. \tag{A.2.23}$$

Define the $L \times W$ matrix $\boldsymbol{Y}_1$ by

$$\boldsymbol{Y}_1 = \boldsymbol{A}\boldsymbol{X}_1\boldsymbol{\Sigma}^{-1}. \tag{A.2.24}$$

It then follows from Eq. A.2.20 that

$$\boldsymbol{Y}_1^H\boldsymbol{Y}_1 = \boldsymbol{I} \tag{A.2.25}$$

which implies that the columns of $\boldsymbol{Y}_1$ are orthonormal. Define $\boldsymbol{Y}_2$ as the $L \times (L - W)$ matrix whose columns are the orthonormal complement of the columns of $\boldsymbol{Y}_1$ and form the matrix $\boldsymbol{Y}$ according to

$$\boldsymbol{Y} = [\boldsymbol{Y}_1, \boldsymbol{Y}_2]. \tag{A.2.26}$$

Because the columns of $\boldsymbol{Y}$ are all orthonormal, $\boldsymbol{Y}$ is unitary and

$$\boldsymbol{Y}_1^H\boldsymbol{Y}_2 = \boldsymbol{O}. \tag{A.2.27}$$

Finally, Eqs. A.2.26 and A.2.17, we write

$$\boldsymbol{Y}^H\boldsymbol{A}\boldsymbol{X} = \begin{pmatrix} \boldsymbol{Y}_1^H \\ \boldsymbol{Y}_2^H \end{pmatrix} \boldsymbol{A}[\boldsymbol{X}_1, \boldsymbol{X}_2] = \begin{pmatrix} \boldsymbol{Y}_1^H\boldsymbol{A}\boldsymbol{X}_1 & \boldsymbol{Y}_1^H\boldsymbol{A}\boldsymbol{X}_2 \\ \boldsymbol{Y}_2^H\boldsymbol{A}\boldsymbol{X}_1 & \boldsymbol{Y}_2^H\boldsymbol{A}\boldsymbol{X}_2 \end{pmatrix}. \tag{A.2.28}$$

Using Eqs. A.2.20 and A.2.24, Eq. A.2.28 relation is simplified to

$$\boldsymbol{Y}^H\boldsymbol{A}\boldsymbol{X} = \begin{pmatrix} \boldsymbol{\Sigma}^{-1}\boldsymbol{X}_1^H\boldsymbol{A}^H\boldsymbol{A}\boldsymbol{X}_1 & \boldsymbol{Y}_1^H\boldsymbol{O} \\ \boldsymbol{Y}_2^H\boldsymbol{Y}_1\boldsymbol{\Sigma} & \boldsymbol{Y}_2^H\boldsymbol{O} \end{pmatrix} = \begin{pmatrix} \boldsymbol{\Sigma} & \boldsymbol{O} \\ \boldsymbol{O} & \boldsymbol{O} \end{pmatrix} \tag{A.2.29}$$

which is the result we sought. The case where $M > L$ is treated in a similar fashion.

A.2.2 The Pseudoinverse

The pseudoinverse of a matrix is based on the SVD is very useful when discussing minimum norm solutions to least-squares problems. Assume the SVD the rank-W $L \times M$ matrix $\boldsymbol{A}$ is given by

$$\boldsymbol{Y}^H\boldsymbol{A}\boldsymbol{X} = \begin{pmatrix} \boldsymbol{\Sigma} & \boldsymbol{O} \\ \boldsymbol{O} & \boldsymbol{O} \end{pmatrix}.$$

The *pseudoinverse* of $\boldsymbol{A}$ is denoted by the matrix $\boldsymbol{A}^{\#}$ where

$$\boldsymbol{A}^{\#} = \boldsymbol{X} \begin{pmatrix} \boldsymbol{\Sigma}^{-1} & O \\ O & O \end{pmatrix} \boldsymbol{Y}^{H}$$

and

$$\boldsymbol{\Sigma}^{-1} = \text{diag}(\sigma_1^{-1}, \sigma_2^{-1}, \ldots, \sigma_W^{-1}).$$

There are two special cases to consider. For the case where $L > M$ and $W = M$ (*i.e.*, $\boldsymbol{A}$ is of full column rank), it can be shown that

$$\boldsymbol{A}^{\#} = (\boldsymbol{A}^H \boldsymbol{A})^{-1} \boldsymbol{A}^H.$$

For the case where $M > L$ and $W = L$ (*i.e.*, $\boldsymbol{A}$ is of full row rank), it can be shown that

$$\boldsymbol{A}^{\#} = \boldsymbol{A}^H (\boldsymbol{A}\boldsymbol{A}^H)^{-1}.$$

Whether or not $(\boldsymbol{A}^H \boldsymbol{A})$ is invertible, the pseudoinverse possesses the following important property. Consider again the equation

$$\boldsymbol{A}\boldsymbol{w} = \boldsymbol{b}.$$

The least-squares solution to this equation is the vector $\hat{\boldsymbol{w}}$ which minimizes the sum of squared errors

$$(\boldsymbol{b} - \boldsymbol{A}\hat{\boldsymbol{w}})^H (\boldsymbol{b} - \boldsymbol{A}\hat{\boldsymbol{w}}).$$

The the least-squares solution is given by

$$\hat{\boldsymbol{w}} = \boldsymbol{A}^{\#} \boldsymbol{b}.$$

If $\boldsymbol{A}$ is not of full column rank, the solution is not unique. However, of all solutions to the least-squares problem, $\hat{\boldsymbol{w}}$ is the one with minimum Euclidean norm. In other words, if $\bar{\boldsymbol{w}}$ is also a least-squares solution, it must be that

$$||\bar{\boldsymbol{w}}|| \geq ||\hat{\boldsymbol{w}}||.$$

A.3 Probability and Stochastic Processes

A random variable x is a variable which can assume a continuum of values randomly. We will use the notation x to denote the random variable and the notation x to indicate a value which x assumes. The qualitative manner in which x assumes possible values is typically indicated by the *probability distribution function* $F(x)$. The distribution $F(x)$ is interpreted as meaning

$$F(x) = Pr(\mathsf{x} \leq x), \tag{A.3.1}$$

i.e., the probability that x is less than or equal to the value x. Obviously, $F(x)$ is always nonnegative and can never be greater than unity. The *probability density function* $f(x)$ is defined by

$$f(x) = \frac{\partial F(x)}{\partial x} \tag{A.3.2}$$

and thus satisfies

$$F(x) = \int_{-\infty}^{x} f(z)\, dz. \tag{A.3.3}$$

The probability density $f(x)$ is also nonnegative and satisfies

$$\int_{-\infty}^{\infty} f(x)\, dx = 1. \tag{A.3.4}$$

The *expectation* of a random variable x is denoted by $\mathcal{E}[\mathsf{x}]$ and is computed as

$$\mathcal{E}[\mathsf{x}] = \int_{-\infty}^{\infty} x f(x)\, dx. \tag{A.3.5}$$

The expectation is also known as the *mean* and gives a measure of the average value which x will assume. The expectation of x^2 ,

$$\mathcal{E}[\mathsf{x}^2] = \int_{-\infty}^{\infty} x^2 f(x)\, dx \tag{A.3.6}$$

is known as the *mean squared* of x. Similarly, the *variance* of x is defined by

$$var[\mathsf{x}] = \int_{-\infty}^{\infty} (x - \mathcal{E}[\mathsf{x}])^2 f(x)\, dx. \tag{A.3.7}$$

The variance gives a measure of the dispersion of values which x assumes about the mean value $\mathcal{E}[\mathsf{x}]$. Comparing Eqs. A.3.6 and A.3.7, the mean-squared value and the variance will be equal only if x has zero mean.

The previous ideas can be extended to more than on random variable. If $\mathsf{x}_1, \mathsf{x}_2, \ldots, \mathsf{x}_N$ are random variables, the *joint probability distribution* function

$$F(x_1, x_2, \ldots, x_N)$$

describes the distribution of random variables according to

$$F(x_1, x_2, \ldots, x_N) = Pr(\mathsf{x}_1 \le x_1, \mathsf{x}_2 \le x_2, \ldots, \mathsf{x}_N \le x_n). \tag{A.3.8}$$

We will frequently use the vector $\mathbf{x}$ to denote the collection of random variables. Similarly, the joint probability density is given by

$$f(x_1, x_2, \ldots, x_N) = f(\boldsymbol{x}) = \frac{\partial F(\boldsymbol{x})}{\partial x_1 \partial x_2 \cdots \partial x_N}. \tag{A.3.9}$$

The mean of the random vector $\mathbf{x}$ is a vector given by

$$\mathcal{E}[\mathsf{x}] = \int_{-\infty}^{\infty} \boldsymbol{x} f(\boldsymbol{x})\, d\boldsymbol{x} \tag{A.3.10}$$

where the integral is to be interpreted as a multiple integral over the entire N-dimensional probability density function. The *covariance* is then defined by

$$cov(\mathsf{x}) = \mathcal{E}[(\boldsymbol{x} - \mathcal{E}[\mathsf{x}])(\boldsymbol{x} - \mathcal{E}[\mathsf{x}])^T]. \tag{A.3.11}$$

Two important probability distributions are the uniform distribution and the Gaussian distribution. A uniform random variable has a flat probability density over the range $a \le x \le b$ and the density is given by

$$f(x) = \frac{1}{b-a}, \quad a \le x \le b. \tag{A.3.12}$$

The Gaussian probability density function is given by

$$f(x) = \frac{1}{\sqrt{2\pi}\sigma} \exp\left[-\frac{(x-m)^2}{2\sigma}\right]. \tag{A.3.13}$$

It is simple to show that the mean of x is given by m and the variance is given by σ^2. The Gaussian distribution is also known as the *normal* distribution. For multiple random values, we have the multivariate Gaussian distribution which has probability density

$$f(\boldsymbol{x}) = \frac{1}{\sqrt{(2\pi)^N |\boldsymbol{C}|}} \exp\left[-\frac{1}{2}(\boldsymbol{x} - \boldsymbol{m})^T \boldsymbol{C}^{-1} (\boldsymbol{x} - \boldsymbol{m})\right] \tag{A.3.14}$$

where N is the number of random variables. Again, it can be shown that the mean of $\mathbf{x}$ is $\boldsymbol{m}$ and the covariance is given by $\boldsymbol{C}$

A.3.1 Stochastic Processes

A discrete-time stochastic process is simply defined as an *ensemble* of discrete-time sequences, any one which might be observed. It is typical to denote a stochastic process by two indices, k and n. The first index denotes the time and the second denotes the observed sequence of the ensemble. For a given time k, the value of $x(k;n)$ over the entire ensemble will be a random variable. Individual sequences from the ensemble are known as *realizations* of the stochastic process. In general, there is a joint probability distribution for the entire process $x(k;n)$, and expectations are implicitly understood to be taken with regard to this joint distribution.

The expected value of the process at time k is denoted by $\bar{x}(k)$ where

$$\bar{x}(k) = \mathcal{E}[x(k)]. \tag{A.3.15}$$

The majority of applications which will be important to us are concerned with second-order properties of the stochastic process. That is, we will examine pairs of observations. The *autocovariance* of the random process is a two-dimensional sequence given by

$$c_{xx}(k_1, k_2) = \mathcal{E}[(x(k_1) - \bar{x}(k_1))(x(k_2) - \bar{x}(k_2))] \tag{A.3.16}$$

where k_1 and k_2 are time indices. Similarly, the *autocorrelation* is given by

$$r_{xx}(k_1, k_2) = \mathcal{E}[x(k_1)x(k_2)]. \tag{A.3.17}$$

In general, the autocorrelation and autocovariance sequences will depend on both indices k_1 and k_2. It is simple to show that the autocorrelation and the autocovariance are related by

$$c_{xx}(k_1, k_2) = r_{xx}(k_1, k_2) - \bar{x}(k_1)\bar{x}(k_2) \tag{A.3.18}$$

so that if the process has zero mean for all times k, the autocovariance and the autocorrelation will be identical.

For two stochastic processes, the autocovariance and autocorrelation can be extended to the concepts of crosscovariance and crosscorrelation. If $x(k;n)$ and $y(k;n)$ are two stochastic processes, the crosscovariance is defined by

$$c_{xy}(k_1, k_2) = \mathcal{E}[(x(k_1) - \bar{x}(k_1))(y(k_2) - \bar{y}(k_2))] \tag{A.3.19}$$

and

$$r_{xy}(k_1, k_2) = \mathcal{E}[x(k_1)y(k_2)]. \tag{A.3.20}$$

The random processes are said to be *uncorrelated* if the crosscorrelation is equal to zero for all k_1 and k_2.

A stochastic process $x(k;n)$ is called *wide-sense stationary* (WSS) if the mean in a constant for all time and if the autocorrelation (and hence the autocovariance) is a function only of the difference $k_2 - k_1$. Two stochastic processes $x(k;n)$ and $y(k;n)$ are called *jointly* (WSS) if the same holds for the crosscorrelation. It is necessary that the individual processes be WSS in order for them to be jointly WSS. To summarize, the mean of a WSS process is given by

$$\bar{x}(k) = \bar{x}, \quad \text{a constant}$$

and the autocorrelation sequence is a *one-dimensional* sequence $r_{xx}(l)$ where

$$r_{xx}(l) = \mathcal{E}[x(k)x(k+l)].$$

A.3.2 Ergodicity

The preceding development has assumed that we have access to the probability distribution for the entire *ensemble* of possible realizations of a WSS stochastic process $x(k;n)$. In practice, this distribution may not be known and hence the mean and autocorrelation must be estimated. The concept of *ergodicity* is important to understand before estimates can be made. Loosely speaking, a process is ergodic if a single realization of the process assumes the behavior of all elements of the ensemble over a wide enough time interval. This allows ensemble averages to be replaced with time averages. More formally, a process is ergodic if its statistics can be determined from a single realization via time averages with probability 1. The use of time averages drastically simplifies the characterization of a random process.

Consider estimating the mean of a WSS stochastic process $x(k;n)$ using the temporal average of a single realization $x(k)$. It is desirable that the estimate should converge to the true mean of the process so that

$$\lim_{N\to\infty} \frac{1}{2N+1} \sum_{k=-N}^{N} x(k) = \bar{x}. \tag{A.3.21}$$

It can be shown that the limit exists if and only if the variance of the time average approaches zero, *i.e.*,

$$\lim_{N\to\infty} \frac{1}{2N+1} \sum_{k=-2N}^{2N} \left[1 - \frac{|k|}{2N+1}\right] c_{xx}(k) = 0 \tag{A.3.22}$$

where $c_{xx}(k)$ is the true *ensemble* autocovariance sequence. If Eq. A.3.22 holds, the process is said to be *ergodic in the mean.*

Similarly, it would be desirable to be able to compute the autocorrelation sequence of the process using a time average of lagged products $x(k)x(k+l)$. The time average satisfies

$$\lim_{N\to\infty} \frac{1}{2N+1} \sum_{k=-N}^{N} x(k)x(k+l) = \mathcal{E}[x(k)x(k+l)] = r_{xx}(l) \tag{A.3.23}$$

if and only if

$$\lim_{N\to\infty} \frac{1}{2N+1} \sum_{k=-2N}^{2N} \left[1 - \frac{|k|}{2N+1}\right] c_{zz}(k) = 0 \tag{A.3.24}$$

where $c_{zz}(k)$ is the ensemble covariance of the process $x(k)x(k+l)$. The covariance sequence $c_{zz}(k)$ involves fourth-order moments of the process $x(k;n)$. If Eq. A.3.24 holds, the process is called *autocorrelation ergodic.* Proving autocorrelation ergodicity is in general extremely difficult so that it must frequently be assumed. In practice, a number of processes encountered will be both mean and autocorrelation ergodic. This will allow the second-order statistics of the process to be estimated from temporal averages of a single realization of the process.

References

[Aka69] H. Akaike. Power spectrum estimation through autoregression model fitting. *Ann. Inst. Stat. Math*, 21:407–419, 1969.

[Aka74] H. Akaike. A new look at the stastical model identification. *IEEE Trans. Automatic Control*, AC-19:716–723, 1974.

[Ale86] S. T. Alexander. *Adaptive Signal Processing: Theory and Applications.* Springer-Verlag, New York, 1986.

[Ant79] A. Antoniou. *Digital Filters: Analysis and Design.* McGraw-Hill, New York, 1979.

[BBC76] M. G. Bellanger, G. Bonnerot, and M. Coudreuse. Digital filtering by polyphase network: Application to sample rate alteration and filter banks. *IEEE Trans. Acoustics, Speech, and Signal Processing*, pages 109–114, April 1976.

[Bel88] M. G. Bellanger. *Adaptive Digital Filters and Signal Analysis.* Marcel Dekker, New York, N.Y., 1988.

[BJ76] G. E. P. Box and G. M. Jenkins. *Time Series Analysis: Forecasting and Control.* Holden-Day, San Francisco, 1976.

[Bla85] R. E. Blahut. *Fast Algorithms for Digital Signal Processing.* Addison-Wesley, Reading, Massachusetts, 1985.

[Bra86] R. N. Bracewell. *The Fourier Transform and Its Applications.* McGraw-Hill, New York, 1986.

[Bri88] E. O. Brigham. *The Fast Fourier Transform and Its Applications.* Prentice Hall, Englewood Cliffs, NJ, 1988.

[BT58] R. B. Blackman and J. W. Tukey. *The Measurement of Power Spectra from the Point of View of Communications Engineering.* Dover, New York, 1958.

[Bur75] J. P. Burg. *Maximum Entropy Spectral Analysis.* PhD thesis, Dept. of Geophysics, Stanford University, 1975.

[Bur77] C. S. Burrus. Index mappings for multidimensional formulation of the DFT. *IEEE Trans. Acoust., Speech, and Signal Process.*, ASSP-25:239–242, 1977.

[Cap69] J. Capon. High-resolution frequency-wavenumber analysis. *Proc. IEEE*, 57:1408–1418, 1969.

[CB84] R. V. Churchill and J. Brown. *Introduction to Complex Variables and Applications.* McGraw-Hill, New York, 1984.

[CG85] C. F. N. Cowan and P. M. Grant. *Adaptive Filters.* Prentice-Hall, Englewood Cliffs, N. J., 1985.

[Che66] E. W. Cheney. *Introduction to Approximation Theory.* McGraw-Hill, New York, 1966.

[Chi78] D. G. Childers, editor. *Modern Spectrum Analysis.* IEEE Press, New York, 1978.

[Chu92] C. K. Chui. *An Introduction to Wavelets.* Academic Press, Boston, 1992.

[CK84] J. M. Cioffi and T. Kailath. Fast, recursive-least-squares transversal filters for adaptive filtering. *IEEE Trans. Acoust. Speech, and Signal Process.*, ASSP-32:304–337, 1984.

[CMK83] G. Carayannis, G. Manolakis, and N. Kalouptsidis. A fast sequential algorithm for least-squares filtering and prediction. *IEEE Trans. Acoust., Speech, and Signal Process.*, ASSP-31:1394–1402, 1983.

[CR83] R. E. Crochiere and L. R. Rabiner. *Multirate Digital Signal Processing.* Prentice-Hall, Englewood Cliffs, New Jersey, 1983.

[CT65] J. W. Cooley and J. W. Tukey. An algorithm for the machine computation of complex Fourier series. *Mathematics of Computation*, 19:297–301, April 1965.

[Dau90] I. Daubechies. The wavelet transform, time-frequency localization, and signal analysis. *IEEE Trans. on Information Theory*, pages 961–1005, September 1990.

[Dau92] I. Daubechies. *Ten Lectures on Wavelets.* SIAM CBMS-NSF Series in Applied Mathematics, Philadelphia, PA, 1992.

[Dep88] E. F. Deprettere. *SVD and Signal Processing: Algorithms, Applications, and Architectures.* Elsevier Sciencxe Publishers, Amsterdam, The Netherlands, 1988.

[Doo53] L. J. Doob. *Stochastic Processes.* Wiley, New York, 1953.

[Dur60] J. Durbin. The fitting of time-series models. *Rev. Inst. Int. Statistics*, 28:233–243, 1960.

[EF86] E. Eleftheriou and D. D. Falconer. Tracking properties and steady state performance of RLS adaptive filter algorithms. *IEEE Trans. Acoust., Speech, and Signal Process.*, ASSP-34:1097–1110, 1986.

[EMT69] P. M. Ebert, J. E. Mazo, and M. C. Taylor. Overflow oscillations in digital filters. *Bell Sys. Tech. J.*, 48:2999–3020, 1969.

[FL78] D. D. Falconer and L. Ljung. Application of fast Kalman estimation to adaptive equalization. *IEEE Trans Communication*, COM-26:1439–1446, 1978.

[Fri82] B. Friedlander. Lattice methods for spectral estimation. *Proc. IEEE*, 70:990–1017, 1982.

[Gab46] D. Gabor. Theory of communications. *Journal of the Institute of Electrical Engineering*, 93:429–457, 1946.

[Gar88] W. A. Gardner. *Statistical Spectral Analysis: A Nonprobabilistic Theory.* Prentice Hall, Englewood Cliffs, NJ, 1988.

[GKM75] D. Graupe, D. J. Krause, and J. B. Moore. Identification of ARMA parameters of time series. *IEEE Trans. Automatic Control*, AC-20:104–107, 1975.

[GM74] A. H. Gray Jr. and J. D. Markel. A spectral flatness measure for studying the autocorrelation method of linear prediction of speech. *IEEE Trans. Acoust., Speech, and Signal Process.*, ASSP-22:207–217, 1974.

[God74] D. N. Godard. Channel equalization using a Kalman filter for fast data transmission. *IBM J. Res. Dev.*, 18:267–273, 1974.

[Goo71] I. J. Good. The relationship between two fast Fourier transforms. *IEEE Trans. on Computers*, C-20:310–317, 1971.

[GR73] R. A. Gabel and R. A. Roberts. *Signals and Linear Systems.* John Wiley and Sons, New York, 1973.

[Gri78] L. J. Griffiths. An adaptive lattice structure for noise-cancelling applications. In *Proc. of the ICASSP*, pages 87–90, Tulsa, Oklahoma, 1978.

[GS58] U. Grenander and G. Szego. *Toeplitz Forms and Their Applications.* University of California Press, Berkeley, California, 1958.

[Har78] F. J. Harris. On the use of windows for harmonic analysis with the discrete Fourier transform. *Proc IEEE*, 66:51–83, 1978.

[Hay86] S. Haykin. *Adaptive Filter Theory.* Prentice-Hall, Englewood Cliffs, New Jersey, 1986.

[Her70] O. Hermann. On the design of nonrecursive digital filters with linear phase. *Electronics Letters*, 6:328–329, 1970.

[Hon85] M. L. Honig. Echo cancellation of voice-band data signals using RLS and gradient algorithms. *IEEE Trans. Communication*, COM-33:65–73, 1985.

[HS70] O. Hermann and Schuessler. Design of nonrecursive digital fitlers with minimum phase. *Electronics Letters*, 1970:329–330, 1970.

[HS81] L. L. Horowitz and K. D. Senne. Performance advantage of complex LMS for controlling narrow-band adaptive arrays. *IEEE Trans. Acoust., Speech, and Signal Process.*, ASSP-29:722–736, 1981.

[Jac79] L. B. Jackson. Limit cycles in state-space structures for digital filters. *IEEE Trans. Circuits and Systems*, CAS-26:67–68, 1979.

[Jac85] N. A. Jacobson. *Basic Algebra I.* W.H. Freeman and Company, New York, 1985.

[Jay82] E. T. Jaynes. On the rationale of maximum entropy methods. *Proc. IEEE*, 70:939–952, 1982.

[JLK77] L. B. Jackson, A. G. Lindgren, and Y. Kim. Optimal synthesis of second-order state structures for digital filters. *IEEE Trans. Circuits and Systems*, CAS-26:149–155, 1977.

[JN84] N. S. Jayant and P. Noll. *Digital Coding of Waveforms.* Prentice-Hall, Englewood Cliffs, New Jersey, 1984.

[JW68] G. M. Jenkins and J. D. Watts. *Spectral Analysis and its Applications.* Holden-Day, Inc., San Francisco, 1968.

[Kai74a] T. Kailath. A view of three decades of linear filtering theory. *IEEE Trans. Information Theory*, IT-20:146–181, 1974.

[Kai74b] J. F. Kaiser. Nonrecursive digital filter design using the i_0 – sinh window function. *Proc. IEEE Symposium on Circuits and Systems*, pages 20–23, 1974.

[Kai80] T. Kailath. *Linear Systems.* Prentice-Hall, Englewood Cliffs, New Jersey, 1980.

[Kay83] S. M. Kay. Recursive maximum likelihood estimation of autoregressive processes. *IEEE Trans. Acoust., Speech, and Signal Process.*, ASSP-31:56–65, 1983.

[Kay88] S. M. Kay. *Modern Spectral Estimation, Theory and Application.* Prentice-Hall, Englewood Cliffs, New Jersey, 1988.

[KL80] V. C. Klema and A. J. Laub. The singular value decomposition: its computation and some application. *IEEE Trans. Automatic Control*, AC-25:164–176, 1980.

[KM79] S. M. Kay and S. L. Marple. Sources and remedies for spectral line splitting in autoregressive spectrum analysis. *IEEE Conference on Acoustics, Speech, and Signal Processing*, pages 151–154, 1979.

[KM81] S. M. Kay and S. L. Marple. Spectrum analysis–a modern perspective. *Proc. IEEE*, 69:1380–1419, 1981.

[Knu69] D. E. Knuth. *The Art of Computer Programming*, volume 2. Addison-Wesley, Reading, Massachusetts, 1969.

[Kol41] A. N. Kolmogorov. Interpolation und extrapolation von stationaren zufalligen folgen. *Bull. Acad. Sci. USSR Ser. Math.*, 5:3–14, 1941.

[KT83] R. Kumaresan and D. W. Tufts. Estimating the angles of arrival of multiple plane waves. *IEEE Trans. on Aerospace and Electronic Systems*, AES-19:134–139, 1983.

[Kum82] R. Kumaresan. *Estimating the Parameters of Exponentially Damped or Undamped Sinusoidal Signals in Noise.* PhD thesis, University of Rhode Island, 1982.

[KVM78] T. Kailath, A. Vieira, and M. Morf. Inverses of Toeplitz operators, innovations, and orthogonal polynomials. *SIAM Review*, 20:106–119, 1978.

[KWK85] S. Y. Kung, H. J. Whitehouse, and T. Kailath. *VLSI and Modern Signal Processing.* Prentice-Hall, Englewood Cliffs, New Jersey, 1985.

[LAKC84] H. Lev-Ari, T. Kailath, and J. Cioffi. Least-squares adaptive lattice and transversal filters: a unified geometric approach. *IEEE Trans. Info. Theory*, IT-30:222–236, 1984.

[Lev47] N. Levinson. The wiener RMS error criterion in filter design and prediction. *J. Math. Phys.*, 25:261–278, 1947.

[Lin84] D. Lin. On digital implementation of the fast kalman algorithm. *IEEE Trans. Acoust., Speech, and Signal Process.*, ASSP-32:998–1005, 1984.

[LL85] S. Ljung and L. Ljung. Error propagation properties of recursive least- squares adaptation algorithms. *Automatica*, 21:157–167, 1985.

[LM80] S. W. Lang and J. H. McClellan. Frequency estimation with maximum entropy spectral estimators. *IEEE Trans. Acoustics, Speech, and Signal Processing*, ASSP-28:716–724, 1980.

[LMF81] D. T. L. Lee, M. Morf, and B. Friedlander. Recursive least squares ladder estimation algorithms. *IEEE Trans. Acoust., Speech, and Signal Process.*, ASSP-29:467–487, 1981.

[LMP85] F. D. Ling, D. Manolakis, and J. G. Proakis. New forms of LS lattice algorithms and an analysis of their round-off error characteristics. *Proc. ICASSP*, pages 1739–1742, 1985.

[LO88] J. S. Lim and A. V. Oppenheim, editors. *Advanced Topics in Signal Processing.* Prentice Hall, Englewood Cliffs, NJ, 1988.

[LP84] F. Y. Ling and J. G. Proakis. Generalized multichannel least squares lattice algorithm based on sequential processing. *IEEE Trans. Acoust., Speech, and Signal Process.*, ASSP-32:381–389, 1984.

[Luc66] R. W. Lucky. Techniques for adaptive equalization of digital communications systems. *Bell Sys. Tech. J.*, 45:255–286, 1966.

[Lue69] D. G. Luenberger. *Optimization by Vector Space Methods.* Wiley, New York, 1969.

[Mak75] J. Makhoul. Linear prediction: a tutorial review. *Proc. IEEE*, 63:561–580, 1975.

[Mak77] J. Makhoul. Stable and efficient lattice methods for linear prediction. *IEEE Trans. Acoust., Speech, and Signal Process.*, ASSP-25:423–428, 1977.

[Mal89] S. Mallat. A theory for multiresolution signal decomposition: the wavelet representation. *IEEE Trans. on Pattern Analysis and Machine Intelligence*, pages 674–693, July 1989.

[Mar87] S. L. Marple. *Digital Spectral Analysis with Applications.* Prentice-Hall, Englewood Cliffs, New Jersey, 1987.

[Maz79] J. Mazo. On the independence theory of equalizer convergence. *Bell Sys. Tech. J.*, 58:963–993, 1979.

[MG76] J. D. Markel and A. H. Gray, Jr. *Linear Prediction of Speech.* Springer-Verlag, New York, 1976.

[Mil74] K. S. Miller. *Complex Stochastic Processes: An Introduction to Theory and Applications.* Addison-Wesley, Reading, Mass., 1974.

[ML78] M. Morf and D. T. Lee. Recursive least squares ladder forms for fast parameter tracking. *Proc. 1978 Conference on Decision and Control*, pages 1362–1367, 1978.

[MLP87] D. Manolakis, D. F. Ling, and J. G. Proakis. Efficient time-recursive least-squares algorithms for finite-memory adaptive filtering. *IEEE Trans. Circuits and Systems*, CAS-34:400–408, 1987.

[MMR78] W. L. Mills, C. T. Mullis, and R. A. Roberts. Digital filter realizations without overflow oscillations. *IEEE Trans. Acoust., Speech, and Signal Process.*, ASSP-26:334–338, 1978.

[MMR81] W. L. Mills, C. T. Mullis, and R. A. Roberts. Low roundoff noise and normal realizations of fixed- point IIR digital filters. *IEEE Trans. Acoust., Speech, and Signal Process.*, ASSP-29:893–903, 1981.

[MN82] G. A. Mian and A. P. Nainer. A fast procedure to design equiripple minimum-phase FIR filters. *IEEE Trans. on Circuits and Systems*, pages 327–331, 1982.

[MP73] J. H. McClellan and T. W. Parks. A unified approach to the design of optimum FIR linear phase digital filters. *IEEE Trans. Circuit Theory*, CT-20:697–701, 1973.

[MPR73] J. H. McClellan, T. W. Parks, and L. R. Rabiner. A computer program for designing optimum FIR linear phase digital filters. *IEEE Trans. Audio and Electroacoustics*, AU-21:506–526, 1973.

[MR76] C. T. Mullis and R. A. Roberts. Synthesis of minimum roundoff noise fixed point diigital filters. *IEEE Trans. Circuits and Systems*, CAS-23:551–562, 1976.

[MR79] J. H. McClellan and C. M. Rader. *Number Theory in Digital Signal Processing.* Prentice-Hall, Englewood Cliffs, New Jersey, 1979.

[Mue73] K. H. Mueller. A new approach to optimum pulse shaping in sampled systems using time-domain filtering. *Bell System Technical Journal*, pages 723–729, May-June 1973.

[NDM84] Y. Neuvo, C.-Y. Dong, and S. K. Mitra. Interpolate finite impulse response filters. *IEEE Trans. Acoustics, Speech, and Signal Processing*, pages 563–570, June 1984.

[Nob69] B. Noble. *Applied Linear Algebra.* Prentice-Hall, Englewood Cliffs, NJ, 1969.

[Nut76] A. H. Nuttall. Spectral analysis of a univariate process with bad data points, via maximum entropy and linear predictive techniques. *Tech. Report TR-5303, Naval Underwater Systems Center*, March 1976.

[Nyq28] H. Nyquist. Certain topics in telegraph transmission theory. *AIEE Trans.*, pages 617–644, 1928.

[Opp78] A. V. Oppenheim. *Applications of Digital Signal Processing.* Prentice-Hall, Englewood Cliffs, New Jersey, 1978.

[Orf85] S. J. Orfanidis. *Optimum Signal Processing, an Introduction.* Macmillan, New York, 1985.

[OS75] A. V. Oppenheim and R. W. Schafer. *Digital Signal Processing.* Prentice-Hall, Englewood Cliffs, New Jersey, 1975.

[OS89] A. V. Oppenheim and R. W. Schaefer. *Digital Signal Processing.* Prentice-Hall, Englewood Cliffs, New Jersey, 1989.

[OWY83] A. V. Oppenheim, A. S. Willsky, and I. T. Young. *Signals and Systems.* Prentice-Hall, Englewood Cliffs, New Jersey, 1983.

[Pap65] A. Papoulis. *Probability, Random Variables, and Stochastic Processes.* McGraw-Hill, New York, 1965.

[Par62] E. Parzen. *Stochastic Processes.* Holden-Day, San Francisco, California, 1962.

[PFTV86] W. H. Press, B. P. Flannery, S. A. Teukolsky, and W. T. Vetterling. *Numerical Recipes.* Cambridge University Press, Cambridge, 1986.

[PK83] L. Pakula and S. M. Kay. Simple proofs of the minimum phase property of the prediction error filter. *IEEE Trans. Acoust., Speech, and Signal Process.*, ASSP-31:501–502, 1983.

[PL76] A. Peled and B. Liu. *Digital Signal Processing.* Wiley, New York, New York, 1976.

[PM88] J. G. Proakis and D. G. Manolakis. *Introduction to Digital Signal Processing.* Macmillan, New York, 1988.

[RG67] C. M. Rader and B. Gold. Effects of parameter quantization on the poles of a digital filter. *Proc. IEEE*, 55:688–689, 1967.

[RG75] L. R. Rabiner and B. Gold. *Theory and Applications of Digital Signal Processing.* Prentice-Hall, Englewood Cliffs, New Jersey, 1975.

[RG78] L. R. Rabiner and B. Gold. *Digital Processing of Speech Signals.* Prentice-Hall, Englewood Cliffs, New Jersey, 1978.

[Ris78] J. Rissanen. Modeling by shortest data description. *Automatica*, 14:465–471, 1978.

[RM87] R. A. Roberts and C. T. Mullis. *Digital Signal Processing.* Addison-Wesley, Reading, Massachusetts, 1987.

[RR72] L. R. Rabiner and C. M. Rader, editors. *Digital Signal Processing.* IEEE Press, New York, New York, 1972.

[RV91] O. Rioul and M. Vetterli. Wavelets and signal processing. *IEEE Signal Processing Magazine*, pages 14–38, October 1991.

[SA79] E. H. Satorious and S. T. Alexander. Channel equalization using adaptive lattice algorithms. *IEEE Transactions on Communications*, COM-29:899–905, 1979.

[SB84] M. J. T. Smith and T. P. Barnwell III. A procedure for designing exact reconstruction filter banks for tree structured subband coders. *IEEE International Conference on Acoust., Speech, and Signal Proc.*, pages 27.1.1–27.1.4, March 1984.

[Sch83] R. O. Schmidt. *A Signal Subspace Approach to Multiple Emitter Location and Spectral Estimation.* PhD thesis, Stanford University, 1983.

[Sha48] C. E. Shannon. The mathematical theory of communication. *Bell Syst. Tech. J.*, 27:379–423,623–656, 1948.

[SK88] R. D. Strum and D. E. Kirk. *First Principles of Discrete Systems and Digital Signal Processing.* Addison-Wesley, Reading, Massachusetts, 1988.

[Sle78] D. Slepian. Prolate pheroidal wave functions: Fourier analysis and uncretainty – V: the discrete case. *Bell System Tech. Journal*, pages 1371–1430, May-June 1978.

[Sol89] V. Solo. The limiting behavior of LMS. *IEEE Trans. Acoust., Speech, and Signal Process.*, ASSP-37:1909–1922, 1989.

[SP81] E. H. Satorius and J. Pack. Application of least squares lattice algorithms to adaptive equalization. *IEEE Trans. Communications*, COM-29:136–142, 1981.

[Swi79] D. N. Swingler. A comparison between Burg's maximum entropy method and a nonrecursive technique for the spectral analysis of deterministic signals. *J. Geophysical Research*, pages 679–685, February 1979.

[Vai87] P. P. Vaidyanathan. Quadrature mirror filter banks, M-band extensions and perfect-reconstruction techniques. *IEEE ASSP Magazine*, pages 4–20, July 1987.

[Vai90] P. P. Vaidyanathan. Multirate digital filters, filter banks, polyphase networks, and applications: a tutorial. *Proc. IEEE*, 78:56–93, 1990.

[Vai93] P. P. Vaidyanathan. *Multirate Systems and Filter Banks*. Prentice Hall, Englewood Cliffs, NJ, 1993.

[Wel67] P. D. Welch. The use of fast Fourier transform for estimation of power spectra: a method based on averaging over short, modified periodograms. *IEEE Trans. Audio Electroacoustics*, AU-15:70–73, 1967.

[WH60] B. Widrow and M. E. Hoff Jr. Adaptive switching circuits. *IRE WESCON Conv. Rec.*, 4:96–104, 1960.

[Wid56] B. Widrow. A study of rough amplitude quantization by means of Nyquist sampling theory. *IRE Trans. Circuit Theory*, CT-3:266–276, 1956.

[Wie49] N. Wiener. *Extrapolation, Interpolation, and Smoothing of Stationary time Series with Engineering Applications*. MIT Press, Cambridge, Massachusetts, 1949.

[WK85] M. Wax and T. Kailath. Detection of signals by information theoretic criteria. *IEEE Trans. Acoustics, Speech, and Signal Processing*, ASSP-33:387–392, 1985.

[Wol54] H. Wold. *A Study in the Analysis of Stationary Time Series*. Almqvist and Wiksell, Stockholm, 1954.

[WS85] B. Widrow and S. D. Stearns. *Adaptive Signal Processing*. Prentice-Hall, Englewood Cliffs, New Jersey, 1985.

[Zem65] A. H. Zemanian. *Distribution Theory and Transform Analysis: An Introduction to Generalized Functions, with Applications*. McGraw-Hill, New York, 1965.

Index